Advanced Practice
PSYCHIATRIC NURSING

Ann Wolbert Burgess, CS, DNSc, FAAN
van Ameringen Professor of Psychiatric
    Mental Health Nursing
University of Pennsylvania School of Nursing
Philadelphia, Pennsylvania

APPLETON & LANGE
Stamford, Connecticut

Copyright © 1998 by Appleton & Lange
A Simon & Schuster Company

98 99 00 01 02 / 10 9 8 7 6 5 4 3 2 1

Prentice Hall International (UK) Limited, *London*
Prentice Hall of Australia Pty. Limited, *Sydney*
Prentice Hall Canada, Inc., *Toronto*
Prentice Hall Hispanoamericana, S.A., *Mexico*
Prentice Hall of India Private Limited, *New Delhi*
Prentice Hall of Japan, Inc., *Tokyo*
Simon & Schuster Asia Pte. Ltd., *Singapore*
Editora Prentice Hall do Brasil Ltda., *Rio de Janeiro*
Prentice Hall, *Upper Saddle River, New Jersey*

ISBN 0-8385-0181-8

9 780838 501818

90000

Library of Congress Cataloging-in-Publication Data

Advanced practice psychiatric nursing / [edited by] Ann Wolbert
   Burgess.
       p.   cm.
     ISBN 0-8385-0181-8 (pbk. : alk. paper)
     1. Psychiatric nursing.   2. Nurse practitioners.   I. Burgess, Ann
   Wolbert.
     [DNLM: 1. Psychiatric Nursing.   WY 160 A2445 1997]
   RC440.A34   1997
   610.73'68—dc21
   DNLM/DLC
   for Library of Congress   97-11817
                                                                        CIP

Acquisitions Editor: Sally J. Barhydt
Development Editor: Barbara Severs
Production Editor: Maria T. Vlasak

Cover art: Photomicrograph of a crystalline lattice of serotonin (neurotransmitter).
Copyright © Dennis Kunkel, University of Hawaii.

PRINTED IN THE UNITED STATES OF AMERICA

CONTENTS

▪ ▪ ▪ ▪ ▪ CONTRIBUTORS

Kathleen M. Andolina, RN, MS, CS
Consultant
The Center for Case Management, Inc.
South Natick, Massachusetts

Gerri Collins Bride, RN, MS, ANP
Assistant Clinical Professor
Department of Community Health Systems
School of Nursing
University of California, San Francisco
San Francisco, California

Jeanne Brince, MSN, RNCS
Advanced Practice Nurse
Visiting Nurse Association of Greater
    Philadelphia
Philadelphia, Pennsylvania

Advanced Practice Psychiatric Nurse
The Health Annex at the F.J. Myers Youth
    Access Center
Philadelphia, Pennsylvania

Verna Benner Carson, RN, PhD, CS-P
National Director of Behavioral Health
Staff Builders Home Health & Hospice
Baltimore, Maryland

Linda Chafetz, RN, DNSc
Associate Professor
Department of Community Health Systems
School of Nursing
University of California, San Francisco
San Francisco, California

Lilli Ann Ciesielski, RN, MSN, CS
Geropsychiatric Clinical Nurse Specialist
Collaborative Assessment and Rehabilitation
    for Elders Program (CARE)
University of Pennsylvania School of Nursing
    Penn Nursing Network
Philadelphia, Pennsylvania

Ina Cochran, RN, MSN, CS
Geriatric Nurse Practitioner/Care Manager
Collaborative Assessment and Rehabilitation
    for Elders Program (CARE)
University of Pennsylvania School of Nursing
    Penn Nursing Network
Philadelphia, Pennsylvania

Beth Vaughan Cole, PhD, APRN
Director of the Division of Social and
    Behavioral Systems in Nursing
University of Utah College of Nursing
Salt Lake City, Utah

Linda S. Cook, RN, PhD, CS
Assistant Professor
Temple University
Philadelphia, Pennsylvania

Margaret Cotroneo, PhD, RNCS
Associate Professor and Chair of
    Psychiatric-Mental Health Nursing
School of Nursing
University of Pennsylvania
Philadelphia, Pennsylvania

Faculty Director
The Health Annex at the F.J. Myers Youth
 Access Center
Philadelphia, Pennsylvania

Lois K. Evans, DNSc, FAAN
Professor and Executive Director
Collaborative Assessment and Rehabilitation
 for Elder Program (CARE)
University of Pennsylvania School of Nursing
 Penn Nursing Network

Director of Academic Nursing Practices,
 School of Nursing
University of Pennsylvania
Philadelphia, Pennsylvania

Lou Everett, RN, EdD, LMFT
Professor and Licensed Marriage & Family
 Therapist
Department of Community and Mental Health
 Nursing and Nursing Services
School of Nursing
East Carolina University
Greenville, North Carolina

Jacqueline Fawcett, PhD, FAAN
Professor
University of Pennsylvania School of Nursing
Philadelphia, Pennsylvania

Linda Flynn, RN, MS
Instructor (Clinical)
University of Utah College of Nursing
Salt Lake City, Utah

Virginia Focht-New, RN, MSN
Director of River Crest Center/Ken-Crest
 Services
University of Pennsylvania
Philadelphia, Pennsylvania

Arthur Freeman, EdD
Chair of Department of Psychology
Philadelphia College of Osteopathic Medicine
Philadelphia, Pennsylvania

Joann H. Grayson, PhD
Professor of Psychology
James Madison University
Harrisonburg, Virginia

Carol R. Hartman, RN, DNSc, CS
Professor Emeritus
Boston College School of Nursing
Chestnut Hill, Massachusetts

Joan Kenerson King, MSN, RN, CS
Director of Mental Health
Visiting Nurse Association of Greater
 Philadelphia
Philadelphia, Pennsylvania

Lenore Kurlowicz, RN, PhD, CS
Postdoctoral Fellow-Geriatric Psychiatry
Department of Psychiatry and Behavioral
 Health
Psychiatric Consultation-Liaison Nurse
Hospital of the University of Pennsylvania
Philadelphia, Pennsylvania

Joyce K. Laben, JD, CS, FAAN
Professor
Vanderbilt University School of Nursing
Nashville, Tennessee

Suzanne Lego, PhD, CS, CGP, FAAN
Private Practice
Pittsburgh, Pennsylvania

Editor
*Perspectives in Psychiatric Care: The Journal
 for Nurse Psychotherapists*

Shelly Lurie, RN, MS, CS-P
Associate Director of Nursing, Faculty
 Associate
The Johns Hopkins University School of
 Nursing
Baltimore, Maryland

Advanced Practice Nurse
Psychotherapist; Private Practice
Baltimore, Maryland

Virginia A. Lynch, MSN, RN, FAAFS
Nurse Educator/Forensic Consultant
Founding President, International Association
of Forensic Nurses
Fort Collins, Colorado

Pamela E. Marcus, RN, MS, CS-P
Private Practice
Upper Marlboro, Maryland

Susan H. McCrone, RN, PhD, CS-P
Associate Professor
University of Maryland
Baltimore, Maryland

Wanda Mohr, RNC, PhD
Assistant Professor
University of Pennsylvania
Philadelphia, Pennsylvania

Freida H. Outlaw, DNSc, RNCS
Assistant Professor and Program Director of
Psychiatric-Mental Health Nursing
School of Nursing
University of Pennsylvania
Philadelphia, Pennsylvania

Advanced Practice Psychiatric Nurse
The Health Annex at the F.J. Myers Youth
Access Center
Philadelphia, Pennsylvania

Patricia Petretic-Jackson, PhD
Associate Professor
Department of Psychology
University of Arkansas
Fayetteville, Arkansas

Albert R. Roberts, MA, DSW
Professor
Graduate School of Social Work
Rutgers—The State University of New Jersey
New Brunswick, New Jersey

Editor-in-Chief
Crisis Intervention and Time-Limited Treatment

Sandra L. Rosen, RN, MSN, CS
Private Practice
Philadelphia, Pennsylvania

Marcia Scoville, RN, MS, CNM
Assistant Professor (Clinical)
University of Utah College of Nursing
Salt Lake City, Utah

E. Wendy Skiba-King, RN, PhD, CS, C
Associate Professor of Clinical Nursing
University of Medicine and Dentistry of
New Jersey
Newark, New Jersey

Private Practice
Somerset, New Jersey

Shirley A. Smoyak, PhD, FAAN
Professor and Director of Public Health
Rutgers—The State University of New Jersey
The Bloustein School of Planning and Public
Policy Program in Public Health
New Brunswick, New Jersey

Charles L. Whitfield, MD
Faculty, Rutgers University Advanced School
of Alcohol and Drug Studies
New Brunswick, New Jersey

Private Practice specializing in trauma recovery
Atlanta, Georgia

Barbara E. Wolfe, RN, PhD, CS
Assistant Professor
Department of Psychiatry
Harvard Medical School
Cambridge, Massachusetts

Clinical Nurse Specialist
Beth Israel Deaconess Medical Center
Boston, Massachusetts

M. Jane Yates, MN, PhD
The Atlanta Center for Cognitive Therapy
Atlanta, Georgia

Beatrice Crofts Yorker, JD, CS, FAAN
Associate Provost for Faculty Relations
Associate Professor of Nursing
Georgia State University
Atlanta, Georgia

Marlene Young, PhD, JD
Executive Director
National Organization for Victims Assistance
Washington, DC

Johanna Yurkow, MSN, RN, CS
Director of Clinical Services
Collaborative Assessment and Rehabilitation
    for Elders Program (CARE)
University of Pennsylvania School of Nursing
    Penn Nursing Network
Philadelphia, Pennsylvania

■ ■ ■ ■ ■ PREFACE

Advanced Practice Nurse (APN) is the umbrella term used by the American Nurses Association (ANA) and the American Association of Critical Care Nurses (AACN) to designate clinical nurse specialists, nurse practitioners, certified nurse-midwives, and certified registered nurse anesthetists. In psychiatric and mental health nursing, nurses are prepared at the graduate level as clinical nurse specialists or nurse practitioners. This text is written for students in psychiatric nursing at the advanced practice level and for nurses who care for patients with a secondary condition of emotional distress.

For more than a decade, the delivery of mental health care has moved from the hospital to the community. The prediction for the beginning of the 21st century is that primary care will redefine health care policy, or that health care policy will define primary care practice. With the emphasis on primary health care, the extension of care into various community-based programs requires that professional nurses be able to assess, manage, and monitor the overall care of people who have emotional and psychiatric problems.

In primary care, one person becomes the organizer and focal manager of care and services for an individual and family. In the ideal health care system, one person would manage both physical illness and mental health problems and would call others in for consultation as needed. In actuality, the delivery of mental health services is quite different from services for physical health. The mechanisms of intervention are far more prescriptive in physical health services because there is a defined etiology, in contrast to the more global disorganizing aspects of mental illness. Further, the nature of mental health interventions at this time is quite different. Excluding medications, other interventions fall into communicative modalities, which are labor intense and less specific in their outcomes. They also require attention and sensitivity by providers as to their own emotional reactions and responses to the client, and clients require more extensive supervision.

Preparation for the primary mental health care provider requires knowledge of the assessment and differential diagnosis of emotional problems. Ideally the primary mental health care provider should have a background in assessment of children, adolescents, adults, and older adults. A primary mental health care provider will need to be knowledgeable regarding legal aspects and rights of patients and third-party payment; assessment of neurological and psychological health; case management in terms of organizing, managing, and monitoring the care plans; psychopharmacology and biological interventions; protocols for use and monitoring of drugs; documented standards; the use of psychosocial interventions; and outcome measurement.

In 1993, the ANA outlined the primary care functions of the psychiatric nurse as follows:

- Conduct mental health promotion activities and education.
- Perform diagnostic and functional assessments.
- Develop treatment plans.
- Administer and/or prescribe drug therapies.
- Provide case management/monitoring services.

- Supervise assisting personnel.
- Provide crisis intervention.
- Conduct psychotherapy.
- Triage psychiatric emergencies.
- Determine levels of care.
- Do consultation/liaison work for hospital patients experiencing emotional or mental disorders.

Our objectives in writing this book are to:

- Relate the principles of community-based case management as it emerges across primary mental health care settings.
- Participate collaboratively with other disciplines and recognize when to seek referral and consultation.

- Describe the ethical and legal implications of advanced practice for nurses, including prescriptive authority.
- Document outcome measures for treatment modalities by type of mental health care problem.

This text aims to develop skills for psychiatric nursing practice, including prescribing and/or monitoring pharmacological needs of patients and identifying outcome results for various mental health modalities. The intent is to speak to the current advanced practice role and to prepare for the inevitable and exciting changes of the new century.

Ann Wolbert Burgess

MERGING THE CNS AND NP ROLES IN ADVANCED PSYCHIATRIC NURSING: PRO AND CON

Linda Chafetz • Geri Collins-Bride • Suzanne Lego

Chapter Overview

- The Case Against Merging the CNS and NP Roles
    The CNS Alone
    The Nurse Practitioner Alone
    The Combined Role
- The Case for Comprehensive Role Preparation
    Advances in Knowledge About Psychiatric Care
    Health Needs of the Severely Mentally Impaired
    Changes in the Profession of Nursing
    Conclusion: A New Mandate for Advanced Practice
        Psychiatric Nursing
- References

Suzanne Lego wrote "The Case Against," and Linda Chafetz and Geri Collins-Bride wrote "The Case For."

THE CASE AGAINST MERGING THE CNS AND NP ROLES

Health care reform has led to the increasing visibility of advanced practice nurses: the clinical nurse specialist (CNS), nurse anesthetist, nurse practitioner (NP), and nurse-midwife. In psychiatric or mental health nursing the concept of the psychiatric nurse practitioner is a new one, spawned by several factors. The downsizing in hospitals has meant the elimination of CNS positions. At the same time, owing to the political acumen of organized nurse practitioners, federal funding has increased for graduate programs preparing NPs. Graduate programs across the country, seeing enrollments drop in CNS programs and rapidly increase in NP programs, have officially converted their CNS programs to NP programs, altering the curriculum to add courses in assessment, health management, and pharmacology.

At the same time, the need for primary health care has become all too evident. Vulnerable mentally ill individuals in public hospitals, shelters, inner cities, poor rural areas, and on the streets lack primary health care. For these reasons, graduate students in psychiatric nursing are being prepared to deliver primary health care including assessment, management, and pharmacological treatment as well as health maintenance and preventive care to psychiatric patients.

A controversy has developed over whether NPs should replace CNSs (who would be phased out), whether CNSs should stay and NPs go (leaving primary care to "generic" primary care providers), whether both should stay, or whether the roles should be combined into a new category called psychiatric/mental health (PMH) advanced practice. Table I–1 gives an overview.

THE CNS ALONE

As the concept of psychiatric nurse practitioner has evolved and graduate programs are designed to prepare them, many psychiatric clinical nurse specialists have been opposed to the idea. (Lego, 1995). They reason that primary care could be provided by physicians and the growing body of generic nurse practitioners. Using the analogy of medicine, psychiatrists are not being trained to give physical examinations and perform the many duties involved in primary care, as well as keep up with their specialty. Some CNSs see the new psychiatric NP as a kind of "generalist/specialist" who would be required to know all there is about primary care and all there is about specialization, and wonder if one person could do all this well.

Because CNSs in PMH have worked so hard to have high educational standards leading to advanced nurse certification, most managed care organizations and insurance companies recognize CNSs as providers, although this varies from state to state. In addition, in many states, CNSs operate independently and need not have a formal collaboration with a physician. This is changing as states develop advanced practice regulations, and in some states CNSs must have a formal collaborative relationship with physicians. This is new to CNSs. NPs, on the other hand, must in most states be either supervised by or collaborate with physicians. Because psychiatric CNSs value independence so much and have relied on internal regulation by the profession, they have been reluctant to give this up and rely on external regulation by state governments.

These battles have been lost. It is clear that each state will have an advanced practice act of some kind, and variation will be based on geographic location. Rural states like Maine, Oregon, and Alabama have regulations that permit independent practice. Advanced practice nurses in states with many medical schools and physicians will have to work more closely with physicians.

It is also clear that nurse practitioners are here to stay. Advanced practice nurses must

TABLE I–1. NURSING ROLES IN ADVANCED PRACTICE

	Advantages	Disadvantages/Liabilities
CNS alone	1. Provides individual, group, and family therapy based on specific theory. 2. Owing to ANCC certification, receives reimbursement from most insurance companies and recognition as providers by most MCOs. 3. Practices independently without the supervision or regulated "collaboration" of physicians, though this is changing in some states.	1. Have not been as well organized politically as NPs and have less political clout. 2. Graduate programs are becoming more scarce than NP programs. 3. Positions in hospitals are dwindling. CNSs must practice privately in group practice.
NP alone	1. Primary care is increasingly becoming synonymous with any health care (Haber & Billings, 1995). 2. Underserved populations will receive better care from NPs (Lego, 1993). 3. Legal entanglements exist when trying to include CNSs in advanced practice legislation (Cronenwett, 1995). 4. "As policy-makers and the public become familiar with the nurse practitioner title, CNSs will become all but invisible" (Caverly, 1995, p. 65).	1. Unless programs are lengthened beyond 2 years, NPs have only a superficial knowledge of specialized theory in psychiatric nursing. 2. Longer programs adversely affect enrollment (Cronenwett, 1995). 3. Psychiatric nurses who want to practice psychotherapy alone, without doing physical exams or care, will leave the field (or will not enter it) for careers in psychology, social work, or counseling.
Combined CNS and NP	1. Many similarities already exist in roles (Soehran & Schumann, 1994). 2. Practice settings for both are expanding and overlapping (Soehran & Schumann, 1994). 3. Unity and an increase in numbers would give more power to advanced practice nurses (Soehran & Schumann, 1994). 4. Many similarities already exist in educational preparation (Soehran & Schumann, 1994). 5. Educational institutions would save money by combining roles into one program (Soehran & Schumann, 1994). 6. Graduates with both credentials would be more marketable (Soehran & Schumann, 1994). 7. In many states they are already combined. 8. The public and other disciplines would be less confused about nursing titles.	1. Scope of practice is different; NPs are generalists who manage illness and promote health, and CNSs are specialists (Cronenwett, 1995). 2. Specialization is watered down, so the APN knows a little bit about a lot of things. 3. The knowledge explosion would make it difficult for the practitioner to keep up with health and disease management, general pharmacology, psychopathology, and psychopharmacology. 4. Same disadvantages as NP alone (see above).

work together politically to achieve more favorable regulations. In Pennsylvania all four groups of advanced practice nurses are working together.

THE NURSE PRACTITIONER ALONE

The elimination of CNS positions in hospitals and the closing of CNS graduate programs could lead to the elimination of the CNS role. It is clear that the concept of the psychiatric NP role is market driven, both by the availability of graduate training funds and the need in the health care industry (insurance companies and hospitals) for less expensive health care providers. The market-driven approach is short-sighted and destructive to any profession. Menand writes, "True professions are self-regulating: they control the nature of their services and they do so by the lights of what is proper for the professions rather than what market conditions demand" (Menand, 1995, p. 17).

Hospitals reason that with nurse practitioners they can get primary care provided for much less money at all hours of the day and night. This is beneficial for hopitals and patients, but how does it affect the profession? Many studies, as well as anecdotal wisdom, tell us that nurse practitioners provide better primary care than primary care physicians. But will psychiatric nurse practitioners? This depends on how they are educated. In some of the new graduate programs, students are taught much about physical assessments, pharmacology, anatomy, physiology, and pathophysiology, but not much of the theory traditionally considered to be core to our specialty. For example, these programs have no organized theoretical courses in psychopathology or individual, group, or family therapy. When I've asked about these deficits, I was told these are a part of the "management" courses or that these will be taught "at the placement." We all know what that means—on-the-job training. Some of these programs use nonpsychiatric patients for a primary care practicum in the first year and psychiatric patients in the second year, thereby reasoning the graduates are psychiatric nurse practitioners.

Other graduate programs are building on a year at the end of the program to learn primary care, or are adding a "postmaster's" extension in primary care. These programs continue to provide courses in the "core" clinical specialization (O'Toole, 1996).

Many CNSs across the country enjoy practicing psychotherapy and have no interest in performing physical tasks. Many are leaving the field, and becoming social workers, psychologists, marriage and family therapists, or counselors.

THE COMBINED ROLE

Those who advocate combining the roles point out that overlap already exists, money in educational programs would be saved, the nurse prepared for the combined role would be more marketable, and the public would be less confused by all the titles in nursing. In addition, there is power in numbers. All of this may be true, but there is more to consider.

First, can one person do all this well? Can the psychiatric advanced practice nurse (APN) provide primary care keeping abreast of all there is to know about assessing and treating disease, health maintenance, general pharmacology and psychopharmacology, and the interactions of drugs, psychopathology, psychotherapy, and theories about human development and behavior? *The psychiatric APN will be the first health profession to claim so much territory.* How could this person keep up with all the new information needed and still have time to practice? The information explosion after all is why we have specialization! It is inevitable that the care this nurse provides will be watered down.

Second, because our patients need primary care, do we simply do away with specialization? Suppose cardiologists as a group decided that because heart disease is caused in large part by poor diet, lack of exercise, and smoking they should eliminate the specialization and prepare primary care cardiologists who only teach good diet, exercise, and smoke-ending techniques. Who would do the highly specific cardiac management and surgery? One might argue, but no one else can *do* these things except cardiologists. Similarly, can what psychiatric CNSs do be done by others, such as social workers or counselors? Can it be done well? Psychiatric CNSs provide high-quality care because of our undergraduate study of general health matters and wellness (Lego, 1993). But, should we abandon our specialization? Specialization does not necessarily mean abandoning a holistic approach.

Autonomy has been maintained in professions by delegating "down" technical tasks. No one confuses a lawyer with a paralegal or a dentist with a dental hygienist. Nursing, however, has failed to gain full respect as a profession because it has not differentiated levels but has rather maintained the stance that a nurse is a nurse (Brannon, 1994). The public sees no difference between the diploma nurse and doctorally prepared nurse. Combining the NP and the CNS is a further example of what some consider an anti-intellectual, self-destructive streak in nursing. By watering down our specialty, following market forces to include primary care, we reduce our professional standing.

Futurists agree that knowledge is the tool that will be marketable in the next century, and that the more specialized one's knowledge, the better. Drucker (1994, p. 68) writes as follows.

> In the knowledge society, knowledge for the most part exists only in application. Nothing the x-ray technician needs to know can be applied to market research, for instance, or to teaching medieval history. The central work force in the knowledge society will therefore consist of highly specialized people. In fact, it is a mistake to speak of "generalists." What we will increasingly mean by that term is people who have learned how to acquire additional specialties rapidly in order to move from one kind of job to another—for example, from market research into management, or from nursing into hospital administration. But "generalists" in the

sense in which we used to talk of them are coming to be seen as dilettantes rather than educated people.

> This, too, is new. Historically, workers were generalists. They did whatever had to be done—on the farm, in the household, in the craftsman's shop. This was also true of industrial workers. But knowledge workers, whether their knowledge is primitive or advanced, whether there is a little of it or a great deal, will by definition be specialized.

> Applied knowledge is effective only when it is specialized. Indeed, the more highly specialized, the more effective it is. This goes for technicians who service computers, x-ray machines, or the engines of fighter planes. But it applies equally to work that requires the most advanced knowledge whether research in genetics or research in astrophysics or putting on the first performance of a new opera.

> Again, the shift from knowledge to knowledges offers tremendous opportunities to the individual. It makes possible a career as a knowledge worker. But it also presents a great many new problems and challenges. It demands for the first time in history that people with knowledge take responsibility for making themselves understood by people who do not have the same knowledge base.

I have been supportive of the nurse practitioner movement since I first learned of it years ago, because I believe the health of the nation will benefit. I do not support the concept of the combined role, because I don't believe one person can know all there is to know about both primary care and specialized care to provide the high level of care that psychiatric clinical nurse specialists have tendered. I believe the move toward "generalizing" the specialist places us in a poor light when viewed by other disciplines.

The best compromise? If psychiatric nurse practitioners are educated to work side by side with psychiatric clinical nurse specialists, I would advocate for having longer NP master's programs that retain the core CNS knowledge, and adding on a year's preparation in primary care.

THE CASE FOR COMPREHENSIVE ROLE PREPARATION

This section presents the case for comprehensive preparation for advanced practice psychiatric nursing that incorporates clinical specialist and primary care competencies. It does *not* advocate wholesale merger of conventional CNS and NP programs, with the dilution of overall content. Instead, it argues for a reconceptualization of the core functions of advanced practice psychiatric nursing to embrace those activities required for autonomous and comprehensive care of the mentally ill: biopsychosocial assessment and diagnosis; psychotherapeutic management of mental disorders with individuals, groups, and families; screening for risk factors and co-morbidities associated with mental disorders; management of common or stable co-morbidity within a comprehensive mental health service plan; and maintenance of an integrated health record.

The arguments for and against comprehensive or "blended" preparation have been presented in a number of recent reports from educators and service providers, including the previous section of this introduction (Cronenwett, 1995; McConnell et al., 1992; Moller and Haber, 1996; Tally and Caverly, 1994; Worley et al., 1990). This literature is often contentious, but a large part of the debate appears to center on whether to maintain the traditional clinical nurse specialist role, which in turn is frequently equated with the practice of psychotherapy. This is an emotionally charged issue for those who fear that a reduced emphasis on therapy may indicate capitulation to market-driven forces.

The place of psychotherapy among advanced practice competencies represents an important concern, but it may be tangential to the question of comprehensive preparation. There is no doubt that a comprehensive or blended curriculum reduces the number of supervised hours that students may complete in specific psycho-

therapeutic modalities. However, core competencies should define the *foundation* for advanced practice roles and not their limits. In this sense they would not prevent further specialization or postgraduate training in specific psychotherapies. If the issue of the therapist role is put aside for a moment, there is actually relative consensus in the literature on the need for at least *some* advanced practice psychiatric nurses to acquire primary care skills for comprehensive services for the mentally ill.

This chapter will consider comprehensive or blended preparation, not as an expedient route to employment or prescriptive authority, but rather as the measured response of a profession to changes that alter its social mandate. These include changes in our knowledge base about psychiatric disorders and their treatment, and changes in the health needs of the mentally ill, determined by their own demography and by their place in emerging systems of managed care. Finally, comprehensive programs represent a reaction to developments within nursing, and to evolving goals of master's-degree-level education.

ADVANCES IN KNOWLEDGE ABOUT PSYCHIATRIC CARE

Changes in our knowledge about the nature and treatment of psychiatric disorders have altered the practice all mental health professions, psychiatric nursing among them. The development of contemporary diagnostic nomenclature provided the common language in psychiatry essential to epidemiological initiatives such as the National Institute of Mental Health Epidemiological Catchment Area (ECA) study and the National Comorbidity Survey (NCS) (Bourdon et al., 1992; Kessler et al., 1994; Sartorius et al., 1993). These provide the beginnings of a map of mental disorders in the United States, within communities and within service sectors. Although this map is tentative and incomplete (for example, work is in progress in the area of childhood disorders), it provides an objective basis for setting priorities for services and training.

In addition to knowledge about distribution of mental disorders, mental health services research provides increasing guidance on their treatment. In 1981, a comprehensive review of the body of research on community treatment programs by Braun and colleagues identified serious problems in the literature as a whole that limited its value in driving program development, including lack of statistical power to detect treatment effects. Today the number of large, controlled studies, including randomized clinical trials, has multiplied, producing predictions of outcome for at least some specific treatments. Comprehensive research reviews, consensus conferences, and the like increasingly provide a basis for published practice guidelines and widely accepted treatment recommendations for some of the most prevalent disorders in the United States (Agency for Health Care Policy and Research, 1993; American Psychiatric Association, 1996; Hirschfield et al., 1994; Laraia, 1996; Reynolds et al., 1993).

Thus, we know from both ECA and NCS reports that the most common psychiatric problems in our general population include mood and anxiety disorders. We also know, on the basis of clinical trials, that effective treatments exist for these problems (e.g., mild to moderate depression, anxiety attacks). When practice guidelines stipulate "effective treatments," they generally refer to new medications that represent important advances in psychopharmacology. Whatever the individual nurse's position on use of medication, newer agents are often safer and more socially acceptable than first-generation drugs, and hence far less likely to be considered as treatments of last resort. Published guidelines and recommendations also include some psychosocial therapies that have shown demonstrable benefits in controlled studies, either in combination with medications or alone; examples are cognitive-behavioral and interpersonal therapies for depression (Agency for Health Care Policy and Research, 1993; Persons et al., 1996) and family psychoeducation in schizophrenia (Gamble and Mindence, 1994; Penn and Mueser, 1996).

Some practice guidelines can be applied safely by primary care providers, particularly medication regimens for mild to moderate disorders (Gonzales et al., 1994). However the literature does not justify a wholesale shift of psychiatric care to the primary care sector. On the contrary, a careful reading of research tends to confirm what has long been suspected by psychiatric clinicians—that even the most common disorders present in more severe, recurrent forms in the mental health specialty sector (Agency for Health Care Policy and Research, 1993), and that common diagnoses tend to co-occur (Bourdon et al., 1993; Kessler et al., 1996). According to the NCS (Kessler et al., 1994), more than half of all lifetime mental disorder occurs among one-sixth of the population with three or more co-occurring disorders. This adds to the complexity of care, even when individual diagnoses are fairly common (anxiety attacks, depression, alcohol abuse). People with diagnoses of more severe and persistent disorders (such as schizophrenia and major affective illness) require extensive specialty sector services to maintain function and to avoid repeated acute care episodes.

Advanced practice nurses require comprehensive skills to meet the complex needs of clients with multiple problems, such as severely mentally ill adults. Proficiency in insight-oriented psychotherapies may be helpful to some clients, but it does not meet their more fundamental needs to understand and manage illness, and to maintain quality of life. These clients require nurses with comprehensive assessment skills (including physical assessment, assessment of mental status, knowledge of laboratory tests, and ability to obtain a complete medical and psychiatric history) that provide the diagnostic basis for treatment planning. They need clinicians who can deliver the supportive and educational interventions recommended in the literature, and who can manage care across systems. Because medication is often the linchpin of treatment, and because psychotropic medications have profound effects on all aspects of health, clients will require advanced practice nurses with thorough preparation in pharmacology. In sum, they will require some of the primary care skills associated with the nurse practitioner role.

HEALTH NEEDS OF THE SEVERELY MENTALLY IMPAIRED

All psychiatric specialists may require some primary care competencies, but nurses working with the most vulnerable subgroups will require the most. Major mental disorders compromise health in every sense. Allebeck (1989) calls schizophrenia a "life shortening disorder," to call attention to the effects of mental illness on survival. Although suicide accounts for much of the premature mortality observed among the severely mentally impaired, a residual amount stems from risk factors associated with psychiatric disability (Simpson and Tsuang, 1996). Cardiovascular disease presents special risk to severely mentally ill adults because of their high rates of cigarette smoking, sedentary activities, and weight gain (Hayward, 1995; Jeste et al., 1996), that is itself an example of the iatrogenic effects of psychotropic medication (Stanton, 1995).

Persons with psychiatric disabilities and with few private resources share many of the health problems associated with unstable housing and unsafe living conditions (Breaky et al., 1989; Gelberg and Linn, 1989). These include infections and infestations, problems related to hygiene and nutrition, and traumatic injuries due to violence. Dependence on congregate living situations increases risk of communicable diseases such as tuberculosis (Kitazawa, 1995; Zolopa et al., 1994). Respiratory problems, asthmatic symptoms, and other disorders related to air quality appear to be on the increase among the urban poor (Bates, 1995; White et al., 1994) and the mentally ill among them.

The mentally ill also present primary care needs related to co-morbidity. Severe mental illness significantly increases the odds of developing a co-occurring substance use disorder (Drake et al., 1996; Regier et al., 1990). Drugs and alcohol are recognized predictors of poor psychiatric outcomes, such as frequent relapse (Bartels et al., 1995; Dickey and Azeni, 1996). They also contribute to a well-known array of medical illnesses. Current reports describe high rates of HIV seropositivity among psychiatric inpatients (Cournos et al., 1994; Empfield et al., 1993) due in large part to intravenous drug abuse (Susser et al., 1996). Less dramatic sequelae of substance abuse may be equally problematic in the future. A cohort of severely mentally ill adults with histories of extensive substance abuse is currently approaching midlife, with serious implications for their future care needs.

Even in the absence of significant co-morbidity, the aging of this population suggests escalating primary care needs. The mentally ill have always grown old, but in the past the most vulnerable among them did so in public hospitals that assumed—for better or worse—the responsibility for their care. During the deinstitutionalization period, elderly state hospital patients often moved directly to other long-term facilities (Chafetz et al., 1983). Currently, a generation of mental health consumers has come of age residing in community settings. As this group accrues the predictable chronic health problems of later adulthood, they will need access to screening, prevention, and care that is integrated with psychiatric regimens and available at a single point of contact with health care services.

More often than not, these clients seek this point of contact for comprehensive services through a mental health program. Mental health staff not only treat psychiatric problems, but also provide access to a range of support services. This is because of their skills in psychotherapeutic management and their ability to establish trusting relationships with individuals who have difficulty communicating or interacting with others. However, many current mental health program staff have backgrounds in social rehabilitation that leave them ill-equipped to deal with medical complexity. They often depend on referrals to community medical providers, fragmenting the overall treatment plan.

Even the best referrals may be difficult for individuals who have difficulty negotiating appointments, articulating their problems clearly, or tolerating questions and physical examination procedures. Nonpsychiatric providers lack the requisite skills and knowledge to guide a symptomatic client through an interview, to determine drug and alcohol use, or to consider a serious psychiatric illness and its treatment in their larger plan of care. Consequently, the severely mentally impaired may receive inadequate care (Jeste et al., 1996; Koryanyi, 1979) or use costly emergency services for preventable crises (Padgett et al., 1995).

Fragmentation of services for mind and body has often been attributed to traditions of different funding sources for medical, psychiatric, and substance abuse services. However, in managed care environments of the future there will be fewer structural impediments to integrated care. Instead, the main obstacle to "seamless" services may be providers without the educational preparation to bridge sectors of care. If we are to remain a relevant force for care of the mentally ill, we will need skills for comprehensive care.

CHANGES IN THE PROFESSION OF NURSING

Advanced practice roles are also changing in reaction to alterations and evolution within the profession of nursing. With restrictions on the duration of inpatient care, many nursing functions have been transferred to community settings. In California, for example, a report entitled *Planning for California's Workforce* predicted a loss of almost 4000 staff nurse positions in acute hospitals during the next decade (California Strategic Planning Committee for Nursing, 1996). Employment opportunities are expected to shift to advanced practice roles in home care and community settings.

Advanced practice psychiatric nurses in these settings cannot rely on the back-up services of a medical center. This means that they will require the ability to at least screen and make safe decisions about general health issues that intrude upon or complicate psychiatric care. This includes having enough familiarity with traditional medical systems to negotiate for urgent care or specialty consultations. Even in cases where primary care skills overlap considerably with CNS competencies, advanced practice nurses will require *credentialing* that allows them to make decisions in the field and act upon them.

At the University of California, San Francisco, we have experimented for several years with a curriculum blending psychiatric and adult nurse practitioner requirements. At present, our psychiatric NP students complete requirements for state and ANA credentialing as adult nurse practitioners (there is no state credential for a psychiatric NP in California). Thus, they have more preparation in primary care than psychiatric NPs who are credentialed for specialty practice in some states. If and when the American Nurses Credentialing Center (ANCC) develops a national examination for psychiatric nurse practitioners, we would reconsider a few of the current ANP requirements, but not many. Our experience to date indicates that comprehensive care of high-risk subgroups (the elderly mentally ill, co-morbid populations) requires thorough training in assessment and management of common or chronic medical illness.

All the same, our comprehensive program differs substantially from the traditional ANP curriculum. First of all it includes all psychiatric specialty core courses. In addition, the psychiatric NP students complete most of their clinical practice requirements in integrated placements that allow them to apply the full complement of their skills—psychiatric as well as medical. For this reason they spend the same amount of time in interaction with the mentally ill as our CNS students (still an option here), and receive comparable process-oriented supervision. Applicants for this comprehensive program come in large part from the ranks of psychiatric inpatient nurses. They envision an expanded role and a new scope of practice, but they maintain a solid commitment to care of the mentally ill. Some of them, particularly younger applicants, are less experienced than prior generations of CNS students. They want course work that will ensure their basic competence as clinicians, before they venture into more complex roles as supervisors or consultants. Some faculty may view these less sophisticated students as an exceptional challenge, but they probably represent the future. With the increasing career choices open to young women, and with more men recruited to nursing programs, we cannot expect students to defer their specialty preparation until they are seasoned clinicians.

CONCLUSION: A NEW MANDATE FOR ADVANCED PRACTICE PSYCHIATRIC NURSING

Our knowledge about psychiatric treatment has developed exponentially over the past decades. Psychiatric services must also adapt to the changing demographic and clinical profile of the mentally ill in community settings. As a profession, we are increasingly recruiting students who see specialty preparation as the debut of a career. Our conceptualization of the advanced practice psychiatric nurse must evolve to remain relevant to health care systems, consumers, and our own profession. Thus, we must reconsider the set of skills that are essential to entry level advanced practice.

These skills would logically correspond to societal expectations for advanced practice nurses in mental health. A growing mental health advocacy movement makes it clear that clients and their families expect clear information about psychiatric disorders and about available treatment options. They expect these from any mental health professional, but given our discipline's traditional emphasis on education and self-care, we probably have special obligations in this area. Clients and families also expect psychiatric providers to possess the level of skill necessary to communicate effectively with persons experiencing a broad range of psychopathology. Even when a treatment plan is essentially pharmaco-

logical, it is our psychotherapeutic skills and our use of self that promote learning, adherence to regimens, motivation, and hope. Because most service plans involve far more than psychopharmacology (and as drug effects are frequently incomplete or disappointing), we also need psychosocial skills with individuals, families, and groups, including techniques to support, manage illness, and prevent relapse. These core competencies could be considered the foundation for training in more long-term or insight-oriented therapies, but they do not include psychotherapy practice.

If blended or comprehensive programs respond to a clear need, should these provide the model for education in advanced practice psychiatric nursing? Or should we also consider programs to prepare nurse psychotherapists as occurring on a parallel track? Much psychotherapy training could be described as multidisciplinary, with similar activities performed by social workers, counselors, psychologists, MDs, and nurse-psychotherapists. Most psychotherapy credentialing or licensing requires extensive practice beyond the master's-degree level. There may be excellent reasons to preserve nurse psychotherapist roles as distinct and to provide a mechanism for their credentialing within the profession of nursing. However, these roles and credentials cannot provide a basis for consistent titling. Given a choice between comprehensive role preparation and therapy training as the bottom line for advanced practice, the arguments for comprehensive preparation outweigh those for requirement of therapy training for the master of science degree, for third-party reimbursement, and for prescriptive authority.

Are there risks in promoting comprehensive or blended preparation? Yes, and they are formidable. It will take clinicians with the courage of their convictions to deliver what they identify as needed services, in systems that would prefer to manage many problems via medication and in primary care. Psychiatric nursing and primary care cultures may be in conflict. For example, speed in evaluation is a value, even an exigence, in many primary care practices. In contrast, we teach psychiatric specialists the art of long and careful assessments that integrate elements of interpersonal process (e.g., establishing trust) into diagnostic encounters. There is a risk that the psychiatric NPS may adapt to the relative structure and clarity of medical-type practice and abandon the commitment to the more intuitive and engaged aspects of mental health nursing.

However, changes also confront our nurse practitioner colleagues, challenging them to rethink their sphere of practice. Nurse practitioner programs were initially created and federally supported to help provide primary care to all people, the underserved in particular. Early programs attracted extraordinary students with the determination to carve out unconventional roles, placing health promotion and protection at the heart of their practice. Today, many NPs work in conventional medical settings where demands for cost-effectiveness constrain their roles and leave little or no time for education and prevention. Nurse practitioners in some settings are also experiencing threats to their autonomy and their recognition as primary care providers, due to corporate decisions about financing of medical care.

Some nurse practitioners may decide that their primary care skills are most valued in settings for vulnerable and medically underserved populations such as severely mentally ill adults, persons with substance use disorders, and the mentally ill with chronic medical disorders. If they do so, they are likely to seek blended preparation. Primary care to many mentally ill clients may be essential, but it is not sufficient to meet their needs for truly comprehensive care, including access to state-of-the-art treatments and services that may resolve or ameliorate their specific problems.

Development of more comprehensive role preparation will require testing, with evaluation of new educational models, and with a willingness from both the specialist and primary care sectors to share knowledge and skills. This collaboration may be easier said than done, given the differences in style and values between CNS (mental health) and NP (medical) sectors, the degree to which both groups may identify with non-nurse providers (e.g., psychotherapists or primary care physicians), and the strong anxiety we all feel about seeing our competencies somehow devalued or diluted. Despite the difficulties, this collaboration is essential if we are to present a meaningful role to consumers, and to assume a significant place in emerging mental health systems. Hopefully, the national leadership will emerge to promote it in the coming decade.

REFERENCES

Agency for Health Care Policy and Research. *Depression in Primary Care*. AHCPR pub. no. 93-0551. Rockville, MD: U.S. DHHS. 1993.

Allebeck P. Schizophrenia: A life-shortening disease. *Schizophr Bull*. 1989;15:81–89.

American Psychiatric Association. *APA Practice Guidelines*. Washington DC: APA; 1996.

Bartels SJ, Drake RE, Wallach MA. Long-term substance use disorders among patients with severe mental illness. *Psychiatr Serv*. 1995;46:248–251.

Bates DV. Observations on asthma. *Environ Health Perspect*. 1995;103(suppl 6):243–247.

Bourdon KH, Rae DS, Locke BZ, et al. Estimating the prevalence of mental disorders in U.S. adults from the Epidemiological Catchment Area Survey. *Public Health Rep*. 1992;107:663–668.

Brannon RL. *Intensifying care: The Hospital Industry, Professionalization, and the Reorganization of the Nursing Labor Process*. Amityville, NY: Baywood. 1994.

Braun P, Kochansky G, Shapiro R, et al. Overview: Deinstitutionalization of psychiatric patients, a critical review of outcomes studies. *Am J Psychiatry*. 1981;138:736–749.

California Strategic Planning Committee for Nursing. *Planning for California's Workforce: A Task Force Report*, Sacramento. 1996.

Caverly S. Clinical specialist or nurse practitioner: An issue of semantics, not true difference. *J Am Psychiatr Nurs Assoc*. 1995;1:61–63.

Chafetz L, Goldman HH, Taube CA. Deinstitutionalization in the United States. *Int J Ment Health*. 1983;11:48–63.

Cournos F, Guido JR, Coomaraswamy S, et al. Sexual activity and risk of HIV infection among patients with schizophrenia. *Am J Psychiatry.* 1994;151: 228–232.

Cronenwett LR. Molding the future of advanced nursing practice. *Nurs Outlook.* 1995;43:112–118.

Dickey B, Azeni H. Persons with dual diagnoses of substance abuse and major mental illnesses: Their excess costs of psychiatric care. *Am J Public Health.* 1996;86:973–977.

Drake RE, Meuser KT, Clark RE, Wallach MA. The course, treatment, and outcome of substance use disorder in persons with severe mental illness. *Am J Orthopsychiatry.* 1996;66:42–51.

Drucker PF. The age of social transformation. *Atlantic Monthly.* 1994;274:53–80.

Empfield M, Cournos F, Meyer I, et al. HIV seroprevalence among homeless patients admitted to a psychiatric inpatient unit. *Am J Psychiatry.* 1993; 150:47–52.

Gamble C, Mindence K. Schizophrenia family work: Mental health nurses delivering an innovative service. *J Psychosoc Nurs Ment Health Serv.* 1994; 32:13–16.

Gelberg L, Linn L. Assessing the physical health of homeless adults. *JAMA.* 1989;262:1973–1979.

Gonzales JJ, Magruder KM, Keith SJ. Mental disorders in primary care services: An update. *Public Health Rep.* 1994;109:251–258.

Haber J, Billings C. Primary mental health care: A model for psychiatric-mental health nursing. *J Am Psychiatr Nurs Assoc.* 1995;1:154–163.

Hirschfeld RM, Clayton PJ, Cohen I, Faucett J. Practice guidelines for the treatment of patients with bipolar depression. *Am J Psychiatry.* 1994; 151 (suppl):40.

Jeste DV, Gladsjo JA, Lindamer LA, Lacro JP. Medical comorbidity in schizophrenia. *Schizophr Bull.* 1996;22:413–420.

Kessler RC, Nelson CB, McGonagle KA, et al. The epidemiology of co-occurring addictive and mental disorders: Implications for prevention and service utilization. *Am J Orthopsychiatry.* 1996; 66:17–31.

Kessler RC, McGonagle KA, Nelson CB, et al. Lifetime and twelve month prevalence of DSM-III psychiatric disorders in the United States. Results from the National Comorbidity Survey. *Arch Gen Psychiatry.* 1994;51:8–19.

Kitazawa S. Tuberculosis health education: Needs in homeless shelters. *Public Health Nurs.* 1995;12: 409–416.

Koryanyi EK. Morbidity and rate of undiagnosed physical illness in a psychiatric population. *Arch Gen Psychiatry.* 1979;36:414–419.

Laraia MT. Current approaches to psychopharmacological treatment of depression in children and adolescents. *J Child Adolesc Psychiatr Nurs.* 1996; 9:15–26.

Lego S. Nurse psychotherapists: How are we different? *Perspect Psychiatr Care.* 1993;11: 144–147.

Lego S. A psychiatric nurse practitioner is not a clinical nurse specialist. *J Am Psychiatr Nurs Assoc.* 1995;1:61–63.

Menand L. The trashing of professionalism. *Academe.* May–June, 1995;16–19.

McConnell SD, Inderbitzzin LB, and Pollard WE. Primary health care in the CMHC: a role for the nurse practitioner. *Hosp Community Psychiatry,* 1992;43: 724–727.

Moller MD, Haber J. Advanced practice psychiatric nursing: The need for a blended role. *Online J Issues Nurs.* August 1, 1996;1–9.

O'Toole AW. Designing a graduate program in psychiatric-mental health nursing. In S. Lego (Ed) *Psychiatric Nursing: A Comprehensive Reference.* Philadelphia: Lippincott. 1996;432–440.

Padgett DK, Streuning EL, Andrews H, Pittman J. Predictors of emergency room use by homeless adults in New York City: The influence of predisposing, enabling, and need factors. *Social Sci Med.* 1995;41:547–556.

Penn DL, Mueser KT. Research update on the psychosocial treatment of schizophrenia. *Am J Psychiatry.* 1996;153:607–617.

Persons JB, Thase ME, Crits-Cristoph P. The role of psychotherapy in the treatment of deoppression: review of two practice guidelines. *Arch Gen Psychiatry,* 1996;53:284–290.

Regier DA, Farmer ME, Rae DS, et al. Comorbidity of mental disorders with alcohol and other drug abuse: Results from the Epidemiological Catchment Area Study. *JAMA.* 1990;264:2511–2518.

Reynolds CF, Lebowitz BD, Schneider LS. The NIH consensus development conference on diagnosis and treatment of depression in late life. *Psychopharmacol Bull.* 1993;29:83–85.

Sartorius N, Kaelber CT, Cooper JE, et al. Progress toward achieving a common language in psychiatry: Results from the field trial accompanying the WHO classification of mental and behavioral disorders in ICD-10. *Arch Gen Psychiatry*. 1993;50: 115–124.

Simpson JC, Tsuang MT. Mortality among patients with schizophrenia. *Schizophr Bull*. 1996;22: 485–499.

Soehran PM, Schumann LL. Enhanced role opportunities available to the CNS/nurse practitioner. *Clinical Nurse Specialist*. 1994;8(1), 23–27.

Stanton JM. Weight gain associated with neuroleptic medication: A review. *Schizophr Bull*. 1995;21: 463–472.

Susser E, Miller M, Valencia E, et al. Injection drug use and risk of HIV transmission among homeless men with mental illness. *Am J Psychiatry*. 1996; 156:794–798.

Talley S, Caverly S. Advanced-practice psychiatric nursing and health care reform. *Hosp Commun Psychiatr*. 1994;45:545–547.

White MC, Etzel RA, Wilcox WD, Lloyd C. Exacerbation of childhood asthma and ozone pollution in Atlanta. *Environ Res*. 1994;65:56–68.

Worley NK, Drago L, and Hadley T. Improving the physical health-mental health interface for the chronically mentally ill: Could nurse case managers make a difference? *Arch Psych Nurs*. 1990;4: 108–113.

Zolopa AR, Hahn JA, Gorter R, et al. HIV and tuberculosis infection in San Francisco's homeless adults. *JAMA*. 1994;272:455–461.

ADVANCED PRACTICE FOR THE 21ST CENTURY

I

HISTORICAL INFLUENCES ON TODAY'S EDUCATION AND PRACTICE

Shirley A. Smoyak • Wendy Skiba-King

Academic programs have responded to changes in practice settings, the focus of care, and reimbursement patterns by developing an array of hybrid curricula. The new choices include terms such as adult nurse practitioner (ANP) and clinical nurse specialist (CNS), producing the cumbersome hybrid ANP/CNS.

Chapter Overview

- Historical Overview
- Advanced Education
- Clinical Practice
- New Program Choices
- Certification and Licensure Debates
    Licensure
    Certification
    Variation Among States
    Health Care Reform and Workforce Regulation
- Plans for the Future
- References

▶ INTRODUCTION

As the debates about managed care and changes in the financing of health care have captured public attention, it is surprising that several essential facts are absent from the articles, speeches, editorials, and books. The specific debate about the utility of educators focusing on clinical nurse specialists or nurse practitioners curiously lacks the acknowledgment of critical historical events. This chapter provides the background and historical grounding for examining the issues of the educational preparation, practice, and legal regulations affecting nurses prepared at the master's-degree level in psychiatric and mental health nursing.

Historical Overview

Forty years ago when Hildegard E. Peplau developed the first master's degree program to prepare clinical specialists in psychiatric or mental health nursing, deinstitutionalization had not occurred. The great majority of nurses and patients were in hospital settings, largely public institutions, supported by government funds at city, county, state, and federal levels. Dr. Peplau's approach was innovative, creative, and pioneering. The master's program begun in 1955 at Rutgers, the State University of New Jersey, had as its exclusive focus the preparation of clinical specialists who studied theories that described and explained human behavior. Other master's programs focused on the preparation of educators or administrators. At this point in time, there was no "advanced practice" literature in psychiatric nursing or any other nursing specialty. Dr. Peplau's book, *Interpersonal Relations in Nursing*, stood alone in the field as a contribution of a nurse to the understanding of human behavior.

Dr. Peplau had studied with many neo-Freudian psychiatrists and was especially impressed by Harry Stack Sullivan. In the early years of the program, students read most of Sullivan's works, as well as those of Frieda Fromm-Reichman and others. The practice of the students was mainly in state psychiatric hospitals, where overcrowding and abysmal care were the order of the day.

Students learned how to use psychiatric interviewing techniques to help patients discover the roots of their problems, theorized as being in flawed interpersonal relationships. The chief focus was psychodynamic work with individual patients, who were seen daily or several times a week for interviewing sessions. The content of these sessions was analyzed in seminars lasting all day, directed by Peplau. Techniques of group therapy were also introduced, and group sessions were held in make-do rooms on locked units of the hospital wards. The patients in these settings rarely saw their families. Many had been hospitalized for decades.

Physical examination and assessment of physiological needs had been done on admission. In more enlightened settings, an annual (or biannual) physical examination might be performed, usually by a medical intern if the hospital had a teaching contract with a medical school, or by a foreign medical graduate, which was the more usual case. During the 1950s and into the 1960s, state hospitals still maintained medical units to treat physical illnesses and even to deliver babies. Slowly, these units closed and the psychiatric hospitals developed relationships with community hospitals to transfer patients with medical problems to them for treatment. Medical illness was considered an acute episode, rather than a chronic problem needing continuous care. Life expectancy had not yet climbed into the 70s for either men or women, and gero-psychiatry as a subspecialty for psychiatric patients was a relatively new idea. Between 1890 and 1950, half of all of the patients admitted to mental hospitals were 65 or older (personal communication, G Grob, October 29, 1996). Yet this elderly population, with its increased likelihood of medical and psychiatric co-morbidity, did not receive a high priority in research or service interests.

During this same period, the only significant medication, chlorpromazine (Thorazine), was introduced by Smith, Kline and French. Peplau's teaching efforts were enhanced by funding from SKF, which supported workshops, produced a film (the classic *Nurse–Patient Relationship* filmed at Greystone Park Psychiatric Hospital in New Jersey), and published copies of her lecture notes in a monograph commonly referred to as the "Purple Pamphlet." Ironically, Dr. Peplau never included psychopharmacology in her seminars or lectures. Nurses were expected to learn what they needed to know about this drug on their own. If the issue of medications was introduced into the seminar sessions, it was not greeted enthusiastically. The students in training were given the clear message that the appropriate focus of study was interpersonal relationships.

Upon graduation, the clinical nurse specialist (CNS) had to become knowledgeable about psychoactive drugs, because he or she was often in administrative roles, and also had to cope with language and knowledge barriers created by foreign medical graduates. Interestingly, in the literature, the case was often made for keeping the "purity" of the CNS role as simply psychotherapist. To our knowledge, a systematic study never documented which CNSs included pharmacological aspects in their care, which CNSs practiced as psychotherapists exclusively, and which included physiological matters in their practice approaches.

For many years, when master's degree programs in psychiatric nursing were funded by the National Institute for Mental Health (NIMH), program directors were brought together yearly to share their curricular concerns, teaching strategies, and ideas about directions for program development. Although nursing chiefs, beginning with Esther Garrison, suggested that the program directors should develop ways to track and monitor the practices of their graduates, it never happened. At one point, a postdoctoral nurse spent several semesters at NIMH trying to analyze the yearly accountability reports, but no publication resulted from those efforts. A huge knowledge void exists about the practice patterns of master's-prepared nurses. When Congress turned its attention to tightening the federal budget and eliminating waste, funds for graduate professional education underwent some scrutiny; accusations were made that federal money was being spent to train professionals for careers in private practice. Eventually training funds were eliminated when the NIMH was restructured.

According to Jan Chamberlain (personal interview, October 16, 1996), former chief nurse at NIMH who retired in 1988, funding for nurse traineeships peaked in 1969 ($120 million allocated, with nursing's share being $13 million). After that, available grant support declined, until virtually nothing remained by the late 1980s.

In an arena removed from psychiatry, in the mid-1960s, Loretta Ford, RN, and Henry Silver, MD, "invented" the pediatric nurse practitioner. The PNP was an outgrowth of physicians wanting to download the more general aspects of their practices, and nurses wanting to expand theirs. In the 1970s, the National Joint Practice Commission (NJPC) studied issues created by the new collaborative efforts of nurses and physicians. Literature emerged to describe the various patterns of clinical practice with shared jurisdictions. Because psychiatrists tended not to be considered "real doctors," the American Medical Association (AMA) never appointed a psychiatrist to fill one of the eight physician seats on the commission. For the entire 10-year tenure of the

NJPC, Shirley Smoyak was the American Nurses Association-appointed psychiatric nurse. Lacking a psychiatrist counterpart on the commission, the discussions of expanded roles of psychiatric nurses were not as thorough or in-depth as those considering practice areas such as pediatrics, obstetrics, cancer, or cardiac care. The NJPC published *Together: A Casebook of Joint Practices in Primary Care*, which did not capture the variety of actual collaborative relationships in psychiatric practice because of the separation of psychiatry from the AMA.

In separate arenas, some efforts were made to describe and analyze collaborative psychiatric practices. For example, the Group for the Advancement of Psychiatry (GAP), an organization begun by community-oriented psychiatrists who objected to aspects of the American Psychiatric Association, secured funding from the Ittleson Foundation to study the similarities and differences in the work of psychiatrists, psychologists, social workers, and nurses. It became clear that psychiatrists and psychologists had a much clearer picture of their ranks (how many practitioners there were, who graduated when, who was practicing where and how) than did the social workers and nurses. In the chapter describing psychiatric nurses, Smoyak (1987) stated: "While all four of the core mental health professions share roughly the same body of knowledge, the psychiatric nurse is unique in the following respects: (1) Uses biological as well as psychosocial theories in providing holistic health care; (2) Provides continuity of patient care on all shifts and days; (3) Plans, monitors, and executes transitions for patients among modalities, services, and settings; and (4) Defines the jurisdiction of her practice to be the diagnosis and treatment of human responses to actual or potential health problems." Smoyak was appointed to this project by the American Nurses Association Council of Specialists in Psychiatric and Mental Health Nursing, which was very active in the 1960s and 1970s.

In the earliest days of psychiatry, the efforts to develop theories to explain mental illness were largely biological, with foci on structure and gross brain abnormalities. The documentary film *Asylums* (1988) is an excellent overview of shifting scientific ideologies. After World War II, psychiatry was largely dominated by interpersonal directions, theories, and practices. Not until technology enabled researchers in the human sciences to examine brains by imaging and noninvasive viewing techniques did the focus shift once again to biological models and theories. The 1990s were declared to be the "decade of the brain" by the NIMH, impressively influenced by the National Alliance of the Mentally Ill (NAMI), a grass-roots, self-help organization of families of persons who are mentally ill (NAMI, 1996). The focus is definitely biopsychosocial. Note that "bio" comes first.

The following sections of the chapter will provide more description and detail about the educational preparation, practice patterns, and changes in legal regulations.

ADVANCED EDUCATION

Advanced psychiatric nursing had its beginning in 1943 when the National League for Nursing Education (NLNE) established a Committee on Postgraduate Clinical Courses and a subcommittee on psychiatric nursing. Three graduate psychiatric nursing programs were in Seattle, Denver, and the Catholic University of America in Washington, D.C. Prior to 1943, all postgraduate courses were in hospital schools of nursing. Then, postgraduate study took place after the diploma was earned or perhaps after the baccalaureate degree. In 1946 to 1947, the National Organization for Public Health Nursing surveyed all university programs offering mental hygiene programs for public health nurses. By 1947, three universities had established advanced programs for the training of mental health consultants in public health nursing—the University of Minnesota School of Public Health, the University of Pittsburgh, and Teacher's College at Columbia University.

Almost immediately after the NIMH was created by Congress in 1946, the education of mental health professionals became a part of its mission. By 1950, Peplau was serving on the National Advisory Council, which advised the Public Health Service, the National Institutes of Health, and the NIMH on the funding and development of all mental health training programs. That spring, she participated in a two-week funded institute at the University of Minnesota to explore "appropriate curricular content" in the psychiatric and mental health programs at the graduate level (Peplau collection). Callaway (1996) reports that Peplau described this as one of the stormiest conferences she would ever attend. Only 11 graduate programs in mental health existed at that time, and 8 had begun after the NIMH inception. "The directors could not agree on the basic content of graduate work in psychiatric nursing. The major bone of contention was whether or not what graduate nursing did in 'counselling' patients could be called 'psychotherapy' " (Callaway, 1997). While the nursing program directors acknowledged Peplau's emphasis on the nurse–patient relationship as very important, and that "counselling" patients was part of the role of master's-prepared nurses, they feared retribution from physicians should there be a hint that nurses were conducting psychotherapy. It wasn't until the 1960s that the term "psychotherapy" was used openly to describe this portion of the work of psychiatric nurses.

Although Peplau developed the first graduate program devoted exclusively to clinical practice, the idea of "clinical specialist" had been floating about in nursing since the turn of the century. In the very first issue of the *American Journal of Nursing* in October 1900, there was an article by Katherine DeWitt titled "Specialties in Nursing" (Smoyak, 1976). Difficulties with the term "specialist" are identified in the same article. Advanced practice nurse (APN) has evolved as the umbrella term to designate a clinical nurse specialist (CNS), nurse practitioner (NP), certified registered nurse

anesthetist (CRNA), and certified nurse-midwife (CNM); however there is no consensus on a common educational experience either by the degree awarded or the content of the curriculum (Bigbee, 1996). The reluctance to acknowledge and deal with the levels of competence and expertise in the field unfortunately erodes the energies of the people caught in the struggle, and fails to lend clarity for legislators or regulators concerned with protecting the public good.

Until recently, psychiatric or mental health APNs had enjoyed a common curricular denominator, preparation for the psychotherapist role, and a shared expectation that graduate study, with a master's degree, was the appropriate educational level. Graduates were called clinical nurse specialists, and practiced in a wide variety of settings, from acute inpatient units of government hospitals, to facilities caring for patients with long-standing chronic illnesses, to different types of community settings. The patient populations for whom they cared spanned birth to death. CNSs worked with individuals, groups, and families. The modalities, clinical strategies, and techniques that they used were selected from intrapsychic, interpersonal, and systems theorists.

It was not until reimbursement realities entered the health care delivery arena that CNSs considered the NP role. Nurse practitioner programs started out as certificate programs, in continuing education settings, and varied considerably in scope and depth. Early programs were as short as a few months. The common core course content was physical assessment and the diagnosing of departures from health, or identification of diseases. Most programs included content that taught the student basic skills in treating uncomplicated, common diseases.

The American Medical Association published a position statement, "Medicine and Nursing in the 1970s," which stated that the AMA "recognizes the need for and will facilitate the expansion of the role of the nurse in providing patient care" (p. 1881). Further, this statement noted that "as there is a marked overlap in the technical areas common to medical and nursing practice, the same act may be clearly the practice of medicine when performed by a physician and the practice of nursing when performed by a nurse." Ten years later, however, the AMA reemphasized that physicians must be "the captain of the ship" and withdrew its financial and organizational support from the National Joint Practice Commission.

In the 1970s, the NJPC had attempted to bring consensus about what the new intersecting roles of medicine and nursing should look like, how the new dimensions of these nurse practices should be regulated, and how curricula in both medicine and nursing should shift to prepare for these changes (Bates, 1972; Hoekelman, 1974; Smoyak, 1976, 1977). Eventually, the physical assessment skills found their way into basic baccalaureate curricula, and advanced skills needed to treat people with a variety of illnesses, in primary care settings, were found at the graduate level, in programs often leading to a master's degree.

Some CNSs pragmatically took physical assessment or psychopharmacology courses to satisfy state requirements for continued professional nurse licensure, secure professional risk/liability insurance plans, or be reimbursed by third-party payors. Changes in reimbursement patterns showed a clear movement toward primary care in community settings.

Academic programs have responded to changes in practice settings, the focus of care, and reimbursement patterns by developing an array of hybrid curricula. The new choices include terms such as adult nurse practitioner (ANP), producing the cumbersome hybrid ANP/Psych CNS. Another new combination is primary psychiatric mental health nurse practitioner, yielding P/MHNP. Practice goals for these new graduates vary considerably. For example, those who complete the ANP/CNS in psychology or mental health could practice in a primary care setting serving a general population, or in a specialized setting serving patients who are seriously and persistently mentally ill.

What might be considered the old, traditional CNS curriculum has kept pace with health care changes, but in a different way. Instead of adding the ANP component, many CNS programs have simply enhanced their curriculum by emphasizing the growing research on the biological basis of mental illness.

The direction that academic programs choose to take tends to vary regionally. This appears to be related to certification requirements, which may differ state by state. For example, Oregon certifies P/MHNPs, but Oregon P/MHNPs who wish national certification are certified as CNSs by the American Nurses Association. The further complexity is that the Oregon Board of Nursing acts as the certifying body, as well as the regulatory board. In other states, the boards of nursing retain the licensure function and leave certifying to specialty groups, as it should be.

In the psychiatric/mental health specialty, individual nurses have always reflected their particular interests and strengths. Taylor (1995), associate editor of the *Archives of Psychiatric Nursing*, the official journal of the Society for Education and Research in Psychiatric/Mental Health Nursing (SERPN), contends that flexibility and the ability and willingness to competently perform a variety of tasks is requisite for success in a managed care environment. When programs, rather than individuals, attempt to change their curricular directions without first achieving consensus on what the new expectations will be in order to incorporate environmental, political, and economic shifts, chaos is likely to result. Academic institutions move slowly compared to individual practitioners. Moreover, graduate nurse faculties have different philosophies and beliefs about what is right or wrong, current or faddish, prudent or ill-founded, and to achieve consensus among them about curricular programs would be almost impossible. The reason for the difficulty is that no central coordinating or authorizing mechanism or institution guides the direction of graduate study in nursing. The NIMH formerly performed this consensus-generating function, by supporting annual meetings of program directors. The NIMH has now been subsumed under NIH, and clinical services and training have been reorganized under the Substance Abuse and Mental Health Services Administration (SAMHSA). SERPN, an organization of program directors that emerged from the earlier NIMH group of program directors, might perform the consensus-generating function. The NLNE, later the National League for Nursing (NLN), has never been considered as a consensus-generating body for psychiatric nursing. The American Psychiatric Nurses' Association (APNA) recently convened a Congress on Advanced Practice in Psychiatric Nursing, but there was not a focus on how graduate education should be altered to assure graduates that their practice skills will be relevant in the real world (APNA News, September, 1996).

It is difficult for psychiatric nurses who are prepared at the baccalaureate level and want to pursue graduate study to know what graduate program will meet their needs. In 1990, Forbes and associates published survey results comparing the CNS and NP core curricula. The American Nurses' Association Council of Clinical Nurse Specialists and the Council of Primary Health Care Nurse Practitioners cooperated to conduct the study. Of the 147 schools with graduate nursing programs, 108 (73.5%) responded. A total of 317 programs were described in the analysis, but unfortunately were not categorized by specialty. For the 60 NP and 195 CNS programs analyzed, the significant differences were that NP programs placed greater emphasis on pharmacology, primary care, physical assessment, health promotion, nutrition, and history-taking in their curricula. CNS programs focussed on secondary or tertiary settings.

To respond to health care policy changes, the newer APN programs in psychiatric nursing are incorporating the skills and knowledge needed to practice within the primary care model. Analyzing the existing graduate programs is a formidable task. An old debate resurfaces with a new twist. Historically, new graduate nurses were advised to get one or two years of medical/surgical experience before entering a specialty. In these times, should those nurses seeking to become psychiatric or mental health CNSs first become proficient as adult nurse practitioners? Dual programs tend to organize their curriculum with the NP component in year one and the CNS in year two. The faculty is divided in a similar fashion. For example, informational literature provided by one such graduate program tells applicants that students are assigned an academic advisor at admission and that dual majors have two advisors. The NP and the CNS courses are separate; integration is left to the novice. Although this may well yield creative, innovative practice strategies, no data accurately describes what graduates do, and how they are received upon completion of their programs. Outcome studies of these new programs have yet to be developed.

Applicants to psychiatric APN programs are disheartened and confused as they see hospital-based CNSs moving away from direct patient services to administrative positions in case management. An old fear reemerges that administrators view a CNS as frosting on the cake, but not essential. When budgets get tight or reduced, the CNS is often the first to be downsized, with the rationale that they are really administrators and clinical finances must be allocated for direct patient care. Some suggest that the CNS credential alone is insufficient, and that NP skills are also necessary. The titles of new graduates vary greatly; designations in the NLN tables for master's programs use the titles nurse practitioner and advanced clinical practice, rather than CNS.

Full-time enrollments of NPs have increased, while those of advanced clinical practice have decreased. In 1991, only 17 nurses (1.0%) were enrolled full time in NP psychiatric or mental health programs. By 1994, there were 112 (2.1%). The total enrollments in NP programs were 1793 in 1991 and 5317 in 1994.

CLINICAL PRACTICE

The Psychiatric CNS maintains a high degree of autonomy. Practice protocols do not require physician collaboration (the one exception for some states is prescriptive authority).

The Nurse Practitioner "movement" was greatly influenced by the fact that the focus of clinicians, policymakers and insurers had turned to considering ways to provide needed care to underserved or unserved populations, living in rural areas or inner cities. As Talley and Caverly (1994) point out, "[t]he Master's degree clinical nurse specialists had begun practicing in psychiatric and medical-surgical nursing during the 1950s, yet the nurse practitioner, with education and training in providing primary care, became the highly visible exemplar of advanced nursing practice." NPs were highly valued by both clinicians and administrators for their ability to deliver primary care services in varied settings. When they were first conceived by Ford and Silver, the expectation was that they would assist physicians in offices. As they gained experience, they functioned more independently and moved farther out into community settings, sometimes not working directly with a physician for extended periods of time. As their independence grew, and their responsibilities expanded, their practices came under scrutiny and state laws were changed to incorporate their expanded practices. Some states have included the authority for nurses to prescribe medications, with or without physician supervision or collaboration. Some states grant full prescribing authority, while others authorize prescribing only by protocol or formulary. As of 1994, more than 40 states allowed some type of prescription writing by advanced practice nurses, primarily NPs. In 20 of these states, there was formal inclusion of advanced practice nurses in their laws (Pearson, 1994).

The AMA Board of Trustees is engaged in producing a document tentatively titled "Principles Guiding AMA Policy Regarding Supervision of Medical Care Delivered by Advanced Practice Nurses in Integrated Practice" (AMA, 1996). Offered as documentation of the draft statement are tables that list states with statutes requiring physician collaboration for integrated practice with APNs, with statutes requiring physician collaboration for APN prescribing, where NPs and APNs can practice and independently prescribe controlled substances (with no MD involvement), where NPs and APNs can practice and prescribe with minimal relationship with MDs, as well as a summary of state legislation on the scope of RN practice.

Some articles by nurses describe NP "fever," a trend wherein CNSs are returning to school to become NPs. Some CNSs make that decision based on personal preference and practice interests; others, however, fear that they may become "frosting," or not essential, if they are not primary care providers. The philosophies of others have shifted toward a broad biopsychosocial skill base. Tusaie-Mumford (1994), in an article in the *Journal of Psychosocial Nursing*, describes how she sought skills at the master's level that would increase her knowledge base in physical aspects of care. She took advanced physical assessment courses along with NPs but was prepared as a CNS. Tusaie-Mumford described the acute anxiety she had experienced when she concluded that a patient with chronic mental illness was having increased delusions as he told her about people dancing in his chest. The patient actually had cardiac problems.

New practices in psychiatric and mental health nursing came quietly and without opposition at first. Growing interest in the biological basis of mental illness, coupled with the nation's preoccupation with health care reform, shifted the focus from educational preparation to clinical practice. Indeed, even SERPN, whose role in psychiatric and mental health curricula is well established, has been focused on health care delivery issues rather than education. In 1993, SERPN, APNA, and the Association for Child and Adolescent Psychiatric Nursing (ACAPN) collaborated with the American Nurses' Association to prepare a mental health policy document for the health care reform team in the first term of the Clinton administration. The document, *Health Care Reform: Essential Mental Health Services* (Krauss, 1993), detailed service issues. Education of the providers who would implement such a comprehensive mental health care system was not addressed.

NEW PROGRAM CHOICES

Education for advanced practice psychiatric nursing includes graduate programs that blend the clinical specialist and nurse practitioner roles and programs that prepare nurses for either the CNS or NP role.

The term "blended-role advanced practice nurse" describes those nurses who graduated from programs providing CNS and NP concentrations, both didactic and clinical, within the individual student's program of study. The graduate is eligible to sit for both the clinical nurse specialist and the adult nurse practitioner certification examinations. The NP component deals with primary health care skills and the CNS concentration is the specialty. These programs vary in length, but most offer between 40 and 57 credits. The core competencies for all advanced practice nurses are included in the various curricula; however, the emphasis given to each is determined by the particular program. It is important to note that although schools may offer both CNS and NP content, they don't necessarily portray themselves as preparing blended-role advanced practice nurses. Some schools offer a choice to students who may elect either a CNS or an NP track.

During the first year, students in both tracks take the same core advanced practice curriculum; in the second year, the emphasis is either CNS or NP. This differs from the blended curriculum in that not all students are being prepared for dual certification. Only those who are "co-admitted" are prepared in both roles. In addition to the two professional role titles, there are two academic degree options. Decisions that a typical applicant is faced with include specialty area; CNS or NP; and MN or MS degree. Although the academic degree earned does not specify the role of CNS or NP, it may influence role enactment. Most schools have a course titled "role theory" or "role

seminar," but not all programs acknowledge the role differences. Language used in these courses tends to be "advanced practice nurse." There are exceptions; one of the schools offering the most extensive menu of courses purposely brings students from the various degree and track options together for this course. Course objectives specifically address the sharing, networking, and collaboration with colleagues within psychiatric and mental health nursing. This approach not only acknowledges differences but promotes variety and creativity in role enactment. This is reminiscent of early CNS programs which acknowledged, supported, and prepared students for various practice settings. CNS programs are still preparing a significant number of advanced practice nurses.

The specialty is clearly continuing to attract nurses; CNS enrollments are up, and the newer NP option is developing alongside its predecessor. The rhetoric declaring the demise of CNSs is clearly at the opinion level and not supported by data. The current state of affairs of educational preparation in our specialty is both stable and dynamic. The best components of the original CNS programs are still available, as the newest NP curriculum is marketed. The choices are fascinating, as they are described in this book's Introduction.

CERTIFICATION AND LICENSURE DEBATES

LICENSURE

Licensure, conducted by a government or regulatory agency, is a process whose aim is to protect the public by assuring that a given individual is safe to practice her or his profession. A current licensure debate is under way, with the National Council of State Boards of Nursing insisting that it must set, at a national level, standards for testing nurse practitioner skills and knowledge. Some states had passed laws requiring a second licensure for nurse practitioners, thus adding requirements that no other profession has. This ill-founded requirement now has spawned a new level of debate, misconstruing the intents of licensure and certification.

CERTIFICATION

The New Jersey Society of Clinical Specialists in Psychiatric/Mental Health Nursing was the first organization to institute the certification process for its members. It was begun in 1974, preceding the American Nurses Association (ANA) process by 4 years. The group had attempted to get the ANA to respond to efforts to begin the certification process, but when the ANA prolonged the launch and insisted that nonmaster's nurses should also be certified, the group went ahead at the state level.

Certification was generally understood as a process directed by the profession, whereby it examined its members and validated their continued excellence in practice, thus assuring the public. The ANA's insistence on certifying nonmaster's nurses produced great confusion.

Currently, the ANA, through the American Nurses Credentialing Center (ANCC), certifies generalists in psychiatric nursing (associate and baccalaureate graduates, as well as diploma graduates). As of October 1995, there were 19,145 certified generalist RNs. By 1998, a generalist will have to be baccalaureate prepared. However, there is no certification process for NPs, who are master's prepared. The ANCC only certifies CNSs. As of October 1995, there were 6030 adult specialists in psychiatric and mental health nursing, and 770 child and adolescent specialists.

VARIATION AMONG STATES

The variety of ways that master's-prepared nurses have been academically prepared further complicates licensure and certification. Nurse practitioners may practice in some states, with only the first-level license. Other states require a second-level license. Some states have given prescriptive authority to nurse practitioners, but vary in their requirements of whether a nurse practitioner must have a formal, collaborative agreement with a physician. In some states, CNSs have prescriptive authority (with or without a second-level license) and in other states they do not. Some states that allow CNSs to write prescriptions require formal collaborative arrangements with a physician; others do not. For example, in New York, a psychiatric NP has full prescriptive authority if there is a formal, collaborative agreement with a physician, but a CNS cannot prescribe. Across the river, in New Jersey, both CNSs and NPs can prescribe, but formal, collaborative physician agreements and state education requirements exist.

HEALTH CARE REFORM AND WORKFORCE REGULATION

Safriet (1992), in a widely discussed article on archaic and discriminatory regulatory barriers, made the case for the increased use of advanced practice nurses in all types of delivery settings. The regulation of health care workers has developed over the course of the last century into 50 discrete, separate, so-called systems, producing a picture that is more colored mud than a mosaic. The certification processes add to the murkiness of the picture, as they are largely handled by voluntary systems.

The Pew Health Professions Commission (1995) highlighted the problem in its introduction to *Reforming Health Care Workforce Regulation.* "The lack of uniformity in language, laws, and regulations between the states limits effective professional practice and mobility, confuses the public, and presents barriers to integrated delivery systems and the use of telemedicine and other emerging health technologies." Safriet (1994) writes that "since health and illness are for the most part biologically and physically based, with some psychological and emotional components, it is not at all clear why licensure laws—that is, proxies for competency—should vary according to political boundaries rather than competency domains."

The Pew document offers ten recommendations; each is salient to the nursing profession and would ensure a much more coherent situation for both professionals and the people whom they serve. For example, the first recommendation says, "States should use standardized and understandable language for health professions regulation and its functions to clearly describe them for consumers, provider organizations, businesses, and the professions." Several of the recommendations clearly address the need to separate licensure from certification.

Drafts of this report were circulated at the same time that the National Council of State Boards of Nursing was threatening to impose its version of standards for practice, offering as a rationale the current diversity in paths toward certification for NPs and CNSs. The American Nurses Credentialing Center, along with the American Academy of Nurse Practitioners, the National Certification Board of PNP/N, and the National Certification Corporation for the Ob/Gyn Specialties, have formed a coalition to resist these efforts, which they describe as unilateral and preemptive (correspondence, summer 1996).

PLANS FOR THE FUTURE

To plan and implement effective change, psychiatric nurses must "move out of the box" and look beyond their specialty for new alignments, networks, and collaborative bodies. For example, Cronenwett (1995) reports on the development of the American Board of Nursing Specialties, beginning in 1988 with the support of the Josiah Macy, Jr., Foundation. National nursing leaders worked together to create a unified approach to standards for professional certification programs. The results of this work were reported in *Nursing Outlook* by Hartshorn (1990). Cronenwett reports that in 1990, eight organizations, collectively representing about 65 percent of all certified nurses, became charter members of the American Board of Nursing Specialties. Their

plan includes providing that a specialty nursing practice certification require a baccalaureate degree by the year 2000 and that advanced specialty nursing practice require a graduate degree or an appropriate equivalent.

Ideally, a plan will be constructed whereby the majors players—official consortia representing schools, practices, and regulatory bodies—will be brought together to study and propose changes such as those identified and described in the Pew report. The time is now.

REFERENCES

American Medical Association. Principles guiding AMA policy regarding supervision of medical care delivered by advanced practice nurses in integrated practice. Board of Trustees Report by N. Dickey, to Reference Committee C., Chicago, 1996.

Asylums. Stone Lantern Films; 1988.

Bates B. Changing roles of physicians and nurses. *Wash State J Nurs.* Spring 1972:3–10.

Bigbee JL. History and evolution of advanced nursing practice. In: Hamric A, Spross J, Hanson C, eds. *Advanced Nursing Practice: An Integrative Approach.* Philadelphia: Saunders, 1996.

Callaway BJ. Teacher's college: The academic nightmare (1948–54). In: Callaway BJ, ed. *Hildegard E. Peplau: A Formidable Woman.* (In press.)

Committee on Nursing. Medicine and nursing in the 1970s: A position statement. *JAMA.* 1970;213: 1881–1883.

Cronenwett LR. Molding the future of advanced practice nursing. *Nurs Outlook.* 1995;43:112–118.

Forbes KE, Rafson J, Sprouss JA, Kozlowski D. Clinical nurse specialist and nurse practitioner core curricula survey results. *Nurse Pract.* 1990;15:43–48.

Ford LC, Silver HK. The expanded role of the nurse in childcare. *Nurs Outlook.* 1967;15:43–45.

Hartshorn, JC. A national board for nursing certification. *Nurs Outlook.* 1990;39:226–229.

Hoekelman R. Nurse physician relationships: Problems and solutions. Commencement address, St. Luke's Medical Center, Chicago, June 26, 1974.

Krauss JB. The mental status of health care reform. *Arch Psychiatr Nurs.* 1994;8:1–2.

Krauss JB. *Health Care Reform: Essential Mental Health Services.* Washington, DC: American Nurses Publishing; 1993.

McBride A. Psychiatric-mental health nursing in the twenty-first century. In: McBride A, Austin J, eds. *Psychiatric-Mental Health Nursing: Integrating the Behavioral and Biological Sciences.* Philadelphia: Saunders; 1996.

NAMI. Update. *NAMI Advocate.* 1996;18:1.

National League for Nursing. *Graduate Education in Nursing: Advanced Practice Nursing. Nursing Data Source.* New York: NLN; 1994, 1995.

Pearson LJ. Annual update of how each state stands on legislative issues affecting advanced nursing practice. *Nurse Pract.* 1994;19:11–53.

Peplau HE. *Interpersonal Relations in Nursing.* New York: Putnam; 1952.

Peplau collection. Archival material on HE Peplau. Boxes 17 and 18, Schesslinger Library, Radcliffe College.

Report of the Task Force on *Reforming Health Care Workforce Regulation: Policy Considerations for the 21st Century.* San Francisco: Pew Health Professions Commission; 1995.

Roueché B, ed. *Together: A Casebook of Joint Practices in Primary Care.* Chicago: NJPC/Educational Publications and Innovative Communications; 1977.

Safriet BJ. Impediments to progress in health care workforce policy: License and practice laws. *Inquiry.* 1994;31:3107.

Safriet BJ. Health care dollars and regulatory sense: The role of advanced practice nursing. *Yale J Regulations.* Summer 1992:417–488.

Smoyak S. Psychiatric/mental health nursing. In: Committee on Governmental Agencies, Group for the Advancement of Psychiatry (GAP). *Psychiatry and the Mental Health Professionals: New Roles for Changing Times.* Report no. 122. New York: Brunner/Mazel, 1987;170–182.

Smoyak S. Problems in interprofessional relations. *Bull NY Acad Med.* 1977;53:51–59.

Smoyak S. Specialization in nursing: From then to now. *Nurs Outlook.* 1976;24:676–681.

Talley S, Caverly S. Advanced-practice psychiatric nursing and health care reform. *Hosp Commun Psychiatr.* 1994;45:545–547.

Taylor C. "Jack of all trades and master of one." *Arch Psychiatr Nurs.* 1995;9:231–232.

Tusaie-Mumford K. My side: Nurse practitioners or clinical nurse specialists? *J Psychosoc Nurs Ment Health Serv.* 1994;32:48.

CHAPTER 2

ADVANCING PSYCHIATRIC NURSING IN A REFORMING HEALTH CARE SYSTEM

Margaret Cotroneo • Joan King • Freida Hopkins Outlaw • Jean Brince

*B*eing able to handle the demands of collaborative networks that include insurers, managers, and other providers requires an approach to psychiatric nursing that is open to negotiation for the benefit of clients, but capable or resisting the temptation to be wholly compromised in order to "belong."

Chapter Overview

- Directions and Emerging Patterns
- Strengths and Resources of Psychiatric Nursing
    Leadership Strengths of Psychiatric Nurses
- Looking to the Future
- The Health Annex: An Integrative Approach to Family and Community Health Care
    Psychiatric Services at the Health Annex
    Case Example
- Critical Issues of Implementation
    Cost
    Team Building
    Strategic Planning
- Education and Training for Integrated Primary Health Care
- Summary
- References

This project is supported by a grant from the Division of Nursing, Department of Health and Human Services.

► INTRODUCTION

Achieving parity of mental and physical health is basic to any effort to move health care in the direction of prevention and health promotion. The most feasible path to reaching the goal of parity may lie in re-linking mental health to physical health in managed care models of primary health care. In Nursing's Agenda for Health Care Reform (ANA, 1992) the point is made that community-based primary care settings will become an essential consumer pathway to mental health services. As providers, care managers, health promoters and educators, and client advocates with family systems expertise, psychiatric advanced practice specialists are a necessary component of all primary health care. As such, they must heighten their visibility and position themselves for success in the complex integrated delivery systems that may represent the future of health care in America.

Psychiatric nurses have been caught up in the health care reform dialogue fueled by President Clinton's campaign promise (Health Security Act, 1993). Any reform of the health care system, however, is complicated because it is inextricably bound to the nature, kind, quality, and consequences of the relationships between providers, users, insurers, managers, and regulators (Boyle and Callahan, 1995). Although a patchwork of changes have clearly moved our health care delivery system along the path of managed care, modifying relationships has proven the harder task and the one most resisted. Consider the competing vested interests that managed to derail the most recent attempts at health care reform on the federal level. Consider further the fact that barriers to practice in the form of reimbursement policies, prescriptive privileges, and staffing privileges still restrict advanced practice nurses' direct access to patients (Baradell, 1994; Heffernan, 1995; Safriet, 1992).

Traditional medical hierarchies have dominated our health care delivery system, with the physician at the top of the hierarchy and other providers "extending" the reach of the physician. A large infusion of technology has been required in order to maintain this system. Furthermore, traditional modes lack the necessary base in the family and the community that completes the process of delivering care. Managed care has challenged traditional modes of service delivery in the physical health arena. Traditional modes, however, had long been challenged in mental health, which is accustomed to interdisciplinary collaboration in providing a continuum of services. What may be new for mental health providers are collaborative mixes that include providers of physical health care (internists, family medicine and general practice physicians, obstetricians and gynecologists, pediatricians, nurse practitioners, nurse midwives, and community health nurses). Increasingly, these providers are coming together under the umbrella of primary health care, but it is unclear how they will work together, from both inter- and intradisciplinary perspectives. A great challenge to nursing is developing models of collaboration in which advanced practice nurses from different fields work together in settings where nurses have greater autonomy. The way in which advanced practice psychiatric nurses position themselves in this transition will have a great effect on where they find themselves once some stability and balance are restored to the health care system.

Biopsychosocial approaches would appear to be the natural domain of advanced practice psychiatric nurses if they are willing to step up to the plate. A reading of the history of the specialty indicates that community care has been underrepresented by clinicians (Church 1987; Fox, 1992).

We will attempt to describe the leadership strengths that advanced practice psychiatric nurses need to bring to the evolving primary health care system. We will then describe our approach to the effective use of psychiatric nurses within a specific primary health care nursing center. We will also describe the special competencies required to practice in a managed primary health care environment.

DIRECTIONS AND EMERGING PATTERNS

Some clear directions are emerging in the mental health field that will deeply affect the domains of practice, education, and research in psychiatric nursing. •

• Continued managed care penetration of the health care market with major changes in Medicare and Medicaid.
• Continued emphasis on increasing access to services, holding the line on costs, maintaining quality, and increasing collaboration.
• A need for providers who can deliver services across the continuum of care, including prevention, risk assessment, early intervention, emergency care, partial hospitalization, treatment, referral, care management, 24-hour coverage, specialty services, and in-home services.
• Less emphasis on credentials and more emphasis on areas of competence; greater blurring of the functional boundaries that separate providers.
• Emphasis on distinct and specific competency areas, including children and adolescents, substance abuse, older adults, the physically dis-

abled, the chronically mentally disabled, pain management, and violence prevention.
• Establishment of cost-effective provider mixes in multidisciplinary groups or clusters within complex delivery systems.
• Integration of mental health services into primary health care settings.
• Emphasis on market factors, such as the range of quality services, consumer satisfaction, and staffing based on supply and demand.
• Integrated, collaborative delivery of services to meet the needs of families and communities.
• A limited fee-for-service market in which providers offer specialized and supportive services that target divorcing families, adoption, fertility, adjustment problems, and problems associated with medical conditions.
• Renewed interest in contracts and ethics.

In the evolving managed health care environment, with its emphasis on primary care, a biopsychosocial family systems approach may serve as the conceptual framework and the vehicle for moving away from traditional mental health carve-outs (Blount and Bayona, 1994; McDaniel et al., 1995). This approach emphasizes the relational, contextual nature of health care by viewing mental health care as instrumental in prevention and health promotion and in the treatment of acute, episodic, and chronic illness. An integrated approach to health care delivery is supported by the body of psychiatric, family systems, and biomedical literature demonstrating relationships between family variables and health (Campbell, 1986; Campbell and Patterson, 1995; Rolland, 1994); behavior and disease (Goldstein and Niaura, 1992); behavior and immune system changes (Ader and Cohen, 1993; Kiecolt-Glaser and Glaser, 1986; Kiecolt-Glaser et al., 1988); and bodily responses to stress (Wolff et al., 1950). The movement toward integration is evidenced in the expansion of the category "psychological factors affecting medical illness" in the fourth edition of the *Diagnostic and Statistical Manual of Mental Disorder* (DSM-IV; American Psychiatric Association, 1994).

However, an integrated approach, although reasonable, presents an implementation challenge in a managed care environment, because initially it involves a higher cost investment. Moreover, measurable outcomes may not be available for 3 to 5 years. The success of the biopsychosocial family systems approaches may well depend on the development of integrated reimbursement systems to fund them, and so that outcomes can be documented, the development of management information systems sensitive to clinical data reflective of these approaches. Success may also depend on the ability of mental health providers to make the case for a more systemic, family-based, and community-responsive approach to primary health care itself. If primary health care is dominated by an individual rather than a systemic orientation, it will be as unfriendly to mental health as the traditional medical model has been.

Although the movement toward breaking down artificial and costly barriers between physical and mental health services is constructive, there may also be less desirable outcomes. In many managed care organizations the primary care provider bears financial responsibility for minimizing the use of expensive "specialists" by providing for as many patient needs as possible in the office. It has been reported that over 70 percent of all patients with diagnosed mental health disorders are never seen by a mental health professional and are treated only in primary care (McDaniel et al., 1995). This leads to the use of psychotropic medications as the first line of treatment, as opposed to an assessment done by the mental health expert, combined with treatment options and medication as appropriate.

It is the bias of the authors that an integrated system of primary health care more adequately reflects the real living situations of clients. Moreover, we believe that these approaches are best implemented by having psychiatric nurses attached to specific primary care practices, seeing families in the office and in the home, and functioning as systems consultants to other providers.

Psychiatric nurses are very well positioned to function in integrated primary care settings.

Their leadership skills are reflective of the more egalitarian, cooperative, interdisciplinary peer models in which they were trained. Primary care settings are still, to a large extent, medical settings; psychiatric nurses would attempt to bring all aspects of care together under a biopsychosocial approach.

STRENGTHS AND RESOURCES OF PSYCHIATRIC NURSING

As primary care has been pushed to the foreground of health care, nursing has needed to emphasize advanced practice as distinct from entry level practice (AACN Bulletin, 1993). This emphasis has given rise to confusion among nurses themselves, as well as confusion among our colleagues in other disciplines, regarding the qualifications and educational preparation for the new advanced practice functions.

Advanced practice psychiatric nurses are now, by virtue of their educational preparation, a heterogeneous group of clinicians, equal in terms of status but differentiated in strengths and competencies, who will have to work collaboratively with each other and with other nurse providers in the evolving health care environment. The primary care nurse practitioner, advanced practice psychiatric nurse, pediatric nurse practitioner, nurse-midwife, and community health nurse can increase their decision-making power by remaining focused on what they need to accomplish together rather than developing practice agendas in isolation. The emphasis on collaborating across competencies has led many of us who are both clinicians and educators to reconsider the practice agenda of psychiatric nurses in a system that emphasizes primary care.

In a reforming health care system that attempts to increase access to high-quality comprehensive and continuous care, the key players have already changed. The relationship between the provider and the user of health care services is no longer the primary relational configuration.

The managers and insurers of health care are positioned as interpreters and monitors of that relationship, both in the public and private sectors. Being able to handle the demands of collaborative networks that include insurers, managers, and other providers requires an approach to psychiatric nursing that is open to negotiation for the benefit of clients but capable of resisting the temptation to be wholly compromised in order to "belong."

LEADERSHIP STRENGTHS OF PSYCHIATRIC NURSES

What leadership strengths must psychiatric nurses bring to the primary care arena?

Biopsychosocial Orientation

Psychiatric nurses share the wider nursing framework of prevention and health promotion and the nursing focus on an integrated whole. They have been part of, and provided leadership in, the history of mental health and illness and the transition from concepts of insanity to concepts of mental health (Church, 1987). Those who have continued to develop the more relational, contextual nature of their practices while integrating the new findings that accrued from the "decade of the brain" will likely find themselves in the most advantageous position in a health care delivery system that has an increased demand for those skills. A biopsychosocial base provides the psychiatric nurse with a unique ability to meet the challenges of co-morbidity, particularly in the elderly population. The challenge for psychiatric nurses will be to develop links to primary care settings in the community.

Collaborative History Across Disciplines and Professional/Client Barriers

The practice of psychotherapy with individuals, couples, families, and groups has enabled psychiatric nurses to gain direct access to patients and third-party reimbursement, thereby rendering them competitive in the larger mental health field (Fox, 1992). In this development, they benefited significantly from an infusion of federal grants (Church, 1987). In assuming the role of primary therapist, clinical specialists gained a measure of authority over their practices that freed them from the bonds of medical hierarchies and exposed them to interdisciplinary models of practice.

The ability to collaborate across disciplines, from the social worker to the physician, from the dietician to the chaplain, has been the key to succeeding in meeting client needs. For the psychiatric nurse this ability to collaborate has been strengthened by training and working closely with other disciplines to serve the needs of clients. Although not all psychiatric nurses are trained in systems theory, many are and function with their colleagues with that philosophy and the skills inherent in it.

Experience as Client Educators and Advocates

Client advocacy is historically a critical element in the training of psychiatric nurses. The belief that one works from an approach to care that focuses on strengths rather than deficits, and which creates opportunities by which the client and family can assume self-care and self-mastery, is a tremendous asset in a managed care environment. In that arena, psychiatric nurses and insurers are speaking the same language, but perhaps for different reasons.

History of Independent Practice

With the increased funding of master's programs by the National Institute of Mental Health, psychiatric nurses had the opportunity to practice with more autonomy as providers. The training in psychotherapy that these master's programs provided was the vehicle toward independent practice (Fox, 1992). In a report to State Nurses' Associations, Sarah Stanley, senior American Nurses' Association policy analyst, noted that "the psychiatric-mental health clinical nurse specialist is one of the earliest advanced nurse providers in the primary health care arena, one of the first to develop national certification and an early pioneer of standard development for the specialty practice. The psychiatric-mental health nurse is the only mental health provider of the twenty-four hour care required by patients" (ANA, 1993).

Implicit in their roles as clinical specialists was the professional expectation that they would assume responsibility for the assessment, plan of care, and treatment for their clients. That assessment covered not only the client's mental status, but physical status and family and community relationships as well. Evidence exists for the cost-effectiveness of services and equivalent or better clinical outcomes when nurse psychotherapists provide care (Baradell, 1994; Fagin, 1992). As providers experienced in delivering services across the continuum of mental health and illness, advanced practice psychiatric nurses can lay claim to the primary health care arena (Baradell, 1994; Haber and Billings, 1993).

LOOKING TO THE FUTURE

The Institute of Medicine defines primary health care as the "provision of integrated, accessible health care services by clinicians who are accountable for addressing a large majority of personal health care needs, developing a sustained partnership with patients, and practicing in the context of family and community" (1996). This definition embodies, in our view, the path to the future of the specialty. Moving forward will require some immediate attention to a number of key areas: partnerships with other providers and groups of providers within and outside of nursing; working in networks or clusters of providers; including clients and their families and communities as partners; and developing collaborative models for training providers to work in primary care settings.

We believe that psychiatric nursing has a significant role to play in the evolving health care environment, but only if its practitioners are willing to move in a countercultural direction; that is, away from the remedicalization of mental health care and toward the biopsychosocial family systems approaches. This movement would require a turning away from our conflicts over what to call ourselves in order to focus on nurturing and marketing the competencies that will add value to the health care system as it develops.

THE HEALTH ANNEX: AN INTEGRATIVE APPROACH TO FAMILY AND COMMUNITY HEALTH CARE

The Health Annex at the F. J. Myers Recreation Center is a nursing center that applies a biopsychosocial family systems approach to health care. This is accomplished by integrating physical and mental health care, which are delivered in a family and community context by an interdisciplinary mix of providers. The Health Annex is a practice of the Penn Nursing Network, a group of nurse-managed practices operated by the School of Nursing of the University of Pennsylvania. The practice is located in an underserved inner-city area of Philadelphia. Its aim is to deliver comprehensive primary care services to children, adolescents, adults, and older adults under both managed care and fee-for-service contracts.

The composition of the staff reflects the mission of the center, which is to provide both physical and mental health services to clients from the community. The faculty director is a psychiatric advanced practice nurse, and the practice director is an adult nurse practitioner who functions as on-site administrator and provider of clinical services. Additionally, a family primary care nurse practitioner, a nurse midwife, and two psychiatric advanced practice nurses provide direct patient services. The support staff includes two community outreach workers, a building services staff member, and two administrative assistants. The nurse-managed practice negotiated with a physician to provide collaborative medical services and has developed links to several large major integrated health care delivery systems to be used as referral sources for clients.

This model assumes that the primary context of health is the family and the community. The staff is philosophically committed to the inclusion of as many community voices as possible in the planning and provision of services. To operationalize this goal, the Health Annex has established close working relationships with the local community through the establishment of a community advisory board. It also has a working relationship with the advisory board of the recreation center and with a variety of other local community organizations. The center has also established ongoing relationships with local politicians, since many of the community's problems have political and public policy implications. A state representative sits on the community advisory board of the Health Annex.

The Health Annex has responded to requests from various organizations by providing a comprehensive community health fair once a year, an extensive immunization drive, and educational programs directed at specific populations in the community, such as an asthma program and a diabetes prevention program. The staff also provides crisis mental health consultation related to acts of violence that affect the entire community. Additionally, the Health Annex staff provides health-related programs for the schools in its service area. Examples of successful programs include an 8-week wellness program given in collaboration with school nurses in an elementary school. This program was targeted to boys who were at least 25 pounds overweight. Several of the boys were at least 50 pounds overweight and many already had related medical problems, such as hypertension and uncontrolled asthma. All of the boys shared that they had problems with sadness or anger because of being teased about their weight. The Health Annex staff also facilitates an adolescent group in an area middle school. Both of these programs were requested by the schools.

The Health Annex serves a community in which 85 percent of the population is of African descent, and the staff reflects the ethnic and racial composition of the community. A deliberate effort was made to hire community residents.

The Health Annex is also committed to interdisciplinary education. Nursing students at all levels and from multiple specialty areas have received clinical training on site. It also serves as a training site for business, social work, pharmacy, dental, and medical students.

A vision supporting the necessity of services that advanced practice psychiatric nurses can provide in primary health care settings has been reported in documents prepared by the American Nurses' Association (ANA, 1993) as well as other current literature (Haber and Billings, 1993; Talley and Caverly, 1994). The staff of the Health Annex supports this vision, believing that the clients and families that they serve, many of whom are disadvantaged, will derive maximum benefit from comprehensive, integrated primary care approaches that include mental health. There is a dearth of research, however, regarding approaches to providing comprehensive, integrated primary health care in poor, underserved urban settings.

In an effort to ensure that the primary health care delivered at the Health Annex was comprehensive, and to generate partial reimbursement for the services of the advanced practice psychiatric nurses, a creative delivery system was jointly developed by the project director from the University of Pennsylvania School of Nursing and the nursing coordinator of psychiatric services for the Visiting Nurse Association of Greater Philadelphia. The advanced practice nurses who provide the mental health services at the Health Annex are subcontracted from the Visiting Nurse Association of Greater Philadelphia (VNAGP). By partnering in this way, resources are linked and expertise in both primary care and community-based home care can be brought to the practice. The decision to do this project jointly was based on a belief that primary mental health care must include both an on site and a community/home component, thereby widening the lens through which the clients and their families are seen.

Both of the advanced practice psychiatric nurses at the Health Annex are master's prepared in the specialty and are certified by the ANCC. At this time, Pennsylvania is one of the states where advanced practice psychiatric nurses and nurse practitioners are denied prescriptive authority; therefore, the advanced practice nurses at the Health Annex must collaborate closely with the consulting physician about their patients' medication needs. Medication monitoring and education remain important components of the advanced practice role on site and in the home.

Widening the scope of practice in nursing to include both the biological and behavioral components in the provision of care to clients has been an agenda of many nursing scientists for well over a decade (McBride and Austin, 1996). In a review of research studies on the identification and treatment of child and adolescent mental health problems in primary health care settings, Richardson and colleagues (1996) found that primary care providers severely underdiagnose and undertreat these problems. The Health Annex population is comprised mostly of young mothers, children, and adolescents. Richardson and associates (1996) further postulate that the critical factor relative to whether a child or adolescent receives mental health treatment is directly related to whether their mental health needs are identified by the primary health care provider. Early recognition and treatment of child and adolescent mental health problems prevents needless suffering, decreases the severity of the impairment, and contains the cost of treatment.

At the Health Annex, the boundaries between physical and mental health are blurred, and the term "primary health care" automatically includes both areas. During intake, all clients are assessed initially by the mental health nurse and the nurse practitioner, regardless of the presenting problem. The advanced practice psychiatric nurse uses a Health Risk Assessment form developed at the center. In addition to the standard health assessment questions, informa-

tion is gathered about issues that are usually not assessed by health care providers, such as home and community safety. "Do you feel safe in your home?" and "Do you have a gun in your home?" are examples of questions that assess how safe patients think they are in their homes and community. Questions that assess the mental status of the patient are also included in the initial health risk assessment. For example, the assessment includes questions about the patient's mood, stress, and coping skills. The risk assessment tool has assisted the advanced practice nurses to identify many patients who need psychiatric services whose needs may have otherwise gone undetected or been uncovered only when the problem became more pronounced. A multigenerational genogram is done by the advanced practice psychiatric nurse on each new patient. The genogram is used to gather information about multigenerational medical, social, relational, and psychiatric patterns found among families.

PSYCHIATRIC SERVICES AT THE HEALTH ANNEX

At the Health Annex patients have the choice of receiving basic health care and mental health care in the same setting. Advanced practice psychiatric nurses are the mental health providers of choice for the Health Annex practice because they bring the neurobiological, behavioral, and psychosocial aspects of care together with a holistic perspective that addresses the challenges of daily living.

A mental health package is provided that includes mental health prevention/promotion, basic treatment/outpatient care, care management services, and primary care integration.

Basic Mental Health Services
• Evaluation, diagnosis, treatment, and/or referral of persons with depression, anxiety, severe and persistent mental disorders, substance abuse, childhood emotional disorders, intrafamilial abuse, and eating disorders. Persons

diagnosed with substance abuse problems are referred out for specialized treatment, although the team does provide primary health care, family support services, and care management services when not provided elsewhere.

- Outpatient individual, group, and family treatment for individuals with a DSM-IV diagnosis.
- Brief counseling, problem solving, psychoeducational interventions, health teaching, comprehensive family-based treatment planning, and family management/support services.
- Crisis intervention and triaging of psychiatric emergencies.
- Management of medication therapies; mental health status monitoring.
- Care management services for patients with serious mental health problems.
- Home visits when appropriate.
- Support groups routinely offered for patients and family members as needs are identified. These include healthy relationships, sexuality, violence, career and education for teens; stress management and assertiveness; parenting and grandparenting; bereavement and loss; substance abuse; caring for a disabled or chronically ill family member; obesity; and wellness and nutrition.
- Identification and follow-up of mental disorders related to medical conditions.
- Individual, group, and family treatment of children with attention deficit/hyperactivity disorders or conduct disturbance disorders referred by counselors from the area schools.
- Geriatric mental health assessment and treatment, including medication monitoring, reassurance calls, and home visits as appropriate.

Primary Care Integration Services

- Routine collection of family genogram data on all primary care patients. The genogram is an interview format that is used as a clinical tool for developing a systematic comprehensive clinical assessment, including assessment of risk factors.
- Routine primary mental health assessments of individuals in at-risk groups. These in-

clude people diagnosed with diabetes or other chronic illnesses; single mothers with young children; teen parents; addicted parents and their children; victims of family and community trauma, particularly children, adolescents, and young adults who have lost family members and friends to violence; families with a mentally retarded or physically disabled child; families with allergic or asthmatic children; older adults living alone; unemployed males; women at risk for cancer; and HIV-positive individuals.

- Monitoring/managing care of members of the same family.
- Education and consultation with other primary care providers both on site and in the community to help them identify and refer individuals and families with mental health care needs or those in need of health education.
- Participation with other community resources in linking services. These include neighborhood antidrug, antiviolence, antigraffiti programs; school-based health programs; targeted programs of the city health department such as HIV and other sexually transmitted disease testing and lead poisoning screening; walk-in pregnancy testing; stroke risk assessment; breast cancer screening; and programs aimed at homelessness and suicide prevention.
- Community health education and promotion programs, including an annual health fair. Community outreach activities in neighborhood schools, churches, a nursing home, community shelters, and a youth access center.
- Identification of the cultural, environmental, and community factors that impede the physical and emotional well-being of patients and families, and participation in community efforts to design responses. An example is parents and children who recently witnessed drug-related violence in southwest Philadelphia.
- School-based primary prevention programs at the neighborhood schools. An example is the Big Girls Wellness Program, which targeted obese girls.

► CASE EXAMPLE

Ms. A walked into the Health Annex one summer afternoon wearing a bathing suit and a pair of shorts, complaining of pains in her head and appearing quite agitated. Because Ms. A was so persistent about the need to have her physical problem assessed, her first contact was with the nurse practitioner (CRNP). However, because the nurse practitioner and the psychiatric nurse (CNS) had observed the client in the waiting room, they decided to do her health assessment together. In the course of doing the physical assessment, the client again became agitated and began to verbalize a history of sexual abuse and the effect it had had on her life. The CNS and the CRNP worked together to manage the client's distress, complete the physical assessment, and do a psychosocial assessment. They developed a comprehensive treatment plan that emphasized the psychosocial aspects of her care, and determined that the CNS would manage her care. An outreach worker was also assigned to work with the client to help her sign up for food supplements and food stamps, a heating allowance, and medical assistance. Home visits were by the CNS and the outreach worker as appropriate, until the client could be engaged in an ongoing wellness group that met weekly at the center.

Additional Services

Additional services include ongoing clinical outcome studies and education and supervision of students from all the health disciplines.

The Health Annex treatment approach is guided by clinical pathways, practice guidelines, and measurable goals. The provider, client, family, and community are viewed as a functional whole—a network of resources. The case vignette above illustrates the practice.

Maintaining both on site and home and community-based perspectives is intended to serve several functions. Institutions create a culture of their own that tends to become exclusive. In mental health this has meant that, despite the intent of providers to care for clients in their own context, the reality has been that clients come to providers. This method of delivering care was based on some practical considerations but also grew out of the medical, deficit-oriented models

of care more prevalent in the culture. Moving the mental health provider into the home and the community works to develop a more contextual, resource-oriented model of care. The provider who enters the home has access to the experiences of clients in their daily lives. The provider can see the roaches in the kitchen, the sick grandmother on the second floor, the lack of running water, and the drug dealers on the corner, as well as what the clients and families identify and use as resources. This immersion in the client's reality assists the provider in helping the client identify and achieve realistic goals by involving the client's own perspective in planning.

This integrated role also gives providers, who are of necessity more facility-based, eyes and ears in the community. This will help the center to stay truly community based and to plan programs that are realistic and meet community health needs.

CRITICAL ISSUES OF IMPLEMENTATION

COST

The biopsychosocial family systems approach requires a provider mix of advanced practice nurse specialists who can work together as a functional, collaborative whole. Although evidence supports the cost-effectiveness of using advanced practice nurse providers to deliver physical or mental health care (Baradell, 1994; Fagin, 1992), we do not yet have enough experience with the cost factors involved in these integrated approaches when they are implemented by nurse specialist providers in a primary health care setting. Evidence suggests that integrated models of care improve outcomes (DeGruy, 1995). In medical practice, specialty care has been linked to improved quality. However, it has also been linked to escalating costs (Wright, 1993). Primary health care has been viewed as a way to decrease the cost of health care, maintain quality, and increase access (Institute of Medicine, 1996; Wright, 1993). However, in the current managed care environment, the data on quality relative to cost are mixed and not yet conclusive. Outcome study data are needed to carefully assess both direct and indirect costs and benefits, both in the short and long term, including benefits to other family members.

In order to experiment with integrated approaches, a practice will need multiple funding streams to sustain itself until adequate reimbursement packages can be developed. In addition to start-up grant funding from the Division of Nursing, Department of Health and Human Services, the Health Annex practice is financed through fee-for-service, managed care contracts, subcontracting arrangements for specified services, and foundation support.

Reimbursement for the range of mental health services delivered on site has proven difficult. Traditional mental health carve-out provider networks in our area have been closed to new providers except for highly specialized services, such as group therapy with selected populations (substance abusers, adolescents). In addition, barriers to Medicaid and Medicare reimbursement for psychiatric nurses limits the services we can offer to our patients. The faculty has been working to educate managed care companies so that they might be willing, in the future, to consider capitation rates that reflect integrated delivery of physical and mental health services.

TEAM BUILDING

Although increased attention has been paid to interdisciplinary collaboration, little has been paid to nurse-to-nurse linkages. Nurses have had little experience working in nursing centers with providers who represent different specialties within the discipline. Each Health Annex provider has had to learn more about the other's vantage point on health care. The nurse-midwife, community health nurse, psychiatric nurse, and primary care nurse practitioner have been operating within the framework of responsibility for their own specialty. Now they are being asked to take responsibility for the whole. We have learned that this more egalitarian, shared responsibility approach does not come naturally to nurses who have been accustomed to working within medical hierarchies. Team building is the essential base for implementing a biopsychosocial family systems approach and is a key management skill that can make the difference in the success of an integrated approach.

STRATEGIC PLANNING

Budgets, business plans, and a concern for costs, quality outcomes, and patient satisfaction are not matters for which nurses have had to assume primary responsibility. In a primary care nursing center that relies on managed care contracts, nurses are accountable for the effectiveness of the practice in meeting both its economic and its care delivery goals. To help advanced practice nurses work effectively in the evolving health care environment, the University of Pennsylvania School of Nursing, in collaboration with the Wharton School of Business, has designed a series of course offerings, under the umbrella of a Nursing Executive Institute, to help advanced practice nurses and nurse executives to build their practices and programs on financially solid foundations.

EDUCATION AND TRAINING FOR INTEGRATED PRIMARY HEALTH CARE

It is already clear that integrated primary health care is a complex process of health care delivery and will require a restructuring of the education and training of advanced practice psychiatric nurses as well as other health care providers. The mental health providers practicing at the Health Annex have identified the following factors as critical components of educational preparation for practice in an integrated primary health care setting.

- Expertise in making complex clinical judgments based on rapid, comprehensive assessments. This includes using mental status exams, health risk assessment instruments, genograms, DSM-IV, psychiatric interviews, and other appropriate diagnostic instruments.
- Ability to diagnose and treat acute, episodic, and severe mental disorders, including medication management and monitoring and referral for psychiatric evaluation.
- Population-based health knowledge, including basic tenets of health education, health promotion, and preventive interventions in communities.
- Understanding of the various functions of the mental health care provider in primary care settings: community outreach, primary therapist, care manager/monitor, consultant, educator, and team member.
- Skill in applying family therapy approaches, group, cognitive, and brief psychotherapeutic methods.
- Knowledge of psychopharmacology and the biological basis of mental illness.

- Basic physical assessment skills including basic understanding of the major physical illnesses that affect the community and the interactions between physical illness and mental health.
- Knowledge of child development and parenting, including the skills to engage children and adolescents in primary health care programs.
- Knowledge of managed care and reimbursement issues, business planning and budget, quality assurance and outcome measures, and the infrastructure and systems of care delivery.
- A continuous practicum experience in a community-based, primary care setting so that students can experience responsibility for a caseload of clients and families over time.
- An interdisciplinary supervision experience so that students can meaningfully exchange views with other providers.
- Knowledge of issues of culture, awareness of one's own ethnicity and biases, and ability to work across cultures to differentiate issues of health from issues of culture.
- Research competency to identify and document cost-effective and quality client outcomes.

Clearly, the list given reflects the experience of one setting. However, it is offered as a place to begin a needed dialogue with the field of psychiatric health nursing, a dialogue that focuses on ways to move forward in the evolving health care system.

SUMMARY

As providers, care managers, health promoters and educators, and client advocates with family systems expertise, psychiatric advanced practice specialists are a necessary component of all primary health care. Their ability to function independently, yet collaboratively; to assess mental health, yet consider physical health; and to advocate for and help clients gain self-mastery gives them a unique role in the evolving health care system. Advanced practice psychiatric nurses must have the flexibility, courage, and skills to pursue new directions.

REFERENCES

Ader R, Cohen N. Psychoneuroimmunology: Conditioning and stress. *Annu Rev Psychol.* 1993;44:53.

Aiken L. Charting nursing's future. In: Aiken L, Fagin C, eds. *Charting Nursing's Future. Agenda for the 1990s.* Philadelphia: Lippincott; 1992:3–12.

American Association of Colleges of Nursing. AACN Issue Bulletin: In Search of the Advanced Practice Nurse. Washington DC: the AACN. 1993; 3:1–4.

American Nurses' Association. *Health Care Reform: Essential Mental Health Services. Executive Summary.* Department of practice, economics, and policy. Washington, DC: American Nurses' Association; 1993.

American Nurses' Association. *Nursing's Agenda for Health Care Reform.* Washington, DC: American Nurses' Association; 1992.

American Psychiatric Association. Diagnostic and Statistical Manual of Mental Disorders. 4th ed. Washington, DC: American Psychiatric Association; 1994.

Baradell JG. Cost-effectiveness and quality of care provided by clinical nurse specialists. *J Psychosoc Nurs.* 1994;32:21–24.

Blount A, Bayona J. Toward a system of integrated primary care. *Fam Systems Med.* 1994;12: 171–182.

Boyle PJ and Callahan D. Managed care in mental health: the ethical issues. *Health Affairs.* 1995; 14(3), 7–22.

Campbell TL. Family's impact on health: A critical review and annotated bibliography. *Fam Systems Med.* 1986;4:135–328.

Campbell TL, Patterson JM. The effectiveness of family interventions in the treatment of physical illness. *J Marital Fam Ther.* 1995;21:545–583.

Church O. From custody to community in psychiatric nursing. *Nurs Res.* 1987;36:48–55.

DeGruy F. Overview of collaboration research. *Working Together.* Newsletter of the Collaborative Family Health Care Coalition. Fall 1995:3–4.

Fagin C. Cost effectiveness of nursing care revisited 1981–1990. In: Aiken L, Fagin C, eds. *Charting Nursing's Future. Agenda for the 1990s.* Philadelphia: Lippincott; 1992:13–28.

Fox JC. Psychiatric nursing: directions for the future. In Aiken L, and Fagin C, eds. *Charting Nursing's Future: Agenda for the 1990s.* Philadelphia: Lippincott, 1992:216–234.

Goldstein MG, Niaura R. Psychological factors affecting physical condition: Cardiovascular literature review. *Psychosomatics.* 1992;33, 134.

Haber J, Billings CV. Primary Mental Health Care: A vision for the future of psychiatric-mental health nursing. *Council Perspect.* 1993;2:1–3.

Heffernan L. Regulation of advanced practice nursing in health care reform. *J Health Hosp Law.* 1995; 28:73–84.

Institute of Medicine. *Primary Care. America's Health in a New Era.* Washington, DC: National Academy Press; 1996.

Jenkins M, Sullivan-Marx E. Nurse practitioners and community health nurses. *Nurs Clin North Am.* 1994;29:459–470.

Kiecolt-Glaser JK, Glaser R. Psychological influences on immunity. *Psychosomatics.* 1986;27:621.

Kiecolt-Glaser JK, Kennedy S, Marikoff S, et al. Marital discord and immunity in males. *Psychosom Med.* 1988;50:213–229.

McBride AB, Austin JK. *Psychiatric-Mental Health Nursing. Integrating the Behavioral and Biological Sciences.* Philadelphia: Saunders; 1996.

McDaniel S, Campbell TL, Seaburn DB. Principles for collaboration between health and mental health providers in primary care. *Fam Systems Med.* 1995;13:283–298.

Redefining psychiatry: Implications for practice, training and recruitment. *Bull Menninger Clin.* 1994;58.

Richardson LA, Keller AM, Selby-Harrington ML, Parrish R. Identification and treatment of children's mental health problems by primary care providers: A critical review of research. *Arch Psychiatr Nurs.* 1996;10:293–303.

Rolland JS. *Families, Illness, and Disability.* New York: Basic Books; 1994.

Safriet B. Health care dollars and regulatory sense: The role of advanced practice nursing. *Yale J Regulation.* 1992;9:417–488.

Talley S, Caverly S. Advanced-practice psychiatric nursing and health care reform. *Hosp Commun Psychiatr.* 1994;45:545–547.

White House Domestic Security Council. *The President's Health Security Plan.* New York: Random House; 1993.

Wolff HG, Wolf S, Hare CE, eds. *Life Stress and Bodily Disease.* New York: Williams & Wilkins; 1950.

Wright RA. Community-oriented primary care. The cornerstone of health care reform. *JAMA.* 1993; 269:2544–2547.

CHAPTER 3

CONCEPTUAL MODELS AND THERAPEUTIC MODALITIES IN ADVANCED PSYCHIATRIC NURSING PRACTICE

Jacqueline Fawcett

If the premises and foci of the conceptual model of nursing and the therapeutic modality are not congruent, the modality should be revised so that it fits the model.

Chapter Overview

- Defining the Differences
- The Value of Conceptual Models to Advanced Practice
- How Conceptual Models Are Used in Advanced Psychiatric Nursing
- Johnson's Behavioral System Model
- Neuman's Systems Model
- Roy's Adaptation Model
- Linking Conceptual Models and Therapeutic Modalities
- Conclusion
- References
- Appendix: Overview of Three Conceptual Models of Nursing
    Dorothy Johnson's Behavioral System Model
    Betty Neuman's Systems Model
    Callista Roy's Adaptation Model

Portions of this chapter are adapted with permission from Fawcett J. Analysis and Evaluation of Conceptual Models of Nursing. *3rd ed. Philadelphia: Davis; 1995.*

► INTRODUCTION

Clinicians must take the lead in implementing systems of nursing knowledge based on appropriate linkages between conceptual models of nursing and therapeutic modalities. The links, and ultimately the systems of nursing knowledge, will determine the direction of advanced psychiatric nursing practice.

DEFINING THE DIFFERENCES

A **conceptual model** is an abstract, general frame of reference about the phenomena within a particular discipline, such as nursing. Nursing conceptual models are, as Reed (1995) points out, "archetypes of nursing practice" (p. 81). More specifically, each conceptual model of nursing presents a distinctive perspective of the recipient of nursing, who can be an individual, family, or community; the environment of the recipient and the environment where nursing occurs; the recipient's state of health; and the definition, goals, and process of nursing.

Among the best-known conceptual models of nursing are Johnson's Behavioral System Model, King's General Systems Framework, Levine's Conservation Model, Neuman's Systems Model, Orem's Self-Care Framework, Rogers's Science of Unitary Human Beings, and Roy's Adaptation Model. The content of each is detailed in the primary sources (Johnson, 1990; King, 1990; Levine, 1991; Neuman, 1995; Orem, 1995; Rogers, 1990; Roy and Andrews, 1991). The content and documented uses of the models in nursing research, education, administration, and practice are described in *Analysis and Evaluation of Conceptual Models of Nursing* (Fawcett, 1995). Three of the conceptual models—Johnson's Behavioral System Model, Neuman's Systems Model, and Roy's Adaptation Model—are discussed later in the chapter.

A **therapeutic modality** is a relatively specific, concrete formulation that describes a precise process of treating a person with a psychiatric disorder. Examples of therapeutic modalities in advanced psychiatric nursing include crisis intervention, cognitive therapy, and family therapy. These and most other therapeutic modalities employed by advanced practice psychiatric nurses are grounded in the discipline of medicine and the clinical specialty of psychiatry.

A therapeutic modality is more limited in scope than a conceptual model. Whereas each conceptual nursing model deals with a broad range of phenomena, each therapeutic modality addresses only one approach to assessment and/or intervention for a person with a psychiatric disorder. For example, Roy's Adaptation Model encompasses the entire nursing process within the context of a broad array of physiological and psychosocial responses to diverse environmental stimuli. Crisis intervention, in contrast, is a particular modality used to help a person overcome a specific instance of psychological disequilibrium (Parad, 1965).

Advanced practice in all clinical nursing specialties carries with it the strong temptation to emulate medical practice. In fact, "the lure of following the medical model is sanctioned and well rewarded in some settings" (Hawkins & Thibodeau, 1993, p. 11). The temptation must, however, be resisted. Moreover, in our evolving health care system, it is crucial that advanced practice nurses not be regarded as a way to fill a medical care gap. As Smith (1995) pointed out,

"Advanced practice nursing is not filling the gap with medical care where it does not exist; it is filling the existing gap in health care with the core of nursing practice" (p. 2).

THE VALUE OF CONCEPTUAL MODELS TO ADVANCED PRACTICE

The use of conceptual models fosters advanced nursing practice that is focused on "the whole client within the context of her/his significant environment, [and that focuses on] mobilizing person-family-community strengths and resources for health and healing" (Smith, 1995, p. 2). Indeed, the essence of advanced nursing practice is the application of knowledge that is formalized in nursing's conceptual models (Parse, 1995).

Conceptual models of nursing are the foundation for advanced psychiatric nursing practice; they delineate the scope of that practice and identify the recipient of nursing, the relevant environment, the aspects of health to be considered, and the steps and substance of the nursing process. As such, the models move advanced psychiatric nursing practice away from an emulation of psychiatric practice and foster autonomy from medicine and a coherent purpose of practice (Bélanger, 1991; Bridges, 1991; Ingram, 1991). Furthermore, conceptual models specify innovative goals for advanced psychiatric nursing and introduce ideas that are designed to improve that practice (Lindsay, 1990) by facilitating the identification of relevant information, reducing the fragmentation of care, and improving the coordination of care (Chalmers, cited in Chalmers et al., 1990). In particular, conceptual models positively affect advanced psychiatric nursing practice "by enabling well-coordinated care to take place, by providing a basis for the justification of care actions and by enabling nurses to talk nursing" (Chalmers, cited in Chalmers et al., 1990, p. 34), to think nursing (Perry, 1985), and to "help nurses better communicate what they do" (Neff, 1991, p. 534) and why they do it.

HOW CONCEPTUAL MODELS ARE USED IN ADVANCED PSYCHIATRIC NURSING

Johnson's Behavioral System Model, Newman's Systems Model, and Roy's Adaptation Model focus on phenomena that are of particular interest to advanced practice psychiatric nurses. They have been applied in situations that typify advanced practice nursing. Overviews of the three conceptual models are presented in the appendix to this chapter.

A conceptual model influences advanced psychiatric nursing practice in four areas:

- Standards for nursing practice
- Patient classification systems
- Clinical information systems
- Quality monitoring programs

Each model identifies certain standards for nursing practice or a particular care plan. The clinical information systems that may be influenced include the admission data base, nursing orders, care plan, progress notes, and discharge summary (Christmyer et al., 1988). In addition, each conceptual model identifies criteria for evaluation of the outcomes of nursing intervention. It is evident that a conceptual model may be systematically reflected in all nursing documentation tools. How three conceptual models can guide the development of patient classification systems and quality monitoring programs will now be described.

JOHNSON'S BEHAVIORAL SYSTEM MODEL

Johnson's Behavioral System Model has been used to guide the development of a psychiatric patient classification system. Indeed, the Patient Classification Instrument (PCI) was directly derived from this model (Auger and Dee, 1983; Dee and Auger, 1983). The PCI operationalizes each behavioral subsystem (attachment, dependency, ingestive, eliminative, sexual, aggressive, achievement) as critical patient behaviors. Specific critical patient behaviors are linked to specific nursing interventions and categorized according to the level of nursing required.

In category I, patient behaviors appropriate for the patient's developmental stage and adaptive to the environment are linked with nursing interventions that provide general supervision; maintain and support healthy, developmentally appropriate behaviors; and reinforce independent behaviors. In category II, patient behaviors that are inconsistent, in the process of being learned, and maladaptive to the environment, along with behaviors that may or may not be appropriate for the patient's developmental stage, are linked with nursing interventions that provide moderate or periodic supervision, modify maladaptive behaviors and maintain newly adaptive ones, and structure the environment to provide limits on behavior. These interventions are carried out in the context of group settings, and include implementation of the medical treatment regimen.

In category III, patient behaviors that are severely maladaptive to the environment and not appropriate for the patient's developmental stage are linked with nursing interventions that provide direct supervision, modify maladaptive behaviors, teach new behaviors, reinforce adaptive behaviors, structure the environment to provide limits on behavior, and include implementation of the medical treatment regimen. In category IV, patient behaviors from category III that are of acute intensity, duration, and/or frequency, as well as behaviors that represent self-destructive acts or aggression toward others, are linked with nursing interventions that provide one-to-one supervision and that are directed toward the reduction of the intensity, frequency, and/or duration of the maladaptive behaviors and the protection of the patient.

The PCI can be used to direct the entire nursing process, from problem determination to evaluation of post-treatment behaviors, and is an especially effective way to document the outcomes of nursing interventions based on

Johnson's Behavioral System Model (Poster, 1989). Dee and Auger (1983) explained that use of the PCI has resulted in many practical benefits.

> The assessment of patient behaviors . . . [is] systematically and comprehensively reviewed within the framework of the behavioral subsystems. . . . The correlated nursing care actions with patient behaviors has assisted in both the planning and the intervention phases of the [nursing] process by identifying a broad range of general areas of potential nursing activity. . . . The use of a model also provides an objective means for evaluating the quality of nursing care. . . . Instead of evaluating patient outcomes for groups based on medical diagnoses, it becomes feasible to evaluate outcomes for groups of patients based on common behavioral problems or nursing treatment approaches (p. 23).

NEUMAN'S SYSTEMS MODEL

Quayhagen and Roth (1989) developed an innovative approach to assessment based on Neuman's Systems Model that is appropriate for advanced practice psychiatric nurses to use. They identified psychometrically sound clinical research instruments that are appropriate measures of the model's physiological, psychological, sociocultural, developmental, and spiritual variables, as well as of the external environment. The instruments form a protocol that can be used for the comprehensive assessment of patients and families and the evaluation of the efficacy of primary, secondary and tertiary prevention interventions.

Physiological variables are assessed using the Cornell Medical Index, sections A to L (Brodman et al., 1949). Psychological variables can be assessed with instruments such as the Mental Status Questionnaire (Kahn et al., 1960), the Cornell Medical Index, sections M to R (Brodman et al., 1949), the Brief Symptom Inventory (Derogatis and Spencer, 1982), the Self-Rating Depression Scale (Zung, 1974), the Coping Strategies Inventory (Quayhagen and Quayhagen, 1988), and the Life Events Questionnaire (Chiriboga and Dean, 1978).

Sociocultural variables are assessed using instruments such as the Family Mutual Aid and Interaction Index (Cantor, 1976), the Marital Satisfaction Scale (Gilford and Bengtson, 1979), Faces II (Olson et al., 1985), the Decision Power Index (Blood and Wolfe, 1960), and the Role Conflict Scale (Kopelman et al., 1983). Assessment of developmental variables is accomplished through the use of a genogram (Wright and Leahey, 1987) and basic demographic information such as age, education, and marital status. Spiritual variables are assessed with the Religiosity subscale of the Coping Strategies Inventory (Quayhagen and Quayhagen, 1988). The external environment may be assessed with the Home Assessment Checklist (Tideiksaar, 1983) and the Community Assessment Guide (Rauckhorst et al., 1980).

The many instruments identified by Quayhagen and Roth (1989) would not necessarily be used with each patient or family. Rather, instruments that are appropriate for the particular clinical situation should be used. If, for example, a patient has symptoms of anxiety, the State-Trait Anxiety Inventory (Spielberger et al., 1970) could be used. Furthermore, as Quayhagen and Roth pointed out, special concerns or problems could be assessed with other instruments. For example, caregiver burden could be assessed using the Burden Interview (Zarit et al., 1980). The important points made by Quayhagen and Roth are that instruments typically used for research purposes can also be used for clinical assessments, and that multiple instruments are needed for comprehensive assessments based on Neuman's System Model.

ROY'S ADAPTATION MODEL

Roy's Adaptation Model has been used to develop exceedingly comprehensive patient care standards, a documentation system, and a quality

monitoring program (Weiss and Teplick, 1995). Although the work reported by Weiss and Teplick focuses on perinatal nursing, it can easily be adapted for use in psychiatric nursing.

Weiss and Teplick explained that the patient care standards, which identify desired patient outcomes and specific nursing interventions used to achieve the desired outcomes, serve as standard plans of care for specific patient populations. Each element of each standard of care reflects an element of a concept of Roy's Adaptation Model (for example, oxygenation from the physiological response mode; body image from the self-concept response mode).

The documentation system, in the form of flow sheets, facilitates recording nursing assessments and interventions, as well as progress toward desired patient outcomes. Weiss and Teplick (1995) explained that the model was used to organize the flow sheets, and that the "items listed on the documentation flow sheets correspond directly with the desired patient outcomes and nursing intervention strategies listed in the patient standard of care" (p. 40)

The quality monitoring program, which uses specific quality assessment tools for each patient population, is a direct extension of the patient care standards. As Weiss and Teplick explained,

> because documentation flows directly from the standards of care, information on all indicators is easily accessible, and compliance with recording [on the flow sheets] on each indicator is very high. Ongoing assessment of patient adaptations and targeted nursing interventions through monitoring of compliance with progress and outcome standards provides a mechanism for identification of patient care problems and opportunities for improvement (p. 41).

Roy's Adaptation Model has also been used as a blueprint to develop the Comprehensive Sexual Assault Assessment Tool (CSAAT), which was designed to provide a standard method of documenting sexual assault and to facilitate nationwide collection of standardized research data (Burgess and Fawcett, 1996; Burgess et al., 1995). The initial CSAAT items were selected from tools currently used by sexual assault nurse examiners. The items were then categorized according to the concepts of the model (focal and contextual stimuli; regulator and cognator coping mechanisms; physiological, self-concept, role function, and interdependence response modes). New items were written to represent concepts of the model not already addressed by existing items. The CSAAT encompasses four major areas for data collection: investigative data, victim forensic data, legal/services information, and psychosocial assessment for post-traumatic stress disorder (PTSD).

LINKING CONCEPTUAL MODELS AND THERAPEUTIC MODALITIES

Advanced psychiatric nursing practice requires a conceptual model and one or more therapeutic modalities. Linking the model and modalities is crucial if nurses are to achieve the social mission of nursing rather than that of medicine (Johnson, 1987). Whall (1980) developed a strategy to link conceptual models of nursing with therapeutic modalities. She proposed that the underlying philosophical premises and pragmatic focus of both the conceptual model and the therapeutic modality should be examined for congruence. If the premises and foci of the model and modality are congruent, they may be linked and used as a system of nursing knowledge. If, however, they are not congruent, the modality should be revised so that it fits with the model. Whall (1980) emphasized that inasmuch as the conceptual model is the more abstract starting point and the foundation for nursing practice, the therapeutic modality—not the model—is reformulated.

For example, the modality of strategic family therapy (Madanes, 1981) requires refor-

mulation to be logically congruent with Roy's Adaptation Model. One area of reformulation is the addition of physiological mode responses required by Roy's model; this domain is completely neglected in strategic family therapy.

Several appropriate linkages between conceptual models of nursing and therapeutic modalities are given in books by Fitzpatrick and associates (1982) and Whall (1986). For example, Roy's Adaptation Model of Nursing has been linked with crisis intervention (Fitzpatrick et al., 1982) and with Madanes' (1981, 1984) strategic family therapy (Whall, 1986). Roy's Adaptation Model has also been linked with music therapy (Hamer, 1991) and group therapy (Kurek-Ovshinsky, 1991). Neuman's Systems Model has been linked with contextual family therapy (Goldblum-Graff and Graff, 1982).

CONCLUSION

This chapter was based on the assertion that conceptual models of nursing are the foundation for advanced psychiatric nursing. When therapeutic modalities are linked to a nursing model, practice is based on a nursing perspective, rather than a purely medical or psychiatric perspective.

REFERENCES

Auger JR, Dee V. A patient classification system based on the behavioral system model of nursing, part 1. *J Nurs Admin.* 1983;13:38–43.

Bélanger P. Nursing models—A major step towards professional autonomy. *AARN Newsletter.* 1991; 48:13.

Blood RO, Wolfe DM. *Husbands and Wives: The Dynamics of Married Life.* New York: Free Press; 1960.

Bridges J. Working with doctors: Distinct from medicine. *Nurs Times.* 1991;87:42–43.

Brodman K, Erdmann AJ, Lorge I, et al. The Cornell Medical Index: An adjunct to medical interview. *JAMA* 1949;140:530–534. (Revised, 1974.)

Burgess AW, Fawcett J. The Comprehensive Sexual Assault Assessment Tool (CSAAT). *Nurse Practitioner: American Journal of Primary Health Care.* 1996;21(4), 66, 71–72, 74–76, 78, 83, 86.

Burgess AW, Fawcett J, Hazelwood RR, Grant CA. Victim care services and the Comprehensive Sexual Assault Assessment Tool (CSAAT). In: Hazelwood RR, Burgess AW, eds. *Practical Rape Investigation.* Boca Raton, FL: CRC; 1995.

Cantor MH. The configuration and intensity of the informal support system in a New York City elderly population. Paper presented at the 29th annual scientific meeting of the Gerontological Society of America, New York, 1976.

Chalmers H, Kershaw B, Melia K, Kendrich M. Nursing models: Enhancing or inhibiting practice? *Nurs Standard.* 1990;5:34–40.

Chiriboga DA, Dean H. Dimensions of stress: Perspectives from a longitudinal study. *J Psychosomat Res.* 1978;22:47–55.

Cristmyer CS, Catanzariti PM, Langford AM, Reitz JA. Bridging the gap: Theory to practice. Part 1, clinical applications. *Nurs Manag.* 1988;19:42–50.

Dabbs ADV. Theory-based nursing practice: For our patients' sake. *Clin Nurse Specialist.* 1994;8:214, 220.

Dee V, Auger JA. A patient classification system based on the behavioral system model of nursing, part 2. *J Nurs Admin.* 1983;13:18–23

Derogatis LR, Spencer PM. *The Brief Symptom Inventory (BSI): Administration and procedures manual, 1.* Baltimore: Johns Hopkins University School of Medicine, Clinical Psychometric Research Unit; 1982.

Fawcett J. *Analysis and Evaluation of Conceptual Models of Nursing.* 3rd ed. Philadelphia: Davis; 1995.

Fitzpatrick JJ, Whall AL, Johnston RL, Floyd JA. *Nursing Models and Their Psychiatric Mental Health Applications.* Bowie, MD: Brady; 1982.

Gilford R, Bengtson V. Measuring marital satisfaction in three generations: Positive and negative. *J Marital Fam Ther.* 1979;41:387–398.

Goldblum-Graff D, Graff H. The Neuman model adapted to family therapy. In: Neuman B., ed. *The Neuman Systems Model: Application to Nursing Education and Practice.* Norwalk, CT: Appleton-Century-Crofts; 1982:217–222.

Grossman M, Hooton M. The significance of the relationship between a discipline and its practice. *J Adv Nurs.* 1993;18:866–872.

Hamer BA. Music therapy: Harmony for change. *J Psychosoc Nurs Ment Health Serv.* 1991;29:5–7.

Hawkins JW, Thibodeau JA. *The Advanced Practitioner: Current Practice Issues.* 3rd ed. New York: Tiresias Press; 1993.

Ingram R. Why does nursing need theory? *J Adv Nurs.* 1991;16:350–353.

Johnson DE. The behavioral system model for nursing. In: Parker ME, ed. *Nursing Theories in Practice.* New York: National League for Nursing; 1990.

Johnson DE. Evaluating conceptual models for use in critical care nursing practice. *Dimensions Crit Care Nurs.* 1987;6:195–197. Editorial.

Kahn RL, Goldfarb AI, Pollack M, et al. Brief objective measures for the determination of mental status in the aged. *Am J Psychiatry.* 1960;117:326–328.

King IM. King's conceptual framework and theory of goal attainment. In: Parker ME, ed. *Nursing Theories in Practice.* New York: National League for Nursing; 1990.

Kopelman RE, Greenhaus HH, Connolly TF. A model of work, family and interrole conflict: A construct validation study. *Organization Behav Hum Perform.* 1983;32:198 215.

Kurek-Ovshinsky C. Group psychotherapy in an acute inpatient setting: Techniques that nourish self-esteem. *Issues Ment Health Nurs.* 1991;12:81–88.

Levine ME. The conservation principles: A model for health. In: Schaefer KM, Pond JB, eds. *Levine's Conservation Model: A Framework for Nursing Practice.* Philadelphia: Davis; 1991.

Lindsay B. The gap between theory and practice. *Nurs Standard.* 1990;5:34–35.

Madanes C. *Behind the One-way Mirror.* San Francisco: Jossey Bass; 1984.

Madanes C. *Strategic Family Therapy.* San Francisco: Jossey Bass; 1981.

Neff M. President's message: The future of our profession from the eyes of today. *Am Nephrol Nurs Assoc J.* 1991;18:534.

Neuman B. *The Neuman Systems Model.* 3rd ed. Norwalk, CT: Appleton & Lange; 1995.

Olson DH, Portner J, Bell R. *Marriage and Family Inventory Project: Faces II.* St. Paul: University of Minnesota; 1985.

Orem DE. *Nursing: Concepts of Practice.* 5th ed. St. Louis: Mosby Year Book; 1991.

Parad H. *Crisis Intervention.* New York: Family Service Association of America; 1965.

Parse RR. Nursing theories and frameworks: The essence of advanced practice nursing. *Nurs Sci Q.* 1995;8:1. Editorial.

Perry J. Has the discipline of nursing developed to the stage where nurses do "think nursing"? *J Adv Nurs.* 1985;10:31–37.

Poster EC. Behavioral category ratings of adolescents on an inpatient psychiatric unit: The use of the Johnson behavioral system model. In: Brackston A, Cooper-Pagé L, Edwards S, et al, eds. *Proceedings: Putting It All Together.* Ottawa: University of Ottawa; 1989:99. Abstract.

Quayhagen MP, Quayhagen M. Alzheimer's stress: Coping with the caregiving role. *Gerontologist.* 1988;28:391–396.

Quayhagen MP, Roth PA. From models to measures in assessment of mature families. *J Prof Nurs.* 1989;5:144–151.

Rauckhorst LM, Stokes SA, Mezey MD. Community and home assessment. *J Gerontol Nurs.* 1980;6: 319–327.

Reed PG. A treatise on nursing knowledge development for the 21st century: Beyond postmodernism. *Adv Nurs Sci.* 1995;17:70–84.

Rogers ME. Nursing: Science of unitary, irreducible, human beings: Update 1990. In: Barrett EAM, ed. *Visions of Rogers' Science-based Nursing.* New York: National League for Nursing; 1990.

Roy C, Andrews HA. *The Roy Adaptation Model: The Definitive Statement.* Norwalk, CT: Appleton & Lange; 1991.

Smith MC. The core of advanced practice nursing. *Nurs Sci Q.* 1995;8:2–3.

Spielberger C, Gorsuch RL, Lushene RE. *STAI manual for the State-Trait Anxiety Inventory.* Palo Alto: Consulting Psychologists; 1970.

Tideiksaar R. *Home Assessment Checklist.* New York: Mt. Sinai Medical Center, Ritter Department of Geriatrics and Adult Development; 1983.

Weiss ME, Teplick F. Linking perinatal standards, documentation, and quality monitoring. *Neonat Intens Care.* 1995;8:38–43, 58.

Whall AL. *Family Therapy Theory for Nursing: Four Approaches.* Norwalk, CT: Appleton-Century-Crofts; 1986.

Whall AL. Congruence between existing theories of family functioning and nursing theories. *Adv Nurs Sci.* 1980;3:59–67.

Wright LM, Leahey M. *Families and Chronic Illness.* Springhouse, PA: Springhouse; 1987.

Zarit SH, Reever KE, Bach-Peterson J. Relatives of the impaired elderly: Correlates of feelings of burden. *Gerontologist.* 1980;20:649–655.

Zung WWK. The measurement of affects: Depression and anxiety. In: Pinchot P, Olivier-Martin R, eds. *Psychological Measurements in Psychopharmacology. Vol. 7: Modern Problems of Pharmacopsychiatry.* New York: S. Karger; 1974.

Overview of Three Conceptual Models of Nursing

DOROTHY JOHNSON'S BEHAVIORAL SYSTEM MODEL

Focus is on the person as a behavioral system, made up of all the patterned, repetitive, and purposeful ways of behavior that characterize life. Seven subsystems carry out specialized tasks or functions needed to maintain the integrity of the whole behavioral system and to manage its relationship to the environment:

1. *Attachment or affiliative* function is the security needed for survival as well as social inclusion, intimacy, and formation and maintenance of social bonds.
2. *Dependency* function is the succoring behavior that calls for a response of nurturance as well as approval, attention or recognition, and physical assistance.
3. *Ingestive subsystem* function is appetite satisfaction in terms of when, how, what, how much, and under what conditions the individual eats, all of which are governed by social and psychological considerations as well as biological requirements for food and fluids.
4. *Eliminative* function is elimination in terms of when, how, and under what conditions the individual eliminates wastes.
5. *Sexual* functions are procreation and gratification, with regard to behaviors dependent upon the individual's biological sex and gender role identity, including but not limited to courting and mating.
6. *Aggressive* function is protection and preservation of self and society.
7. *Achievement* function is mastery or control of some aspect of self or environment, with regard to intellectual, physical, creative, mechanical, social, and caretaking (of children, partner, home) skills.

The **structure** of each subsystem includes four elements:

1. *Drive or goal.* The motivation for behavior.
2. *Set.* The individual's predisposition to act in certain ways to fulfill the function of the subsystem.
3. *Choice.* The individual's total behavioral repertoire for fulfilling subsystem functions, which encompasses the scope of action alternatives from which the person can choose.
4. *Action.* The individual's actual behavior in a situation. Action is the only structural element that can be observed directly; all other elements must be inferred from the individual's actual behavior and from the consequences of that behavior.

Three **functional requirements** are needed by each subsystem to fulfill its functions:

1. *Protection* from noxious influences with which the system cannot cope.

2. *Nurturance* through the input of appropriate supplies from the environment.
3. *Stimulation* to enhance growth and prevent stagnation.

Nursing practice is directed toward restoration, maintenance, or attainment of behavioral system balance and dynamic stability at the highest possible level for the individual. The nursing diagnostic and treatment process has four steps:

1. *Determination of the existence of a problem* in behavioral subsystem functions or structural elements.
2. *Diagnostic classification of problems* as internal subsystem problems or intersystem problems.
3. *Management of nursing problems* through three types of treatments: (a) *fulfilling subsystem functional requirements* by protecting the patient from overwhelming noxious influences, supplying adequate nurturance, and providing stimulation; (b) *imposing external regulatory or control mechanisms on behavior*, such as setting limits for behavior, inhibition of ineffective behavioral responses, and assisting patients to acquire new behavioral responses; and (c) *changing the structural elements of the subsystems* by altering set through instruction or counseling and adding choices through teaching new skills.
4. *Evaluation of the efficacy of nursing treatments* by comparing the extent of behavioral system stability and balance before and after the treatments.

Betty neuman's systems model

Focus is on the wellness of the client system in relation to an environmental stressor and reactions to that stressor. The **client system**, which can be an individual, family or other group, or community, is a composite of five interrelated variables:

1. *Physiological variables.* Bodily structure and function.
2. *Psychological variables.* Mental processes and relationships.
3. *Sociocultural variables.* Social and cultural functions.
4. *Developmental variables.* Developmental processes of life.
5. *Spiritual variables.* Aspects of spirituality on a continuum from complete unawareness or denial to a consciously developed high level of spiritual understanding.

The client system is depicted as a central core, which is a basic structure of survival factors common to the species, surrounded by three types of concentric rings:

1. *Flexible line of defense.* The outermost ring; a protective buffer for the client's normal or stable state that prevents invasion of stressors and keeps the client system free from stressor reactions or symptomatology.
2. *Normal line of defense.* Lies between the flexible line of defense and the lines of resistance; represents the client system's normal or usual wellness state.
3. *Lines of resistance.* The innermost concentric ring; involuntarily activated when a stressor invades the normal line of defense. They attempt to stabilize the client system and foster a return to the normal line of defense. If effective, the system can reconstitute; if ineffective, death may ensue.

Environment is all internal and external factors or influences surrounding the client system:

1. *Internal environment.* All forces or interactive influences internal to or contained solely within the boundaries of the defined client system; the source of *intrapersonal stressors.*
2. *External environment.* All forces or interaction influences external to or existing outside the defined client system; the source of *interpersonal and extrapersonal stressors.*

3. *Created-environment*. Subconsciously developed by the client as a symbolic expression of system wholeness; supersedes and encompasses the internal and external environments. Functions as a subjective safety mechanism that may block the true reality of the environment and the health experience.

Nursing practice is directed toward facilitating optimal wellness through retention, attainment; or maintenance of client system stability. There are three steps of the nursing process:

1. *Nursing diagnosis*. Formulated on the basis of assessment of the variables and lines of defense and resistance making up the client system.
2. *Nursing goals*. Negotiated with the client for desired prescriptive changes to correct variances form wellness.
3. *Nursing outcomes*. Determined by means of evaluation of the results of three types of prevention as intervention modalities.

The three types of prevention are as follows:

1. *Primary prevention*. Action required to *retain* client system stability; selected when the risk of or hazard from a stressor is known but a reaction has not yet occurred. Interventions attempt to reduce the possibility of the client's encounter with the stressor or strengthen the flexible line of defense to decrease the possibility of a reaction when the stressor is encountered.
2. *Secondary prevention*. Action required to *attain* system stability; selected when a reaction to a stressor has already occurred. Interventions deal with existing symptoms and attempt to strengthen the lines of resistance through use of the client's internal and external resources.
3. *Tertiary prevention*. Action required to *maintain* system stability; selected when some degree of client system stability has occurred following secondary prevention interventions.

CALLISTA ROY'S ADAPTATION MODEL

Focus is on the responses of the human adaptive system to a constantly changing environment. **Adaptation** is the central feature of the model. Problems in adaptation arise when the adaptive system is unable to cope with or respond to constantly changing stimuli from the internal and external environments in a manner that maintains the integrity of the system. **Environmental stimuli** are categorized as:

1. *Focal*. The stimuli most immediately confronting the person.
2. *Contextual*. The contributing factors in the situation.
3. *Residual*. Other unknown factors that may influence the situation. When the factors making up residual stimuli become known, they are considered focal or contextual stimuli.

Adaptation occurs through two types of innate or acquired coping mechanisms used to respond to changing environmental stimuli:

1. *Regulator subsystem*. Receives input from the external environment and from changes in the person's internal state and processes the changes through neural-chemical-endocrine channels to produce responses.
2. *Cognator subsystem*. Also receives input from external and internal stimuli that involve psychological, social, physical, and physiological factors, including regulator subsystem outputs. These stimuli then are processed through cognitive/emotive pathways, including perceptual/information processing, learning, judgment, and emotion.

Responses take place in four modes:

1. *Physiological mode*. Concerned with basic needs requisite to maintaining the physical and physiological integrity of the human system; encompasses oxygenation, nutrition,

elimination, activity and rest, protection, the senses, fluids and electrolytes, neurological functions, and endocrine functions.

2. *Self-concept mode.* Deals with people's conceptions of the physical self (body sensation and body image) and personal self (self-consistency, self-ideal, and the moral-ethical-spiritual self).

3. *Role function mode.* Concerned with people's performance of roles on the basis of their positions within society.

4. *Interdependence mode.* Involves the willingness and ability to love, respect, and value others; and to accept and respond to love, respect, and value given by others; concerned primarily with relationships with significant others and social support systems.

The four modes are interrelated. Responses in any one mode may have an effect on, or act as a stimulus in, one or all of the other modes. Responses are judged as *adaptive*, promoting the integrity of the person in terms of the goals of the human adaptive system, including survival, growth, reproduction, and mastery; or *ineffec-* *tive*, not contributing to the goals of the human adaptive system.

Nursing practice is directed toward promoting adaptation in each of the four response modes, thereby contributing to the person's health, quality of life, and dying with dignity. The nursing process encompasses six steps:

1. *Assessment of behavior.* Collection of data regarding adaptive system behaviors; determination of adaptive and ineffective responses; setting priorities for further assessment.

2. *Assessment of stimuli.* Identification of the focal and contextual stimuli that influence adaptive system behaviors.

3. *Nursing diagnosis.* Judgments regarding adaptation status.

4. *Goal setting.* Statement of behavioral outcomes of nursing intervention.

5. *Nursing intervention.* Management of environmental stimuli by increasing, decreasing, maintaining, removing, or otherwise altering or changing relevant focal and/or contextual stimuli.

6. *Evaluation.* Judgments regarding the effectiveness of nursing intervention.

With permission from Fawcett J. Conceptual models and theories of nursing. In: Thomas CL, ed. Taber's cyclopedic medical dictionary *18th ed. Philadelphia: Davis; 1997.*

INTEGRATING MENTAL HEALTH IN A NURSE-MANAGED REHABILITATION PROGRAM FOR OLDER ADULTS

Johanna Yurkow • Lois K. Evans • Ina Cochran • LilliAnn P. Ciesielski

*T*he geropsychiatric clinical nurse specialist (GPCNS) has a multidimensional role in the CARE Program that facilitates successful holistic rehabilitation by identifying and addressing relational, behavioral, or other mental health barriers to treatment.

Chapter Overview

- CARE Program
    Structure, Services, and Providers
    Client Description
- Mental Health Integration Model
    Program Process
    Care Management
    Interdisciplinary Team Collaboration
    Geropsychiatric Clinical, Consultative, and
        Educational Services
- Case Example
- Summary
- References

Especially among older adults, the line between physical and mental health is often inseparable, with one fundamentally affecting the outcome of the other (Cohen, 1996). Although the prevalence of most mental disorders in community-dwelling elderly people nearly parallels that in other age groups, it is also true that elders with medical illness and functional disabilities have higher rates (Blazer, 1990; Blazer et al., 1987; NIH Consensus Development Conference, 1996; Parmalee et al., 1989, 1991). The complex effects of specific mental disorders, particularly depression and depressive symptoms, on functional recovery following surgery or medical illness are increasingly well-documented (Harris et al., 1988; Kennedy et al., 1990; Mossey et al., 1990). Thus it is not surprising that in rehabilitation settings, where older adults with serious medical and functional disabilities are treated, attention to these interdependent relationships of emotional and physical well-being are of paramount importance if functional and quality-of-life outcomes are to be achieved (Kemp, 1986).

Unfortunately, in many ambulatory rehabilitation settings, the importance of the role of mental health in older adults is neither acknowledged nor addressed. When clients do not achieve treatment goals in a timely fashion, they are often labeled "unmotivated" and discharged as "treatment failures" (Kemp, 1986). Yet motivation in rehabilitation is increasingly understood to be related to such factors as sense of self-efficacy, relationship with therapist, and emotion (Resnick, 1996), all factors that are potentially subject to intervention.

It was, in part, to address this gap in care by providing a more holistic program of rehabilitation and health care services for the frail elderly that the Collaborative Assessment and Rehabilitation for Elders (CARE) Program was developed (Evans et al., 1995). Modeled after the British interdisciplinary day hospital, which provides intermittent comprehensive care to community-residing older adults, the CARE Program was envisioned as playing a key role in eliminating fragmented care for frail elders. An important signature of this care has been the integration of health, rehabilitative, and mental health services, uniquely using advanced practice nurses in a collaborative, interdisciplinary team approach. This chapter briefly describes the CARE Program and its model of service integration, and then illustrates the model with a case example.

CARE PROGRAM

STRUCTURE, SERVICES, AND PROVIDERS

The CARE Program is one component of the academic practice of the University of Pennsylvania School of Nursing, the Penn Nursing Network, and is operated in collaboration with the university's School of Medicine and Health System. As a nurse-managed academic practice, the executive director is a member of the School of Nursing standing faculty, and the director of clinical services is a master's-prepared gerontologic nurse practitioner (GNP). The advanced nursing practice team is completed by GNPs, who also serve as care managers, and a geropsychiatric clinical nurse specialist (GPCNS). All clinicians serve as preceptors for students from the nursing undergraduate and master's-level geropsychiatric nursing and geriatric nurse practitioner programs, as well as from a broad range of health care disciplines.

CARE Program personnel include the executive director, director of clinical services, gerontologic nurse practitioner/care manager, medical director (geriatrician), geropsychiatric clinical nurse specialist, physical therapist, physical therapy aide, occupational therapist, speech-language pathologist, social worker, consultant physiatrist, business manager, program assistant, and administrative support staff.

Clinical staff and faculty from the relevant rehabilitation departments in the health system, two departments in the school of medicine, and the school of nursing form an interdisciplinary team, directed by the GNP/care manager, that provides a broad range of services on a day-to-day basis.

Services provided in the CARE Program include nursing, care management, mental health and family therapy, physical therapy, occupational therapy, social work, speech-language pathology, medical consultation, nutritional counseling, blood and urine laboratory tests, physiatric consultation, orthotics/prosthetics, podiatry, and continence. Primary care and podiatry services are provided in the adjoining geriatric primary care clinic.

For each client, a GNP also serves as care manager, coordinating, monitoring, and providing care in close collaboration with team members as well as with the medical director and the client's own primary care provider. Certified under Medicare as a comprehensive outpatient rehabilitation facility (CORF), the CARE Program demonstrates the kind of self-supporting clinical service that a school of nursing can implement as part of its academic practice in collaboration with other components of a health system.

The Program is located near the campus in a renovated building that previously served as a residence for retired older women. The building also houses additional geriatric nursing, medi-

cine, and psychiatric services, fostering a unique opportunity for a level of multidisciplinary planning and coordination of services not often available in other settings. The physical space used by the Program also enhances close interdisciplinary team communication and planning. Once the dining room in a Victorian residence, the space is largely open, with partitioned areas available for physical examination and treatment, family meetings, and private interviews.

CLIENT DESCRIPTION

The average age of CARE Program clients is 78 years, with a range of 49 to 97. Most are women (74%), nonwhite (69%), and single (76%). Many (35%) live alone or with their adult children (33%). The average length of stay in the program is 7 weeks, with a range of 1 to 29 weeks. For most clients, referral is initiated by a physician (48%) and from an outpatient setting (66%). The majority of clients are referred from University of Pennsylvania providers of geriatric acute, outpatient, and home care services. The most common health problems of clients include degenerative joint disease, diabetes, stroke, and depression. Nearly all clients receive nursing and physical and occupational therapy services, and about 75 percent are also seen by the GPCNS.

MENTAL HEALTH INTEGRATION MODEL

PROGRAM PROCESS

The CARE program is designed for chronically ill older adults who live in the community and need more than simple outpatient rehabilitation services, yet are not appropriate candidates for inpatient rehabilitation (Evans et al., 1995). Clients who present a complicated picture of nursing, rehabilitative, medical, and psychosocial problems are best served by this Program. The client's illness and function are often found to be complicated by current or lifelong psychosocial factors, making assessment, intervention, and achievement of outcomes challenging. Clients who are newly bereaved and despondent are less likely to eat appropriately, move adequately, or take medication consistently, all affecting their ability to function in a manner that positively affects quality of life. Severe pain from degenerative joint disease and chronic shortness of breath from chronic obstructive pulmonary disease often leads to a life of social isolation, restricted activities, and depressive symptoms. In still other clients, lifelong mental health problems, such as incomplete grieving, recurrent depression, or bipolar disease, may impede successful rehabilitation. Psychosocial issues such as inadequate support, stressful family relationships, inconsistent nutritional supplies, or inadequate housing are problems that must also be addressed to allow the individual to function optimally.

In light of the interrelationship between mental and physical functioning, the highly refined skills of the interdisciplinary team are required to create a plan of treatment that best facilitates improvement. The CARE Program was designed to demonstrate best practices related to the integration of physical and mental health services for older adult clients, and to test the impact of the Program on overall improvement in function and well-being. This is accomplished through specialized roles and a system of staffing and communication that encourages formal as well as informal collaboration at all levels of client care. The components of the model have evolved to successfully integrate the provision of more holistic care to these clients through three interrelated components: the *care management role* of the GNP; the *collaborative practice role* of the interdisciplinary team; and the combined *clinical, consultation and educational roles* of the GPCNS. These will be described later in the chapter.

CARE MANAGEMENT

The Program is unique in its utilization of the master's-prepared GNP as a care manager, responsible for overall coordination and monitoring of client care. This ensures that assessments have been completed and referrals made in a timely and appropriate manner, that the team is communicating about and making appropriate adjustments in the plan of care, that the client receives services that are needed, and that the primary and specialist care providers are kept informed of the client's progress. On referral to the Program, the GNP/care manager assesses health state and social and relational functioning. This includes the client's perspective of personal problems, goals, and issues that may interfere with progress of rehabilitation. Assessments are completed for speech, hearing, language, nutrition, cognition, and mood by the GNP using standardized tools. These data are used to initiate appropriate referrals and are also available to team members as they make their initial assessments and develop the plan of care.

INTERDISCIPLINARY TEAM COLLABORATION

On the initial preadmission visit, the client is also seen by the physical and occupational therapists to determine level of dysfunction and attainable rehabilitation goals. The team then meets formally to discuss the client and develop the plan of care. Subsequent biweekly meetings afford the team an opportunity to revise the treatment plan and discuss discharge needs. The team meeting is facilitated by the GNP/care manager. Each clinician speaks to discipline-specific treatments and outcomes. For example, occupational therapy may focus on activities of daily living, such as dressing, toileting, and other aspects of self-care; physical therapy will speak to balance and ambulation ability; nursing may address continence, medication compliance, and individualized education needs. Also addressed at the meeting are interdisciplinary problems, including pain management, program compliance, and hygiene, as well as psychosocial issues that may surface during treatment sessions or interviews. Such issues may concern home environment, relationships, services, or elder mistreatment. The

Omaha Classification System of client problems (Martin and Scheet, 1992) is used to facilitate interdisciplinary aspects of care. This system encourages development and implementation of interdisciplinary interventions whereby all clinicians address the same problem; it also eliminates the fragmentation typically found in multidisciplinary records.

Informally, during therapy sessions with individual clients, team members have immediate access to one another for collaboration. At times, more than one clinician may evaluate a client simultaneously. For example, an individual experiencing chest pain during timed ambulation exercises may be assessed by both the physical therapist and the GNP. This allows immediate consultation without delay in treatment, ultimately providing the client with a seamless program of services.

GEROPSYCHIATRIC CLINICAL, CONSULTATIVE, AND EDUCATIONAL SERVICES

Mental health services in the Program are provided by a geropsychiatric clinical nurse specialist (GPCNS). Thus, all clients have access to mental health services as needed. A client may be referred directly to the GPCNS at the time of admission by the referring provider based on the individual's history or a recently identified mental health need. Otherwise, any client may be referred for mental health services by the medical director or GNP/care manager when indicated by formalized screening results or treatment team observations. Any team member has the option of recommending mental health services for a client based on issues related to psychosocial need, program compliance, barriers to treatment related to cognition and mood, or problems related to other behaviors. Clients are automatically referred for mental health screening if they present with a score of less than 24 on the Folstein Mini-Mental State Exam (Folstein et al., 1975) or 11 or above on the Geriatric Depression Scale (Yesavage et al., 1983). These scores fall within the abnormal range (for cognitive function and depression, respectively) and represent a potential for interference with the program of rehabilitation. Addressing these issues early in the Program lessens client and provider frustration, improves client compliance, assures that needed services are provided, and shortens the overall length of stay.

The GPCNS has a multidimensional role in the Program that facilitates successful, holistic rehabilitation by identifying and addressing relational, behavioral, or other mental health barriers to treatment. Three of those role components are especially relevant here:

- *Clinical role.* Evaluating clients for mental health issues; referring clients and serving as liaison to appropriate psychiatric services; providing brief individual, couples, or family therapy when indicated; co-facilitating treatment and support groups.
- *Consultation-liaison role.* Acting as a consultant to staff members regarding family and organizational systems issues and problematic client behaviors.
- *Staff education role.* Educating about psychiatric disorders and family therapy.

These roles are well within the scope of practice for the advanced practice psychiatric nurse (ANA, 1994), but have seldom been discussed in relation to this client population.

Evaluation of client outcomes as they are influenced by advanced practice nursing interventions is extremely important for advancing the science of nursing as well as for public policy initiatives (Brooten and Naylor, 1995; Burns et al., 1996). As part of its continuous quality improvement activities, the CARE Program measures improvement in individual client outcomes at time of discharge using valid and reliable clinical indicators (such as the Geriatric Depression Scale). In addition, client status is evaluated at 1 and 3 months postdischarge, using a telephone follow-up format. A formal program evaluation is under way, with funding from the National Institute for Nursing Research, which is expected to have implications for public policy (Sochalski, 1996).

▶ CASE EXAMPLE

JR is an 81-year-old man who was referred to the CARE Program by a home health agency for functional problems related to degenerative joint disease of the lumbar spine and postherpetic neuralgia of the upper extremities. Additional medical diagnoses included hypertension, diabetes mellitus, congestive heart failure, and chronic obstructive pulmonary disease. He presented with complaints of back pain over the past 5 years accompanied by progressively difficult ambulation. He had begun to use a walker some 3 months before on discharge from the hospital where he had undergone treatment for "shingles." He reported that walking was further limited by bilateral knee pain (left > right) and chronic shortness of breath. He demonstrated an ambulation distance of only 25 feet before onset of extreme fatigue, pain, and shortness of breath. The referring provider did not order mental health services, and neither did JR report concerns in this area. In fact, JR denied any history of depression, previous counseling, or hospitalization for mental health needs.

The eldest in a large family, JR was born and raised in a large urban area, and had an eighth-grade education. As an adult, he had worked at various factory jobs. Although he had enjoyed singing in the church choir, woodworking, and small appliance repair nearly all his life, he now reported no leisure-time activities. Widowed for 15 years, JR had one daughter who lived nearby. He was living alone in a two story home with the downstairs arranged to accommodate a hospital bed and commode. He was receiving home health aide services for 2 hours on four days a week, with his daughter providing assistance the remainder of the week. He was also receiving home-delivered meals 7 days a week. He reported that his referral to the CARE Program was related to back pain and based on his need for therapy to improve ambulation and, ultimately, the ability to care for himself.

Mental status testing on admission using the Mini-Mental State Exam revealed a score of 29/30 with a deficit in recall after 3 minutes. His Geriatric Depression Scale score was 11/30 indicating mild depression. JR reported life dissatisfaction, restricted interests, and emptiness along with feeling helpless, worthless, and hopeless; he also had difficulty in self-motivation and decision-making. JR was referred to the GPCNS for mental status evaluation because of the Geriatric Depression Scale score. Just prior to evaluation by the GPCNS, the occupational therapist reported during a team meeting that JR was reluctant to fully participate in therapy and at times appeared unmotivated, although he was thought to have significant potential for improvement. This observation was confirmed by the physical therapist as well, and thought to be a potential source of frustration for client and clinicians alike. This was identified as an aspect of JR's behavior that would potentially interfere with achieving his rehabilitation goals.

JR was evaluated by the GPCNS and was found to have no cognitive impairment on interview. He denied feeling depressed, but reported feeling hopeless concerning his deteriorating physical functioning. He reported nighttime awakening for urination with easy return to sleep. He denied suicidal/homicidal ideations, anhedonia, poor appetite, or fatigue. He was diagnosed with an adjustment disorder with depressed mood and prescribed weekly psychotherapy by the GPCNS.

JR was seen weekly throughout the 8 week program of treatment. On subsequent visits with the GPCNS, JR revealed feelings of sadness related to increased disability and resultant restricted lifestyle. It was also identified that he perceived his relationship with his daughter to be tied to his need for care: He saw potential improvements in function as likely to decrease the number of visits by the daughter. With help, he was able to identify how this negative thinking would impede progress in the treatment program. Family-of-origin issues related to unrealistic expectations also surfaced as contributing to stalls in rehabilitation. He was able to identify himself as a perfectionist based on his relationship with his own father; throughout his life he had learned to hold himself to these same high expectations. As a result, he was less than enthusiastic about any improvement short of a full functional recovery. He was eventually able to see how this "all or nothing" attitude would negatively affect his success in rehabilitation.

Family counseling was also provided for JR and his daughter. The daughter was able to identify her own anger at her father for not working to his potential. JR's high expectations of his daughter were discussed in the context of his desire for an immediate and unconditional response to his needs. JR's daughter, who also cares for her own grandchildren, reported feeling "trapped" and, as she watched her father deteriorate, concerned about who would be there to provide care for her as she herself aged. Beginning work on the multigenerational transmission process was initiated by examining family myths. The GPCNS assisted the team both formally in plan of care conferences and through informal dialogue to understand the issues underlying JR's behavior and to respond effectively. At a later time, concepts related to family-of-origin issues and multigenerational transmission process (Bowen, 1985) were elaborated in a more general inservice program.

JR was able to progress well while in the program, aided by his work with the GPCNS. Physically, he made significant gains. At discharge he was preparing his own meals and incorporating new knowledge about his diet provided by the GNP/care manager. Exertional shortness of breath decreased through improved endurance and the use of a rolling walker. He demonstrated an improved technique in the use of his inhaler, which had a significant impact on his ability to ambulate unencumbered. Urinary incontinence, which had a large functional component, improved with better physical function. An interdisciplinary approach to pain management—physiatric consultation, physical therapy exercises, occupational therapy energy conservation and joint protection training, and nurse-initiated medication management—facilitated a significant reduction in back and knee pain that had previously impeded JR's mobility. He was now independent in all aspects of personal care and was able to ambulate 250 feet safely and independently. On discharge, his Geriatric Depression Scale score had improved to 4/30. He no longer complained of life dissatisfaction or emptiness. He denied feeling helpless or worthless, and described a renewed motivation related to his function and life in general. JR reported that a helpful psychotherapeutic experience had empowered him to integrate a new ability to formulate reasonable expectations for both himself and his daughter. These gains had been maintained at least 3 months after discharge when the follow-up interview was conducted. He had begun to attend a senior center shortly after discharge. Finally able to provide care for himself in a more independent manner, JR has begun to develop a relationship with his daughter based on issues other than personal care tasks.

SUMMARY

The interplay between physical and mental health and illness in the elderly is especially apparent in a rehabilitation setting where improvement in functional independence and quality of life are programmatic goals. Mental health dysfunction can contribute to excess disability in the medically ill elderly; functional disabilities can also contribute to worsened emotional function, particularly depression. To make a positive impact in one aspect of an individual's health, other areas of dysfunction that may impede overall improvement must first be identified. Significant and life-sustaining change in self-care and lifestyle requires that all aspects of the client's well-being be evaluated and addressed in conjunction with each other. Integrating and offering mental health services to older adults within an overall comprehensive treatment program makes the services more accessible and acceptable to the client. The continuing refinement of the advanced practice nursing role, particularly the nurse-to-nurse collaborative process, will be important in the future provision of high-quality care to frail older adults. The outcomes achieved with clients in the CARE Program confirms that, when given an opportunity, age is not a deterrent to an individual's ability to change and grow.

REFERENCES

American Nurses Association. *Statement on Psychiatric Mental Health Clinical Nursing Practice and Standards of Psychiatric Mental Health Clinical Nursing Practice.* Washington, DC: American Nurses Publishing; 1994.

Blazer D. *Emotional Problems in Later Life.* New York: Springer; 1990.

Blazer D, Hughes DC, George LK. The epidemiology of depression in an elderly community population. *Gerontologist.* 1987;27:281–287.

Bowen M. *Family Therapy in Clinical Practice.* New York: Jason Aronson; 1985.

Brooten D, Naylor MD. Nurses effect on changing patient outcomes. *Image: Int. J Nurs Sch.* 1995;27:95–99.

Burns M, Moores P, Breslin E. Outcomes research: Contemporary issues and historical significance for nurse practitioners. *J Am Acad Nurs Pract.* 1996;8:107–112.

Evans LK, Yurkow J, Siegler EL. The CARE Program: A nurse-managed collaborative outpatient program to improve function of frail older people. *J Am Geriatr Soc.* 1995;43:1155–1160.

Folstein MF, Folstein SE, McHugh PR. Mini-mental state: A practical guide for grading the cognitive state of patients for the clinician. *J Psychiatr Res.* 1975;12:189–198.

Harris RE, Mion LC, Patterson MB, Frengley JD. Severe illness in older patients: The association between depressive disorders and functional dependency during the recovery phase. *J Am Geriatr Soc.* 1988;36:890–896.

Kemp B. Psychosocial and mental health issues in rehabilitation of older persons. In: Brody SS, Ruff GE, eds. *Aging and Rehabilitation.* New York: Springer; 1986.

Kennedy GJ, Kelman HR, Thomas C. The emergence of depressive symptoms in late life: The importance of declining health and increasing disability. *J Comm Health.* 1990;15:93–104.

Martin KF, Scheet NJ. *Omaha System.* Philadelphia: Saunders; 1992.

Mossey JM, Knott K, Craik R. The effects of persistent depressive symptoms on hip fracture recovery. *J Gerontol.* 1990;4:M163–M168.

NIH Consensus Development Conference. *Depression in Late Life: Diagnosis and Treatment.* Bethesda, MD: DHHS; 1991.

Parmalee PA, Katz IR, Lawton MP. Relation of pain to depression among institutionalized aged. *J Gerontol.* 1991;46:P15–P21.

Parmalee PA, Katz IR, Lawton MP. Depression among institutionalized aged: Assessment and prevalence estimates. *J Gerontol.* 1989;44:M22–M29.

Resnick B. Motivation in geriatric rehabilitation. *Image: Int J Nurs Sch.* 1996;28:41–45.

Sochalski, J. Outcomes of a nurse-managed geriatric day hospital. NIH NINR grant no. R07 NR 00090-01. 1996.

Yesavage JA, Brink TL, Rose TL, eds. Development and validation of a geriatric depression screening scale: A preliminary report. *J Psychiatr Res.* 1983; 17:37–49.

CHAPTER 5

A COLLABORATIVE MODEL OF ADVANCED NURSING PRACTICE

Beth Vaughan-Cole • Marcia Scoville • Linda Flynn

*A*fter the nurse-midwife or nurse practitioner assesses a woman for abuse and the woman states that she has been or is currently being abused, the provider asks for additional information to clarify if the client is in immediate danger. The client is asked whether she would like to be referred to a psychiatric nurse. She is given a brief explanation of the services of an advanced practice psychiatric nurse, and a referral form is completed.

Chapter Overview

- The Nursing Clinic in Context
- Collaborative Practice Identifying Mental Health Problems
- Collaborative Practice With Women With a History of Sexual Abuse
- References

► INTRODUCTION

A model of collaborative practice among certified nurse-midwives, nurse practitioners, and advanced practice psychiatric nurses is sponsored by the University of Utah College of Nursing. Within the model a plan has been developed for working with women who have been sexually abused.

The focus of the collaboration has been through a faculty practice. Many nursing faculty are interested in continuing their clinical practice. They value the skills and intellectual knowledge that they have developed in their careers, and their commitment to their profession encompasses teaching as well as practice and research. Within the many gyrations and explorations of health care reform, nursing colleges have ventured into the realm of health care delivery services.

THE NURSING CLINIC IN CONTEXT

There are four reasons that this faculty practice has been sponsored by the University College of Nursing. One reason is to enhance the teaching mission by providing learning environments where students can observe nurses practicing as faculty would like them to learn to practice. Often the learning environments for students are less than ideal, and faculty members feel frustrated in teaching cutting-edge nursing practice in a setting where the nursing care does not demonstrate the best of nursing practice.

A second reason for colleges of nursing to develop a health care delivery service is to research, study, and write about cutting-edge nursing practice. Not all nursing practice settings have been supportive of nursing studies. Some institutions offering nursing services have been unable to foster and support nursing's professional agenda. Nursing employment has been under the control and restrictions of non-nursing personnel. Some practice environments have blocked or limited nursing's access to populations of patients, interfered with legitimate scholarly inquiry, and actively discouraged research efforts. Therefore, to enhance student learning with clinical practice, nursing colleges have developed their own teaching sites with faculty practice clinics and services.

A third reason that colleges of nursing have supported health care delivery services is to generate income. Some colleges have been able to generate significant income activities. As funding for higher education has either peaked or has reached the limits of many legislatures to respond, colleges are having to seek additional avenues to increase their financial resources.

The fourth reason for colleges to sponsor nursing services is to demonstrate nursing's efficacy. In this era of health care reform, nursing care is often seen as a service embedded in other services. Unable to articulate the unique contributions of nursing to service delivery, colleges of nursing are carving out limited services in order to articulate and demonstrate specific aspects of nursing practice. Such aspects as cost-effective practice, improved client outcomes, and alternative practice methods are possible reasons for establishing a service run by nurses.

For these reasons and additional philosophical commitments, the University of Utah College of Nursing has supported the faculty practice called Birth Care Health Care throughout its 18-year development. The practice environment has evolved from a small certified nurse-midwifery (CNM) faculty practice. The CNM faculty was successful in providing clients with the option of an out-of-hospital birth experience for most of those years, by contracting for privileges at a series of free-standing birth centers, as well as in hospitals. As their practice grew, the need for a pediatric care provider afforded an opportunity for a pediatric nurse practitioner on faculty to join the practice. A critical decision to address the frequent problems women were having with diagnosis and treatment of depression, anxiety, and mood disorders led to the inclusion of psychiatric and mental health advanced practice faculty joining the practice. The inclusion of a family nurse practitioner created a primary care nurse-managed center.

This unique collaborative nursing practice model has proven to be a watershed of clinical practice and research opportunities. Early in the CNM experience, there was thought to be an increased incidence of women with a history of childhood sexual abuse seeking the practice for reproductive health care. This population has been demonstrated to have a number of needs frequently unmet in traditional medical women's health care environments. The CNMs provide care within the framework of philosophical commitment to women's choice, client education, informed consent, nonintervention, culturally and individually sensitive flexible care, and feminist empowerment models of care. They usually are female providers. This environment is attractive to women with a history of childhood sexual abuse, whether recognized and treated or undiagnosed and sometimes unconscious.

The Birth Care Health Care nurse providers were in a unique position to enjoy that coalescing of curiosity and experience that can lead to research questions, where research and practice can work together. The practitioner-researchers are studying the effects of a history of sexual abuse on the health of women and their families. The immediate need to identify symptoms, risks, and therapeutic provider interactions with these women has supplied a focus for collaborative practice and cooperative research.

Reimbursement mechanisms are self-pay, through insurance, and as is the case in many regions, through contracts with managed care companies. The management office is proactive in joining the lists of providers, where available. Birth Care Health Care, Inc., is part of the University of Utah Hospital clinics and network of services. Faculty from the University of Utah College of Nursing are part of the college's faculty practice organization. In addition, nurse faculty with advanced practice licenses can be part of the Health Sciences Center Faculty Practice Organization (FPO). This FPO seeks out and negotiates contracts for health care services. Birth Care Health Care is a recognized service within these contracts.

COLLABORATIVE PRACTICE IDENTIFYING MENTAL HEALTH PROBLEMS

A concerted effort has been made in the past two decades to study and present the prevalence of mental health problems, and their incidence, diagnosis, and treatment in primary care settings. A large multisite Epidemiologic Catchment Area (ECA) study (Robins et al., 1984) reports a point prevalence in western industrialized nations of major depressive disorders as 2.3 to 3.2 percent for men and 4.5 to 9.3 percent in women. Major depressive disorders represent a lifetime risk for men of 7 to 12 percent and for women of 20 to 25 percent. For dysthymic disorders there is a lifetime risk of 4.1 percent for women and 2.2 percent for men. Panic disorders are estimated to occur in 1.6 to 2.9 percent of women and in 0.4 to 1.7 percent of men (Katon, 1993). Although these prevalence statistics touch on only a few of the mental health problems, they do not identify the incidence of dual diagnoses or multiple diagnoses.

In one study (Rowe et al., 1995), researchers gave a self-administered health-habits questionnaire to 1898 patients at 88 sites. They reported a total of 21.7 percent of women and

12.7 percent of men met the DSM-III-R criteria for depression in the month prior to completing the survey. Their lifetime rates for depression were 36.1 percent for women and 23.3 percent for men. And their conclusion, stated powerfully, was that one in 5 women and one in 10 men who see their primary care physicians have recently been depressed. In a study by Fifer and associates (1994) it was reported that 10 percent of eligible patients screened in clinic waiting rooms had unrecognized and untreated anxiety disorders. The dramatic statistics of Rowe and coworkers (1995) confirmed previous studies. The prevalence of depression among patients in primary care settings is nearly twice that among the general population. Two recent articles in medical journals outline identification and management strategies for primary care intervention in mental health problems (Olfson et al., 1995).

In an attempt to develop a model of health care that offers both physical and mental health care, the providers at Birth Care Health Care developed a strategy for identification, referral, and treatment. The PRIME-MD: Primary Care Evaluation of Mental Disorders tool was developed by Robert L. Spitzer and Janet B. W. William of the Biometrics Research Department, New York State Psychiatric Institute, working with an executive committee of primary care physicians, including Mark Linzer, who developed a self-learning program that can be purchased. This tool was reported in the December 14, 1994, issue of *Journal of the American Medical Association.*

PRIME-MD was chosen for its ease in administration and its discrimination of five common mental health problems (mood, anxiety, alcohol, eating, and somatoform disorders). New clients are screened for mental health problems by asking them 25 questions. These questions are currently being asked by the CNMs and family nurse practitioner of all adult clients. Depending on the answers to these first 25 questions, the provider may ask additional questions from the eating, mood, somatoform, anxiety, or alcohol modules. If the equipment were available, the patient questionnaire could be put on a computer and programmed to follow up with the next line of questioning. At this time, when the provider detects a mental disorder from PRIME-MD or through interview, the client is referred to the psychiatric nurses. Although not all clients referred accept an appointment with the psychiatric advanced practice nurse, they are given the opportunity. About 70 percent of those referred attend one or more counseling sessions.

COLLABORATIVE PRACTICE WITH WOMEN WITH A HISTORY OF SEXUAL ABUSE

The incidence of women who have been sexually abused is generally reported as 27 percent or about one in four women (Finkelhor et al., 1990). Wescott (1991) states that 74 to 96 percent of female survivors of sexual abuse are left with physical and/or emotional sequelae. Some of the long-term effects of sexual abuse include sexual and relationship problems, depression, low self-esteem, communication difficulties, a sense of vulnerability and isolation, feelings of shame or guilt and anger or hostility, dissociation, promiscuity, dependency, somatization, chronic pelvic pain, and preterm labor (Bachmann et al., 1988; Edwards and Donaldson, 1989; Kitzinger, 1992; Lowery, 1987; Reiter et al., 1991). The physical and psychological impact of a history of abuse on the lives of many women can first become apparent and create problems during the childbearing years.

Because of the sexual context of pregnancy, childbirth, and breastfeeding, and because of the location and musculature involved in the birthing process, words, actions, or situations may unexpectedly trigger memories and experiences of childhood or previous sexual abuse and unleash a flood of suppressed feelings. Such psychological triggering may precipitate problem behaviors that interfere with adaptation to pregnancy, childbirth, and postpartum adjustment (Courtois and Riley, 1992; Rose, 1992; Satin et al., 1992).

Holz (1994) stated that early identification of sexual abuse affords the health care provider and the client an opportunity to incorporate strategies in the treatment plan that build trust, use mental health resources, decrease trauma during physical exams and interventions, and provide educational instruction to meet associated needs relative to abuse.

Toomey and associates (1993) studied the relationship of sexual and physical abuse to pain and psychological assessment variables in chronic pelvic pain clients. They found that their study correlated with other studies in finding that childhood abuse, especially when it involved pelvic or abdominal abuse, was represented in clients with chronic pain syndromes. In a study of chronic pelvic pain, Peters and co-workers (1991) found that 20 percent of the clients had a history of childhood sexual abuse or rape.

Stevens-Simon and associates (1993) identified a history of past physical or sexual abuse as one of the five contributing characteristics to preterm labor among pregnant adolescents. Their study reinforced the idea that the unresolved psychosocial stress associated with abuse could adversely affect women during pregnancy, childbirth, and the postpartum period.

Van der Leden and Raskin (1993) found that psychological symptoms associated with traumatic events hinder optimal health participation and practices. Assessing for sexual abuse as part of standard health care practice, and addressing the physical and psychological issues of sexual abuse, is a vital factor in promoting healing and proving health care to adult survivors.

Nurse authors (Cole et al, 1996; Limandri and Tilden, 1996; McFarlane et al., 1992) as well as physician authors (Gremillion and Kanof, 1996); strongly support assessment for a history of abuse before a clinical examination. Often women have never been asked about abuse, and many women do not openly state that they have been victims of sexual abuse unless asked (Finkelhor et al., 1990; Furniss, 1993). Some women have vivid memories but do not disclose the information because they are frightened, ashamed, or depressed. Others deny the negative connotations of the abuse to protect their perceived and actual relationships. For many, the repressed memories of abuse remain hidden until they are stimulated by changes in sexual intimacy or during pregnancy and childbirth (Bachmann et al., 1988; Courtois and Riley, 1992; Lowery, 1987; Rose, 1992).

Primary care providers at Birth Care Health Care screen all women for current and past emotional, physical, and sexual abuse. A research study was undertaken to develop a usable and effective tool for assessing abuse. The authors of this chapter modified the Abuse Assessment Screening tool developed by McFarlane and associates (1992) to include a question about childhood sexual abuse and whether the client would like to be referred for counseling if there is a current or past history of abuse. This tool became the Modified Abuse Assessment Screen (Fig. 5–1).

After the nurse-midwife or nurse practitioner assesses a woman for abuse and the woman states that she has been or is currently being abused, the provider asks for additional information to clarify whether the client is in immediate danger. The client is asked if she would like to be referred to a psychiatric nurse. She is given a brief explanation of the services of an advanced practice psychiatric nurse, and a referral form is completed. If the client does not want to be referred at that time, the provider can supply a list of emergency services or other community services, should the client be interested.

If the advanced practice psychiatric nurse is available on site, the nurse provider can check and see if the psychiatric nurse is available for an introduction. This often facilitates the first appointment with the psychiatric nurse. Otherwise the referral form is placed in a box for the psychiatric nurse to follow up with a phone call and the setting of an appointment. In a review of records for one year, the incidence of a previous history of sexual abuse noted in the client record was 33 percent. Not all of the clients who reported abuse asked for mental health counseling.

Provider introduction to client: This issue of domestic violence and childhood sexual abuse are of increasing concern to health care providers as they seek to serve their clients. I am going to ask you questions about this area.

(Please circle YES or NO for each question, as appropriate.)

1. Have you ever been emotionally, physically, or sexually abused?   **YES   NO**

2. When you were a child (under the age of 18), can you remember having any experience you would now consider sexual abuse—
   a. like someone trying or succeeding in having any kind of sexual intercourse with you or anything like that?   **YES   NO**
   b. involving someone touching or grabbing, or kissing, or rubbing or anything like that?   **YES   NO**
   c. involving someone taking nude pictures of you, or someone performing some sex act in your presence or anything like that?   **YES   NO**
   d. involving oral sex or sodomy or anything like that?   **YES   NO**

3. **WITHIN THE LAST YEAR,** has anyone forced you to have sexual activities?   **YES   NO**
   3a. If yes, who (Circle all that apply)
   Husband   Ex-husband
   Boyfriend   Ex-boyfriend
   Parent   Step-parent
   Sibling   Other relative
   Stranger   Mutiple (Group/Gang/Cult)
   Other (specify)

4. **WITHIN THE LAST YEAR,** have you been hit, slapped, kicked, or otherwise physically hurt by someone?   **YES   NO**
   4a. If yes, who (Circle all that apply)
   Husband   Ex-husband
   Boyfriend   Ex-boyfriend
   Parent   Step-parent
   Sibling   Other relative
   Stranger   Mutiple (Group/Gang/Cult)
   Other (specify)

If no to all of the previous questions, then this is the end of the questions. Thank you.

If yes to any of the questions please continue with questions 5 to 7

5. **Please circle all forms of abuse that have occurred in the past year.**
   a. None
   b. Threats of abuse including use of a weapon
   c. Slapping, pushing; no injuries and/or lasting pain
   d. Punching, kicking, bruises, cuts and/or continuing pain
   e. Beating up, severe contusions, burns, broken bones
   f. Head injury, internal injury, permanent injury
   g. Use of weapon; wound from weapon

6. Have you received counseling for the abuse?   **YES   NO**

7. Would you like to be referred for counseling services?   **YES   NO**

Thank you

The MAAS is an expansion of the Abuse Assessment Screen (AAS) developed by the Nursing Research Consortium on Violence and Abuse.

Modified by Beth Vaughan-Cole, PhD, APRN; Marcia Scoville, CNM, APRN; and Linda T. Flynn, MS, RN
University of Utah College of Nursing   12/95

Figure 5–1. Modified Abuse Assessment Screen.

In a review of a majority of the referrals that included an element of sexual abuse, four treatment issues predominated: depression, dissociation, sexual adjustment in couples, and maternal/infant adjustment. The literature supports these categories as significant areas of concern for adult women who have been sexually abused as children.

Lowery (1987) indicated that psychological symptoms such as depression and personality disorders may be external symptoms of untreated sexual abuse. According to a study by Hall and colleagues (1993), women who have experienced severe physical or sexual abuse are four and a half times more likely to have severe depression. In their study of 206 women, 51 percent indicated severe depressive disorders and 70 percent of those women indicated some form of physical or sexual abuse as children. Managing depression during and after pregnancy is a serious issue for women who were sexually abused as children.

Women who were frequently and violently abused may develop dissociation as a way of coping with the abuse. Assessment for dissociation is critical. Some women are very clear that they dissociate and others are not. Just inquiring about the phenomenon allows some women the opportunity to acknowledge this experience and prepare for their delivery. Pregnant women who dissociate may have difficulty participating in the delivery process and with the postpartum adjustment. Courtois and Riley (1992) noted that abuse survivors often need more extensive education and training in dealing with the physical aspects of pregnancy and childbirth. The labor and birthing processes may prompt flashbacks from the original abuse that may lead the woman to use familiar defenses, such as dissociation, in order to cope with the physical and psychological pain. Use of positive affirmations and relaxation techniques may help women remain in touch with their bodies and cope with the pain, thus permitting their active participation in the process of childbirth.

Wood and associates (1990) found that female adult survivors of childhood sexual abuse had more indications of sexual dysfunction and difficulties forming close relationships. They were generally more dissatisfied with their roles as wives and mothers. Developing safety and trust around sexual expression was not an easy process for these women because their own personal histories interfered with the logical progression of developing close personal relationships. Abused women feared intimate relationships and associated sexual activity with pain and lack of control (Bachmann et al., 1988).

The fourth area of assessment and intervention is related to maternal/infant attachment. In an article by Rose (1992) and in an unpublished article by Boullie (1993), women who had been sexually abused reported having difficulty in attachment and adjustment with their newborns. Prior to delivery an infant is often cherished in the minds of abused women, but after the infant is born, its many demands heighten the inadequate parenting experiences of their own childhood. Breast feeding is difficult and may not be successful. Responsiveness to the infant's needs and demands may be not met. Preparation of high-risk mothers for postpartum adjustment is a serious and important task of psychotherapy during the prenatal stage. Cole and Woolger (1989) found that most of the survivors of incest expressed frequent concerns about parenting and feared that they would be bad parents. Without positive models for loving and providing parental control, these women may lack strategies for being responsive to their children's dependency on them and may experience anxiety and anger in certain child-rearing situations. Some women report resentment and hostility toward the demands their children make on them, and were unaware that they reflected their own disappointment in their lost childhoods.

Advanced practice psychiatric nurses and other mental health providers need to assess and address these mental health issues in pregnant women who have been sexually abused during childhood. Preventive education and treatment interventions are important in preventing severe postpartum depression, encouraging mental integration, and improving marital functioning and maternal/infant attachment and adjustment. Obviously, the goals of treatment would be individualized to meet the needs of each client.

During the first client interview with the psychiatric advanced practice nurse, the client is asked for permission to share information between the therapist and the nurse-midwife or nurse practitioner. A consent form is signed by the client. The exchange between the nurse providers allows for coordinated services and a concerted effort to prepare the client for her delivery and postpartum adjustment.

The cooperative exchange and referral services within the collaborative practices of nurse-midwives and advanced practice psychiatric nurses provide the needed physical and mental health services for assessing and caring for survivors of sexual abuse, especially during the childbearing years.

REFERENCES

Bachmann G, Moeller T, Benett J. Review: Childhood sexual abuse and the consequences in adult women. *Obstet Gynecol.* 1988;71:631–641.

Boullie P. *The nurse-midwifery care of women molested as children.* Unpublished master's project, University of Utah, Salt Lake City, 1993.

Cole BV, Scoville M, Flynn LT. Psychiatric advance practice nurses collaborate with certified midwives in providing health care for pregnant women with histories of abuse. *Archives of Psychiatric Nursing.* 1996;10:229–34.

Cole P, Woolger C. Incest survivors: The relation of their perceptions of their parents and their own parenting attitudes. *Child Abuse Negl.* 1989;13:409–416.

Courtois C, Riley C. Pregnancy and childbirth as triggers for abuse memories: Implications for care. *Birth.* 1992;19:222–223.

Edwards P, Donaldson M. Assessment of symptoms in adult survivors of incest: A factor analytic study of the responses to childhood incest questionnaire. *Child Abuse Negl.* 1989;13:101–110.

Fifer SK, Mathias SD, Patrick DL, et al. Untreated anxiety among adult primary care patients in a health maintenance organization. *Arch Gen Psychiatry.* 1994;51:740–750.

Finkelhor D, Hotaling G, Lewis I, Smith C. Sexual abuse in a national survey of adult men and women: Prevalence, characteristics, and risk factors. *Child Abuse Negl.* 1990;14:19–28.

Furniss K. Screening for abuse in the clinical setting. *AWHONN's Clin Issues.* 1993;4:402–406.

Gremillion DH, Kanof EP. Overcoming barriers to physician involvement in identifying and referring victims of domestic violence. *Ann. Emerg. Med.* 1996;27:769–73.

Hall L, Sachs B, Rayens M, Lutenbacher M. Childhood physical and sexual abuse: Their relationship with depressive symptoms in adulthood. *Image Nurs Sch.* 1993;25:317–323.

Holz K. A practical approach to clients who are survivors of childhood sexual abuse. *J Nurse Midwifery.* 1994;39:13–18.

Katon W. *Panic Disorder in the Medical Setting.* Rockville, MD: U. S. Department of Health and Human Services, Public Health Services, National Institutes of Health, National Institute of Mental Health; 1993.

Kitzinger J. Counteracting, not reenacting, the violation of women's bodies: The challenge for perinatal care givers. *Birth.* 1992;19:219–220.

Limandri BJ, Tilden VP. Nurses' reasoning in the assessment of family violence. *Image J Nurs Sch.* 1996;28:247–252.

Lowery M. Adult survivors of childhood incest. *J Psychosoc Nurs* 1987;25:27–31.

McFarlane J, Parker B, Soeken K, Bullock L. Assessing for abuse during pregnancy: Severity and frequency of injuries and associated entry into prenatal care. *JAMA* 1992;267:3178–8.

Olfson M, Weissman MM, Leon AC, et al. Psychological management by family physicians. *J Fam Pract.* 1995;41:543–550.

Peters A, van-Dorst E, Jellis B, et al. A randomized clinical trial to compare two different approaches in women with chronic pelvic pain. *Obstet Gynecol.* 1991;77:740–744.

Reiter R, Shakerin L, Gambone J, Milburn A. Correlation between sexual abuse and somatization in women with somatic and nonsomatic chronic pelvic pain. *Am J Obstet Gynecol.* 1991;164:104–109.

Robins LN, Helzer JE, Weissman MM, et al. Lifetime prevalence of specific psychiatric disorders in three sites. *Arch Gen Psychiatry.* 1984;41:949–958.

Rose A. Effects of childhood sexual abuse on childbirth: One woman's story. *Birth.* 1992;19:214–218.

Rowe MG, Fleming MF, Barry KL, et al. Correlates of depression in primary care. *J Fam Pract.* 1995; 41:551–558.

Satin A, Ramin S, Paicurich J, et al. The prevalence of sexual assault: A survey of 2404 puerperal women. *Am J Obstet Gynecol.* 1992;167:973–975.

Spitzer RL, Williams JBW, Kroenke K, et al. *PRIME-MD: Primary Care Evaluation of Mental Disorders.* Pfizer, Inc; 1995.

Spitzer RL, Williams JBW, Kroenke K, et al. Utility of a new procedure for diagnosing mental disorders in primary care. *JAMA.* 1994;272: 1749–1756.

Stevens-Simon C, Kaplan D, McAnarney E. Factors associated with preterm delivery among pregnant adolescents. *J Adolesc Health.* 1993;14: 340–342.

Toomey T, Hernandez J, Gittelman D, Hulka J. Relationship of sexual and physical abuse to pain and psychological assessment variables in chronic pelvic pain patients. *Pain.* 1993;53:105–109.

Van Der Leden M, Raskin V. Psychological sequelae of childhood sexual abuse: Relevant in subsequent pregnancy. *Am J Obstet Gynecol.* 1993;168: 1336–1337.

Wescott C. Sexual abuse and childbirth education. *Int J Childbirth Ed.* 1991;6:32–33.

Wood D, Wiesner M, Reiter R. Psychogenic chronic pelvic pain: Diagnosis and management. *Clin Obstet Gynecol.* 1990;33:179–195.

CHAPTER 6

CASE MANAGEMENT FOR ADVANCED PRACTICE PSYCHIATRIC NURSING

Kathleen M. Andolina

*C*linical case management refers to a system-based program that is outcomes oriented, provider driven, and patient centered. Advanced practice nurses functioning in these models for case management occupy a variety of roles in organizations of all sizes.

Chapter Overview

► INTRODUCTION

As multiskilled professional service providers, advanced practice nurses who are often clinical specialists in psychiatric nursing are educated in advanced clinical concepts, research, organizational management, and consultation skills. Advanced practice nurses (APNs) are not to be overlooked as candidates for high-level operational executive positions, including those positions developing case management services.

Case management, at the turn of the century, referred to activities performed by local police to secure food and fuel for indigent people. Today, trends in economic and health care systems have changed the context but not necessarily the coordinating activities that form the basis of case management. Case management is concerned with securing access, continuity, and high-quality health care for all people with complex health care needs. Psychiatric clients are often the most challenging populations, as patients often present with multiple needs. The requirement to manage chronic, serious mental illness, along with uneven individual and community resources, provide the context for psychiatric case management today.

As 50 years of explosive growth in health care slows down, complex care populations will require all the finesse of expert providers and resource managers to achieve health care goals. As payers pressure hospital systems to improve quality and lower costs, hospital systems will pressure providers to do the same. A resurgence of interest in case management services has resulted. Today's best systems and providers understand that to maintain effective and efficient health care outcomes for the most costly and challenging populations, they must have coordinating authority to design care before, during, and beyond the discrete episode of care. Although case management is a strategy used to guarantee cost and quality goals, *professional* case management adds the extra dimension of value. This chapter addresses different approaches to case management programs and the opportunities and directions that case management provides for advanced practice psychiatric nurses.

WHAT IS THE VALUE OF VALUE?

The emphasis on value in health care delivery is beginning to enter into health care design discussions. In the past, the emphasis was on cost or quality; increasingly, both payers and consumers of health care are coming to realize that the balance between the two is key. Finding that balance is the goal of numerous organized and emerging health care representative groups. In mental health, consumer groups are increasingly finding that there is a willingness to listen to their voices at critical times in health care design. Although much of this inclusion has been mandated through legislative gains, consumer groups have been busy developing anti-stigma, alternative treatment, legal assistance, and access initiatives. These first steps are essential to harnessing the economic power and influence required to achieve value goals.

For general population care, value is also beginning to revolve around inclusion of mental health goals. For example, advanced practice nurses and other professional women gathered in 1996 in New York to discuss and debate the concept of "health" for women. They conducted focus sessions with women who had had a variety of life and professional experiences. The sessions eventually resulted in a vision statement inclusive of psychosocial aspects and interventions necessary to accomplish "health." If this group, by chance or design, continues to grow and represent significant numbers, they could become an economic force in acquiring health care resources that are compatible with their vision of value.

Although these specialized initiatives for value have made gains, the greatest opportunity currently for maximizing value occurs through expert management of outcomes at the closest point of actual care. Advanced practice clinicians, as diversely trained and clinically expert providers, have the skills and knowledge required to innovate case management systems that will achieve the best outcomes for the cost within realistic time frames.

► CASE EXAMPLE

Ann, an APN home care nurse, is able to assume community-based case manager functions that complement the skills of the nonprofessional case manager assigned to Tim. Tim, a 34-year-old man with schizophrenia, was just released from the hospital. His parents have died and he has no supports or relatives to care for him. He wants to live alone with his cat. His house has been neglected and is in serious need of repair. At each session at his home, Ann deftly assesses the environment, his nutrition, hygiene, mental status, physical adjustment to psychotropic medications, how he gets and spends his money, his ability to care for his cat, his level of knowledge regarding self-care and medication, and the status of his trust and alliance with providers and systems, all within the single session. It doesn't matter that the payer only reimburses the visit for care activities that support the medical plan of care (medications and management of side effects). Later, during a phone call to Peg, Tim's state-assigned case manager, Ann finds that Peg is going on vacation for 2 weeks and even when she returns will not be able to set up time with Tim until the end of the month. Peg has been coordinating contact with the community medical care provider. She will be having Joe cover for her until she returns. Ann sets up a plan to continue to coordinate Tim's goal for primary care and sets about contacting the public health center; his blood pressure was high the last visit and he was sweating profusely on a cool day. He was more anxious than usual. The next time she sees Tim she will be sure to discuss carefully how he will manage getting to the doctor and what barriers would prevent him from keeping the appointment. Upon Peg's return, Tim had successfully made his first medical appointment and had averted a need for a potential hospitalization. His escalating anxiety was related to physical complications of a glucose metabolism problem for which he was now being treated.

CASE MANAGEMENT

Case management is a strategy for coordinating patient access to services, maintaining continuity, and improving the efficiency of current care delivery. Case management is often devised as a discipline-neutral role, but when assumed by a particular discipline, it cannot help but to take on the flavor of that profession. Designers of case management roles who understand this fact can direct certain disciplines to case management roles that make the most use of their skills. Advanced practice psychiatric nursing has the opportunity to bring its unique view to case management and to fully flex opportunities to enhance patient outcomes.

Although there is no single model for case management design on advanced practice levels, there must be consensus as to what case management is to achieve. A key question that can assist APNs to determine the case management focus is this: "Is the role (or system) about improving the processes of care or improving patient outcomes?" How this question is answered determines the shape that case management programs take. The former focus requires APN strategizing for systems efficiency goals, whereas the latter requires attention to actual and sustained health maintenance for patient populations.

MODELS FOR APN CASE MANAGEMENT

PAYER CASE MANAGEMENT

Definitions of case management abound, and often reflect the definers' interests or constituency. For example, in payer case management, case managers hired by payers (insurance companies, health maintenance organizations) provide a service that assists high-cost patients to move quickly through the system of care and prevents future expensive episodes of care. Payer case management is performed by people who may or may not be medical professionals, who often work from distant, off-site locations and may manage client care through telephone communications with the direct care providers (psychiatrists, direct providers) or their representatives (office staff, discharge planners, care coordinators). The APN as a payer case manager, working off site, is in a good position to seek assessment information, match it to payer criteria, and catalyze the provider team to appropriate use of resources (hospital days, numbers of visits). The APN can determine information requirements, develop resource use guidelines, and clarify admission and discharge/transfer criteria for the providers and referral sources that providers will use. In addition, the advanced practice provider often understands the complexities that work to delay expected client movements through a system (Table 6–1). The APN is in a better position to judge when to extend benefits to providers to manage complex care patients (e.g., when providers are attempting to place a frail elder with both psychiatric and functional disabilities, but who resides in a community where few nursing homes will accept psychiatric patients).

APNs in payer case management roles are also in a position to develop quality improvement projects aimed at improving provider–payer communication, patient information systems, and access solutions, as well as to monitor internal payer responsiveness. For example, when providers have complaints about payer case managers or the communication process, an APN payer case manager can develop a mutual quality improvement audit system, collect data, form an improved process, test it, and continuously improve it. An APN would also ensure that providers are included in the information and solution-finding process.

CASE ADMINISTRATION

Case administration, a "cousin" of case management, represents another model for APNs interested in independent practice, boundary spanning, and patient advocacy. In this model, the indepen-

TABLE 6–1. COMPLEXITIES THAT DELAY CLIENT MOVEMENT THROUGH SYSTEMS

Patient/family	Axis II or personality disorder pathology, lack of home-based caregiver or no back-up, patient/family requires more teaching, lack of financial resources to gain access to necessary community supports, alternate funding will require an extensive application process, patient/family abusive situations requiring investigation, language or cultural barriers, patient/family motivation lacking, inability to participate in care, fear of patient, indecision, physical/mental illness of dependent family member, extenuating circumstances (e.g., death in the family, therapist vacation).
Provider	Community provider disagrees with discharge plan, refuses to support placement plan; lack of adequate discharge planning.
System	Lack of beds, access barriers, prohibitive costs in setting up spectrum of services required by populations of patients, poor communications (internal and external).
Community	Home placement barriers such as environmental, electrical, safety, or other unmodifiable risk; no local agency or resources for discharge; inadequate agencies or poor follow-up outcomes; referral agency requires additional support and education to manage referred patients; agencies do not take psychiatric patients.

dent clinical specialist partners with patients and their families to provide a health care system "navigation service" with the precise needs of the client as the focus. The client or family independently contracts for case administration services with the APN to define and advocate for client needs, with both a cost and quality focus. The context for using case administration usually involves extremely complex clients, families who are emotionally and financially drained, and numerous care-delivery systems working at cross purposes. The model, developed by Joyce Shields, an independent clinical specialist and founder of Aftercare Resources Associates in Belmont, Massachusetts, emphasizes a number of principles that hinge on expert clinical management.

- Respond to the family's anxiety as quickly as possible.
- Discuss financial concerns early.
- Educate the patient and family about the management of regression and how to master it.
- Keep the family informed.
- Review past transitions—what worked and what did not.
- Anticipate and manage anger and rejection (from client, family, providers).
- Maintain an empathic stance.
- Watch for the more subtle family response (e.g., regressions, undoings).

- Work with providers to focus and anticipate client needs.
- Define the "work" in terms of what the client is supposed to learn while using the service plan.

Insurers and other payers who seek a balanced cost, quality solution for patients requiring expensive service plans would have interest in this advanced practice service.

CLINICAL CASE MANAGEMENT

Clinical case management refers to a system-based program that is outcomes oriented, provider driven, and patient centered. APNs functioning in these models for case management occupy a variety of roles in organizations of all sizes. Director of case management, director of outcomes planning, or vice-president for clinical and nursing services are typical titles for these executive-level roles. APNs may also be known as coordinators for case management or case management project managers and might report to directors, vice-presidents, or other executive-level leaders. In project manager roles, the APN assumes leadership for a system-wide or product line case management project. The project manager oversees case manager role development, clinical pathways projects, and cost/quality improvement projects that will enhance population outcomes. As the project gains momentum, the importance of top-level inclusion often necessitates moving the project to director-level status. In executive-level case management, the case management project expands from a limited to a system-wide focus and includes oversight of all case management initiatives, including psychiatry case management programs.

An example of a systems level role is that of the director of patient outcomes planning at Southshore Hospital in South Weymouth, Massachusetts. Michael Hartley, as the director, typifies the APN in an executive role. The role requires Hartley to assure interdisciplinary accountability for patient outcomes across the continuum of services. This is provided through the implementation of over 50 pathways called patient outcome plans, or POPs. In addition, he sits on key collaborative decision-making and strategic planning committees where he participates in policy-making decisions and presents cost/quality analyses of any variances to the outcomes. The reports often point to discoveries about population care and the variances that commonly sidetrack results. The most important element of his job involves catalyzing people and systems to achieve outcomes despite those variances. He reports that being a clinical specialist in psychiatric mental health nursing has prepared him well for these executive responsibilities. APNs, as systems thinkers and managers, understand the dynamics of interpersonal and institutional change and resistance to change. This is advantageous to early identification and strategizing around resistance while preserving relationships and the important collaborative connections necessary to achieve case management success.

THE APN AS CASE MANAGER

The APN as a clinical case manager may have been a psychiatric consultation-liaison nurse, nurse manager, or assistant nurse manager who now assumes greater authority in shaping an interdisciplinary team to manage a particular population of clients with cost or quality issues. The case manager may assume leadership in managing a particular high-volume diagnostic group such as patients with depression, chronic mental illness, or dual diagnosis. The case manager in these instances assumes a number of activities that assist in achieving patient outcomes. These activities may include reviewing the admission assessments and customizing the careplans, placing patients on appropriate maps or pathways, being present at team conferences, negotiating accountability for complexities as they occur, working collaboratively with the discharge planners and community service providers, and maintaining data on individual as well as aggregate outcomes achievements.

APNs require a minimum of supervision, making them efficient service providers. They work particularly well in mature organizations using product line care delivery designs. In product line systems, resources are consolidated around certain products (e.g., behavioral health) and clinicians report to the leadership (often a partnership of service director and physician) within the particular product line. APNs as case managers, however, may need to mobilize resources in another product line (such as primary care) if a client requires those services to achieve expected results in behavioral health. APNs have the system savvy to move within product lines or other complex matrix models and communicate to numerous managers while mobilizing the system to achieve those goals. Although other clinicians may assume roles called "case management," the assistance provided is often one dimensional, (such as facilitating or expediting discharge planning). APN case managers change systems. They engineer improvements in care delivery by mobilizing systems that support the real inventors of quality care processes, the direct care providers.

For example, an APN case manager for depression patients found that change of shift reports between nursing staff were often focused on information about patient actions during the day but had little to do with the goals for hospitalization. She worked with the nurses to redesign the guideline for the change of shift report, and developed a form that complemented the out-comes stated on the depression pathway. In addi-tion, she collaborated with the charge nurses and nurse managers to collect exemplars of critical thinking in response to the changed format. She collected the exemplars and integrated them into ongoing education for all staff to develop critical thinking and variance management skills while working with depressed patients.

The standards for clinical case manage-ment, at a minimum, involve assessment and co-ordination. Bower, however, provides the gold standard for clinical case management:

> Case Management is a clinical system that focuses on the accountability of an identi-fied individual or group for coordinating a patient's care (or group of patients) across a continuum or episode of care; insuring and facilitating the achievement of quality and cost outcomes; negotiating, procuring and coordinating services and resources needed by patients/families; intervening at key points (and/or at significant variances from the usual pattern of care) for individ-ual patients; addressing and resolving pat-terns in consistent issues that have a nega-tive quality-cost impact; and, creating opportunities and systems to enhance out-comes (Bower, 1995; Zander, 1996).

This definition underscores the reliance on criti-cal thinking and action taking as essential to pro-fessional case management roles. APN case managers, when placed in authorized positions close to patient care, provide the critical thinking and follow-through necessary to guarantee cost, quality, and value goals.

RELATED FORMS OF CASE MANAGEMENT

CARE MANAGEMENT

Often referred to as care coordination, care man-agement is not case management, but case man-agers function within local care climates and are required to understand the care delivery systems. Care management is defined by Bower (1995) as "the process and system developed to organize and orchestrate the care of all patients within spe-cific geographic areas in such a way that it is di-rected toward meeting desired/anticipated unit-based goals within an appropriate length of stay and resource utilization." Care management refers to the routines, norms, values, and care-delivery mechanisms that exist for each disci-pline or service attending to clients in a service area (e.g., unit, floor, program area). A more for-mal example of a care coordination model is the primary nursing model and how it is specifically practiced on a mental health admission unit. High-functioning care management actually re-duces the need for high numbers of case man-agers. When all providers are functioning at maximum authority and accountability and have the proper resources to achieve cost/quality goals, then case managers find they can focus on ad-vanced functions. Rather than case finding and assessing a patient's progress through the system, the focus is placed on managing at points of com plexity, extending outcomes study into pre- and post-acute care, continuity and access planning, and aggregate analysis of quality and cost data. An investment in good care management benefits systems and allows case managers to become complex population experts.

SKILLED (COMMUNITY) CASE MANAGEMENT

Skilled case management refers to the activity of coordinating resources/services for home care pa-tients. Activities usually involve ensuring that the care provided meets the criteria for reasonable and necessary care and that the rationale for home care services can be defined as medically neces-sary. Skilled case management is usually trig-gered by extensive lengths of service time where a patient is requiring mental health home care ser-vices. The case manager would review the chart and speak with providers to determine the acute nature of the service. If the condition requiring mental health services appears to be of a chronic, stable nature, then efforts are made to transition care needs to less intense services, agencies, or primary care. An APN assuming skilled case management responsibilities may assist in developing a pathway program. Pathways for mental health home care have been developed for depression, anxiety, and schizophrenia, among other disorders (Andolina, 1996; Maturen, 1992).

INTEGRATED CASE MANAGEMENT

Case management programs or roles provide organizations with the opportunity to combine departments in ways that serve populations. For example, Montclair Baptist Hospital in Birmingham, Alabama, has integrated fiscal services, quality improvement, and case management into one service and calls it "integrated case management" (Clements and Love, 1993). This presents advantages to both the system and patients through pooling of expert resources and coordinating knowledge to manage complex care populations.

HOSPITAL-BASED CASE MANAGEMENT

Hospital-based case management simply means that the location for case management services is hospital based. It is sometimes refered to as "within-the-walls" case management (Cohen, 1993).

SOCIAL CASE MANAGEMENT

Case management provided by social workers recognizes their unique knowledge in managing difficult psychosocial issues in high need populations. Social case management is key in providing access to public assistance programs, conducting complex family work, and providing comprehensive community service planning.

NURSING CASE MANAGEMENT

Nursing case management refers to case management of patient groups and outcomes, but is organized with a focus on continuity of the nursing care plan and multidisciplinary collaboration. Early models included nursing case management as an advanced version of primary nursing at New England Medical Center in Boston in the mid-1980s (Zander, 1986).

EPISODE-BASED CASE MANAGEMENT

An episode of care is defined as all the services and care elements involved in managing a particular instance of illness. Episode-based case management begins with the identification of the need for enhanced coordination of resources and services and continues until the individual no longer requires facility services for that health problem (Bower, 1995).

CONTINUUM-BASED CASE MANAGEMENT

In this form of case management, the continuum of care refers to the spectrum of services provided by an organization until the particular health issue is resolved. This often challenges organizations to expand their services into pre-episode services (early detection/prevention) and post-episode services (health maintenance). Additionally, case managers are required to either declare their areas of accountability and negotiate the hand-off of responsibilities to another case manager or span all the boundaries within the defined continuum. This model brings into focus the need for a comprehensive outcomes plan that addresses activities required for primary, secondary, and tertiary prevention; health promotion; timely access to services; and health maintenance.

OUTCOMES PLANNING FOR CASE MANAGEMENT

The health care delivery climate for all services, including psychiatric services, is one of increasing pressure to define outcomes. Defining and describing outcomes remains a difficult task in psychiatric care and different disciplines tend to come at the task in different ways. For example, a psychiatrist may define outcomes based on data from studies with rigorous research designs and control groups. A nurse may refer to outcomes in descriptive but measurable statements based on experience with the nursing care planning process. A psychologist may use symptom scales or other measurement instruments to define the results of an intervention.

At the direct care level, providers form opinions about expected outcomes through synthesizing the assessment data and engaging in the treatment planning and evaluation process. Complicating this process is inundation with outcomes measures from multiple sources (Table 6–2). A model to guide the selection and timing of outcomes will assist providers in outcome decisions. The outcome planning model (Fig. 6–1) offers a conceptual model that attempts to rem-edy the fragmented approach to outcome planning. In the model, outcomes are arranged into categories with the client and family at the center of concern. The categories illustrate clinical concerns that many measures, indicators, or goals fit into. The six general categories include symptom relief/alleviation, functioning, self-care or appropriate supervision, well-being, access, and complication management. When the model is superimposed on the spectrum of levels of care (Figs. 6–2 and 6–3), the resulting intersection indicates outcomes that tend to be emphasized at that level.

Models such as these are a rich source for focus in nursing research. Information about use and application of the models is necessary. Further study could answer questions such as these: What are the definable steps for arriving at stable, replicable, and generalizable outcomes measures? Would the outcomes sort into the predicted categories or into others? What is the purpose of

TABLE 6–2. SOURCES OF OUTCOMES MEASURES FOR BEHAVIORAL HEALTH

Public and regulatory	State Departments of Mental Health Offices for Mental Health Health Care Financing Organization (HCFA)
Expert	American Psychiatric Association Agency for Health Care Policy and Research National Institute of Mental Health American Academy of Child and Adolescent Psychiatry
Accreditation and report cards	National Quality Assurance Committee (NCQA) Healthcare Employer Data and Information Set (HEDIS 3.0) Joint Commission for Accreditation of Health Care Organizations (JCAHO)
Metric measurement systems	Kennedy J. Axis V sub-scales. In: *Fundamentals of Psychiatric Treatment Planning.* American Psychiatric Press; 1996, Washington, D.C. SF-36, BASIS 32, GEMA, Delametrics, Psychsentinel, SCL-90, OCQ, YOQ, COMPASS.
Specialty organizations	Substance Abuse and Mental Health Services Association Center for Mental Health Services
Advocacy and access oriented	National Association for the Mentally Ill "Parity" bills National Institute of Mental Health: "Depression, Awareness, Recognition and Treatment" (D/ART) campaign

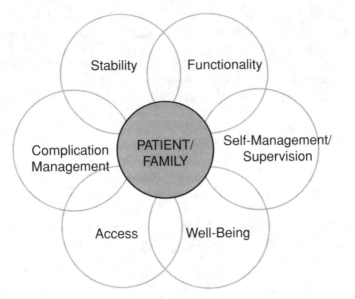

Andolina, The Center for Case Management, (1996)

Figure 6–1. Outcome planning model and domains for describing categories of outcomes.

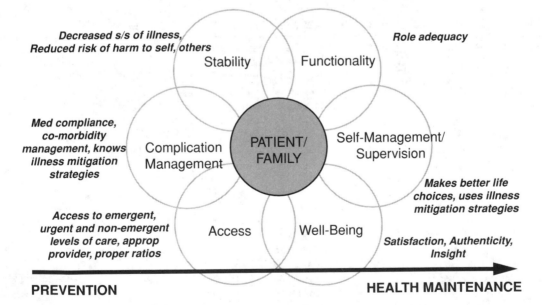

Andolina, The Center for Case Management, (1996)

Figure 6–2. Subdescriptions of outcomes can be further defined within the domains. The prevention/ health maintenance progression is superimposed on the model to illustrate where domains relate to wellness interventions.

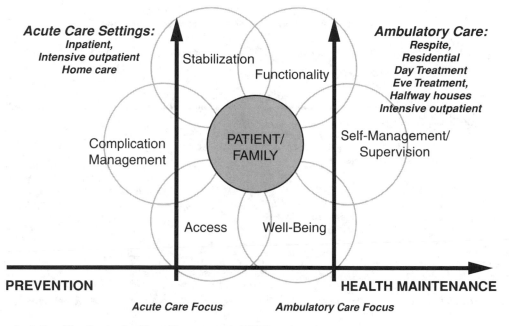

Andolina, The Center for Case Management, (1996)

Figure 6–3. Intersection of the levels of care and correlating settings. Acute care settings in an outcomes planning model emphasize outcomes related to stabilization, management of complications, and access. Ambulatory settings emphasize improved functioning, self-maintenance, and enhanced well-being outcomes.

the client-centered context? How can organizations use the model to develop meaningful and relevant interventions? How does an outcome planning model assist to achieve healthier populations and communities?

Whatever models emerge as influential to the practice of case management, APNs can be instrumental in research design, self-study, and assuring that a comprehensive and balanced approach is used when forming outcomes plans.

IMPACT OF CONTINUITY ON CASE MANAGEMENT DESIGNS

While services, providers, and levels of care have multiplied, the continuity between them has not always been maintained. Whether it is the closure of large state-sponsored care facilities, resulting in displaced patients, or increased num-

bers of primary care providers willing to carry behavioral health patients in their general practices, the resulting fragmentation and potential for losing clients between the cracks is inevitable. This fragmentation has resulted in a greater need for continuity plans. Case management is an obvious strategy for providing the glue where it is needed for populations of clients using many levels of care within the spectrum of services available (Fig. 6–4).

Behavioral health leaders are finding that care delivery system redesign is more the norm than the exception to the rule. Ultimately these designs will need to account for the multiple levels within and across the organization and continuums of care. The potential for discontinuity is inevitable and poses a significant problem now and in the near future. Case managers are boundary spanners who orchestrate care services, piecing them together and providing

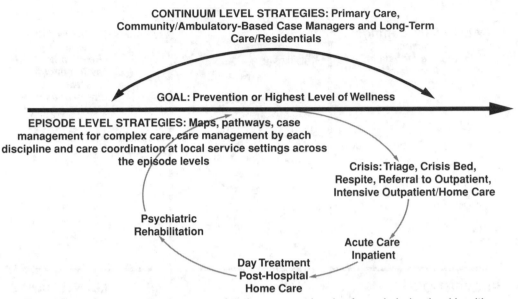

Figure 6–4. Care coordination strategies that support levels of care in behavioral health.

the glue for continuity, while keeping a firm eye on the bigger picture. Advanced practice nurses have the discriminating ability to assess system complexities and effectiveness during periods of fragmentation, allowing accurate appraisals of system readiness to meet patient needs.

PROFESSIONAL ISSUES AFFECTING CASE MANAGEMENT

Issues affecting the profession will influence the shape of case management roles and systems. A general climate of economic uncertainty, with concerns about job viability and job security, can impact the pace at which case management roles and programs are expanded into an organization. Additional complications for nursing may arise from other work issues. These include reporting to non-nursing leadership positions and potential role erosion through cross-training and roles substitution programs (for example, unlicensed assistive personnel administering medications to clients in residential placements). Role erosion, in particular, can have a devastating effect on professional confidence. A general sense of expendability may exist in organizations going through these, as well as other, redesign efforts. Tragically, this can contribute to inertia and a less-than-enthusiastic embracing of "new role designs." Although it is difficult to become energized within this climate, APNs have the ability to apply structure to chaotic situations, form long-term plans, and maintain a visible presence of value in health care delivery.

CASE MANAGEMENT AND OTHER CARE COORDINATION STRATEGIES

In complex systems of care, case management is one of several strategies in providing coordinated care to psychiatric clients. These strategies include pathways/CareMap programs, resource management (utilization review and allocation programs), program management (special organization of care for particular programs such as dual diagnosis programs, post-traumatic stress disorder programs, and pastoral care), and care management. Table 6–3 provides several patient descriptions and illustrates how an advanced practice nurse accountable for case managing complex care patients comprehensively develops the case management (or care coordination plan). In these clinical vignettes, it should be observed how clinical case management might work with these other strategies to benefit short-term and long-term outcomes both for system and client.

EDUCATION OF APN CASE MANAGERS

Although educational preparation has provided much of the necessary skill to promote advanced practice nurses as leaders in case management, the basic clinical curriculum needs to be enhanced. APNs would benefit through inclusion of courses on cost accounting, data management, systems management, and practice-based research designs in the curricula. Each of these areas would provide the APN with a rich repertoire of skills and knowledge required to manage tomorrow's complicated systems and populations. Although it is increasingly popular to add nurse practitioner tracks to clinical specialist frameworks, educators may be building only half the bridge (although a spectacular one) if they do not include content related to systems thinking and role positioning and design in complex organizations. The goal must be oriented towards preparing APNs as systems managers fully capable of positioning themselves in mental health organizations. Until the ideal integrated curriculum exists, advanced practice nurses in mental health can continue to seek certifications, separate degrees (as with the Villanova School of Nursing Case Management Program), and, of course, on-the-job training.

EVALUATION OF APN CASE MANAGERS

Evaluation of the APN case manager can be approached in a number of ways. One method evaluates the APN based on whether or not the role achieved expectations for improved patient outcomes. In this instance the evaluation is based on how the following question is answered: Were cost and quality outcomes for the patient for whom the case management services were provided improved and sustained? If yes, then the role is successfully being implemented. If no, then the reasons for the shortcomings must be evaluated. Were expectations for cost and quality out of alignment with the realities of the population or resources available? Was the role designed in a hasty, haphazard manner without much thought to the conflicts and redundancies with other roles? Was there a lack of authority to implement the role properly? Was the APN mismatched or unqualified for the job responsibilities?

Another approach to APN evaluation is through a competency appraisal system. Skills associated with case management can be stated and progressively acquired through experience, apprenticeship, peer consultation, describing and collecting exemplars from actual practice of the role, and mentoring. A sample competency format is given in the next section.

CASE MANAGER COMPETENCIES AND INDICATORS

The APN case manager uses the nursing process to assess, plan, intervene/coordinate, and monitor/evaluate.

- Quickly assimilates data from numerous sources, including chart reviews, participation in care planning sessions, and data research related to population case types.
- Ascertains and remedies data gaps and determines what other data are necessary to arrive at a comprehensive assessment.

TABLE 6-3. EXAMPLES OF CARE COORDINATION STRATEGIES TO MANAGE BEHAVIORAL HEALTH CLIENTS IN AN ACUTE LEVEL OF CARE

Patient	CareMap/Path	Care Management	Case Management	Other Strategies
1. Jose, 34 y.o. Hispanic male who speaks broken English. He is psychotic, refusing meds. Goals include encouraging him to voluntarily take meds. *Variances/Complications* Broken English, refusing meds, restraining order (wife).	Start on the Major Mental Illness/Psychosis pathway (describes the basic standard of care and outcomes for patients with acute psychosis and major mental illness). Customize pathway to address cultural, communication, and legal issues.	*Psychiatry:* Responsible for initial and ongoing risk assessments as necessary, including necessity of using Tarasoff warning. Takes medical history and establishes the medication management plan. *Nursing:* Observes response to milieu, interpersonal relationships, risk assessments. Structures milieu to include activity and destimulation strategies, varies the medication offering strategy, obtains med teaching tools in Spanish. *Social Work:* Evaluates family stressors, behaviors leading up to restraining order, and finances and need for assistance. Identifies community resources, secures Spanish interpreters. *Rehabilitation:* Establishes appropriate group participation goals, evaluates potential for ed/voc when psychosis abates.	*Case Manager:* Oversees development of maps for acute psychosis. For this individual patient, serves as the community resource expert, works collaboratively with social service on discharge planning. *Long-term Case Management Projects:* Does community policing education related to major MI, goal to educate police as to approach, psychiatric interventions, community resources, cultural issues, and to achieve earlier intervention and access to psych services. Affiliates with a Hispanic liaison to educate staff related to sociocultural issues and community outcomes.	*Unit-based Care Coordinator:* Reviews all the patient assessments, makes sure that appropriate patients are placed on the maps, sees that staff documents on the map, and documents any variances in the progress notes. Ensures that the map reflects the individual patient care needs. Attends team meetings or ensures that the variances from plan are communicated to the team. Keeps track of who specifically is accountable for managing the identified variances.
2. Linda, 39 y.o. female with major mental illness. Hospitalized for affective instability, increasing anxiety, acting out, and suicidal ideation. She is needy and irritable.	Start on the Major Mental Illness/Psychosis pathway. Customize pathway to address her physical needs and attention-seeking behaviors.	*Psychiatry:* Does risk assessment, develops target symptom list and medication plan, takes med history. *Nursing:* Observes interpersonal response and times of increased neediness, does risk assessment, provides structure as negotiated with patient, teaches how to use support and PRNs to manage affect.	*Case Manager:* In collaboration with the MDs, creates links to primary care physician and evaluates primary care issues and concerns. *Long-term Case Management Project:* Develops a liaison program for primary care physicians treating "problem" or complex care patients. Program will offer care planning and community support input.	*Unit-based Care Coordinator:* Same as above. Establishes and monitors integrated primary care program for effectiveness on specific cost and quality goals.

Patient	CareMap/Path	Care Management	Case Management	Other Strategies
Variances/Complications Obesity and diabetes, regresses into needy and attention-seeking behaviors, along with occasional escalations, assault potential.		*Social Work:* Evaluates family, significant others. Contacts housing manager, other community service provider, and invites to team meetings. *Rehabilitation:* Evaluates potential for ed/voc. Sets group structure with patient, identifies group goals, affect management, and coping strategies.		
3. Paul/Paula. This male pt. has been taking hormones and is seeking medical care for an eventual sex change operation. He/she has long unkempt hair, is unshaven and disheveled. Speaks little and remains isolated in the milieu. *Variances/Complications* Gender issues, unclear status of the medical treatment, interpersonal relationships.	Started on the Major Mental Illness/Acute Psychosis pathway. Customize to gender issues and milieu management needs.	*Psychiatry:* Determines the medico-psychiatric plan of care. Evaluates the endocrine/medication management plan, psychodynamic history, psychiatric diagnostics. *Nursing:* Observes response to milieu, interpersonal relationships, teaching r/t issues of illness recovery and rehabilitation. Monitors for adverse medication effects. *Social Work:* Evaluates family/significant others, community resources for trans-gender people with mental illness.	*Case Manager:* Works collaboratively with the social worker on DCP issues as necessary. *Long-term Case Management Project:* Obtains information on gender change and educates caregivers on biopsychosocial issues (or obtains articles, or arranges for speaker to educate staff). Follows trends on number of patients admitted with gender issues and major mental illness for evaluation as a specialty program or care planning process.	*Unit-based Care Coordinator:* Reviews all the patient assessments, makes sure that appropriate patients are placed on the maps, sees that staff documents on the map, and documents any variances in the progress notes. Oversees the customizing of the maps, attends team meetings or communicates the variances the team. Keeps track of who specifically is accountable for managing the variances.

(continued)

TABLE 6–3. *CONTINUED*

Patient	CareMap/Path	Care Management	Case Management	Other Strategies
4. Raymond, 24 y.o. male with schizoaffective disorder with cocaine abuse. He is irritable and reactive to redirection, grandiose and easily prone to rage. His residential placement is in jeopardy. *Variances/Complications* Able to ask for PRNs when anxious or angry, but in denial r/t his illness. States that he misses cocaine.	Place on the Dual Diagnosis pathway. Customize to cocaine use, discharge planning problems.	*Psychiatry:* Does risk assessment for hospital and community levels of care, med plan. *Nursing:* Engages pt. in therapeutic contracting on management of cocaine cravings and rages. Handles teaching, risk assessment, daily structure. Monitors and supports pt. interest in self-care goals. *Social Work:* Evaluates family, significant others, and degree of support. Evaluates residential capability to manage pt. Begins to form an alternate discharge plan. *Rehabilitation:* Evaluates coping, motivation, and substance abuse potential.	*Case Manager:* Oversees the development of dual diagnosis pathway. Individually with this patient, establishes alternative discharge plan if residential placement is unlikely and state hospital admissions are increasingly difficult to obtain. *Long-term Case Management Project:* Creates links to state mental health programs, corrections, community policing, substance abuse providers. Establishes a program of early detection, residential staff development in patient management issues, and easy access to acute level of care services.	*Unit-based Care Coordinator:* Same as above. Establishes program for dual diagnosis patients who have limited resources.

CareMap tools available: depression, major mental illness/psychosis, dual diagnosis, bipolar, cognitively impaired, and generic.

- Identifies appropriate patients for case management and determines where in the service plan or area that case management will start.
- Continues to use the nursing process to proactively develop backup options for common complications or barriers to achieving desired patient outcomes.
- Uses or develops maps/pathways when appropriate to case-managed patients.
- Knowledgeable about the cost, discharge planning, or other outcomes that pathways are managing and determines additional outcomes as necessary.
- Designs process(es) to enhance outcomes where negative system variances are detected.

Accesses internal and external resources for coordinating care.

- Uses referral lists and known resources when available and appropriate to the patient.
- Identifies the history associated with the referral resources and the outcomes they manage (if known).

Maintains quality standards appropriate to the case type, role, and system.

- Integrates existing practice guidelines into case management plans or pathways.
- Leads a practice guideline task force to resolve conflicting practice patterns.
- Searches and obtains outcome standards from a variety of sources related to case type(s).

Knowledgeable about regulations and standards related to the case types.

- Integrates local, state, and federal regulations related to case type care.
- Teaches other collaborative care providers about regulatory requirements.

Establishes, invents, and maintains effective communication systems.

- Uses resources that provide supervision, second opinions, or different assessments to situations that present as problematic.

- Recognizes complex care patients requiring second opinions and seeks those opinions.
- Critically appraises or uses feedback to improve patient care outcomes.

Self-monitors and measures performance within the role.

- Maintains data base on case-managed patients and periodically monitors data for cost, quality, or clinical trends.
- Stays apprised of local and national trends in case management.
- Develops a quality monitor measuring satisfaction with case management services.

As in any role evaluation, the barriers to role performance must be taken into consideration. At times, the barriers may have more to do with the system than the actual performance of the person occupying the role. Typical barriers include lack of authority to implement necessary role functions; role overload characterized by too many task responsibilities and too few supports (e.g., educational or technological, or lack of access to information, people, or expertise); and role confusion such as may occur when there is difficulty determining who best would qualify as the case manager.

SUMMARY

Mental health care continues to make strides in status as a full partner with primary health care in maintaining the health of individuals, populations, and communities. At the same time it too struggles with the economic changes brought on by managed care. The continued demand for psychiatric services and access to skilled providers will fuel the demand for expert psychiatric case management. Case management offers a place for advanced practice psychiatric nurses to parlay their unique skills into careers beyond traditional tracks. If the past is any indication of the future, advanced practice nurses will continue to shape the face of health care in essential and meaningful ways, bringing with them great skills, rich traditions, complex knowledge, and focused energy. As the value formula gains acceptance and momentum in health care designs, APNs will be one resource health care will not want to do without.

REFERENCES

Andolina K. Center for Case Management. South Natick, MA, 1996.

Bower KA. Case management designed for the care continuum. In: Zander K, ed. *Managing Outcomes Through Collaborative Care: The Application of Care Mapping and Case Management*. Chicago: American Hospital Publishing; 1995:167–167.

Clements F, Love K. Responsive restructuring: Decision support for coordinated care and financial integration. In: Zander K, ed. *Definition and the New Definition: A Decade of Looking Forward*. South Natick, MA: Center for Case Management; 1993: 93–95.

Cohen EL, Cesta TG. *Nursing Case Management*. St. Louis: Mosby; 1993:36–46.

Maturen V. *Care Map and Comap Tools for Home Health*, Oak Park, Il.: VNA First, Inc., 1992.

Shields J. *Aftercare Resources*, Belmont, MA, 1996.

Zander K. Case management: Cost, processes and quality outcomes. In: Zander K, ed. *Definition and the New Definition: A Decade of Looking Forward*. South Natick, MA: Center for Case Management; 1996:5–7.

Zander K. Towards a fully integrated CareMap and case management system. In: Zander K, ed. *Definition and the New Definition: A Decade of Looking Forward*. South Natick, MA: Center for Case Management; 1996:87.

CHAPTER 7

PSYCHIATRIC HOME HEALTH SERVICES

Verna Benner Carson

The advanced practice psychiatric nurse must continue to articulate the broad dimensions of the role, to conduct research that demonstrates the clinical and cost effectiveness of nurses as primary providers of psychiatric care, and to lobby Congress and the Health Care Financing Administration to change the laws that govern Medicare.

Chapter Overview

- Current State of Psychiatric Home Care
- The Advanced Practice Nurse as Therapist and Expert Clinician
- Plan of Care
    Assessment
    Analysis of Data: Nursing Diagnoses
    Expected Outcomes and Goals
    Implementation
    Evaluation of Care
- The Advanced Practice Nurse as Consultant
- The Advanced Practice Nurse as Program Developer
- Vision for Future Role of the Advanced Practice Psychiatric Nurse
- References

► INTRODUCTION

Psychiatric home care is a relatively new specialty in the United States. Although Medicare began to reimburse home care agencies for psychiatric nursing services in 1979, it was not until the 1990s that the specialty experienced any significant growth (Carson, 1996). The growth in psychiatric home care is largely due to two factors: the increasing numbers of elderly who need psychiatric care and an interest among payors to explore cost-effective treatment alternatives to the more costly inpatient and partial hospitalization modalities. Psychiatric home care is cost effective. Studies have demonstrated not only a cost savings of as much as 70 percent when compared to inpatient costs, but also clinical efficacy in maintaining patients in the community for longer periods of time (Health Care Today, 1996; Lima, 1995).

In order to provide psychiatric home care, a home health agency (HHA) must submit the resumes of each of its psychiatric nurses to its Medicare intermediary for approval. The resumes are screened to see if the nurse meets the required educational and clinical criteria required by Medicare. Medicare's criteria include a master's degree in psychiatric nursing, a bachelor's degree in nursing with a minimum of 1 year of inpatient adult/geriatric psychiatric nursing experience, or a diploma or associate arts degree with a minimum of 2 years of inpatient adult/geriatric psychiatric nursing experience.

If the HHA works with managed care organizations (MCOs), the HHA may have to submit information on the whole agency and/or on each nurse in order to be credentialed and become part of the MCO's panel of providers. MCOs that require this process only credential master's-prepared nurses who are also certified as advanced practice nurses. There is a paradox in relation to both the Medicare and MCO credentialing processes; although they both identify the master's degree and certification as important, neither recognizes in clinical practice the advanced level of skill that this nurse brings to clinical situations. Medicare makes no distinction between the practice or the reimbursement of the master's-prepared psychiatric nurse and less educationally prepared nurses.

MCOs vary in the types of referrals that are made to psychiatric home care. Sometimes referrals are made for psychiatric services where the patient or family definitely require the skill level of the advanced practitioner; other times the referrals are made for psychiatric services easily provided by the generalist in psychiatric nursing. In clinical practice, the recognition and appropriate use of the advanced practice nurse is done within individual HHAs. These skills are needed in two areas: (1) psychotherapy for adults, families, children, or adolescents; and (2) consultation for a variety of consultees including other home-care providers, physicians, hospital staff, community mental health professionals, and school personnel. Furthermore, the advanced practice nurse is usually charged with ongoing program development and refinement in response to changing needs of patients as well as changing needs of the health care system. Because the Medicare home care regulations do not recognize the independent roles of the advanced practice psychiatric nurse to deliver psychotherapy and to order prescriptions, every home care patient must be under the care of a physician who not only orders all prescriptions, but also signs the plan of care that specifies the mode of psychotherapy.

This chapter explores the current state of psychiatric home care and the ways in which the role of the advanced practice psychiatric home care nurse is operational-

ized. In addition, this chapter presents a vision regarding the future role of the advanced practice psychiatric home care nurse.

CURRENT STATE OF PSYCHIATRIC HOME CARE

Psychiatric home care began as a service to assist the elderly with psychiatric diagnoses to successfully transition from the hospital to home. Even today, as many as 85 percent of all referrals for psychiatric home care services are for this population. The primary diagnoses seen in home care are the affective disorders, especially major depression (Carson, 1995, 1996). The seriously and persistently mentally ill of all ages are the next most frequent type of referral, with approximately 11 percent diagnosed with schizophrenia. Children and adolescents, usually presenting with attention deficit disorder and/or oppositional defiant disorder as well as major depression, represent no more than 1 percent of all psychiatric home care referrals nationwide. The remaining 3 percent of referrals are made up of patients with anxiety disorders and those who are dually diagnosed with either a substance abuse disorder and another psychiatric disorder or with a medical diagnosis (such as cancer) and a psychiatric diagnosis.

In 1993, Medicare reported that 41,800 patients, or 1.5 percent of all patients receiving home visits, were treated for "mental disorders," which includes codes 290 to 320 in the *International Classification of Diseases*, ninth edition (HCFA, 1993). In 1994, the number of patients increased to 60,600, or 1.9 percent of the total patient group receiving home care services. In its reporting, Medicare does not identify the number of patients represented by specific diagnoses.

The MCOs are referring even fewer patients for psychiatric home care. Several of the large behavioral health MCOs reported that no more than 0.0025 percent of the patients who received psychiatric care were receiving psychiatric home care (personal conversations with MCO representatives, 1996).

These numbers represent a small percentage of the potential patients who could benefit from psychiatric home care. Many who could benefit are not referred. The limited use of psychiatric home care is largely attributed to the current system of insurance coverage for the mentally ill. Most health care plans severely limit the benefits available to patients diagnosed with psychiatric disorders; the coverage usually has co-payments, many restrictions on the type and amount of services allowed, and a low lifetime cap. Many people who require care beyond the limits of their policies are transferred to the public mental health system. In 1990, 28 percent of funds for care of the mentally ill came from state and local governments; for physical health care the comparable figure was 14 percent. An additional 26 percent of funds for the care of the mentally ill came from Medicare, Medicaid, Veteran's Affairs, and other federal programs. Managed care organizations, with their focus on limiting health expenditures, have traditionally either ignored the needs of the seriously and persistently mentally ill entirely, relegating their care to the public health system, or they have subcontracted the care of this population to companies whose sole focus is the mentally ill. This adversely affects the risk pool, allows less money to provide care, and leads to the provision of less care. In the current health care arena, with Medicare and Medicaid programs still viable, MCOs have had little impetus to explore cost-effective care alternatives for the seriously and persistently mentally ill. They can continue to shift the burden of this care to federal and state-funded programs.

The future growth of psychiatric home health services is projected to be explosive. This projection is based on three factors: national trends that promise to convert the interest of MCOs to actively embrace psychiatric home care, cultural and environmental changes, and the sheer numbers of psychiatric patients who could benefit from in-home psychiatric services.

The national trends

- The shifting of Medicare and Medicaid patients to MCOs. Increasingly, MCOs will no longer be able to refuse to manage the care of the chronic schizophrenic and bipolar patients.
- Shifting Medicaid funding from the federal to state levels. This trend will force states to examine creative ways to manage the health care needs of the psychiatric population. Many states are currently moving these patients into MCOs.
- Parity in mental health care coverage. The push for parity in mental health care (which would eliminate any disparity in medical coverage that insurance companies have between physical and mental health coverage) has gained tremendous momentum. In 1996, an amendment that would have guaranteed parity was tied up in Congress for 6 months before it was finally defeated. This was the furthest that a parity measure has ever gotten in the national legislative process. Parity is law in Maryland and Minnesota.
- Medical cost offsets. A large demonstration project caught the managed care industry's attention. The study found that for chronically medically ill patients using managed psychiatric home care programs, the efficacy of the programs brought across the board declines in medical inpatient, emergency room, outpatient, and pharmacy costs, from a range of 9.5 to 22 percent (Faulkner and Gray, 1995).

The cultural and environmental changes

- The aging of the population. As people age, the need for in-home services, including psychiatric services, increases dramatically.
- The high percentage of elderly who suffer from a major psychiatric disorder, usually depression.
- Demand from advocacy groups, such as NAMI (National Alliance for the Mentally Ill), to provide the least restrictive services for individuals who need psychiatric care.
- The 1996 revision of HM-11 (Medicare's home care regulations) allowing primary physicians to refer to psychiatric home care. This will significantly increase access to this specialty, especially for the elderly who usually avoid seeing psychiatrists for treatment of depression and anxiety disorders (Badgio, 1996).

The numbers of patients who could benefit from psychiatric home care is shown in Table 7–1.

THE ADVANCED PRACTICE NURSE AS THERAPIST AND EXPERT CLINICIAN

As the specialty of psychiatric home care grows, the role of the advanced practice psychiatric home care nurse will undergo further definition and refinement. Today the advanced practice nurse is involved in managing the most challenging patients and families; APN requires the greatest knowledge and skill level. A specific case example (see page 95) illustrates the advanced practice nurse as therapist and expert clinician.

PLAN OF CARE

ASSESSMENT

The assessment involved interviewing Kathleen and her mother, stepfather, and sister; a comprehensive mental status examination of

TABLE 7–1. POTENTIAL HOME CARE REFERRALS[a]

Diagnostic Category	Potential Psychiatric Home Care Referrals
Schizophrenia	600,000
Bipolar disorder	100,000
Anxiety disorders	1,000,000
Depression	2,000,000
Substance abuse disorders	74,250
Childhood and adolescent disorders	1,000,000
Traumatic brain injury patients	10,000
Dementia	2,000,000
TOTAL	6,784,250

[a] Estimates are compilations from the literature and based on a percentage of the number of Americans diagnosed with these illnesses.

Kathleen; evaluation of her developmental level, educational achievement, and functional abilities both in activities of daily living as well as in instrumental activities of daily living; the administration of standardized measures to evaluate Kathleen for depression as well as for obsessive-compulsive behaviors, and the completion of a family genogram. Additionally, the nurse inquired about Kathleen's support system and the the burden of care experienced by her family. The assessment was completed with a full systems review, specifically focusing on Kathleen's diabetes and her seizure disorder.

Kathleen exhibited multiple problems. She displayed outbursts of temper accompanied by physical aggression in a variety of situations including home, school, and in the community. Her mother stated that the motivating factor to

▶ CASE EXAMPLE

Kathleen, an 18-year-old living with her mother, stepfather, and sister, was referred for psychiatric home care as a last resort. The case manager who made the referral stated, "Kathleen has burned out all her therapists; she has been in the hospital four times in the last six weeks; she hits her mother; and we don't know what else to do." Kathleen's diagnoses included the following.

- Axis I: Major depression.
- Axis II: Mild developmental disability.
- Axis III: Insulin-dependent diabetic since age 11, complex seizure disorder.
- Axis IV: Severe psychosocial stressors including problems with primary support group—hits mother; argues with sister; no friends; dependent on mother for all social outlets. Educational problems: struggles with school work; in a class for special needs students; involved in frequent discord with classmates. Occupational problems: history of three terminations from part-time jobs for verbal and physical aggression.

Kathleen's case was so complex that she was assigned to an advanced practice psychiatric nurse. On the initial visit the nurse began the assessment. Although assessment is an ongoing process, the bulk of the data was collected over two home visits.

Kathleen's outbursts was being told "no." Kathleen's primary target for aggression was her mother, who expressed hopelessness, cried throughout the interviews, and stated, "I feel like a battered woman—only my daughter is the abuser." Kathleen's sister expressed ambivalent feelings toward Kathleen. "I love her but I also hate her. She makes mom miserable and keeps us in an uproar all the time." The stepfather's position was "I help out when I'm here but mostly I try to stay out of it." He did not see his role as important in the management of Kathleen.

In addition to the physical outbursts, Kathleen engaged in self-destructive behaviors such as adjusting her insulin and her nutrient intake to produce insulin reactions. On one occasion she ate a 12-ounce bag of chocolate chips and drank a 2-liter bottle of regular soda while at the same time refusing to administer her insulin; on another occasion she fasted from eating her meals and tripled the amount of insulin she was scheduled to administer. It was not uncommon for Kathleen's blood glucose levels to fluctuate between a low of 40 and a high of 400. Kathleen occasionally engaged in head banging, and on one occasion she pulled off the nail on her big toe. When the home care nurse asked Kathleen what motivated her to do these things, Kathleen responded, "Oh, I just wanted to see what would happen."

In addition to these behavioral problems, Kathleen experienced severe learning problems and was assigned to a special class. She was in her senior year of high school and looked forward to graduation. However, school was very difficult; her attention span was short; she had some difficulties with memory; she engaged in very concrete thinking; her ability to express her own feelings was severely limited; and she had no friends.

Kathleen was an insulin-dependent diabetic and had been so since the age of 11. Also at age 11 she was diagnosed with a complex seizure disorder; she experienced three to four seizures a month, usually during her sleep. She was on many medications; throughout the course of her home care treatment, her medications were continually adjusted.

Kathleen expressed considerable sadness and hopelessness over her condition. She indicated her unhappiness with her behavior but couldn't see how she could control or change it. She wondered why God had made her like this and stated, "Everyone would be better off without me." She did not express a suicidal plan, denied that her self-destructive behavior was suicidal, and refused to commit to a "no harm" contract.

ANALYSIS OF DATA: NURSING DIAGNOSES

After analyzing the assessment data, the advanced practice psychiatric home care nurse decided on the following nursing diagnoses:

- Risk for violence, self-directed and directed at others related to inability to express feelings appropriately and to accept limit-setting evidenced by hitting mother, verbal outbursts toward others, and engaging in behaviors that seriously threaten her own well-being.
- Ineffective individual coping related to multiple stressors and evidenced by Kathleen's verbal and physical acting out and self-destructive behaviors.
- Chronic low self-esteem related to long-standing history of minimal accomplishments, evidenced by self-negating verbalizations and feelings of shame, guilt, and despair.
- Hopelessness related to long-term physical and emotional problems, evidenced by symptoms of depression.
- Social isolation related to inability to make friends evidenced by no friends and total dependence on mother for social activities.
- Spiritual distress related to chronicity and complexity of problems evidenced by verbalizations questioning why God had made her.
- Family dysfunction related to chronic stress evidenced by rigid roles, poor communication, and the expression by individual family members of profound isolation.

EXPECTED OUTCOMES AND GOALS

- *Expected outcome:* By the end of 8 weeks Kathleen will be free of violent behaviors, both those directed at self and others. *Short-term goals:* Kathleen will participate in a no-harm contract. Kathleen will participate in a behavioral modification program to address her aggressive acting out toward mother and others. Kathleen will express a desire to live and be able to identify daily goals and at least one long-term goal for her life.
- *Expected outcome:* By the end of 8 weeks Kathleen will display at least three new coping behaviors to deal with her feelings of anger and frustration. *Short-term goals:* Kathleen will practice suggestions for coping and will evaluate the effectiveness of these techniques. Kathleen will verbalize her feelings of frustration and anger.
- *Expected outcome:* By the end of 8 weeks, Kathleen will demonstrate behavior consistent with increased self-esteem. *Short-term goals*: Kathleen will verbalize feelings of self-worth. Kathleen will demonstrate absence of self-negating comments. Kathleen will participate in activities that allow her a sense of accomplishment.
- *Expected outcome:* By the end of 8 weeks, Kathleen will demonstrate hopefulness regarding future life. *Short-term goal*: Kathleen will state on three different occasions something that she is hopeful about.
- *Expected outcome:* By the end of 8 weeks, Kathleen will be involved in social activity apart from her mother. *Short-term goals:* Kathleen will demonstrate socially appropriate behaviors needed to initiate a friendship. Kathleen will choose a community-based activity to investigate. Kathleen will commit to weekly participation in at least one activity apart from her mother.
- *Expected outcome:* By the end of 8 weeks, Kathleen will find hope in her relationship with God. *Short-term goals:* Kathleen will make a positive statement about God. Kathleen will discuss her expectations of her relationship with God.
- *Expected outcome:* By the end of 8 weeks, each family member will express the belief that the family is functioning more effectively. *Short-term goals:* Family members will participate in eight family sessions. Family members will complete homework assignments. Family members will follow communication rules. Family members will express feelings directly to each other rather than through hostile actions and words. Family members will "try on" different roles within the family.

IMPLEMENTATION

The nurse used a variety of therapeutic techniques to address Kathleen's needs and to work toward the goals that were established for care. For instance, the nurse provided instruction to Kathleen and her family about the nature and interaction of Kathleen's various diagnoses, managing the medications that Kathleen was taking, coping techniques, and the impact of chronic stress on both individual and family functioning. She also used behavior modification strategies to set up a plan to assist Kathleen in developing more effective coping behaviors. Implementing the behavioral plan involved engaging the support of Kathleen's family and teaching them the value of responding to Kathleen in a nonreactive and consistent manner. Also, the nurse encouraged Kathleen's sister and stepfather to take charge of the daily monitoring of the behavioral plan. This approach was designed to provide more freedom for Kathleen's mother and to spread the burden of Kathleen's care more equitably among family members.

Supportive therapy techniques were used with each individual to improve self-concept, to communicate a sense of respect for each family member, to provide an empathetic ear for the expression of their stress, and to support and improve their problem-solving abilities. Once a week the nurse met with Kathleen and provided one-on-one supportive therapy designed to improve Kathleen's self-esteem, to instruct regarding expression of feelings and healthy coping techniques, and to discuss Kathleen's expressed spiritual distress. Because Kathleen belonged to a Christian church, the nurse used selected scripture passages to help Kathleen look at how precious she was in God's eyes. One evening a week the nurse met with the whole family and provided family therapy designed to free family members from rigid roles and allow greater support and understanding of each other. A third meeting was held every week with Kathleen, her mother, and usually her sister to evaluate progress and to modify the treatment goals.

The nurse assisted the mother to investigate various community supports such as the Alliance for the Mentally Ill. Kathleen's mother was able to get Kathleen accepted into an after school and weekend treatment program run by the Alliance, where Kathleen interacted with other adolescents. The Alliance also provided vocational support to Kathleen as she approached high school graduation without a clear sense of what she would do following graduation.

The nurse's case management activities included communicating with Kathleen's teachers and guidance counselor as well as linking the various physicians involved in Kathleen's care in a conference call. The connection with school personnel facilitated their understanding of Kathleen's needs and brought them into the behavioral plan. Their support was enlisted to monitor and reward positive coping behaviors that Kathleen displayed in school. The linkage with the physicians provided continuity to Kathleen's care rather than the fragmentation that had characterized it prior to the nurse's interventions. Kathleen was seen by a psychiatrist, a neurologist, and an endocrinologist . . . none of whom had ever conferred about her case. Each of these physicians was engaged in prescribing very strong medications. Once they began talking, they recognized the need to coordinate their efforts, in particular their medication-prescribing activities.

EVALUATION OF CARE

After every contact with Kathleen and her family, the nurse evaluated their progress and made modifications to the care. For instance, she recognized that Kathleen required concrete instruction about feelings. The nurse used pictures of faces displaying a variety of emotions to teach Kathleen what anger, happiness, frustration, sadness, surprise, and fear look like. Then she provided step-by-step instruction on ways to verbalize these feelings and ways to cope with strong negative feelings without hitting and screaming. After 8 weeks the nurse discharged Kathleen and her family. Kathleen was still occasionally engaging in verbal outbursts but had not hit her mother or any one else in 5 weeks. Kathleen's depression was markedly improved; she no longer expressed a desire to die, nor did she engage in self-destructive behaviors. Probably the most significant change occurred in the family's functioning. The stress level was appreciably less; everyone was calmer and much more nonreactive toward Kathleen. Kathleen's mother summed up her feelings in this way, "We are in this together for the first time." The nurse encouraged them to closely monitor not only each other's behaviors but also the emotional climate of the family. She let them know how well they were functioning, but also told them that families who deal with excessive stress may require an occasional "emotional tune-up" to stay on track.

After 24 visits that spanned 8 weeks, Kathleen was discharged with all of the expected outcomes achieved. The care manager at the insurance company expressed delight and also surprise that the psychiatric home care nurse was able to do what many other mental health professionals had been unable to achieve. The nurse responded that the nature of the care was holistic, drawing on the natural supports in the patient's life and included a tapestry of interventions that ranged from traditional nursing activities of monitoring medications, blood glucose levels, and nutritional intake to advanced practice skills of providing family therapy.

THE ADVANCED PRACTICE NURSE AS CONSULTANT

Frequently the advanced practice nurse is called on to do consultations, both internally at the home health agency as well as for external sources. The internal consultations deal with a variety of issues including the evaluation of medical patients for secondary psychiatric problems that are interfering with healing, such as depression or anxiety. The psychiatric nurse is often called upon for a professional opinion regarding staffing issues such as morale and group process. In addition, the advanced practice nurse is frequently looked to for direction on ethical and legal issues that are not as clear cut as they might be in a different type of care setting. External sources that seek the nurse as a consultant are looking for advice regarding the appropriateness of potential referrals for psychiatric home care and for clinical suggestions for managing difficult behaviors in the home setting.

THE ADVANCED PRACTICE NURSE AS PROGRAM DEVELOPER

Psychiatric home care is not a static service but evolves as the needs of patients and payors require modifications and new programs. Most psychiatric home care programs begin by serving the homebound elderly, who are diagnosed with either an affective or anxiety disorder. The expansion into other areas, such as the care of children and adolescents and home detoxification and rehabilitation, requires systematic thought and program development. It is usually the advanced practice nurse who is responsible for this evolution. The nurse is equipped with a theory base and a broad understanding of not only the individual patient and that patient's psychiatric pathology but also an understanding of change theory, the health care system, the expanding role of the nurse, and the research process, including access to literature and other resources. These qualities provide the expertise and "big picture view" that is needed as programs change.

VISION FOR FUTURE ROLE OF THE ADVANCED PRACTICE PSYCHIATRIC NURSE

As the demand for psychiatric home care services increases and pressure builds to determine the most cost-effective ways to manage the care of children and adolescents, the seriously and persistently mentally ill, and the homebound elderly, the role of the advanced practice nurse will become better defined. The nurse's future in psychiatric home care will most likely include recognition of the nurse's prescriptive authority as well as the nurse's ability and appropriateness to independently manage the majority of psychiatric home care patients including ordering the care and signing for the continuance of care. In order for this vision to become reality, the advanced practice psychiatric nurse must continue to articulate the broad dimensions of the role, to conduct research that demonstrates the clinical and cost effectiveness of nurses as primary providers of psychiatric care, and to lobby Congress and the Health Care Financing Administration (HCFA) to change the laws that govern Medicare. The Medicare system currently recognizes the advanced practice psychiatric nurse as an independent practitioner in rural areas where medical care is scarce, but has not extended that recognition to other areas where the nurse is in direct competition with physicians.

As we move into the new millenium, psychiatric home care will emerge as a major component of the psychiatric care continuum, and the advanced practice psychiatric nurse will emerge as a major provider and shaper of that care.

REFERENCES

Badgio H. Psychiatric Health Care Management: A cost effective alternative, *Home Health Line*, January, 1996: 18–23.

Carson VB. Psychiatric home care: Reflecting on the past, evaluating the present, and envisioning the future. *Caring Magazine*. 1996;32:28–34.

Carson VB. Bay Area health care psychiatric home care model. *Home Health Care Nurse*. 1995;13: 26–33.

Faukner and Gray. Behavioral outcomes and guidelines Sourcebook, *New Trends*, Findings and Outcomes, 1995. New York, Penn Plaza.

Health Care Financing Administration, Bureau of Data Management and Strategy. Data from the Medicare Decision Support System: Data Development by the Office of Research and Demonstrations. Washington, DC: HCFA;1994:62.

Health Care Financing Administration, Bureau of Data Management and Strategy. Data from the Medicare Decision Support System: Data Development by the Office of Research and Demonstrations. Washington, DC: HCFA;1993:49.

Lima B. In-home psychiatric nursing: The At-Home Mental Health Program. *Caring Magazine*. 1995; 31:14–20.

CHAPTER 8

LEGAL ISSUES IN ADVANCED PRACTICE PSYCHIATRIC NURSING

Joyce K. Laben • *Beatrice Crofts Yorker*

*I*t is important for nurses to remember that to be liable for malpractice there must be a deviation from the standard of care, not simply patient injury or dissatisfaction.

Chapter Overview

► INTRODUCTION

The legal implications of delivering mental health care must be a part of any advanced practice psychiatric nurse's knowledge base. (As a cautionary note, when a legal issue arises, the content of this chapter should not substitute for the advice of an attorney located in the jurisdiction of the advanced practice nurse.)

A brief history follows of some of the recent trends in mental health law, including discussions of pertinent issues of which advanced practice psychiatric/nurses should be aware. Mental health law did not change from the 19th century until the late 1960s.[1] From the late 1960s and continuing into the 1970s, the U.S. Supreme Court began to provide equal protection and due process to various dispossessed groups. This activity stimulated the interest of law school professors and psychiatrists to teach their students the implications of mental health law. Subsequently, some graduates of law schools went into practices that served the underprivileged, especially the mentally ill who resided in state hospitals.[2] Information on mental health law proliferated, and authors of psychiatric nursing texts began to write about this subject.

Applebaum, a prolific writer on mental health law, describes four different focal points of change that occurred from the late 1960s to the mid-1980s.[3] First, commitment law criteria became more stringent and the number of individuals who could be involuntarily hospitalized decreased. Patients were given the opportunity to participate in commitment hearings and to question and dispute the process.

The second focal point of change was the concept of the duty to protect, which followed the *Tarasoff* decision in California in the 1970s.[4] All mental health professionals should be aware of their duty to warn third parties of a dangerous patient's threats, and to take action to protect the potential victim and consider taking protective measures for the patient. This concept is discussed later in the chapter.

The right to refuse treatment, especially psychotropic medication, has been frequently litigated. Until the 1970s, it was considered almost unthinkable for a patient to challenge a prescribed medication, even though severe irreversible side effects could occur. Many states, either through case law or legislation, mandated procedural requirements for a refusing patient. These procedures could include administrative hearings, independent review by outside consultants, or the presentation of evidence in a judicial hearing.

As the fourth change, reforms in the insanity defense included the requirement that the burden of proof be placed on the defendant rather than the prosecution. Some states adopted the guilty but mentally ill concept rather than not guilty by reason of insanity. More stringent requirements for release and for supervisory controls after discharge of these individuals were instigated.[5]

LEGAL AUTHORITY FOR ADVANCED PRACTICE

As the cost and effectiveness of mental health care is scrutinized by public and private sectors, the use of advanced practice nurses (APNs) to appropriately extend the continuum of care has gained widespread support. Looking to the skills and competency of midlevel providers generated much optimism and research in the early 1970s, when the shortage of primary care physicians became critical. At that time, the prediction of decreasing numbers of primary care physicians caused schools of nursing and physician assistant programs to fill the widening gap in access to care.[6] The decreased access to care, particularly for disenfranchised populations, has resulted in initiatives aimed at educating and training midlevel providers. Rationale for the educational initiatives include the reduced cost of training clinical specialists and nurse practitioners, the rural and urban demography of existing health care providers, and the cost-effectiveness of midlevel providers. In addition, nurses can extend the access to health care through their grounding in home-based care and through provision of care in schools, community health centers, and residential treatment facilities.

HISTORICAL PERSPECTIVE

Nursing licensure was supported by the American Medical Association after all of the states enacted registration acts for physicians. However, it was more difficult for the subsequent health professionals, such as nursing, to define their scope of practice, as it was necessary to avoid encroaching upon the territory already carved out by medical practice acts.

Nursing licensure falls into three general phases. First, between 1903 and 1938, states allowed nursing registration, but it was purely voluntary and nothing prohibited the practice of nurses who were not registered. Beginning in 1938 with New York and ending in 1971, all states had enacted mandatory nursing licensure

acts. During that phase, the American Nurses' Association favored university-based education and nursing began to shed its apprentice form of training. The third phase, beginning in 1971, included the expansion of registered nurse functions and defined the advanced practice of nursing. The legal mechanisms involved in the transition from initial nurse practice acts to the incorporation of the expanded nurse role fell into the following general categories:

- No change in the nurse practice act, but reference to the rules and regulations delineated by state boards of nursing that sanction and define the qualifications for advanced practice nursing.
- Delegation of advanced practice functions by physicians through amendments to medical practice acts.
- Statutory language in the nurse practice act being updated to reflect the various aspects of advanced practice nursing.

The American Nurses' Association prefers the first approach, encouraging broad nurse practice acts that allow for regulation of advanced practice through the profession rather than the legislature.[7] As the states grapple with legally defining advanced nursing practice, most practice acts now include diagnosis, certain treatments, and often some type of prescriptive authority.[8]

CASE LAW

Although psychiatric mental health clinical specialists have not emerged specifically in the case law regarding scope of practice, two landmark cases about the scope of advanced practice nursing may guide nurses who are functioning in an expanded role. The close alliance between psychiatric mental health clinical nurse specialists and other mental health professions has benefited the integrity of advanced psychiatric nursing practice. The certification requirements are similar to those for other psychotherapists, and the standards of practice are based not only on nursing standards but on standards of psychotherapeutic modalities.

Sermchief v Gonzales[9] involved two nurse practitioners who were employed in a federally funded agency that provided lower-income clients with family planning, obstetrics, and gynecology services in three rural clinics. They took cultures for Papanicolaou tests, drew blood for serology, and provided contraceptives. They operated under physician standing orders and protocols that delineated what they could do themselves and what should be referred to a physician.

The nurses were sued by a physician group for practicing medicine without a license, and the physicians who wrote the protocols were charged with aiding and abetting the unauthorized practice of medicine. The nurses and physicians countersued, alleging that stopping their practice was a constitutional violation of their clients' free choice of health care. The case was decided against the nurse practitioners at the trial level; however, on appeal, the Missouri Supreme Court ruled in favor of the NPs. The court concluded that "nurses can assume responsibilities heretofore not considered to be within the field of professional nursing so long as those responsibilities are consistent with . . . specialized education, judgement and skill based on knowledge and application of principles desired from the biological, physical, social and nursing sciences."[10] The court responded to amicus briefs from several health organizations and heard input from consumers that emphasized the need for health care services among the populations served. A nurse educator also testified to the difference between basic nursing preparation and how a master's degree plus certification ensures the ability of advanced practice nurses to carry out diagnosis, prescription, and treatment. The court also stated that there was no evidence showing the nurses' assessment and diagnosis had exceeded the limits set forth by the protocols.

Fein v Permanente Medical Group,[11] a California case, involved a 34-year-old male attorney who sued a nurse practitioner employed in a health maintenance organization for failing to diagnose his impending myocardial infarction and for practicing outside the scope of nursing. The plaintiff had been experiencing chest pain intermittently and made an appointment to be seen in the brief appointment clinic. He voluntarily saw a nurse practitioner who examined him and consulted with the physician, who ordered an x-ray and prescribed Demerol, concluding that he was suffering from a muscle spasm. The next day, the patient continued to have intermittent pain and returned to the clinic to see a different doctor, who ordered an electrocardiogram (EKG). The EKG revealed an acute myocardial infarction and the patient was placed in the intensive care unit.

The court determined that the nurse practitioner had not exceeded the scope of practice, reasoning that when the state legislature amended the Nurse Practice Act they had expressly intended to recognize "the overlapping functions of physicians and nurses and to permit the sharing of functions with organized health care systems which provide for collaboration between physicians and registered nurses."[12] The court, however, allowed the jury to conclude that there was negligence in the failure to administer an EKG (which was available to the nurse practitioner). The ruling was vague about whether advanced practice nurses would be held to the standard of care of a physician or the standard of care of a similarly situated nurse practitioner.

When organized nursing groups expressed concern over the implication that physicians could testify about the standard of care of nurse practitioners, the California Supreme Court clarified that the jury instructions that had held the nurse to a physician standard of care were in error. These two cases together show judicial recognition that there is not a single profession that can claim ownership of functions such as diagnostic reasoning, physical assessment, treatment, and prescription. The court also supported the view that the standard of care of advanced practice nurses should be measured against other advanced practice nurses rather than physicians. [13]

ASSESSMENT OF QUALITY OF CARE

Advanced practice nurses (predominantly nurse practitioners and nurse midwives) have been the focus of many clinical effectiveness studies over the past 25 years. The results have shown at least equal and often superior performance of these groups of nurses relative to physician care in quality, access, and cost.[14] In 1990, the Office of Technology Assessment released a comprehensive study to the Senate Committee on Appropriations on the effectiveness of nurse practitioners, nurse-midwives, and physician assistants in meeting the nation's health care needs. They concluded that "in terms of quality of care, nurse practitioners (NPs) appear to provide care that is of as high quality as that of physicians. . . . There is some evidence that NPs working, according to protocols, may provide services of even better quality than those provided by some physicians."[15] In order to reach this conclusion, the study cited 268 sources, which included measures of outcome and process, patient satisfaction, and physician acceptance.

BARRIERS TO EFFECTIVE USE OF ADVANCED PRACTICE NURSES

As Safreit[16] points out, the simple timing of medical practice acts created a large barrier for other health professionals. For example, North Carolina broadly defines the practice of medicine and prohibits others from engaging in any activity that appears to "treat any human ailment, physical or mental, or any physical injury to or deformity of another person."[17] This illustrates the history of medical preemption that has characterized the "often-tortured efforts" of nursing and other health disciplines to carve out a scope of practice following medical practice acts.[18]

The diversity in titles of advanced practice nurses and their differing levels of statutory de-

pendence or independence of physicians does not help achieve recognition of the expanded role of nurses. In at least 12 states, advanced nurse providers are not regulated by the board of medicine, pharmacists, joint committees, or "mixed regulators."[19]

At least 40 states currently have statutory or regulatory provisions for advanced practice nurses to have some form of prescriptive authority. Many are clearly a delegation of the physician's authority to prescribe, while others are more cognizant of the independent skills and judgment of nurses. This results in a variety of practices by nurses—using protocols with physician signatures, obtaining a physician co-signature, calling in prescriptions, following protocols established by state regulatory boards, or functioning only in statutorily specified practice settings such as public health or government-operated clinics that have institutional policies regarding prescriptive abilities. Advanced practice psychiatric nurses need to be aware that the 1994 *Standards of Psychiatric-Mental Health Practice* include "prescription of pharmacologic agents" under the heading "advanced practice interventions." The *Standards* state that this activity is to be done in accordance with the state nursing practice act.[20] Talley and Brooke provide an excellent overview of the implications of prescriptive authority for advanced practice psychiatric nurses in their 1992 article, which discusses the unique issues faced by psychiatric nurses compared to nurse practitioners or nurses in primary care settings.[21]

As demand for cost-effective, accessible mental health services increases, advanced practice psychiatric nurses should know that legal mechanisms support their expanded role, and both the courts and policy makers see the benefits of removing barriers to independent practice. As the health care agenda proceeds, psychiatric mental health clinical nurse specialists are in an excellent position to advocate for, and demonstrate, their role in a collaborative mental health care system.

INFORMED CONSENT

At the beginning of this century, Supreme Court Judge Benjamin Cardozo wrote, "every human being of adult years and sound mind has a right to determine what shall be done with his own body."[22] Consent has been a tradition in this country for many years, but the concept of informed consent, rather than simple consent, has been more prevalent since the 1960s. From Judge Cardozo's definition, there would be some question as to whether a mentally ill individual would be competent to make a decision relative to his or her treatment.

The elements of informed consent include the right to information concerning a specified treatment, including the material risks and benefits of the treatment; and information on the alternatives to the treatment, including the material risks and benefits. A material risk is something to which a person would attach great importance. For example, tardive dyskinesia, which can be irreversible, would be a material risk that a patient would consider very important.[23]

Grisso and Applebaum evaluated competence to consent to psychiatric and medical treatments. Using reliable instruments, they assessed the abilities of six groups to consent to treatment. The groups included recently hospitalized patients with diagnoses of schizophrenia, major depression, and ischemic heart disease. In addition, three groups of individuals who were not ill and who resided in the community were matched with the hospitalized patients, based on demographic data. The findings included measures as to the person's understanding, appreciation, and reasoning. Patients with mental illness did have more deficits than the physically or medically ill patients and the control groups. Impairments for the patients with schizophrenia were more prominent and consistent than for patients with the diagnosis of depression. Despite this result, the majority of individuals with schizophrenia did not perform substantially worse than other patients or the community group. The mean for the group with schizophrenia was attributed to a minority of this population. This minority demonstrated severe psychiatric symptomatology.

The implications of this study indicate that mentally ill persons with major mental illnesses can take part in decision-making related to their mental illness. Almost 50 percent of the individuals with schizophrenia and 76 percent of the individuals with depression performed sufficiently in all of the "decision-making measures and a significant portion performed at or above the mean for persons without mental illness."[24]

Some of the findings demonstrated that the patient groups responded with better comprehension after the information was provided a second time, rather than after one disclosure. This fact indicates that the mental health professional should consider informed consent about treatment an ongoing process. Individuals with schizophrenia might have a substantial deficit in understanding, especially if there is a thought disturbance such as delusions and hallucinations. Additional assessment or frequent contacts with the individual about treatment, especially when first initiated, should occur as often as feasible. Development of a tool that can be administered in a short period of time was to be investigated.

Regulations for informed consent vary from jurisdiction to jurisdiction. In Ohio, state regulations provide that a treating professional can check a box indicating that informed consent has been given. In addition, a note in the narrative portion of the record must be completed. In one review project of 87 records, 77 had checks in the boxes, but there were only 55 notes recorded. Of these, only 34 were considered to be acceptable. The deficiencies in the other records included failure to record the reason for prescribing the medication, and a lack of discussion of the benefits and risks associated with the drug and the alternatives that are available.[25]

Extreme care with informed consent should be practiced when using the mentally disabled as research subjects. This is especially true with regard to the elderly. Because people are living longer, more individuals are afflicted with Alzheimer's disease and other dementias. There is great pressure to discover medications and interventions to relieve the burden of the disabled and their family members. All advanced practice nurses serving on institutional review boards need to be aware of some of the following issues. Dresser (1996) defines these issues as guidelines:

- Use procedures that will identify subjects who can make decisions for themselves; encourage subjects to share decisions with significant others; health care proxies should be informed of the ethical standards before making decisions about participation in research.
- If an individual objects to involvement in a research project, he or she should be excluded unless a direct benefit can be attributed to participation.
- Subject populations should have representation when reviewing and planning potential research.[26]

Advanced practice nurses should be aware of state statutes, regulations, and case law about informed consent, especially for prescribing medications. The nurse should understand the elements of informed consent and be knowledgeable about the ethical and legal standards related to research. Moreover, the nurse should recognize that ongoing and repeated explanations for the necessity of some treatments might need to be initiated, especially for patients diagnosed with schizophrenia.

COMMITMENT

The three paths to hospitalization in a mental health facility are voluntary, emergency, and judicial or indefinite commitment.[27] An individual who is of age to be legally considered an adult can sign voluntarily into a mental health facility. Unless evidence suggests that he or she is a danger to self or others, requiring involuntary procedures, the person may leave upon request. Voluntary hospitalization is usually a preferable route for inpatient treatment. In some instances, however, the patient's condition precludes this.

EMERGENCY COMMITMENT

Emergency commitment is usually for a limited time and based on the criteria of dangerousness to self or others. When a mental health professional concludes that a person is in need of treatment, the least restrictive alternative should be considered and selected. Availability of an array of alternatives is paramount if the person is to avoid hospitalization. Segal and associates (1996) observed and appraised clinicians' evaluations of 425 patients in seven California county general hospitals. Less restrictive alternatives were present for 61 percent of the patients but were used only 39 percent of the time, missed in 14 percent of the cases, and thought about but not employed in 8 percent of the evaluations. A major point in the article was that, with current cost constraints, a focus should be placed on developing supervised hospital alternatives. Encouragement for clinicians to "engage the patient in treatment" was also emphasized.[28]

For an emergency commitment, the law in some states provides that designated mental health professionals have the authority to sign the initial commitment paper, while others specifically list a physician or psychologist.[29] When advanced practice nurses do sign commitment papers and list symptoms, it is critical that the papers be completed in a manner that a layperson can understand. The nurse should describe the psychotic behavior rather than merely labeling it delusional or hallucinatory. The nurse should recount specifically how the person was dangerous (for example, "Mr. Jones threatened his mother with a knife").

INDEFINITE OR JUDICIAL COMMITMENT

Judicial or involuntary, indefinite commitment is becoming rare in the age of expanding managed care. It continues, however, to be an option. In the 1970s, with the increase in mental health litigation, many cases adopted restrictive mechanisms that limited commitment options. Since that time, especially with large numbers of mentally ill homeless persons on the streets or languishing in local jails, commitment standards have been expanded to include the gravely disabled with "inability to exercise self-control in addition to the terms likelihood of serious harm or dangerousness to self or others."[30] The standard or proof for commitment is clear and convincing evidence. It is more proof than "preponderance of the evidence," which is required in a civil trial for malpractice, and less than "beyond reasonable doubt," as required in a criminal trial.[31]

In an Oregon case, a woman was diagnosed with a form of schizophrenia known as Capgras syndrome. It caused her to believe that people were replaced by look-alikes. She lived in a condominium complex and received Social Security and retirement benefits. She was able to take care of herself, including shopping and managing her money. There were instances where she would refrain from going to the grocery store and would deny her social worker access to her home. Based on this information, a trial court committed her. The appeals court reversed this decision, commenting that evidence was not submitted detailing how many shopping trips she missed or whether she was receiving other health care besides visits from the social worker. Moreover, no information substantiated whether she was considered dangerous. This case clearly points out the importance of delineating the reason for request of commitment.[32]

MANDATORY OUTPATIENT COMMITMENT

Mandatory outpatient commitment is a more recent development. It is usually initiated when a patient is noncompliant with treatment once discharged from an inpatient setting. As in civil commitment for inpatient care, the doctrine of *parens patriae* is the basis for such laws. This legal authority allows the state the authority to protect those who are disabled. According to Torrey and Kaplan (1995), 35 states and the District of Columbia have such laws, but they are commonly used in only 12 states.[33]

Questions have been raised in some instances as to the amount of coercion used by the state and the potential for great intrusiveness into an individual's life.[34] The contrary argument set forth is that this procedure prevents frequent rehospitalization of noncompliant patients and ultimately improves the overall quality of life.[35]

An example of a mandatory outpatient commitment is the following. K.J.L. resided in a residential rehabilitation program after suffering head injuries. He had periods of assaultive behavior toward his nurse and other residents. When he did not take his medication, he became assaultive and aggressive. The court ordered him to undergo 90 days of outpatient treatment subsequent to his discharge, to which he objected. The reason for the outpatient treatment was to insure that K.J.L. took his medication. The state Supreme Court of North Dakota ruled that there was clear and convincing evidence that there was a need for outpatient treatment based on his behavior and diagnosis of organic mental disorder and mood disturbance with a hypomanic state caused by his head injuries.[36]

CONFIDENTIALITY

Advanced practice nurses are well aware of the responsibility for confidentiality in practice. Not as well understood, however, is the concept of privileged communication. Privilege is generally granted by statutory authority and allows the professional, such as an advanced practice nurse, psychiatrist, lawyer, and member of the clergy, to keep information given to them by patients, clients, and parishioners confidential. All 50 states and the District of Columbia have enacted some form of privilege for therapists.[37] This does not necessarily mean that the privilege would extend to an advanced practice psychiatric nurse, so each nurse should be aware of the law in the state where he or she is practicing. In Utah, privilege is extended to "marriage and family therapists, professional counselors, and psychiatric mental health nurse specialists."[38]

The advanced practice nurse needs the authorization of the patient to release information. Privilege exists only in the context of the therapeutic relationship. Instances where the issue might arise would be in a correctional facility where a nurse therapist counseled an inmate who confessed to a commission of a crime for which there had been no conviction. It is important for the nurse to be aware of the statutes in the state where practicing, as not all advanced practice psychiatric nurses have such a privilege.[39]

In a recent U.S. Supreme Court ruling (*Jaffee v Redmond*, 1996), the court stated that, according to the Federal Rule of Evidence 501, social workers do have a psychotherapist–patient privilege. The facts of this case are that Mary Lu Redmond, a former police officer, shot and killed Ricky Allen. A lawsuit was filed by a petitioner for the deceased, Allen, alleging that Redmond had violated Allen's constitutional rights by using unreasonable force in the encounter with him. At the trial, there was disagreement about the facts of the incident. After the death of Allen, Redmond sought counseling services with a social worker. At depositions and the trial, the social worker and Redmond both refused to answer questions and stated they could not recall details of the therapy sessions. The judge in the trial court instructed the jury that it could be concluded that the notes of the therapist must have been unfavorable to the defendant, Redmond. The jury awarded the petitioner a total of $545,000 on state and federal claims.[40]

The Court of Appeals for the Seventh Circuit reversed and remanded for a new trial. On appeal, the U.S. Supreme Court pointed out that the state of Illinois, in which the suit was brought, extended a therapeutic privilege to social workers and supported the confidentiality of the exchange between the social worker and Redmond.

Whether this privilege would extend to the advanced practice psychiatric nurse was not explicitly decided. However, if the state jurisdiction allows privilege for the nurse, it is probable that the *federal* courts would also recognize it. It should be emphasized that not all states recognize a nurse–patient privilege.

DUTY TO PROTECT

All advanced practice nurses should be aware of the duty to warn third parties. The first legal case in which precedent was established that a mental health professional should warn third parties of impending danger from a patient was *Tarasoff v Regents of the University of California* (1974), which was decided more than 20 years ago.[41] The well-known facts of this particular case are that Mr. Poddar was a student at the University of California when he met Ms. Tarasoff. They dated each other during one semester in 1968. She eventually communicated to Poddar that she did not want an exclusive relationship with him. He was distraught over this action and sought counseling from a psychologist at the University. He indicated to the psychologist that he intended to harm Ms. Tarasoff. Campus security was notified and spoke with him and concluded that no further action was needed.

When Ms. Tarasoff returned from a trip out of the country, Mr. Poddar went to her home and killed her. The ruling in a suit filed against the University of California by her family, and later appealed to the Supreme Court of California, stated that the therapist had a duty to warn third parties if a patient presents a danger to a specified individual.

Since this ruling, 23 states other than California have adopted the *Tarasoff* duty.[42] "*Tarasoff* caused controversy yet it has been widely accepted (and rarely rejected) by courts and legislatures in the United States as a foundation for establishing duties of reasonable care upon psychotherapists to warn, control, and/or protect potential victims of their patients who have expressed violent intentions."[43] Numerous jurisdictions have adopted a statutory rule imposing a duty to warn in situations similar to that addressed in *Tarasoff*.[44] Several states have passed statutes exempting mental health professionals from liability if a warning is given. In some instances, nurses are specifically named as being exempt.[45] Advanced practice nurses should be aware of the law in their jurisdictions, including not only warning third parties but also when it is appropriate to hospitalize to protect the public.

REPORTING LAWS

Advanced practice nurses should know whom to contact when child abuse is suspected. Professional nurses have a responsibility to report child abuse in all jurisdictions. This duty is paramount over the responsibility to keep information private and confidential in a therapeutic relationship.

One particular case illustrates the dilemma that mental health professionals could encounter. Ms. Fewell brought a suit against a physician, Dr. Besner, and the St. Vincent Health Center, for infliction of emotional distress. Dr. Besner had informed the county coroner that Fewell had communicated to him that she had suffocated her 4-month-old son. The death had been deemed accidental. After the death, Fewell became depressed and suicidal and was involuntarily hospitalized, at which time she conveyed the cause of death to the doctor. She was subsequently charged with criminal homicide.

The court stated that even though there was a psychotherapist–patient privilege, the child protection laws prevailed over the privileged communication. Fewell had another child at home who could also have been a victim of abuse, and the doctor, although he had no specific duty to report in this instance because he had had no contact with the dead infant, had immunity in this case.[46]

RIGHTS OF PATIENTS

RIGHT TO REFUSE MEDICATION

In the 1970s, lawsuits were filed related to a patient's right to refuse medication. Two prominent cases, *Rogers v Okin* (1979) filed in Massachusetts, and *Rennie v Klein* (1978), filed in New Jersey, caused great consternation in the psychiatric community.[47] An impetus for filing the suits was the irreversible side effects that could result from the use of some neuroleptic medications.

The legal decisions resulted in several different approaches to the problem. The *Rogers* decision decreed that a guardian needed to be appointed for incompetent patients, and that the final decision about treatment should be left to a judge. The standard to be used (Applebaum, 1994) for determination of medication administration was "substituted judgement"—would the person, if competent, consent to the proposed treatment?[48] The logic for the judicial decision making was that antipsychotic medication was an intrusive treatment and only a judge could be an objective arbitrator.

Other jurisdictions relied on review by panels within the various facilities, by independent psychiatrists, by a panel of outside consultants, or by the medical director.[49] Despite the concern of many mental health professionals that the right to refuse medication would greatly impede the delivery of mental health care, this has not proven to be the result. Applebaum reviewed many studies and concluded that "only a small minority of refusals are upheld by the reviewing body; and given the continuing trend toward judicial review, the percentage is likely to become even smaller in the future."[50]

The cases continue to be adjudicated in relation to a patient's right to refuse treatment. In a recent ruling in Connecticut,[51] it was found that a patient, despite his conservator's consent to administration of psychotropic drugs, had the option to have his own ability to give informed consent reviewed by the probate court.[51]

More and more jurisdictions are giving advanced practice nurses prescriptive authority. It is important for the nurse to review the statutory and case law, and the rules and regulations promulgated by the jurisdiction in which he or she is practicing, in order to be aware of the responsibility to a refusing patient. Informed consent by the individual is imperative. Appropriate monitoring for side effects is essential. Possible interactions with other medications and appropriate doses, especially for the elderly, should be explored. Nothing, however, substitutes for a caring, trusting therapeutic relationship where the nurse is willing to listen to complaints about medications and to adjust treatment modalities when appropriate. Consultation and second opinions can also be very helpful.

ELECTROCONVULSIVE THERAPY

Electroconvulsive therapy (ECT), one of the oldest known treatments for depression, continues to cause controversy. "Few other medical treatments have been in use for as long (more than 40 years), yet remain so controversial."[52] A recent article described the growing concern about its use, especially for the elderly.[53] Information about the frequency of its use is hampered by lack of data. Only three states—Texas, California, and Colorado, with Texas having the most stringent requirements—mandate reporting of the numbers of patients who undergo ECT.[54] It is clear from the Texas data that once Medicare pays, the number of treatments increases. The overwhelming majority of recipients are white females over age 65.[55]

For the knowledgeable advanced practice nurse working in a facility where ECT is administered, there are important factors to consider. Knowledge about the regulation of administration of ECT is imperative. California, for example, has stringent requirements for administration, including what data must be disclosed for informed consent.[56] Factors that must be disclosed include the following.

- The need for treatment based on the patient's condition.
- A description of the procedure.
- The proposed frequency of treatments and length of time that will be required.
- The risks and potential side effects (especially memory loss), including whether the risks can be controlled or limited.
- A discussion of the controversy about the effectiveness of such treatment.

- Alternative treatments.
- The reason the physician is recommending this particular treatment.
- The right to refuse treatment at any time.[57]

If the patient is deemed incompetent, the nurse should know the procedure to follow for obtaining consent in the particular jurisdiction. Courts in California are reluctant to consent to ECT for an incompetent person. "Only if a patient utterly lacks comprehension of what is being proposed will he or she be found incompetent."[58] Patients should be free of coercion, and one author recommends that the nurse not be over-reassuring when information is requested by the patient.[59]

Fitzsimmons (1995) lists the pre-ECT assessment that should be completed, including physical examination, electrocardiogram, blood work, and urinalysis. Other tests such as a computed tomography (CT) scan might be requested. Awareness of the recommended procedures by experts is pertinent knowledge for nurses working or supervising in this area. A reference on essential pre-ECT requirements should be available in all hospitals where ECT is performed.[60] Recently, a reported death in Texas indicated that a patient died shortly after administration of shock therapy, and there was no medical history or physical exam in the medical record.[61]

AMERICANS WITH DISABILITIES ACT

The Americans with Disabilities Act (ADA) was passed in 1990. It defines disability as "any physical and mental impairment that limits any major life activity."[62] There are some exclusions, if an individual uses a controlled substance for unlawful purposes or takes prescribed medication without monitoring by a licensed health care provider, there is no disability under the ADA. The ADA also specifically excludes such problems as transsexualism, pedophilia, gender identity disorders that have not resulted from a physical impairment, and kleptomania or pyromania.[63]

Understanding the types of accommodations to implement for the mentally disabled has sometimes been confusing for employers. Compounding the issue is the fact that some clients' vocational counselors persuade the mentally disabled to withhold information about psychiatric hospitalization or treatment for mental illness. Undoubtedly this advice is based on the issue of stigma and the fear that revelation of a mental health problem will affect them at work or in the job market.[64] If the mentally disabled person does not communicate to the employer about the mental illness, it is difficult, however, to make an accommodation. In reviewing three cases of workers with schizophrenia, Kaufman (1993) found that the usual accommodations were flexible work hours, especially if it was necessary to visit the mental health provider; protecting the employee's privacy; and reducing stress when possible and necessary.[65] Advanced practice psychiatric nurses, especially those in management positions, should be aware of the ADA and the kinds of adaptations that can be implemented to ensure a successful work experience for the individual.

FORENSIC EVALUATIONS

Nurses working with forensic patients should be aware of two kinds of evaluations that may be requested by the court when criminal charges have been made: one for competency to stand trial and the other for assessment of criminal responsibility. In the 1990s, these evaluations are frequently performed on an outpatient basis.

COMPETENCY TO STAND TRIAL

To evaluate competency to stand trial, the examiner should assess the defendant's ability to understand what criminal charges have been filed; evaluate if the defendant can appropriately advise the defense attorney and control his or her behavior in the courtroom; assess the individual's understanding of the roles of participants in the legal process, that is, what are the various roles of the participants including the judge, prosecuting attorney, jury, and defense attorney; and evaluate the defendant's knowledge of the con-

sequences of the criminal charges. To assess competency to stand trial, it is recommended that any advanced practice nurse who desires to become involved in this process, or is mandated to do so by virtue of employment, participate in a training course in order to learn how to assess for competency, and to learn the techniques of writing letters to the court and being effective in courtroom testimony.

Since 1972, after *Jackson v Indiana* was decided by the Supreme Court, more and more evaluations have been done in the outpatient setting. Jackson was mentally retarded and had hearing and speech impairments. Consequently, he had great difficulty communicating. He was charged with two counts of robbery for a sum of nine dollars. Because of his inability to communicate, he would never be competent to stand trial. At the time that his case reached the U.S. Supreme Court, he had been hospitalized for three and one-half years. The court ruled that the defendant could not be detained on the issue of competency to stand trial without civil commitment for more than a "reasonable period of time," and that three and one-half years was too long.[66] Because many states had residents confined for long periods of time, states were forced to look at the evaluation process for competency to stand trial.[67]

CRIMINAL RESPONSIBILITY (INSANITY DEFENSE)

The insanity defense relates to the defendant's state of mind at the time of the commission of the offense. Competency to stand trial relates to the ability of the defendant to participate in the defense in the courtroom during the trial. Evaluations by mental health professionals may be regulated by statute or rules and regulations of the various states. Some states do not allow persons other than psychologists or psychiatrists to testify on this issue.[68]

The insanity defense has been a part of the criminal justice system for many years. To convict someone of a criminal offense, there must be intent (*mens rea*). If the person cannot form the requisite intent because of symptoms of mental illness, then there is no guilt.[69] In the United States, many jurisdictions have adopted a modern version of the insanity defense, which essentially states that if the individual is unable, because of mental illness, to understand or appreciate the wrongfulness of the conduct or has an inability to modify conduct as the law requires, he or she will not be held responsible.[70] For example, if voices told a mentally ill defendant to rob a bank, and because of the hallucinations the defendant did not realize that it was wrong to do so, this evidence could be presented to the court by the defense. When the defense raises the issue of insanity, in many instances the prosecution and the defense will present mental health professionals as witnesses. There may be conflicting testimony about the state of mind of the individual on the day of the commission of the crime. It is up to the judge or jury to accept or reject the insanity plea of the defendant.

In a recent case, a defendant raised a battered spouse defense rather than an insanity defense. Clara Hess was convicted of murder. She had refused to submit to examination by government experts about her alleged battered woman's syndrome. The Ninth Circuit Court of Appeals ruled that even though the battered woman's syndrome is not an insanity defense, it is based on psychological and psychiatric evaluation and testing. The court ruled that there could be a requirement that she be examined by government experts without defense counsel present, as well as her known experts.[71]

MANAGED CARE

The need for health care reform has been evident for some time because of rising health care costs. Managed care has been increasingly initiated across the country, and the advanced practice nurse should be aware of the different types of structures for managed care.

The most distinguishing characteristic of the structures is whether they are for profit or nonprofit.[72] The for-profit plans trade shares pub-

licly and are not guided by the rules of charitable organizations.[73] For-profit administrative costs can include large executive salaries and bonuses, depending on the success of the organization. Nonprofit organizations tend to run much lower administrative costs.[74]

Several types of organizations fit under the managed care umbrella. Preferred provider organizations sign contracts with managed care organizations and are paid on a fee-for-service basis, usually discounted. In a group model HMO, the health care provider is a member of a group that contracts with one or several HMOs. The group is paid a capitated rate in advance of providing services. In many instances, the health care provider is paid a specific salary, which can include a bonus or other financial incentives.[75]

In staff HMOs, the health care provider is an employee who receives a salary along with other financial inducements. Before joining any managed care organization, it would be important to inquire if the system is capitated, and if so, the number of covered lives. Are mental health services included in the services provided and are they carved out? It is difficult to assess how many covered lives are sufficient, as rates can vary within even small geographic areas.[76] A major issue in all of these programs is the question of whether care will be withheld to keep down costs. Christensen emphasizes, "If health plan subscribers are educated and involved in their health care, they may be less likely to accept inadequate care, and more likely to understand the financial trade-offs involved in every health care decision".[77]

CONTRACTING

It is important to be informed about certain aspects of a managed care organization before a mental health provider signs a contract to provide services. Obtaining legal consultation to review terms of the contract before signing is imperative. Several aspects of the contract need to be considered: What services are to be provided by the advanced practice nurse? What services can be referred to another subcontractor?[78] Is reimbursement based on fee for service or a capitated rate, and what are the billing procedures and payment provisions? Is there additional remuneration for certain "risk pools" such as the seriously and persistently mentally ill? What are the co-payment and deductible expenses required of patients?[79]

What are the quality assurance and utilization review procedures to which the provider must submit?[80] What are the provisions for renewal or termination of contracts? Are there indemnification and malpractice insurance stipulations? Are there certain requirements for disclosure, such as continued licensing or certification? Is there a noncompete clause within a particular region or area?[81]

An advanced nurse practitioner who wants to become a provider for a managed care company should inquire about panel openings and obtain information about the application process.[82] The provider should confirm that he or she is in compliance with federal and state law, especially any antitrust law that is applicable.

Even though managed care is a challenge to the advanced practice nurse, Haber (1994) recommends that "it makes economic sense to make a friend of the managed care delivery system."[83] She believes that managed care can be an opportunity for advanced practice psychiatric nurses to become providers in the network of services that are being developed. Shore and Biegel (1996) write, "The challenges to all mental health professionals are to prepare themselves to assume responsibility for population-based practice without losing concern for the care of individual patients and to strike a balance between individual professional responsibility and corporate accountability, both of which will be demanded by patients and funding sources."[84]

MALPRACTICE

The area of psychiatric mental health is generally considered a low malpractice risk. Psychiatry does, however, have some clear categories of practitioner and hospital liability. A study by the American Psychiatric Association revealed that 30 percent of psychiatric malpractice claims were for negligent treatment; 20 percent involved medication issues; 11 percent, negligent supervision; 10 percent, improper confinement; 10 percent, misdiagnosis; 6 percent, undue familiarity (sexual misconduct); and the remaining 7 percent such claims as breach of confidentiality, lack of informed consent, abandonment, and negligent electroconvulsive therapy.[85] The leading dollar awards for successfully litigated psychiatric claims are for inpatient suicide, failure to adequately protect a victim from homicide by a psychiatric patient, and patient injury due to negligence.[86] Nurses should be aware that a patient injury or self injury does not automatically mean that a malpractice claim will succeed. The following elements must be met to litigate a malpractice claim.

1. *Duty*. The care provider must have established a relationship with the plaintiff.
2. *Breach of duty*. The care provider must have behaved in a way that falls below the standard of care.
3. *Causation*. This can be factual causation or "proximate cause," meaning that the breach of duty more likely caused the injury than not.
4. *Damages*. The patient must have suffered actual injury, death, or emotional distress. In some cases, a court will award punitive damages if the injury is not significant but the court wants to deter the grossly negligent or willful misconduct of the defendant care providers.[87]

It is also important for advanced practice psychiatric nurses to know that the standard of care used to determine whether a care provider has breached his or her duty is determined in three ways. First, the American Nurses' Association *Statement on Psychiatric-Mental Health Clinical Practice* (1994) would provide guidance.[88] Many legal claims involve questions of nursing practice that are not specifically referred to in the published *Standards*. Thus, the second source of standards of care would be the policies and procedures of the agency. If there is clearly a deviation from a published policy, then there will most likely be a determination of negligence. Nursing administrators should keep in mind this use of policies and procedures and should only publish the essential elements of any policy. Publishing an ideal policy that is not realistic for the agency resources places nurses in a position of appearing negligent if they fail to meet every element of a given policy.

Third, expert witnesses are used to establish the standard of care of a similarly qualified and situated psychiatric nurse. This does not mean that a nurse who is being sued would need to have acted the way that the expert witness would have acted. The expert is simply qualified, based on experience and training, to make a determination of the appropriate standard of care for the qualifications of the nurse defendant. As discussed in the *Fein* case, in some cases a similarly qualified non-nurse mental health care provider may be allowed to address the standard of care. For example, if an advanced practice nurse is functioning as a therapist in a community mental health center, a master's-prepared social worker or even a clinical psychologist might testify regarding the generally accepted standard of care for an outpatient community.

CASE LAW

The majority of successful claims for patient suicide involve inpatient suicide. In general, the courts are reluctant to second-guess the clinical judgment of a psychotherapist who must balance the patient's right to treatment in the "least restrictive environment" with protecting a patient from self-harm. Successful cases involving outpatient suicide have required a strong showing that a reasonable psychotherapist would have made the decision to hospitalize any patient who manifested features identical to those of the patient in question. Advanced practice psychiatric nurses should be familiar with the case law against all mental health professionals (not just

nurses) practicing in similar circumstances. For example, a nurse psychotherapist engaged in independent practice with the ability to hospitalize patients would look at the case law related to psychiatrists who are engaged in psychotherapy and make hospitalization decisions. The same general guidelines would apply to liability for the acts of homicidal patients.

The cases that specifically involve psychiatric nurses as named defendants also tend to involve hospital care. Claims against psychiatric nurses for negligence include an allegation that a multidisciplinary team decision to allow an agitated and disoriented patient out on pass was negligent after the patient threw herself in front of a truck and sustained multiple injuries.[89] The appeals court dismissed the malpractice and negligence claims. Another common claim against nurses is for failure to restrain a confused or debilitated patient who incurs injury. In the case of *Brooks v Coliseum Park Hospital* (1988), a patient with Alzheimer's disease fell while getting out of bed during the night. The plaintiff's nurse expert witness alleged that the nurses should have used siderails on the patient's bed. The psychiatric nurse expert witness for the defendants explained the current treatment philosophies of helping patients attain their maximum level of functioning and of promoting mobility when feasible. She and the physician expert also explained that studies show that siderails may increase injuries in the confused elderly. The court found that the hospital had used reasonable care, and stated that "the mere failure of a hospital to furnish a constant attendant to a patient does not constitute negligence."[90]

Other claims against psychiatric nurses and hospitals have been made for patient elopement,[91] fractured bones as a result of electroconvulsive therapy,[92] failure to supervise unlicensed personnel who perform illegal acts, sexual contact between patients, extended use of physical restraints rather than medication to control psychotic behavior with an adolescent patient,[93] intent to defraud third-party payers by unnecessary or prolonged hospitalization[94,95] and allegations that psychiatric nurses aggravated an adolescent male patient's sexual confusion.[96] Many of these claims were decided in favor of the nurses or the hospitals involved. In conclusion, it is important for nurses to remember that there must be a deviation from the standard of care, not simply patient injury or dissatisfaction, to be liable for malpractice.

One interesting case demonstrates the importance of advocating for a patient when insurance coverage is denied.[97] Joe was 16 years old and hospitalized for depression with suicidal ideation. He was treated by a physician, a nurse therapist, and a social worker. The doctor wanted a blood level of the patient's medication to be drawn on July 13th; however, the patient's insurance was due to run out on July 12th. The parents agreed to guarantee payment for 2 extra days. Subsequently, he was discharged on July 14th. Joe went with his family on vacation and was seen for follow-up on July 22nd and 24th in an outpatient clinic. On July 30th, he failed to make his appointment, and on July 31st he took an overdose of an antidepressant and died.

A suit for wrongful death was brought by Joe's parents against the hospital and the corporation that owned the hospital. Testimony was given that the nurse therapist had been on vacation and upon his return was surprised that Joe had been discharged. An expert witness stated that after study, it was concluded that the discharge was based on expiration of insurance benefits and not on the patient's condition. The jury awarded the parents damages. In this particular case, there was a nurse involved, although he did not have input into the decision to discharge. It is particularly important during these times of cost constraints, if the advanced practice nurse is requesting continued care, either inpatient or outpatient, that an understanding of the appeal process to the insurance company be part of the knowledge base of the nurse, so that the best interests of the patient are taken into consideration.[98]

ERISA AND MALPRACTICE

In 1976, Senator Jacob Javits initiated legislation, the Employment Retirement Income Security Act (ERISA), to protect employee pension plans if the employer's company went bankrupt. Unknown to the health care industry, provisions for health care benefits were added. The legislation "removed self-insured pension and benefit programs from states' jurisdiction."[99] Stone comments that this effectively exempted any plan that was formed under ERISA from a malpractice claim.[100] Claims that are filed and removed from the jurisdiction of state courts have usually been dismissed. Health care providers for these plans should be aware that they may be a target for a suit when providing care for ERISA-exempt organizations. This strategy often leaves the health care provider and not the care plan to bear an "undue share" of the malpractice burden.[101] Kilcullen recommends that ERISA be amended to allow for recovery from the plan if needed health care is withheld.[102]

REFERENCES

1. P.S. Applebaum, *Almost a Revolution: Mental Health Law and the Limits of Change*, New York: Oxford University Press (1994).
2. *Id.*
3. *Id.* at 211.
4. *Tarasoff v. Regents of the University of California,* 592 P.d. 533 (Cal. 1974) or 551 P2d 334 (Cal. 1976).
5. *Supra*, note 1.
6. C. Harrington, S.L. Feetham, P.A. Moccia, G.R. Smith, Health Care Access: Problems and Policy Recommendations. In P.R. Lee & C.L. Estes (eds.), *The Nation's Health*, Fourth Edition, Boston, MA: Jones and Bartlett Publishers (1994).
7. P.S. Chally & B.C. Yorker, Legal Parameters for Expanded Roles in Nursing, *Journal of Neuroscience Nursing* 21:258–260 (1991).
8. N.J. Brent, *The Nurse Practitioner after* Sermchief and Fein: Smooth Sailing or Rough Waters? *Valparaiso Law Review* 21(2) 221–243 (1987).
9. *Sermchief v. Gonzales*, 660 S.W. 2d 683 (Mo. 1983).
10. *Id.* at 190.
11. *Fein v. Permanente Medical Group*, 695 P2d 665 (Cal. 1985).

12. *Id.* at 190.
13. J.A. Smith & M.E. Kelly, Nurses employed as practitioners, anesthetists, midwives, clinical specialists. In C.E. Northrop & M.E. Kelly, *Legal Issues in Nursing*, St. Louis, MO: C.V. Mosby Co. (1987).
14. B.J. Safriet, *Health Care Dollars and Regulatory Sense: The Role of Advanced Practice Nursing*, Yale Journal on Regulation 9(2)417–488 and M. Beck, *Improving America's Health Care: Authorizing Independent Prescriptive Privileges for Advanced Practice Nurses*, University of San Francisco Law Review 29: 951–998 (1995).
15. Abstracts of Case Studies in the Costs and Effectiveness of Nurse Practitioners, 1990: Office of Technology Assessment.
16. *Id. supra*, note 14.
17. North Carolina General Statutes 90-18, 1983.
18. *Id. supra*, note 14 at 442.
19. *Id.*
20. American Nurses Association, *A Statement on Psychiatric-Mental Health Nursing Practice*, Washington, DC: ANA (1994) at 33.
21. S. Talley & P.S. Brooke, *Prescriptive Authority for Psychiatric Clinical Specialists: Framing the Issues*, Archives of Psychiatric Nursing 6(2)71–82 (1992).
22. *Schloendorff v. Society of New York Hospital*, 105 N.E. 92 (N.Y. 1914).
23. J.K. Laben & C.P. MacLean, *Legal Issues and Guidelines for Nurses Who Care for the Mentally Ill*, Owings Mills, MD: National Health Publishing (1989).
24. T. Grisso, P.S. Applebaum, *The MacArthur treatment competence study. III: Abilities of patients to consent to psychiatric and medical treatments*. In (Ed.), Law and Human Behavior, *19* (2)149–174 (1995).
25. M.R. Munetz, G.A. Petersen, *Documenting informed consent for treatment with neuroleptics: An alternative to the consent form*. Psychiatric Services, 47(3)302–303 (1996).
26. R. Dresser, *Mentally disabled research subjects: The enduring policy issues*. Journal of the American Medical Association 276(1), 67–72 (1996).
27. Laben and MacLean, *Supra*, note 23.
28. S.P. Segal, M.A. Watson, P.D. Akutsum, *Quality of care and use of less restrictive alternatives in the psychiatric emergency service*. Psychiatric Services 47(6), 623–627 (1196).
29. Tennessee Code Annotated § 33-6-103, Revised Code of Washington Annotated § 71.05.150.
30. Applebaum, *supra*, note 1 at 49.
31. *Addington v. Texas*, 441 U.S. 418 (1979).
32. In re Sea 904 P2d 182 (Or. Ct. App. 1995).
33. E.F. Torrey, R.J. Kaplan, *A National Survey of the Use of Outpatient Commitment*, Psychiatric Services, 46(8), 778–784 (1995).
34. *Id.*
35. *Id.*
36. In re K.J.L. 541 N.W.2d 698 (N.D. Sup. Ct. 1996).
37. *Jaffee v. Redmond*, 116 S. Ct. 1923 (1996).
38. *Id.*
39. *Myers v. State*, 310 S.E. 2d 504 (GA 1984).
40. *Id. Supra*, note 37.
41. *Tarasoff v. The Regents of the University of California*, 551 P.2d 334 (Cal. 1976).
42. *Bradley v. Ray*, 904 SW 2d 302 (Mo. App. W.D. 1995) see also, *McIntosh v. Milano*, 403 A2d 500 (N.J. 1979); *Peck v. The Counseling Service of Addison County, Inc.*, 449 A2d 422 (Vt. 1985); *Lipari v. Sears Roebuck & Co.*, 497 F. Supp. 185 (D. Neb. 1980); *Petersen v. State*, 671 P2d 230 (Wash. 1983); *Matt v. Burwell, Inc.*, 892 S.W. 2d 796 (Mo. Ct. Of Appeals, 1995).
43. P.F. Lake, Revisiting Tarasoff, 58 Albany Law Review 97 at 98 (1994).
44. *Bradley v. Ray supra* at 309.
45. Tennessee Code Annotated § 33-1-103, California Civil Code § 43.92.
46. *Fewell v. Besner* 664 A.2d 577 (Pa. Super. 1995).
47. *Rogers v. Okin*, 478 F. Supp. 1342 (D. Mass. 1979); *Rennie v. Klein*, 462 F. Supp. 1131 (N. J. 1978).
48. Applebaum, *supra*, note 1.
49. *Id.*
50. *Id.* at 144.
51. *Doe v. E. K. Hunter*, 667 A2d 90 (Conn. 1995).
52. M.S. Kashka, P.K. Keyser, *Ethical Issues in Informed Consent and Ect.*, Perspectives in Psychiatric Care 31(2) 15–21 (1995).
53. D. Cauchon, *Shock Therapy: Patients Often Aren't Informed of Full Danger*, USA Today, December 6, 1995 1A–2A.
54. *Id.*
55. *Id.*
56. D. Whitcomb, *The Regulation of Electroconvulsive Therapy in California: The Impact of Recent*

Constitutional Interpretations, Golden Gate University Law Review, 18 Summer 469–494 (1988).

57. *Id.* and California Welfare & Institutional Code § 5326.2.
58. Id., *supra*, note 56 at 482.
59. Id., *supra*, note 53.
60. L. Fitzsimmons, *Electroconvulsive Therapy: What Nurses Need to Know*, Journal of Psychosocial Nursing, 33(12) 14–17 (1995).
61. Id., *supra*, note 53.
62. 42 U.S.C. § 12102.
63. 42 U.S.C. § 12114, 12211, and J.W. Parry, *Mental Disabilities Under the ADA: A Difficult Path to Follow*, Mental & Physical Disability Law Reporter, 17(1) 100–112 (1993).
64. C.L. Kaufman, Reasonable Accommodation to Mental Health Disabilities at Work: Legal Constructs and Practical Applications, The Journal of Psychiatry & Law, 153–174 (Summer, 1993).
65. *Id.*
66. *Jackson v. Indiana*, 406 U.S. 715 (1972).
67. Laben & MacLean *supra*, note 23 at 129.
68. Laben & MacLean *supra*, note 23 at 124.
69. S. Shah, *Criminal Responsibility in Forensic Psychiatry and Psychology*, Philadelphia: F.A. Davis (1986).
70. *Graham v. State of Tennessee*, 547 S.W. 2nd. 531 (Tenn. 1977).
71. *Hess v. Macaskill*, 67 F.3d. 307 (9th Cir. 1995).
72. K.T. Christensen, *Ethically important distinctions among managed care organizations*, The Journal of Law, Medicine & Ethics 23(3) 223–229 (1995).
73. *Id.*
74. *Id.*
75. *Id.*
76. D.G. Smith, *Evaluating managed care contracts*, Michigan Medicine 22–24 (February, 1996).
77. Christensen *supra*, note 72 at 226.
78. W. Miller, *Legal Consideration in Managed Care Contracting*, Topics in Health Care Financing 20(2) 17–25.
79. *Id.*
80. *Id.*
81. *Id.*
82. J. Haber, *Managed Care: Friend or Foe?* Perspectives in Psychiatric Nursing Care 30(4) 5–6 (1994).
83. *Id.* at 6.

84. M.F. Shore, A. Biegel, *Sounding Board: The Challenges Posed by Managed Behavioral Health Care*, New England Journal of Medicine 11.116–117 (January 11, 1996).
85. B.M. Edenfield, *Psychiatrist's Liability to Third-party Victims for Patient's Acts of Violence: The Status of Law Following Tarasoff*, in Psychiatric Malpractice, Athens, GA: Institute of Continuing Legal Education (1991).
86. B.C. Yorker, *Liability Issues for Nurses Who Work with Psychiatric Mental Health Patients*, Journal of Nursing Law 2(4) 7–20 (1995).
87. W. Prosser, *Handbook on the Law of Torts, Fourth Ed.*, St. Paul, Minn: West Publishing Co. (1971).
88. American Nurses Association, *supra*, note 20.
89. *Kirkland v. State Department of Health*, 489 So.2d 800 (Fla. Dist. Ct. App. 1986).
90. *Brooks v. Coliseum Park Hospital, Inc.*, 369 S.E.2d 319 (Ga. Ct. App. 1988) at 322.
91. *Ahn v. Kim*, 658 A.2d 1286 (N.J. Super Ct. App. Div. 1995).
92. *Myers v. Barringer*, 388 S.E. 2d 615 (N.C. Ct. App. 1990).
93. *Allelo v. Smith*, 641 So.2d 664 (La. Ct. App. 1994).
94. *Craft v. NME Psychiatric Properties, Inc.*, 1993 WL 441816 (E.D. La. 1993).
95. *Supra*, note 9.
96. *Id.*
97. *Muse v. Charter Hospital Winston-Salem, Inc.*, 452 S.E.2d 589 (N.C. App. 1995) and J.K. Laben & E.G. Rudolph, *Nursing Case Law Update: Professional Judgement versus Constraints*, Journal of Nursing Law 3(2) 57–61 (1996).
98. J.K. Kilcullen, *Groping for the reins: ERISA, HMO Malpractice, and the Enterprise Liability*, American Journal of Law Medicine 22(1) 7–50 at 36 (1996).
99. A.A. Stone, *Paradigms, Preemptions and Stages: Understanding the Transformation of American Psychiatry by Managed Care*, International Journal of Law & Psychiatry 18(4) 353–378.
100. *Id. Supra*, note 98 at 48.
101. *Id. Supra*, note 98 at 49.
102. See also for an in-depth discussion. R. Roth, ERISA: The Wildcard in the Health Law Deck, in A.G. Cosfield, Health Law Handbook (1996), Deerfield, IL: Clark Boardman Callaghan.

CONCEPTS AND INTERVENTIONS

II

CHAPTER 9

THE PSYCHIATRIC NURSING INTERVIEW

Ann Wolbert Burgess

Many nurses have conceptual difficulties that interfere with observation. One difficulty involves finding a balance between skeptical inquiry and jumping to conclusions. Another is an almost universal tendency to attribute what transpires during an interview to how well the interview was conducted.

Chapter Overview

- Differences Between Psychiatric and General Nursing Interviews
- Assessment and Nursing Diagnosis
    - The Depressed Patient
    - The Psychotic Patient
    - The Hostile Patient
    - The Somatic Patient
    - The Manic Patient
    - The Demented Patient
    - The Personality Disordered Patient
- The Science of Observation
    - Case Example
    - Active Vigilance
    - Ever-hovering Attention
- Content and Process
    - Case Example
- The A.R.T. of Interviewing
    - Assessment
    - Ranking
    - Transition
    - A.R.T. Sequence
- Specific Psychiatric Interviewing Techniques
- Summary
- References and Suggested Readings

Sections of this chapter are adapted with permission from Reiser DE, The psychiatric interview, In: Goldman HH, ed. Review of General Psychiatry, 4th ed. Stamford, CT: Appleton & Lange; 1995:110–117.

Patient interviewing is a core skill in nursing. Despite technical advances and new medications, communication continues to form the basis of assessment and nursing care. The nurse and patient must talk. Both parties, and especially the nurse, must also listen. No diagnostic test or apparatus can replace the nurse–patient relationship. It creates a therapeutic alliance that is the basis for nursing practice. The primary tool that cements the nurse's relationship with the patient is a sensitive and skilled interview. Integral to that relationship is the nurse's ability to communicate in a way that facilitates problem solving, improved coping, change, and growth.

There was a time when little other than communication was available to a psychiatric nurse for treating patients; antipsychotic drugs, effective antidepressants, and benzodiazepines are relatively recent developments. Although the future holds prospects for even more effective somatic and pharmacologic interventions, communication will no doubt continue to play a central role.

The working alliance is critical to all nursing interventions. Psychiatric patients are often ambivalent about needing professional help. Even though they want assistance with life problems, they may feel defeated and even humiliated by such a need. Although they may want to change behaviors, they nevertheless fear giving up familiar ways of coping. Cultural proscriptions, taboos, and stigma about psychiatry reinforce such attitudes. A patient with a diseased lung or heart usually does not feel shame to the same degree that a patient with alcoholism or psychosis does. For these reasons, the nurse must be sensitive to the importance of empathy, respect, and trust in order to develop a good working alliance with the patient. Regardless of what patients say or how they behave, the nurse should assume that seeking psychiatric help is a distressing and conflict-laden event for all patients (Reiser, 1995).

DIFFERENCES BETWEEN PSYCHIATRIC AND GENERAL NURSING INTERVIEWS

The psychiatric nursing interview differs from the general nursing interview in that the psychiatric patient communicates distressing thoughts or feelings through behavior that may indicate disturbed mental functioning. Depending on the patient's mental health or psychiatric condition, this problem can be small or great, but in all cases, tact and sensitivity are required of the nurse.

Three requirements differentiate the psychiatric nursing interview from the general nursing interview. The psychiatric interview requires multiple evaluations over time, careful observation of the patient, and collateral information.

The psychiatric nursing interview will require multiple evaluations over time. Patients suffering from an acute psychiatric disorder are generally unable to tolerate a lengthy interview at the first meeting. Depressed patients may be too despondent and withdrawn to give coherent details. A manic patient may be more interested in talking about profit projections from her latest scheme to establish a nationwide chain of coffee shops than in reporting that she stopped taking her lithium. Paranoid patients may eye the nurse suspiciously, convinced microphones are hidden in the sleeves of her sweater. In all cases, the nurse must be prepared to stop the interview and resume it when the patient's condition improves.

The more acutely impaired a psychiatric patient is, the more critical the science of observation. Words are not the only source of information during an interview. Nonverbal communication through facial expressions and body language conveys the underlying mood. If a nurse observes a disheveled young woman with clenched fists darting fearful glances around the room, the nurse has observed a great deal although the patient has said nothing.

The nurse must be prepared to seek out ancillary sources of data to complete a psychiatric interview. Patients are usually part of a social network. Important people such as family, friends, and work associates will often visit. It is usually worthwhile to spend some time talking with them, always with the patient's knowledge. Stresses in relationships may underlie psychiatric decompensation. The collateral information from people who know the patient is often invaluable.

Similarly, prior medical records and other sources of potential data (school, military, employment records) may assist in understanding the patient. The patient's confidentiality, dignity, and trust must always be respected, but data obtained from collateral sources may be critical for planning nursing care.

ASSESSMENT AND NURSING DIAGNOSIS

Formulating nursing diagnoses for psychiatric conditions can vary considerably from patient to patient. An individual with a nonpsychotic disorder characterized by anxiety or depression may be able to communicate with no greater difficulty than any other patient. Many psychiatric conditions, however, affect the patient's ability

to communicate and to comprehend reality, as shown in the following examples.

THE DEPRESSED PATIENT

The patient suffering from depression tends to perceive the world in a negative light, to feel bleak and pessimistic. Depressed patients are often in desperate need of hope and reassurance. They may repeatedly ask whether they are bad or if they can be helped. Nonetheless, when reassurance is given, it may be received with quiet skepticism and generally results in only transitory relief.

Depressed persons may be convinced they are being justly punished by God for transgressions. Such beliefs may be delusional in psychotic depressions, such as when patients think they have committed "unforgivable" sins; think that they, or the world, no longer exists (nihilism); or think they are riddled with cancer (somatic delusion). Explaining that such ideas are the result of depression and will go away with treatment offers momentary hope, but is unlikely to change the patients' opinion until improvement occurs (Yates et al., 1994).

THE PSYCHOTIC PATIENT

A patient suffering from a psychotic disorder, such as paranoid schizophrenia, may experience a flood of derogatory and frightening auditory hallucinations. He may be convinced that someone is plotting to poison him and steal all of his belongings. A nurse who walks into his room, extends a hand, and begins with a friendly introduction may be surprised. Instead of smiling back obligingly, the patient may say, "Do not come near me with that poison!"

When delusions are persecutory in nature, the patient may be reluctant or unwilling to talk for fear the nurse is an agent of the persecutory process. With such a patient, the interview may involve only quiet observation. Interacting with such patients often provides stimulation that makes evidence of psychosis more apparent. In addition to grossly distorting reality, acutely psychotic patients are often very frightened. Both of these factors can result in unpredictable and occasionally violent behavior. Although such patients need to be treated with kindness and understanding, precautions are necessary to prevent the patient from acting on delusional thoughts (Yates et al., 1994).

THE HOSTILE PATIENT

Hostile patients usually have histories of angry behavior. Such behaviors may seen in patients with antisocial personality disorder, alcoholism, substance abuse, or a paranoid psychosis, as well as in a patient who is threatening violence even in the absence of a psychiatric disorder.

One sensitive indicator of whether a situation is escalating and becoming dangerous is your emotional intuitive response. If you feel uncomfortable or fearful with the patient, precautions should be taken immediately to ensure your safety. In a hospital setting, if concern is minimal, precautions may involve nothing more than sitting between the patient and an open door, or making sure that other staff are nearby and know you are talking to the patient. When the index of concern is higher, one or more staff may be positioned in the patient's direct view. Such precautions are often a relief to confused, psychotic, or agitated patients because they provide structure and absolve patients of the necessity of making decisions at a time when they may not be in control of their actions (Yates et al., 1994).

THE SOMATIC PATIENT

The patient suffering from various physical symptoms may be quite demanding of staff time. Many patients with psychiatric disorders manifest physical symptoms in which a medical diagnosis is not readily found. The disorders include conversion disorder, hypochondriasis, somatization disorder, and nonspecific complaints associated with depression or anxiety. Such complaints may be the result of a physical illness too early in onset to permit diagnosis, or may be due to the patient's attempt to receive attention.

Somatic complaints need to be categorized as single or multiple. If the somatic complaint is single, a medical evaluation continues until a physical cause has been excluded. If the complaints are multiple and somatization disorder is a possibility, then symptoms must be seriously listened to, but only objective evidence of disease should lead to further medical work-up. It is important to know that some patients have a limited psychological vocabulary and communicate their feelings in physical terms when experiencing emotional distress. This trait, sometimes called affective language, is noted in many cultures worldwide (Yates et al., 1994).

THE MANIC PATIENT

A patient suffering from a manic episode may rush about the hospital ward, or go on many spending sprees in the community, hardly able to heed anyone's advice. The patient may be busy testing all the water faucets on the unit and trying to convince staff that she has a magic formula for converting tap water to liquid gold. Interviewing this patient needs to be done in short periods, gradually increasing her tolerance to sit and talk.

THE DEMENTED PATIENT

A patient suffering from dementia may often be outwardly cooperative. He will sit compliantly, nod when asked if he understands, and smile affably. Unfortunately, he may think it is 1926 and be firmly convinced the nurse is his college professor. He will be unable to remember to come for medications and will require constant, repetitive instructions regarding daily functions of eating, hygiene, medications, activities, and sleep.

THE PERSONALITY DISORDERED PATIENT

The patient with a personality disorder may give a heart-wrenching story about the anguish of insomnia, leading the physician to miss the twinkle in her eye as she asks for a prescription for 100 amphetamine tablets "just like my physician gives me back home."

THE SCIENCE OF OBSERVATION

Many students think of the interview chiefly as something that they do, perform, or conduct, but the interview is also a time to observe, perceive, and take in. The first concept of the interview is active and intrusive; the second is passive and receptive. An essential skill of observation is staying quiet so the patient can talk and so that things can happen that need to be noted. There are two phases to the observation component of the interview: active vigilance and what Freud called ever-hovering attention.

ACTIVE VIGILANCE

Active vigilance begins immediately, as soon as the nurse and patient see each other—not when they have settled down, with names exchanged, and notes taken. In the case example below, the phase of active vigilance began the instant the group walked to the patient's bedside. During this phase of the interview, the nurse should absorb as much as possible, actively and aggressively processing data that come in through all of the senses. How does the patient first greet the nurse? Does he or she offer a hand or sit passively? Does the patient make eye contact? Is the handclasp firm and warm, or is it cold and clammy? Are there any books on the bed or table? What is the patient wearing? What are the first jokes and casual banter uttered by the patient? Are there any unusual sounds or smells in the room?

When the interview formally begins, the phase of active vigilance continues for the first few minutes of the dialogue. The nurse should make an effort to remember everything the pa-

► CASE EXAMPLE

A group of nursing students and their instructor had come to interview a 77-year-old woman in the surgical unit. Flowers and cards were in the room, as well as a framed photograph on the bedside table of a handsome man in his late 50s wearing clothes in the style of the late 1950s. The patient had undergone hip replacement surgery and was in good spirits. When the students entered, the patient asked a visitor, a woman in her mid-40s, to return another time. "I am happy," she said, "to have some young people to talk to." The instructor was then called away, and she urged the students to proceed with a 20-minute interview.

Later, the instructor offered her impressions of the patient, though she had been less than a minute at her bedside. The students were amazed at how much she had been able to observe in that time: that the patient was a widow, because she wore a wedding band and the picture would have been more recent—or there would have been none—if her husband were still alive; that she had grown children and maintained close ties with them, because a greeting to "the kids" (possibly her grandchildren) had gone with the visitor, who said "Good-bye, Mom," and because the patient related so well to the young nursing students; and that she belonged to several clubs and groups, because there were so many flowers and cards—some with a great many signatures—in the room.

tient says. What was the very first thing the patient said? What was the accompanying emotional tone? One patient "joked" at the start of an interview, "Whatever it is they're accusing me of, I didn't do it!" It turned out that this man had been riddled with guilt since the suicide of his son 2 years earlier, which was when his health began to fail. In another case, on approach, a woman said to a nursing student, "I wouldn't have nothin' to offer anyhow! Go away and leave me alone!" This patient turned out to be deeply tormented and embittered by her children's recent decision to place her in a nursing home.

EVER-HOVERING ATTENTION

After the phase of active vigilance, the nurse should shift to ever-hovering attention. Nurses will discover, especially if they have been vigilant in the first few minutes of the interaction, that they can remember the rest of the interview without resorting to detailed notes. Note-taking is in fact discouraged, except in order to jot down a few key facts. A nurse with head lowered over a notepad is not looking at the patient and paying attention.

After the first few minutes, the nurse can simply adopt a relaxed and receptive stance. Listening is essential. The nurse should allow whatever the patient is saying to come into his or her mind freely, and should pay attention to the thoughts, ideas, and random associations that occur while the patient is talking. There will be time for more focused and directive interviewing later.

Many nurses have conceptual difficulties that interfere with observation. One difficulty involves finding a balance between skeptical inquiry and jumping to conclusions. Another is an almost universal tendency to attribute what transpires during an interview to how well the interview was conducted. In the case example, although most of the students were impressed by the instructor's acumen, a few of them were angered by it and felt the instructor had jumped to conclusions. This does happen, and students are right to be cautious. Any conclusions drawn from limited data should be regarded as hypotheses,

not certainties. Nurses should not hesitate to modify or expand their ideas about patients' problems as more data become available. At the same time, they should give the science of observation the benefit of the doubt before dismissing all hunches. To be nonjudgmental and resist premature appraisal is laudable, but nurses cannot afford to ignore the clinical data the nurse–patient interaction so often provides.

The converse of this is that nurses should never assume that the data a patient provides are always perceived by the nurse and the patient in the same way. Just as some interviewers ignore small yet important facts, others erroneously assume that they understand what the patient means, even when the patient uses ambiguous terms. Patients talk about "not being myself lately," being "out of sorts," or "without get-up-and-go." The nurse should never assume that these and similar phrases are automatically clear. "Not being myself" could mean "I'm sexually impotent" or it could mean "I cry all night, and I've just bought a gun to kill myself." It never hurts to ask "What do you mean when you say you are not yourself?" "Out of sorts in what way, specifically?" "What do you mean, no get-up-and-go?" The patient's clarifying responses may startle the nurse, who thought the patient meant something else entirely.

Regarding the nurse's second concern—that he or she is always responsible for how an interview proceeds—only experience will teach that the interview is less influenced by what the nurse does than by the temperament and mood of the patient. It is primarily patients who shape interviews, with the same coping styles, wishes, fears, and conflicts with which they shape (or fail to shape) their lives. This is precisely why the interview provides such valuable data: It replicates the coping pattern and difficulties of the patient.

Nurses are always eager to learn how to correct what they did wrong and to understand what they could have done to make an interview go better. Interviewing technique is important, and nurses are right to ask for constructive criticism. But they must also understand that how an interview goes usually says more about the patient than about the nurse. To assert this principle is not to deny responsibility, but to recognize an important diagnostic principle of psychiatric nursing.

CONTENT AND PROCESS

All interpersonal communication has both a content and a process (Reiser and Schroder, 1980). Everyone is accustomed to focusing on the content of communication, but it is often the process that communicates what is most important. Music offers a good analogy: the content forms the basic notes of communication, while process comprises the rhythm, timing, chord structure, and harmony. Content is the literal "what" that is being said; process is the timing and flow, the all-important way in which something is said.

Although there is process communication in all interactions, its importance obviously varies. If one is asking a store clerk how much something costs, the process is hardly important unless local custom encourages bargaining. In the nurse–patient interaction, process is always important. Regardless of what the problem is, the patient will always have concerns about nurses. "Can this person help me?" "Do they care about me?" "Do they find my problem disgusting?" "Trivial?" "Have they ever seen anyone with my problem before?" The foreman in the illustrative case had an important concern: Would the young nurse treat him with understanding and respect? Although the specifics may vary, the concerns are universal. Addressing them sympathetically will help establish a good working alliance. Because patients can rarely express these concerns directly, they almost always do so through process, though they are not always aware of it.

► **CASE EXAMPLE**

A 51-year-old construction foreman was being evaluated on a neuropsychiatric unit for symptoms of forgetfulness. He had only a sixth-grade education but was highly regarded on the job. He boasted of being a "self-made man." A nursing student was interviewing him. In responding to a question about his family, the patient began to speak derisively about his son, whom he had sent to college but who was now at home. He was collecting unemployment insurance, playing a guitar, and dreaming of riches on the rock scene. "He may have a college degree, but there are things I know that only life can teach!"

The nursing student listened attentively and respectfully, and then said, "It sounds like your son doesn't always respect what you know, what experience has taught you."

"That's right!"

The nursing student then made an important intuitive connection. "I'm probably about the same age as your son," he said. "I hope I don't come across as a know-it-all with you. I'm a student—I told you that. Be sure to let me know if I'm not understanding something."

"No, you're doing all right. You're all right."

Mastering and understanding the process level of communication is an exacting skill that takes time and experience to acquire. The nurse can usually detect the process level of a patient's communications by asking three questions:

- What is the patient telling me about his or her concerns right now?
- What is the patient telling me about his or her feelings right now?
- What is the patient telling me about his or her feelings concerning what is going on between us right now?

In the case example, the nurse understood his patient's concerns as follows. Right now, the patient was saying he was concerned about whether the young student would patronize him. Right now, he was saying that he wanted to be treated with respect, even though he was not an educated man.

Attention to process often answers another key question in the psychiatric interview: Why now? A 46-year-old man with a 20-year history of manic-depressive illness comes to the emergency room markedly depressed. Why now? A young college senior develops a delusion that he is part of an international scheme. Why now?

What has been going on in the patient's life? The answer is always critical. More often than not, it will be found in the process of a patient's communication more than in the content. In the case of one very depressed man, for example, the process level of his communication dwelt extensively on themes of rejection and loss. He even told a sad joke about a man who was a cuckold. This process unfolded while the patient ostensibly disclosed only content. "I've been married 15 years to a good woman." This prompted the interviewer to inquire further about the patient's marriage and enabled him to learn that the patient suspected his wife had started an affair, which was the "why now?" for this patient's illness.

Finally, the concept of process is closely related to the phenomenon of transference. In psychiatric relationships, the intense feelings a patient has toward his or her therapist may be critical. Success in psychotherapy often depends on the skillful handling of these feelings. In certain forms of therapy, such as psychoanalysis and psychoanalytically oriented psychotherapy, an understanding of the patient's transference becomes an integral part of the process of treatment itself. With few exceptions, the nature and extent of the transference will be communicated in process.

THE A.R.T. OF INTERVIEWING

Every psychiatric interview can be divided into three phases: assessment, ranking, and transition (Reiser, 1995; Reiser and Schroder, 1980). This gives the acronym ART.

ASSESSMENT

The assessment phase of the interview is the maximally open-ended, nondirective phase of the nurse–patient interaction. The setting should be a quiet and closed place where nurse and patient can talk in an unhurried manner. Both should be seated at about the same eye level and able to interact in normal tones. If such a setting is not available, an empathetic attitude can go a long way toward overcoming the disadvantage of noise and lack of privacy. In all cases, the nurse should try to ensure the best setting possible under the circumstances.

The nurse should introduce and identify himself or herself, clearly explain the purpose of the meeting, and then invite the patient to begin in as open-ended a manner as possible. Some standard phrases can be used, such as "What sort of trouble have you been having?" or "Tell me about the problem that brings you here." Some nurses simply begin with a look of interest and an inviting gesture of the hand.

It is important to start in an open-ended manner for several reasons. First, an invitation to talk tells the patient "You are important to me. I am interested in everything about you. Everything that concerns you is potentially of concern to me." Communicating this attitude is always important in nursing, but is even more important with patients who have problems with damage to their sense of self-worth and their ability to trust others. Second, the nurse can often discern subtle but important clues to disturbances in thought processes. In response to the open-ended beginning of the interview, does the patient begin to tell his or her story in a logical, goal-directed manner? Or does the patient ramble in a loose and incoherent way about seemingly unrelated concerns? Does the patient start to cry and seem unable to articulate any story at all? Is there inappropriate laughter? Is there a rush of language amounting to pressure of speech? These and similar incongruities of affect and cognitive disturbances can be readily observed if the nurse is appropriately nondirective. If the nurse launches too quickly into a content-intensive checklist style of interviewing, such data may be missed.

A third reason for beginning in an open-ended manner is perhaps most important of all. The nurse may be wrong in assuming he or she knows what is most important in the patient's presentation. If a patient entering an emergency room appears belligerent and paranoid and expresses fears of gangland revenge, the nurse may initially assume that the person suffers from a psychosis of the paranoid type, probably schizophrenia. Yet this conclusion would have to be reassessed if, in the course of an open-ended interview, the patient begins to talk about his activities as a drug dealer and his recent heavy use of cocaine.

During the assessment phase, the patient will raise concerns, describe symptoms, and offer other clues that the nurse will wish to investigate further. These will range from the patient's medical and past psychiatric history to family relations and vocational and financial difficulties. After a time—usually 3 to 10 minutes—the nurse will be ready to begin the second phase of the interview process.

RANKING

During the ranking phase of the interview, the nurse makes decisions about the order in which different areas of inquiry should be examined. During the assessment phase, the patient may introduce half a dozen areas of interest worth pursuing. What comes first? The nurse might rank a given patient's problems as follows: (1) concerns about whether the patient's fear is understood, (2) a 3-week history of depression and suicidal ideation, (3) breakup of a marriage, and (4) loss of job after 20 years.

Within each ranked area, the nurse should proceed from an open-ended, nondirective style to progressively more focused and defined inquiry. The nurse might say, "Tell me more about this feeling of hopelessness." After the patient has attempted to do so, the nurse's inquiry would become progressively more directive: "Have you lost any weight over the past few weeks?" "How many pounds would you say you have lost?" Finally, questions that require the most specific type of responses may be asked: "Would you say you've lost a couple of pounds or 10 pounds in the last 2 weeks?" A good rule in ranking is to let the patient's priorities control whenever possible. The nurse may be eager to elicit data concerning sleeplessness and euphoria or a 20-year drinking history. The patient may be much more troubled by concerns about being hospitalized or perhaps by something else altogether, something concerning the family or changes in employment or health.

TRANSITION

Assessment and ranking are complex clinical skills that develop gradually as experience and knowledge increase; transitions are fairly easy from the first day. A transition consists of telling the patient when and why the subject of the interview is being changed. After the assessment phase, for example, the nurse may say "It sounds like you're very concerned about the effect your drinking is having on your wife. But right now I'd like to hear more about why you think you want to end it all." In this instance, the nurse has properly given assessment of suicidal ideation a very high priority. The nurse ranked this consideration first after listening to many of the patient's concerns and then made a transition by telling the patient exactly what the focus of attention was and why.

Transitions may also be used to return to a more open-ended interview, after a specific line of inquiry has run its course. After a careful review of functional status, the nurse might say, "Now that I've gotten the basics I need concerning your physical health history, perhaps we could return to something you mentioned earlier, that your grandmother was hospitalized once for a psychiatric problem and things didn't go well. Could you tell me more about that?" The line of questioning is usually clear in the nurse's mind, but may not be clear to the patient. Great care must be taken to avoid confusion in changing the topic of inquiry.

A.R.T. SEQUENCE

Although assessment, ranking, and transition have been presented here in sequence, all three actually go on simultaneously. For example, the nurse may come upon a new fact that should immediately be assessed more thoroughly, indicating a need to return to the assessment phase of the interview. As the nurse–patient relationship proceeds, new facts are always emerging that require reassessment and ranking.

SPECIFIC PSYCHIATRIC INTERVIEWING TECHNIQUES

The foundation of good psychiatric interviewing—indeed of all nursing interviewing—is a working alliance between nurse and patient in a spirit of growing mutual trust. No amount of skill in technique can compensate for basic defects in this alliance. Conversely, a patient will usually forgive the nurse any number of mistakes if basic trust is there. The single most potent interviewing technique is empathy, an appreciation of what the patient is going through. It is far more important than any special technique, and more

meaningful to the patient than anything learned from this or any other book. With that understood, the nurse may consider "tricks of the trade" of interviewing. The following list of twelve such interviewing techniques is adapted with permission from Reiser and Rosen (1984).

Technique	Outcome
Attend to patient comfort	Privacy and quiet
Remember the basics	Questioning style
Be natural	Two-way communication
Encourage expression of feelings	Encouragement of affect
Consider patient's developmental stage	Stage of stress/crises
Be aware of patient apprehension	Patient at ease
Be sensitive	Interpretation of feelings
Repeat patient's phrase	Interview stall avoided
Ask direct questions	Suicide assessment
Maintain therapeutic silence	Listening to patient
Use nonverbal language	Reading body language
Go from the general to the specific	Broad-narrow - specific

Attend to Patient Comfort

Paying attention to the patient's comfort is critical. Too often, nurses see patients in crowded institutional settings where dignity, privacy, and comfort are neglected. Nurses and staff converge around the bedside in large groups and literally "talk down" to the supine patient. Introductions are mumbled or omitted altogether. Perhaps some of this is inevitable, but the nurse should be meticulous in such matters. A quiet and private setting should be found, if possible. Nurse and patient should both be comfortable and able to interact at eye level. Perhaps this sort of courtesy should not be called a technique at all, but its benefits for the patient and the interviewing process are so frequently overlooked that it must be underscored.

Remember the Basics

As emphasized in this text, understanding the patient is more important than rigid adherence to classic technique. Nevertheless, a review of a few of the standard interviewing rules and nostrums are helpful.

- Don't ask two questions at the same time. ("Have you ever been bothered by voices or odd beliefs?")
- An open-ended question is usually preferable to a closed-ended one.
- Don't ask questions calling for negative answers. ("You haven't had any experience with voices, have you?")
- Avoid being judgmental. ("Have you had any obscene thoughts?")
- Make liberal use of facilitating remarks. ("I see. Tell me more. How was that for you? Go on.")
- Ask for clarification. ("Can you explain what you meant by that? I'm not sure I exactly followed that.")

Be Natural

Nurses should trust their natural behavioral styles. Experience in living teaches interpersonal skills that are therapeutic in the broadest sense. Unless a nurse has no friends and is avoided by relatives, he or she does have natural talents. Therefore, if a patient tells a joke and the nurse thinks it is funny, the nurse should laugh. If the patient wants to know something about the nurse—for example, place of origin or whether the nurse is married and has children—it is perfectly acceptable to answer. It is an unfortunate myth that the nurse–patient relationship should be unilateral, with the patient telling all and the nurse nothing. In a manner that is not self-conscious and always respectful of the patient's dignity, the nurse should feel free to let the patient get to know him or her, through the facts disclosed and attitudes conveyed by the nurse.

There are times when it is appropriate—indeed indicated—to touch a patient on the hand or shoulder. A nurse should never be afraid to reach out and be human. Touching, however, may be perceived as "phony" if the nurse is naturally reserved. If that is the case, touching should not be forced.

Physical contact is a potent "drug" that, like any drug, may have major side effects. It takes experience to know when to touch and when not to. The nurse should remember that a patient can be "touched" in many ways. An empathetic expression of understanding or a sincere look of concern often touches a patient more deeply than a hand on the shoulder. In communicating, whether through words or by touch, the nurse should be guided by the answer to the question "Am I doing this for my patient?"

Encourage the Expression of Feelings

Some patients are under strong cultural proscriptions against public displays of affect, especially grief and rage. Nurses may have the same attitude and may believe that if a patient starts to cry, for example, something must have gone wrong with the interview. Most psychiatric patients are in emotional states they feel they cannot express—usually rage and sorrow. Almost without exception, they should be encouraged to let these feelings come out. ("There are tears in your eyes. His death has left you very sad, hasn't it?") The only case in which encouraging expression of affect is contraindicated is when a patient is in danger of total loss of control, as signaled by escalating behaviors (louder and louder voice, tenser body). In such circumstances, the nurse should demand that affect be controlled.

Consider the Patient's Developmental Stage

The nurse must always consider the patient in development terms. Growth and development do not cease at age 21. It is often useful to consider the patient's stage of development. Might this depressed 50-year-old woman be suffering from "empty nest syndrome" (depression because the children have all left home)? Might this agitated psychotic young man be struggling with emotional conflicts related to sexual intimacy and separation from his family? A developmental perspective can assist the interviewer in understanding the patient's concerns, especially if the patient and nurse are of widely disparate ages.

Be Aware of Patient Apprehension

The nurse should remember that the patient is likely to be scared. A young man is nervous about meeting the nurse and about the implications of having a psychiatric disturbance. Will the nurse read his mind? Find him unlikable? Is he on a course leading to incurable insanity? Or will the nurse find his problems laughably trivial, not worthy of serious attention or compassion? Inexperienced nurses are often apprehensive in approaching a psychiatric patient, but are usually not nearly so apprehensive as the patient. Awareness of the patient's apprehension may enable the nurse to help more quickly.

Exhibit Sensitivity

Being sensitive is being acutely aware of subtle changes in the patient's mood, thought, or behavior. Think of someone who is suffering from a psychiatric disorder and has developed severe phobic symptoms. The person has become afraid to travel by air, then by car, and now is afraid even to leave home on foot. Which of the following would seem more sensitive or empathic? "Can you describe your reaction to these events?" or "You must feel like a prisoner! How painful for you!" Some clinicians argue against what may seem like putting words in a patient's mouth. Although that is a pitfall to be avoided, the risk is often exaggerated. If a nurse is occasionally wrong about what a patient is feeling, the patient will say so. If the nurse is consistently wrong, something has prevented the formation of an empathic bond with that patient. If the nurse is not sure what the patient is feeling, it is easy enough to ask "What is this like for you?" or "How was that for you?" in order to elicit the patient's affective experience. Nurses miss a good opportunity to interact therapeutically when they do know how the patient is feeling, but fail to communicate their insight to the patient. Using the human quality of sensitivity, nurses are able to communicate to the patient that they know something is on his mind and that they are interested in listening.

Repeat the Patient's Phrases

When an interview bogs down, the nurse can try repeating the patient's last words. This technique was first popularized by the psychologist Carl Rogers (1951), who felt it was maximally nondirective and encouraged patients to proceed in the direction they preferred. Excessive reliance on this technique, however, is counterproductive. The interview should follow the patient's lead, but sometimes the nurse must be directive. Repeating the patient's last words is a technique that can be effective and should be used when needed. Encouraging nods of the head or supportive murmurs can accomplish the same thing. Periods of silence also should be permitted.

Ask Direct Questions

The nurse should go ahead and ask the unaskable. If in touch with his or her own feelings as well as those of the patient, the nurse may realize that a patient is very scared, angry, or depressed. It may even occur to the nurse that the patient is thinking of committing suicide. Fortunately, most do not act on suicidal thoughts, but the patient may feel terribly isolated and alone. Many patients think about death but feel they cannot tell anyone. A similar burden is imposed by other intense affects that patients dread sharing. If a nurse thinks that a patient might be suicidal, the nurse can ask tactfully and respectfully. It is impossible to put the idea of suicide into a patient's head, which is what interviewers sometimes fear. However, it is quite possible and very dangerous to ignore a patient's nonverbal signals. Most people who attempt suicide have seen a health professional recently, often without indicating their intent, and many go on to use medications in the suicide attempt. Thus, in the case of suicide, nurses must always ask the unaskable.

The same principle applies to many other areas. If the nurse suspects alcoholism, drug abuse, child battering, homicide, or some other socially delicate problem, nurses must not be afraid to inquire. Occasionally they may give offense, but less often than one might think. Special note should be made of the subject of sexuality. Despite our "liberated" times, it is surprising how often interviewers overlook inquiring about sexual concerns. Sex is part of being human and is frequently affected by illness, especially psychiatric illness. Usually, however, nurses must inquire firmly if they hope to be of any help in this aspect of the patient's welfare. Ultimately, it is not just suicide and sex but all taboos to which the admonition **ask** applies: fear of death, mutilation, sexual dysfunction, madness, suicide, and homicide. A patient will let the questioner know if he or she should back off. More often, the patient will open up with an outpouring of gratitude and relief.

Use Therapeutic Silence

The nurse must also learn to be quiet. When patients come to a point in their story where they are about to disclose something uncomfortable, they will often fall silent. Silence can be socially awkward, but a psychiatric interviewer must learn to take advantage of it. When a patient falls silent, the interviewer should be silent, too. The pressure does build, and it may seem awkward for a time, but the patient usually goes on to tell the interviewer what is really bothering him or her. Most interviewers would do well to listen more and talk less. If the silence becomes unduly protracted, it may be useful for the interviewer to say something neutral such as "Go ahead. Yes, go on. I'm listening," to relieve awkwardness and encourage the patient to continue.

Be Aware of Nonverbal Language

The nurse should pay attention to body language. Body language is one of many ways in which patients try to communicate. This subject has received considerable attention in both nursing and lay publications, perhaps more than it deserves. Yet body language is an important way in which people express themselves. And unlike the tongue, the body seldom lies.

Body language can be particularly revealing at the beginning of the interview. The nurse can observe how patients position themselves and move, and watch how they sit or stand and seek or avoid eye contact. Body language is a reliable form of communication that everyone uses. The trick, as with other observational skills, lies in being conscious of what is observed.

Go from the General to the Specific

The nurse should start the interview broadly and then narrow the focus. As the earlier discussion of the A.R.T. of interviewing makes clear, it is rarely necessary to focus narrowly on any agenda at the outset of an interview. The patient is best allowed at least 3 to 10 minutes for assessment, the most open-ended phase of the interview. Books about interviewing list many techniques for staying broadly focused or narrowing in. They speak of open-ended versus closed-ended questions or compound versus simple sentences of facilitating responses. As in photography, the nurse should think of technique as a gradual focusing in, from wide-angle shots to narrow-angle close-ups. The nurse's responses during the assessment phase are broadly focused, wide-angle responses consisting of empathetic silences, repeating the patient's last words, identifying the patient's affect ("That must have made you very sad!") and requesting clarification. As the nurse begins to focus in, questions become more directed. "Tell me more about this depression, Mr. Jones." Or "You mentioned that you and your wife have been fighting. Tell me more about what's going on there." As the camera angle narrows progressively, the questions naturally become more constricting: "How long have you been feeling life was hopeless?" "How many pounds have you lost?" At this stage, the emphasis is on specific data, such as chronology of symptoms, their nature and severity, and their relations to other symptoms. The nurse inquires about symptoms and signs directly related to the diagnostic criteria for specific mental disorders. Finally, the nurse may focus in on the most narrowly directed questions of all—those that can only be answered yes or no: "Have you ever had blackouts?" "Have you found yourself thinking that everyone is against you?"

Summary

The twelve interviewing techniques discussed, coupled with an understanding of the distinction between content and process and the A.R.T. of interviewing, should enable a psychiatric nurse to obtain a meaningful story from the patient. The nurse should always remember, however, that technique is invariably secondary to the human dimension of interviewing—above all, establishing empathy, respect, and trust.

REFERENCES AND SUGGESTED READINGS

Reiser DE. The psychiatric interview. In: Goldman HH, ed. *Review of General Psychiatry*. 4th ed. Stamford, CT: Appleton & Lange; 1995:110–117.

Reiser DE, Rosen DH. *Medicine As a Human Experience*. Baltimore: University Park Press; 1984.

Reiser DE, Schroder AK. *Patient Interviewing: The Human Dimension*. Baltimore: Williams & Wilkins; 1980.

Yates WR, Kathol RG, Carter J. Psychiatric Assessment DSM-IV, and Differential Diagnosis. In Stoudemire A, ed. *Clinical Psychiatry for Medical Students*, Philadelphia: Lippincott; 1994.

CHAPTER 10

PSYCHODYNAMIC CASE FORMULATION: SYNTHESIZING ASSESSMENT AND PLANNING TREATMENT

Ann Wolbert Burgess • Carol R. Hartman

---

*I*ncorporating the principles of psychodynamic case formulation into practice guidelines in managed care systems is imperative. As clinicians, we tend to operate from our synopsis of detailed assessment information. It is important, however, not to blindly follow this predetermined pattern, but instead to continuously reevaluate our assessment based on new information about the patient.

Chapter Overview

Whether done formally or informally, the advanced practice nurse synthesizes the individualized assessment data pertaining to a patient and makes a psychodynamic case formulation. This process provides a glimpse of the cognitive filter used by the nurse, and when communicated to others serves as the rationale for the plan and course of treatment.

Traditionally, psychodynamic concepts and assessments have been used to interpret and predict behavior. This chapter will focus on the psychodynamic principles and formulation activities related to the inter- and intradynamics of the patient's psychiatric history and the multiaxial diagnoses. Synthesizing of the information into the psychodynamic case formulation takes time, practice, and supervision.

PSYCHODYNAMIC PRINCIPLES AND THERAPY

DYNAMIC FORMULATION

"Dynamic" refers to the ongoing interaction between self and others or within the self. "Psychodynamic" refers to how these processes and patterns of interaction play a role in the individual's motivation, interpretation, and actions. For purposes of describing the focus of the dynamic interpretation, "inter" refers to the exchange between people and "intra" to the information processing and dialogue within an individual.

During the assessment interview, it is critical to pay careful attention to the presenting symptom(s). The connection between the patient's symptoms on one hand, and past events and situations on the other, are one focus of psychodynamic treatment. This connection relates to three fundamental psychoanalytic principles, outlined by Davanloo (1992, p. 17).

- Releasing the patient's hidden feelings by actively working on and interpreting *resistance*.
- Paying strict attention to the *transference* relationships.

- Linking those relationships to both *current and past relationships*.

Using these connections as a psychodynamic process, the advanced practice nurse is constantly watching for feedback. In the initial stages, feedback consists of increased resistance, but as soon as the core problem is touched on, the patient almost invariably experiences relief and hope, which is reflected in an increased willingness to collaborate as well as in a stronger therapeutic alliance.

Psychotherapy may be viewed as a set of interpersonal transactions. It is a process that may become therapeutic because of the patient's unwitting tendency to cast the advanced practice nurse in the role of a significant other and to enact with him or her unconscious conflicts or maladaptive patterns of behavior rooted in unconscious conflicts. Through participant observation, the advanced practice nurse provides a new model of identification. By understanding the dynamic meanings in the patient's interpersonal behavior and communicating this understanding to the patient, the nurse assists the patient in assimilating aspects of the experience that were unrecognized. This new information gives the patient an opportunity to change interpersonal aspects of behavior.

PSYCHODYNAMIC MODELS

Although there are many theories of personality and psychological theories, the psychodynamic model in American psychiatry began with the work of Sigmund Freud and was modified by the subsequent work of Sullivan, Fromm, Reichman, Erikson, and others. Freud's thesis derived from the "conviction that psychological events, however obscure, were understandable" (Havens, 1965). With his technique of free association, Freud was able to reconstruct childhood experiences, which he believed were the basis of adult psychopathology. In the current use of the psychodynamic model, the developmental impasse or fixation, the early deprivation, the distortions in early relationships, and the confused communication between caregivers and child are viewed as leading to vulnerabilities to certain stresses.

The concept of fixation is one of the basic Freudian explanations of patient conflict. Development is stunted, particularly sexual and aggressive drives and their expression. Through an examination of the process of defenses and personality structure, that is, the organization of superego, ego, and id, assumptions are made regarding the internal dynamics and motivations of an individual. For example, failure to compete in the oedipal structure of attachment to mother and father can lead to passivity in the male and great fear and resentment of the father figure and fear of the forbidden object of the female.

Patients' self-identity and interpersonal behavior are greatly influenced by learning experiences during their formative years. The challenges of growing up are rooted in the prolonged biological and psychological dependency characterizing human development. Accordingly, interpersonal relations with significant others in childhood prove decisive for the child's development. The family's role and function in childrearing include the categories of nurture, structuring the child's personality, basic socialization, enculturation (including language development), and providing models of identification for the child to internalize.

Deficiencies in any of these sectors may result in developmental deficits that at the adult level may be recognized as neurotic (or psychotic) disturbances. At the least, they interfere with the person's adaptive functioning. Psychoanalytic theory holds that because of early deprivations and traumatic experiences, the individual is unable to gain sufficient gratification from his or her contemporary interactions with others and lacks adequate resources (or denies their existence) to mold his or her environment in accordance with legitimate wishes and needs. The person has unrealistic expectations of self and others, and frequently feels frustrated. Patterns of dealing with changing life circumstances are rigid, and although the patient may perceive their maladaptive character, he or she feels unable to change them. Chronic anxieties are a manifestation of a pervasive sense of helplessness resulting, in part, from interpersonal conflicts, but also from unconscious fantasies relating to primitive sexual and aggressive impulses whose vicissitudes are basic to psychoanalytic thinking. In essence, the patient is in a state of conflict and suffers as a result. The dilemma, according to Strupp and Binder (1984, p. 30), often takes the following form.

- The patient does not know the nature of the problem he or she is trying to resolve, having hidden it in order to avoid painful affects.
- Excluding the problem from awareness, however, does not result in its resolution. Instead, the person is forced to return to it because it continually interferes with current interpersonal relationships. Thus, the patient dimly recognizes that there is unfinished business with significant childhood figures, but feels unable to complete it.
- Without realizing it, the patient continually reenacts the original problem with significant persons in his or her life (including the nurse), and in important aspects treats them as if they were the significant others of the patient's past. Because, however, the clock cannot be turned back, there can be no solution.

• Grounded in many respects at an earlier phase of development, the patient is unable to take advantage of opportunities for satisfying interpersonal relationships in the present. This inability contributes to a continual state of frustration and rage.

The contemporary psychodynamic model looks at life events, developmental achievements, and lack of developmental experiences that contribute to an individual's growing up. Integrated development involves a sense of self, emotional control and regulation, positive attachment, a sense of moral awareness and development of right and wrong, and a commitment to actions to uphold socially positive and binding behaviors.

Part of the psychological assessment for case formulation is the determination of what led to the patient's request for help. By listening for the precipitant, one can assess the critical dynamic issue that is distressful to the patient. The issue or reason is called "dynamic" because there is meaning in why it has occurred.

Every situation has a psychodynamic issue. For example, did the precipitant present a threat of loss of love, or a loss of people giving to the person emotionally? Or is the person one who needs to feel good but now feels that he is a bad person? Or is the person one who needs to feel in control but now feels out of control? Or is the person one who needs to win and now feels that she is going to lose? Or is the person one who needs to be admired but no longer feels that anyone admires her?

The same precipitating event could have two different meanings for two different people. For example, someone dies. To one person this means the loss of someone who cared and gave him something he needed. To another person it means that because he had been so angry at the person, he contributed to that person's death and now feels that he is a bad person. He may feel that he could have done more to prevent the death.

When we look at what is presently going on in the life of an individual in terms of case formulation, we are looking at the structure and evolution of that person's behavior in terms of past history and its current interaction with the individual's present life circumstances. We make some assumptions as to how the structures that emanate from early experiences shape the subjective experiences in the here and now and filter incoming information and meaning along with interpretation as to choice and action in the present.

An example would be a woman who has great difficulty forming intimate relationships and establishing reciprocal friendships in her present life, and who manages her emotional life either through withdrawal or extreme emotional outbursts. She presents with a history of early separation from her mother after birth with problems with attachment and bonding with the mother, as reflected in stories told in her infancy where her mother felt she could never please the infant when she tried to care for her later in life. The little girl attached to a father who ruled the house with an iron fist and tended to be very physical in his punishments of his daughter, frequently spanking her when the mother complained about the child's behavior. Then he would gather her in his arms and ask for her forgiveness for his behavior towards her. The little girl had difficulty in behavior in her preschool church school on Sunday. She'd be sent home for being overly active and did not conform to the rules. In growing up in grammar school, she tended to be physically active and a tomboy, much to the chagrin of her mother but to the praise of her father. However, when it came time to further support her athletic prowess by buying baseballs or bats, he withheld them from her and lavished them upon the older brothers.

In high school the young girl found herself very competitive on the girls basketball team but unable to establish positive relationships with the team; rather she had to be the star player, and this resulted in great conflict with the female coach, who often restricted her playing time because of her lack of team involvement. At no time did her father attend any of her sports activities during this period of what she considered most positive experiences. All through grammar school and high school she was unable to establish a best friend. This pattern of loneliness, isolation, and longing for friendship carried through college and into her work situations. At work she found herself in constant conflict with authority figures and in highly competitive relationships with her peers, leading to many unhappy experiences although she was a perfectionist in her work effort.

The traditional psychoanalytic model fits in terms of self-soothing and her intense rage. These emotions were activated in the therapy relationship with the advanced practice nurse as a reenactment of her frustration and highly ambivalent relationship with her mother. It also activated her inability to control as she entered into competitive, passive-aggressive behavior in interpersonal situations. Either she was overinhibited in expressing emotion or she exploded into rages, hurt feelings, and anguish at being treated unfairly.

A contemporary psychodynamic model looks at what she missed in her development, peer relationships, modulation of affect, and building of some positive experiences in evalu

ating herself in a noncritical way. These become the important areas for treatment. The deeper issues of attachment require deeper levels of drive regulation; that is, the origin of her rage and self-soothing are related to the early infant experiences. The therapist may never have an opportunity to deal with these issues.

The use of a timeline assists in determining the psychodynamics of the patient's life. The therapist can ask the patient to put each life event on a timeline and rate each event as to level of stress, either negative or positive. This timeline presents a picture of what has been achieved developmentally and what has not. Has the patient had any positive and pleasurable events? In one case, an 8-year-old boy could not remember anything pleasant from his childhood. The nurse can then ask questions about each event. This format allows the patient to be in control. Patients can think about it; the timeline is in front of them; they are not asked to recollect in detail and reexperience the event; they are recalling and commenting rather than emotionally exploring the event. This gives the nurse and patient some comprehension and a framework upon which to work.

► CASE EXAMPLE

A 10-year-old boy is in a residential treatment setting with aphasia from multiple physical abuse to the head. He has trouble communicating verbally, usually remaining mute in the dayroom. From his history, information was gained about the boy's mother being in a wheelchair as a result of the father's violence. There was a strong possibility that the boy witnessed this domestic violence. One day a wheelchair is left at the nurse's station. Suddenly, the boy gets in the wheelchair and begins wheeling furiously around the ward and yelling loudly. This is his first communication outburst in weeks. Clearly the visual cue of the wheelchair activated memories and moved the boy into aggressive behavior.

From a treatment intervention standpoint, is he acting as the mother or father? As witness to the emotional communication, we can take the behavior as communication from the child and understand it as his means of trying to communicate some aspect of the fragmented history. He is using action and language; he can talk and uses words.

The intervention would be to approach him while he is in the wheelchair, and ask if he is the mama and if he is trying to tell something that scared and frightened him. This interaction would be slowly worked and pieced together until the boy could verbalize in some way.

This vignette gets to some of the dynamics of the early traumatic experience. We are not looking at loss of control because of fixation, but rather at efforts of trying to communicate something that happened in the child's life. This action is not emanating out of fantasy or a sense of guilt over impulses.

CASE FORMULATION

A case formulation is as complete as the information available in the assessment phase. An outline for case formulation includes the following information.

- Summary
- Differential diagnostic considerations
- Best diagnoses
- Missing information
- Treatment plan
- Prognosis

The summary contains assessment information that has been gathered during the psychiatric interview. Diagnostic clues are attended to throughout the interview and prompt the advanced practice nurse to focus or expand the assessment procedure to allow for an adequate differential diagnosis.

The summary information includes identifying data, informant, chief complaint, and history of the present problem. The *identifying data* includes such factors as age, gender, marital status, children, employment, income, religion, and living conditions. The *informant* or patient is described as to reliability as a historian, whether responses to inquiries are marked by inconsistencies, gaps, or confabulation, and the perceived truthfulness of information. The *chief complaint or presenting problem* includes the following information.

- What is the nature of the problem? (What brings the patient in now?)
- What is the problem in interpersonal terms? (Who are the significant persons involved?)
- Is there an immediately identifiable precipitant or trauma? If not, can one be found?
- How did the patient decide to seek treatment now?

The *history of the present illness* includes information regarding the first known onset of distress and what led to the present situation. A clear description is given of symptoms and behavior that presented at the time of evaluation. Is this the first time the problem has appeared? Have there been previous episodes? If so, how were they handled? How long has the patient been aware of the problem?

The second major area of data is derived from the patient's relationships and *significant losses*. It is a dynamic assessment based on relationships that are current as well as those from the recent past and from adolescence and childhood. Assessment is made of the prior history and personality of the individual and of the social history, family history, and developmental history. The separations and/or losses reviewed are those occurring in childhood, adolescence, and adulthood. Such losses or separations might include parental separation or divorce, death of a parent or caretaker, birth of siblings, frequent moves, patient's own separation or divorce, or the death of a spouse or other loved one. Other significant life disruptions include serious injury or illness to self or significant other and job or career disruptions.

Also included are *past medical history* and data related to a review of systems, habits, physical and neurological examination, mental status examination, and diagnostic tests.

Third, *assets and strengths* are assessed in the present and over time with a projection into the future. This is represented by the treatment plan and the prognosis. The final aspect of the formulation is prognosis. Expected outcomes of the treatment strategies are noted within the framework of expectations of the impact of biological, psychological, and social factors operative now and in the future.

The primary focus of the psychodynamics of multiaxial diagnoses is analyzing the interaction of biology with behavior and cognition. Critical in examining disruption in thought and behavior are physical health, present and past, and internal and external exposure to toxins, either from self-medication with drugs and alcohol or unintentional mixing of medications or ingestion of lead. The organization of this disruption is matched according to diagnostic criteria already established.

Evaluation continues with consideration of familial history of similar patterns of behavior and cognition. Further considerations include trauma of both a physical and psychological nature. Biological disruption has now been identified not only with axis I disorders but also with axis II disorders, which fall under consideration of biological instability. The avoidance patterns and deficits as well as excesses often definitive of the personality disorders have to be considered not only from a behavioral learning matrix but also from a traumatic and biological consideration, which is most often explored through family history.

Stability of defensive patterns and coping patterns are examined in light of historical, biological, and social environmental and psychological triggers arising out of habitual patterns. The dynamics arising out of the psychiatric history are tied in with the clinical findings making up the multiaxial diagnoses. Of particular importance is the understanding of the developmental history derived from the psychiatric history. However, the dominance of the current presentation of symptoms and their organization and understanding drive the multiaxial diagnoses. Furthermore, this information is more forthcoming and can be supported by a variety of neurological and psychological tests.

The psychiatric history is often usefully conceptualized as a timeline of events, experiences, and levels of adaptation, which in turn is related to a timeline of family history and development facilitated by a genogram. Conceptual models of personality development, learning, and patterns of psychosocial adaptation prevail in the analysis of data collected in this aspect of the assessment. The multiaxial diagnostic information also informs and shapes an understanding of the behaviors and cognitions being explained by this aspect of the assessment.

The interactions between and within these major systems of information are guided by levels of presumptions of cause and effect, as well as by assumptions of the mechanisms contributing to the disruption of behavior and the dynamics restricting the change of behavior. Repetition, deficits, control, and flexibility become the important areas of focus for the most immediate interventions. The strategies are designed to address these problems at biological, sensory, and cognitive levels (thoughts, feelings, images, beliefs supported by these dimensions).

The case formulation is now a summary of the key arguments of causality and rationale for treatment intervention based on the conclusions drawn from analysis of all of the assessment data up to the time of the report. This point is important, because it is critical to constantly review the formulation within the gathering of ongoing information, such as responses to treatment and other ongoing life events, as well as to conduct further evaluation of past history information and a systematic review of the multiaxial diagnoses.

Based on these three major areas, information is assessed through evaluation of diagnostic criteria, leading to the multiaxial diagnoses. There is evaluation of the individual's presentation according to criteria for clinical disorders (axis I), trait characteristics for evaluation of personality disorders (axis II), physical illnesses (axis III), psychosocial and environmental problems (axis IV), and level of present functioning (axis V). In presenting the case formulation, the severity, chronicity, and dangerousness are noted as well as the clinical multiaxial diagnoses. The nature of the history of the disorders is noted, as is response to treatments.

Next, different diagnostic considerations are reviewed, as well as gaps in information. Following this step, the best diagnoses are offered with consideration of both the psychiatric history and multiaxial evaluation. This is followed by a presentation of the contributing factors, in which there is a blend of the psychiatric history and the biological behavioral consideration of the multiaxial diagnoses. Missing information is noted. The treatment plan notes the level of focused intervention strategies—biological, behavioral, psychological, social, and environmental.

A diagnosis is made which is comprised of the diagnostic formulation, based on a summary statement of the multiaxial diagnoses and its psychodynamic interaction with the psychiatric history. A summary of a treatment plan and a prognosis comprise the case formulation.

PITFALLS IN CASE FORMULATION

Sometimes, in the press of time allocated to assessment and planning, only partial consideration of all of the dimensions of a case formulation is made. This can occur because staff become focused on the most immediate issues, which often center on axis I considerations and the immediate safety and potential for harm to others. It is important for the case formulation to include preparation for discharge from an acute setting back to the community.

An example of failure to do this involved a mother of three children with a long and complex history of bipolar disorder and numerous hospitalizations. Stability of symptoms was always difficult, and the toll it was taking on her family was alluded to but never fully evaluated. In her last hospitalization, she was discharged home after 2 days of symptom remission. The condition presented to her by her husband was that she was to move to an apartment by herself, if she wished to avoid a divorce. The day she returned home, she committed suicide in her car by carbon monoxide poisoning in the family garage.

The above example represents the limits of case formulation under the pressure of time and the short-sighted goals of a service system. In the example, the emphasis of the service system was on the symptom stabilization of the patient. Once this was done, she was released home to her husband. What was not assessed at this hospitalization was the burnout factor within the marital and family situation that would have led to reconsideration about the decision to release the patient. The husband could no longer tolerate the family disruption and had communicated directly with the patient that she would have to move into an apartment or he would divorce her. The impact of this decision was neither noted nor evaluated, nor was the case reformulated taking this new information into account. Within the context of managed care systems, there is a tendency to follow prescribed guidelines for practice and treatment, and individual shifts in the personal and interpersonal dimensions of the patient are not consistently reevaluated with new information. With this in mind, one has to recognize not only the organizing aspects of case formulation but also the limitations to this organization when it is not updated with the inclusion of new and changing information and dynamics. Even though developing the psychodynamics of a case requires time and thoughtful consideration, the insights gleaned are usually critical for treatment.

► CASE EXAMPLE OF HENRY

To better understand the psychodynamics of a case formulation, a complex case of a serial killer will be described. This case is presented for several reasons. First, the repetitive pattern of this man's killing had its origins of development in early childhood experiences. The dynamics set into play in those early experiences shaped his views of himself and others in his world. What emerged in his lifeline of relationships was a deep preoccupation with sex and power as well as the social experience of humiliation and shame. This evolved patterning was clearly revealed in his initial confession to police for the murders of 11 women.

Second, this was the first convicted black serial murderer who killed black women he knew. Previously, serial killers were white and targeted strangers. Third, one of the authors (AWB), examined him for trial and testified as to his mental illness, childhood history, and the development of his obsessional murderous fantasies. Fourth, serial killers are not born, but rather, they develop. Background histories always include chronic childhood abuse, which supports the argument for preventive intervention early in the lives of children at risk. Fifth, such cases show that even the most public of crimes are motivated by personal issues (de Becker, 1997) and as noted in the research of Ressler, Burgess, and Douglas (1988) on sexual homicides, the crime scene will have behavioral footprints.

► THE CONFESSION

All it took was a prayer. In June 1992, a detective investigating a missing person and looking for the roommate who was the reporting person, met with Henry, manager of the fast food restaurant where the roommate worked. Henry advised the detective that the roommate was his girlfriend and she was living with him. However, because that violated work policy, he wished that fact to be kept quiet. Then he gave the detective her address. Over the next several years, the detective saw Henry approximately 5 or 6 times at Henry's various workplaces, and they exchanged social greetings. On March 17, 1994, Henry was brought to a police station for questioning in connection with a murder. The detective was brought in to interview Henry because of their prior relationship, and went over the evidence indicating that a bank card used by Henry belonged to a murder victim. The detective said that he felt Henry was involved in the murder. They talked about Henry's drug habit and the murder and how wrong it was. The detective asked Henry if it was okay to say a prayer, to which Henry agreed. The detective then held Henry's hand and together they prayed for guidance and forgiveness in this serious matter and the opportunity to confess. Henry cried during the prayer, then asked for a pencil and paper and wrote out the names of his 11 victims.

The explanation of how Henry was capable of such violent acts lies in an understanding of two critical factors: (1) the early formative dynamic life events that shaped his thinking and fantasies about sex, aggression, and females, and (2) the life stresses that weakened his psychological defenses and triggered his acting on murderous fantasies.

▶ EARLY FORMATIVE EVENTS

When Henry finished describing in detail his killing of the 11 women over 18 months, he spontaneously added, "There is no way that I can say why I did what I did because I really don't know. Like when I was a little kid, my mom used to ask why I would steal and I couldn't explain it . . . I could never say that it was abuse from childhood because I don't think that I was abused no more or no less than any other kid who grew up the way I grew up. I got my ass cut up sometimes on a daily basis, sometimes for things I didn't do. You just learn to expect that, but I was first sexually active way before I even knew about sex. I was about four or five years old and the women that I was having intercourse with were like sixteen and I really didn't know what I was doing . . . I really didn't experience sex until my junior year in high school . . . I remember when I was about eight years old seeing several guys rape a girl and they got off scot-free. They walked away and the charges were dropped in court . . . then the first time I'd ever heard something about somebody being raped and killed was that same girl's sister. She was raped and strangled to death . . . It was her husband or boyfriend and it seems like ever since I heard that, raped and strangled to death, it always stuck in my mind, raped and strangled to death."

In this brief soliloquy, Henry identifies key formative events: physical abuse by mother, sexual abuse by teenage girls, seeing a gang rape, and hearing of the rape-strangulation of the rape victim's sister.

▶ HISTORY

Henry, a 31-year-old African American, was the second child born to his mother, Lottie, and her married lover, John. John, a high school science teacher was 20 years older than Lottie and never provided financial support for the children. When John learned of the second pregnancy, he said he could understand one mistake but not two. He left town and his teaching position shortly after the birth of Henry.

Henry was raised in abject poverty and in an oppressive matriarchal environment. He lived with his mother, great-grandmother, and sister in a four-room shack with no running water, indoor plumbing, or electricity. A bucket that served as a toilet was kept in Henry's bedroom and he had the task of emptying the bucket in the outhouse, a task he was ashamed for other children to see.

In analyzing the intricate dynamics between mother and son, it is important to note the chain of disappointments that the mother suffered at the hands of the men in her life. Beginning with her own father who abandoned her at birth, Lottie was later robbed of the only person with whom she was able to bond, her mother. Her mother's marriage to a new stepfather and the resulting birth of her youngest brother proved tragic. Not only was Lottie replaced by this newest brother as the favored child, but within three months, her mother died of a massive coronary; Lottie was 13 years old. Lottie was told not to grieve or express her loss and to take over the mother's duties. Her emotional development was stymied; her older brother was physically abusive to her and one of his friends tried to rape her.

Within two years of her mother's death, at age 15, Lottie was seduced by her teacher who filled the role of surrogate father and lover in exchange for a vow of silence, not unlike relationships involving fathers and daughters. At the time of Henry's birth, the father's name was withheld, although the midwife said that everyone knew John was the father. When Lottie was again abandoned by a parental figure (John) it was yet again because of a male child. Her son Henry became the object onto which the mother projected her feelings of rage toward men who had caused her pain. Although Lottie was physically abusive to her daughter, grandmother and Henry, he bore the brunt of the abuse.

In many ways, Henry paid for the wrongs that had been done to his mother by the men in her life. She made him pay through a process of control, abuse, and intimidation. She had no control over her father, her teacher, or a second married lover who abandoned her after 10 years when she became pregnant for a third time, even though she elected to have an abortion. To the degree that she abdicated control of her life to these men, she regained it through psychological maneuvering of her son.

Henry's earliest memories are of his toilet training and his mother beating him when he failed to "make potty." She needed him trained by age two so that she could place him in daycare in order to work. The beatings were inconsistent and inflicted at random; the children were beaten with anything the mother could get her hands on, including extension cords, a water hose, and tree limbs. When Henry was beaten with the race tracks of his cherished set of racing cars, he said he grew to hate the car set. He would throw out the pieces of track to avoid being beaten by them, but his mother would retrieve them and beat him for throwing them away. There was a pattern to the beatings: the children would lie on the bed, trapped in such a manner to avoid escape. Sometimes Henry knew the trigger to the beating; other times he would not. He had trouble controlling bowel movements; his mother thought he soiled on purpose and would beat him. He recalled many times rushing to get home before his mother so that he could wash his soiled underwear before she saw them. Henry's soiling continued until age 10 or 11.

Henry's mother was proud of her control over her children, stating they were scared of nothing—only lightning and their mama. The beatings were frequent and when the mother would physically tire of beating, she would have the children beat each other. If Henry did not hit his sister hard enough, the mother would threaten to beat him more. This action sanctioned Henry's physical abuse to his sister. Henry was also called dumb, stupid, clumsy and other degrading names whenever he displeased his mother. Henry was an object of ridicule for both his mother and sister. His sister would dress him in girls' clothing, and he was also jeered for his dark complexion. His mother would remark that he was "the blackest thing in my family."

The mother's second boyfriend came into Henry's life when he was about 2 years old and stayed for about 10 years. This man had a positive relationship with Henry, taking him fishing, to the ballpark, and other sports events. The break-up of this relationship coincided with Henry's believing that his father was coming to visit. The visit never happened, and Henry's mother later said she did not want or expect him to visit. This revelation called into question the mother's deliberate blocking of Henry's access to his father.

Henry's sexual exposure began around age 4 when an 11-year-old girl forced him under a car where she removed her underclothes and had him lay on top of her. They were caught, and Henry remembered the girl being whipped. He expected a beating, but his mother only laughed at him because the girl was so ugly. That sexual encounter led to many others. Girls ranging from seven to twelve years older than Henry exploited him over a ten-year period. The activities included oral sex and fondling. His mother recounted that the girls would make up rhymes, "We have the buns and Henry makes our buns rise." The mother's boyfriend's comment was that Henry was the only boy in the neighborhood and it was natural for him to "service the girls."

Henry's preoccupation with sex, aggression, and females was evidenced by the many magazines that he was exposed to from young childhood through adolescence. He described reading his mother's magazines including confession, detective, and pornography. In addition to the molestation, Henry witnessed a high school girl gang raped by a group of high school boys when he was 8 years old; the girl's sister was raped and strangled several months later.

Henry molested a 5-year-old girl when he was 13 years old in the same way the older girls had abused him. The girl's mother told Lottie, who acted as though it was no big deal, stating, "He's gotta get it from somewhere."

To the outside world, Henry presented a picture of buoyancy, a contradiction to the inner turmoil he felt. School was a place where Henry did fairly well. His mother was less successful in controlling him in school activities. When she tried to keep him from playing school sports because of a prior shoulder injury, he joined the cheerleading squad, as the only male. It provided an opportunity to travel with the team and independence from his mother. A former teacher and coach of the cheerleading squad remembered Henry's deportment as exemplary and his camaraderie with the members of the squad. He "was like a big brother to the girls." Henry was said to have a good sense of responsibility and was hard working. His school grades fluctuated but when he graduated, he ranked 80 in a class of 126, completing high school with a cumulative of 2.02. During his high school years, Henry participated in the School Bus Driver Program, 4-H program, and served on the Vocational Center Student Council. He was a newspaper staff photographer and was commended for his outstanding service to his community.

Despite the positive activities, Henry's mother still exercised control over his life. On the night of his high school graduation, he was forced to keep a midnight curfew; his sister, two years before was allowed to stay out until 3 a.m. Henry attended a state college where in the first academic semester he attempted 13 credits, but only earned five, scoring a cumulative of .64. For spring semester, he entered a technical school pursuing studies in Nuclear Engineering Technology and earned a cumulative of 2.5 grade point. He lived at home for the school year, and his mother would check his car odometer to be sure he was driving only to and from school. He had wanted to attend the college his sister attended, but his mother refused.

Henry's military record was excellent. He enlisted in the Navy in December 1984. All reports describe him as an outstanding seaman; he was ranked above average. He was selected for advancement to third class petty officer and qualified for a sea service ribbon. He reported witnessing the deaths of seven persons in an aircraft crash. He left the service in December 1988 and had earned an overall trait average of 3.76, out of a possible 4. Henry's exemplary career was cut short when he broke into a garden supply store, thus losing his security clearance. He was given the option of being honorably discharged or facing criminal charges. He chose discharge.

Henry's employment history from 1988 to his arrest in 1992 showed a steady decline from his military performance. He was fired from his first job at a radio station for stealing tape recorders and CDs. He then worked as a security guard at a department store where he was fired for suspected larceny. At his next employment, he worked 18 months but was fired for excessive absenteeism. His remaining jobs were at fast food restaurants. He had been unemployed several weeks before his capture.

▶ PARTNERSHIPS

Henry's first romantic involvement began in tenth grade. This first girlfriend and first sexual partner was to become his wife. During high school, Henry was sexually active with other girls. His relationship with his girlfriend fluctuated and during one separation he met another woman whom he decided to marry; however, his mother discouraged him, stating the girl did not have a promising future. He returned to the first girlfriend, who in the interim, had had a child that she claimed was conceived during a rape. When they married, Henry declared he wanted a child of his own, but his wife refused and the relationship deteriorated. His wife asserted that whenever they had sex, she was reminded of the rape. He suggested they go for marriage counseling and she refused; the couple separated.

Upon dissolution of his marriage, Henry returned to his mother's new house, one that he had helped pay for. Henry's mother stated that for the first time, Henry began answering her back, which caused problems. Henry tried a reconciliation with his wife, but when he failed, he took an overdose of pills. He was not encouraged to seek professional help; rather, Henry recalled his mother slapping his face because he stayed in his room moping over the breakup of his marriage.

Henry began dating again but his mother constantly discouraged him, referring to his girlfriends as "whores and sluts." She also searched his car, wallets, and dresser drawers. Lottie complained that Henry did not play around with her as he once did, e.g., she would hold him down and playfully try to kiss him. Henry told her to get herself a man because he was tired of playing that role. She was dismayed with his attitude because she said she was supporting him while he was not working steadily. Other people who were interviewed commented on the inappropriateness of the intimacy Lottie shared with her son.

During Henry's childhood he suffered four accidents that left him unconscious for a short time. About age 7 he fell out of a tree; age 10 he was hit in the head with a bat; age 13 he was in a bicycle accident, and age 14 he had a skate board accident.

He reported a history of polydrug abuse, including LSD, cocaine, and marijuana; beginning at a very young age up until age 30 he drank an average of 16 to 18 beers a day. While in the service, he was treated for secondary syphilis and he was circumcised to treat painful erections.

Intellectual testing indicated a full scale IQ of 92 on the WAIS-R, which is in the average range of functioning. Neurological testing indicated impairment on measures of sustained auditory attention and cognitive flexibility, consistent with mild frontal lobe impairment. This impairment was believed to be consistent with a history of possible multiple mild closed head injuries in addition to his history of alcohol and drug abuse.

▶ THE CONSEQUENCES

By age 14, Henry became aware of his sexually aggressive fantasies. Part of these secret fantasies were grounded in the sexual acts from his own exploitation and the gang rape he witnessed, and part were from his ruminations over the visual images he retained from the magazines he coveted.

His confessions to the murders had a patterned script. He methodically repeated how he administered the choke hold; he rendered the victim unconscious; he performed sexual acts and had intercourse. But there was no detailing of the sexual acts, in contrast to the detailing of killings and robberies. He would go back to the crime scenes of his first four victims, an example of the unreality of what he did. He questioned himself: did it really happen; did I really kill them?

Henry is a mass of contradiction. He says he rapes his victims but forensic evidence is inconclusive or absent, and he left all but one of his victims totally dressed. He says he wiped the crime scene of fingerprints but left many footprints. He left the biggest clue, the victim; he left his signature, the ligatures. He took a taxi and pawned stolen jewelry, giving his name. He denied involvement in the crimes but talked to police and admitted two murders the police knew nothing about.

▶ CASE SUMMARY

Henry's method of committing crimes reflected the abusive events in his early life with females; however, in the repetition of the traumatic events, he switched his role from victim to perpetrator and put the females in the role of victim. He is alert for any behavior that is reminiscent of the control that the girls had over him when he was younger, such as calling him names and criticizing or teasing him. He also related how some of his victims were like sisters. His crimes were like a map to his personal history with cross streets and landmarks. Henry was street wise, and after the first murder, one of the women he dated (Henry's term for a prostitute) told police that they should make Henry a prime suspect. The police discredited her because of her work, but she too was street wise. She knew what Henry was capable of, given the structure of his fantasies. Henry admitted that, while in the service, he visited many prostitutes, raped and did not pay them. He also had a rape charge pending at the time of his first murder; a charge that he strongly denied. Clearly, there were early warnings that if addressed might have spared 11 lives.

▶ DIFFERENTIAL DIAGNOSIS

Extensive neurological and physical evaluations were done to rule out genetic neurological contributions to his symptoms and violent behaviors. These evaluations revealed no gross abnormalities in these areas. Extensive psychological testing in conjunction with the physical findings ruled out psychotic disorders, major depressive disorders, and anxiety disorders. A conclusion was arrived at that the anxiety and depression were manifestations of axis II personality disorder traits.

► BEST DIAGNOSIS

The best fit diagnosis was Personality Disorder Not Otherwise Specified. There are features of more than one personality disorder (mixed personality), and together they cause clinically significant distress or impairment in one or more important areas of functioning. Compounding this diagnosis is incarceration and the fact that Henry is facing execution.

► MISSING INFORMATION

An extensive psychiatric history was taken. The impact of early traumatic and negative experiences on aggressive behavior is not fully known. The other information is how his brain functions when stimulated to a point that he acts aggressively.

Aggressive patterns and mental illness are present in at least three generations of his family, but information on Henry's father and his family is missing.

► TREATMENT PLAN

Continuation of medication.

Continuation of psychotherapy that directs attention to supportive work as well as gradual uncovering of associative information to violent behavior.

Evaluation of eating disorder.

Suggest a program of diet and exercise.

Psychotherapy. Some of the areas to explore related to the murders are as follows. The first murder was of a prostitute. He is puzzled. "How come I killed her because I didn't even know her? There was no reason for her to die." After they had sex (vaginal, oral, anal), the prostitute said, "Is that [anal sex] the way you like it?" That question threw him into a rage; he picked up a stone and bashed her head.

A treatment issue would be to take him back in time to the rage and ask: "What was it you heard her say to you? What made you so angry? Was it the sound of her voice or her words?"

The next four murders were of women Henry knew. He was not aware that he was necessarily going to murder them. He was aware of robbing and raping them, and says he murdered them so as not to be identified by them. He raises the issue, "I don't know where rape and murder end." He reveals he had keys made after stealing a key from his former girlfriend. A treatment issue would be to ask if the women ever confronted him about his using their keys or cars without permission. When confronted with the violation of their boundaries, what happened? It would be important to find out how he thinks about these women.

Did these women upset him? Did he think about how he might get even with them? What does his view of them as "sisters" mean in terms of his "big brother" relationship style?

Going back to his childhood and the exploitation, did the neighborhood girls get away with their behavior or did the boy always get blamed?

With the next five murders, Henry knew he was going to rape and murder. A treatment issue would be to ask how he knew this. He no longer said he was just going to rob and rape them. One victim had two young boys; did that make a difference?

By appealing to his narcissism, ask how he understands the killing. The nurse could say, "I'm going to ask you questions and if it bothers you, tell me— it may be a clue to understanding." Usually, the women said something to enrage him. Henry began to move to ligatures after the fifth victim. Of the tenth victim he says, "I had no intention of killing," but he had a pillowcase with him. The last victims involved the use of towels. The nurse could ask when he decided to take towels. How did he understand the towel, especially during childhood? Children were present in two of the killings and he tied a towel around one boy's neck. What does the towel mean? What does he mean when he states, in his confession, that boy would grow up without a mother?

In some killings, Henry tried to cover up the rapes. He did not want to focus on his sexual behavior. Was the murder a covering of the sexual issue? With some victims, the rage broke through. A treatment issue would be to try to get back to his terror and rage with early abuse by older girls.

▶ PROGNOSIS

Prognosis is very poor and Henry will always be dangerous. The lesson to be learned from Henry's life is to understand it for prevention and education.

CASE FORMULATION AND DIAGNOSTIC CLUES

Diagnostic clues have an interpersonal emphasis. Interpersonal transactions are emphasized because they provide a common psychological stage on which problematic life dramas are repeatedly played out (Strupp and Binder, 1984, p. 68). In essence, psychological activity, structure, and organization involve a life story or script. Many aspects of life stories or scripts are frequently, or even typically, unconscious (Strupp and Binder, 1984, p. 69). The concept of cyclical psychodynamic patterns (Anchin and Kiesler, 1982; Strupp and Binder, 1984, p. 72; Wachtel, 1982; Wender, 1968) best reflects the patient's self-defeating persistence and inflexibility of maladaptive and stereotypic interpersonal interactions. The causation is described as early trauma and unfortunate developmental circumstances that continue to exert an influence on later behavior, much as a series of billiard balls set into motion with the cue.

Developmentally, what one sees with Henry is that he has developed in such a way that character is critical. In the trait development we note great divergence of descriptions. People who knew him as a boy and young adolescent said he had an easygoing personality, was humorous and a class clown. He received positive school comments and achieved merits in the Navy. However, as an adult, and especially as he increased his drug use, he was described as moody and hot tempered.

The traits of character influence how we treat people, relate to them, like them. Put this all together and we talk about character and personality. We have different levels by which we say a person has character: emotion and reaction, judgment and intellect, relationships with people, and morality, or right and wrong.

Many things go into this development of character, including genetics, conditions under which a person is reared, and the social context that gives support or guidance to or detracts from the development of the individual. There is an individual commitment to trying to do the right thing. When we look at Henry we begin to see deviations in his development of character to do the right thing. We see struggles with trying to do the right thing, such as by going into the service. His struggle there was with using his intellect and positive abilities. Undermining his ability to do the right thing was the fact that he cannot regulate his emotion around doing the right thing. He has no insight into the development of relationships with people; he doesn't even have an idealized concept of a complete relationship. His concept is full of shoulds and should nots that have nothing to do with reality. This comes out in how he thinks a woman should respond to him or treat him. He has severe criteria, and if there is any transgression of the criteria he feels it justifies the rage and punishment he inflicts. In the process of this abusive behavior, particularly in the area of sexual encounters and exchanges through adolescence and into the adult years, these criteria have provided justification for the murder of women. He claims to have confined this to a group of women towards

whom it was easy to rationalize violent behaviors. But then the violence extended to women who were his friends, acquaintances, or like sisters.

A diagnosis in the DSM-IV is limited to those states that have clear definitive parameters and that have been studied in populations of patients. The group of serial killers is not large enough to study for determination of a clinical diagnosis. In this type of situation, we rarely find anyone who has a clear pattern of mental illness associated with their killing, and we cannot force them into a diagnostic category. We find alterations in thoughts, feelings, and behavior. Henry's ability to manage emotional arousal is peculiar and is compounded by his faulty thinking. He is compelled to kill.

The severity of the aggression and the repetition of murder directed the assessment to a thorough evaluation of biological contributors, as well as psychosocial contributors. Seizure disorders, gross abnormalities of the nervous system, and physical disorders that would contribute to aggressive acts had to be ruled out. The aggression and acts had to be evaluated as to whether they arose out of psychotic disorders or were a manifestation of post-traumatic stress disorder and flashbacks, or atypical mood and psychotic disorder.

Severe personality disorders had to be evaluated, in particular sociopathic, borderline, dissociative identity, and obsessive compulsive personality disorders. A careful physical evaluation was done to rule out the role of drug abuse and other toxic conditions.

Psychosocial and environmental stressors were evaluated as to triggering factors in the expression of murderous rage. These included stresses in key interpersonal relationships, work relationships, and social connections. An evaluation of Henry's level of functioning at the time of the murders was assessed and compared to his functioning prior to committing the first murder.

Diagnosis
The diagnostic clues led to the evaluation of presenting symptoms that met or did not meet

criteria for the DSM-IV. The primary outcome of multiaxis assessment was that of Personality Disorder Not Otherwise Specified. At trial, testimony was given that Henry was diagnosed as having a severe mental illness given the nature of his murderous fantasies and acts; that there was no specific category for him in the DSM as he was an emotional condition unto himself. That he, in fact, contained many pieces of the DSM, specifically features of various personality traits and disorders to include the following.

Obsessive-compulsive personality: Henry is preoccupied with control. The obsessions drive the compulsion to kill. The obsession is noted in the crime scene patterns. The victims are known black women, with whom he has a psychological connection and even an emotional bond and where he is in a position of control. The fantasy does not include women who have control over him, e.g., mother, sister, ex-wife, girlfriend.

Henry provides no logic for the killings. He has an elaborate ritual of killing that is built on an irrational perception. He had to kill the same each time. The obsession or fantasy drives the behavior or killing. The rage breaks through and he can not control it; it controls him. He cannot stop. He has intent and can plan the killing but he does not have the choice not to kill. In his confession he repeatedly said, "It was like a switch was turned; I couldn't stop." It is like the compulsive handwasher, who cannot stop the washing.

Borderline personality: Henry describes unstable interpersonal relationships, mood swings, and impulsivity. He exhibits great sensitivity to slight and rejection. He describes a victim teasing him; he explodes and kills her.

Anti-social personality: Henry shows a pattern of disregard for and violation of the rights of others. He steals from his employment. There is the breakdown of inhibition to steal and to take from people where value is not the issue.

Schizoid personality: There is a pattern of detachment from social relationships and a restricted range of emotional expression. Henry also exhibits bizarre thinking in the content of his fantasies.

Paranoid personality: There is a pattern of distrust and suspiciousness in other's motives. Some of this suspicion is heightened because of the drug abuse while some is grounded in reality that he is afraid of being caught. He does not know who he can trust.

Narcissistic personality: There is a pattern of grandiosity, a need for admiration and a lack of empathy that is manifested in his self-aggrandizement, sense of entitlement and sensitivity if people say no to him or do not give him what he wants. He was offended by his wife saying she was raped; he felt betrayed and preoccupied with himself rather than any concern for her experience.

The Stresses

What one has to understand about Henry is that there is a part of him that worked hard to put together a life, albeit an idealized life, of marriage, family, and a career in the service. He was partially successful, but when adversity challenged his idealized construct of himself and his life, he began to expand his already exploitive behavior toward prostitutes and toward women he knew.

His ability to manage frustration is very poor. He uses an obstacle to his goals as an excuse; he feels justified in getting even with the system; he robs. His underlying hatred of authority is carried out in antisocial acts. He has two things going for him: he can take women whom he considers inferior—prostitutes—and discharge his anger, contempt, and humiliation and demonstrate his dominance with them; and he can gain power over authority by exploiting it, stealing, robbing even while in the role of protecting.

What we have is construction of two fantasy worlds. One is occupied by the monster. The second is the white house, with picket fence and children. Henry tried to initially activate the second fantasy, but was unable to handle the disappointments that occurred in this process. It dipped him into his monster world where he had a fantasy of control. His second world constantly slipped away. His wife claimed to have been raped and that upset him. She was no longer the idealized woman, but tarnished and not in the fantasy. Then she told him that she wanted to leave him and he felt he had been used, exploited, and rejected. His decline into his monster world increased.

The absent father meant there was no protection and no model for the little boy growing up. There was no man there to help him be sensitive to his vulnerability as a child in being exploited. There was no protection against the irrational behavior of the mother; no one protected him from excessive stimulation of aggressive sexually written material. The social community did nothing to intervene and stop either his exploitive behavior or the behavior of those continuing to exploit him.

This was compounded by the fact he was denied participation in what became the idealized world—playing sports, developing wholesome friendships. He was indulged in a peculiar way; there was a dependency and pride taken in him in that he was male and intelligent, but there was no moral construct or mature attachment.

Henry was not born evil; he developed into a killer. He was a little boy, came home, was confused, and met with behavior that diminished his trust in attachment to anyone. The minute he got close, he became dependent. He was striving to have a decent life. The establishment of his terror was his sexual incompetence. He was scared as a little boy and this transfered to impotence.

His greatest fear is of women. He is not consciously aware of that fear; he states he is afraid of his mother, but the fear of women is sexual fear. By his own admission, he could not maintain an erection with the women he killed, and there was inconclusive forensic evidence that he even raped them. He is consciously aware of his humiliation and anger at women, but not his fear.

SUMMARY

Advanced practice nurses need an understanding of psychodynamics for case formulation for several reasons. First, such an understanding will alert the nurse to how the client's behavior is repeated in the treatment relationship, as well as in other relationships. Second, an understanding of psychodynamics assists in giving priorities to the structure of treatment. Third, an understanding gives direction for helping the patient with interpersonal resources. And fourth, from a forensic behavioral standpoint, it suggests characterological footprints in crime behavior and/or crime scene factors.

Advanced practice nurses can increase their skill in psychodynamic case formulation by peer group case consultation, supervision, and continuing education programs. And most importantly, advanced practice nurses must read multidisciplinary journals focusing on psychodynamics as well as consulting with therapists who have expertise in this area.

REFERENCES

Anchin JC, Kiesler DJ, eds. *Handbook of Interpersonal Psychotherapy*. New York: Pergamon; 1982.

Burgess AW, Hartman CR, Ressler RK, et al. Sexual homicide: A motivational model. *J Interpersonal Violence*. 1986;1:251–272.

Davanloo H. *Short Term Dynamic Psychotherapy*. Northvale, NJ: J Aronson; 1992.

de Becker G. *The Gift of Fear*. Boston: Little Brown. 1997.

Havens LL, Emil Kraeplin. *J Nerv Ment Dis*. 1965; 141:16–28.

Strupp HH, Binder JL, eds. *Psychotherapy in a New Key*. New York: Basic Books; 1984.

Wachtel P. Vicious circles: The self and the rhetoric of emerging and unfolding. *Contemp Psychoanal*. 1982;18:259–272.

Wender PH. Vicious and virtuous circles: The role of deviation-amplifying feedback in the origin and perpetuation of behavior. *Psychiatry*. 1968;31:309–324.

CHAPTER 11

TRANSFERENCE AND COUNTERTRANSFERENCE

Carol R. Hartman

*I*n-depth interviews
and self-reported
measurements and
studies have estab-
lished that there is a
parallel process of
excessive emotional
arousal in both victim
and therapist. The fac-
tors that influence this
arousal have led students
of traumatology and
treatment of trauma vic-
tims to construct para-
digms in an attempt to
better understand trans-
ference and counter-
transference.

Chapter Overview

- Case Example
- Transference and Countertransference in Light of Violent Interpersonal Events
- Vicarious Traumatization or Compassionate Fatigue
- Two Models of Countertransference
    - Interactive Processes
    - Survival Strategies
- Application of the Models
- Case Example: Self-sufficient or Dependent? An Important Early Question
- Summary
- References

► CASE EXAMPLE

The call came from a colleague. Could I fill in on a case conference for him at a local clinic? I told him I would be glad to. Several days later a young woman with a tentative voice identified herself on the phone as a doctoral student who was preparing to present a case at the conference. She asked if I would like to know a little about the patient. The following story emerged.

The student was asked to take Mr. M.'s case when he first came to the clinic complaining of depression. His estranged wife had died 6 months earlier and he was critical of himself for not having done more to help her. He had been an active alcoholic in past years and he was concerned that his mental state was pushing him back toward drinking. His wife's death was still under investigation because her body had been found in her car in the woods outside of town. It was not clear whether she had committed suicide or had been murdered.

The student was at the end of her rotation and was, of necessity, terminating work with Mr. M. She was not sure how to proceed with him and what should be the next areas of work. Her presentation and her sense of working with him tended to be amorphous. When pressed, the student revealed that she thought she had been working well with him and thought that she liked him. In the previous month, however, she had presented his case at another conference and the experience had been devastating for her. She had been very involved in assisting Mr. M. to establish a life for himself since the death of his wife. She presented to the conference the sense that he was self-defeating in his behavior; that is, resistant to following through with behavior that could be beneficial to him, and potentially self-destructive in that he had become involved with a younger woman who is a recovering alcoholic. At the presentation, the consultant and group had focused on whether the student had talked with Mr. M. about the fact that his estranged wife might have been murdered and his feelings about them even though he was not a suspect.

The student was alarmed by the case review, feeling she had missed the most important aspect of the case and not sure now if the patient was lying to her or withholding information. Her supervisor was upset about the conference. The supervisor had worked diligently with the student, but had gone on leave from work as she was expecting a baby. The student was surprised at the intensity of her emotional reaction and what she had revealed to the new consultant. She let me know she was "afraid" that a new consultation would open her up to more criticism and a sense of humiliation. When asked how much of the last conference dealt with trauma and its impact on the therapeutic relationship, the student stated that she was not sure. The conference before her last case presentation had focused on spousal abuse, which she thought set the stage for the consultant's and group's reactions, but she felt little had really been said about the impact of traumatic life events on the therapeutic relationship. We agreed that this would be the focus of the case conference, and it was scheduled for one week from the day of the student's call.

This example reminds us that as nurse therapists, we do not work in a vacuum and that our objectivity is constantly challenged. Whether in the role of therapist, supervisor, or consultant, the complex aspects of human encounters require us to examine our models of practice. Since the 1970s, there has been increased documentation of interpersonal violence and cruelty as a strong associative factor in all forms of mental disorders, and the need to understand how these events are activated within helping relationships cannot be denied (Danieli, 1980; Eth and Pynoos, 1985; Friedman et al., 1995; Giller, 1990; Gleser et al., 1981; Hinshaw and Atwood, 1984; Norbeck, 1986; Pynoos and Nader, 1988; Solomon, 1990).

The following pages examine the concepts of transference and countertransference as being driven by the violent events in the background of the patients we offer to help, necessitating a broader view of these linked phenomena.

TRANSFERENCE AND COUNTERTRANSFERENCE IN LIGHT OF VIOLENT INTERPERSONAL EVENTS

The focus on transference and countertransference as essential aspects of therapeutic management and outcome originated with Freud's work on psychoanalysis in 1910 to 1912. Transference was held to be the reenactment within the therapeutic relationship between the analyst and patient of patterns of relating to primary people in one's past. The strong positive or negative emotional response of the analyst to the patient, whether overt or covert, was seen initially as a "nuisance" to the analyst. Basically it was to be

kept to the realm of a private reaction, with the focus on the analyst "interpreting" the transference reactions of the patient.

The analyst's noncommittal stance was considered critical to the work and to the purity of the information coming from the patient. As early as 1924, however, analysts and students of therapy believed the therapeutic relationship was anything but a one-sided projection emanating from the patient (Sullivan, 1953). Patients often dropped out of therapy and complained about the nonresponsive therapeutic stance of the therapist. The noncommittal stance was viewed with suspicion, anger, and frustration. Analysts who regard a noncommittal stance as essential to the purity of the analytic process argue to this day with others who view the interactive reactions between a patient and therapist as normal reactions. Among those who view the reactions as a normal process, debate revolves around the extent to which the therapist's reaction is a focus of the therapy session and the extent to which an avoidance of the therapist's reactions undermines understanding the patient and leads to premature abandonment of therapy by either the patient or the therapist, or to exploitive dynamics between therapist and patient (Racker, 1968; Slatker, 1987).

Today this link between transference and countertransference is strongly forged by what has been learned regarding the impact of interpersonal violent acts upon victims. There are alterations in attachment, perception, memory, and information processing of new interpersonal events because of changes in personal schema regarding the self and others, as well as basic alterations in the fundamental mechanisms of emotional regulation, memory, and interpersonal learning. These changes give rise to behaviors and actions on the part of both the patient and therapist that can reach extreme dimensions. Emotional arousal within the therapist to the trauma story and the trauma engagement patterns of the patient results in levels of stress that override the biological flight or fight systems of the therapist, causing changes that affect the therapist's responsive patterns. When this happens, the phenomenon of vicarious traumatization, secondary traumatization, or compassionate fatigue has occurred.

VICARIOUS TRAUMATIZATION OR COMPASSIONATE FATIGUE

When a patient reveals his or her trauma story, several characteristics are important in considering its impact on the therapist. First, the type of stressor and its complexity is a powerful factor in whether the therapist is overburdened physiologically and psychologically. Whether the event is natural or human in origin plays a role in the emotional arousal dimensions associated with the story. Death, injury, mutilation, abuse, torture, and exploitation, as well as the grotesqueness of the events, increase emotional arousal in the therapist and tax the therapeutic empathetic position. The cycle of life in which the victim and therapist meet can contribute to emotional intensity. The role the victim played in the event, moral dilemmas occurring during the event (for example, a child forced to abuse another child), the degree of psychological ensnarement of the victim by the perpetrator, and the psychological sensory load of events (e.g., witnessing gross body mutilation) increase affective responses to the trauma story. The duration, severity, and frequency of exposure and/or exploitation add to the emotional dimensions of a trauma story, as does the degree of community involvement. In some parts of the world, for example, young women who have been captured by government troops, raped and tortured upon interrogation, and then released, may go to a clinic in which the providers themselves may be at risk of being picked up and investigated for assisting the victims, increasing the stress of listening to the trauma story. All of these factors in both the victim and the victim's story interact with factors in the therapist.

The defensive style and disposition of the therapist, personal beliefs, religious values, ideological systems, and preconceptions must accommodate the trauma story. When there is conflict, there is cognitive dissonance with additional emotional arousal in the therapist. Personal historical data in the life and experiences of the therapist interact with the victim's trauma story; for example, therapists who survived physical and sexual abuse as children listening to accounts from patients of early sexual and physical abuse. Theoretical assumptions about personality, life cycle and development, and lifestyles all interact with the trauma story and the new personal arousal information generated by the story, and as well as with behavioral engagement patterns. For example, when the pleadings of a patient for the therapist's protection against critical and exploitive managers in a work setting correspond with the therapist experiencing work difficulties in a clinic, the emotional ante goes up for the therapist. Experience with trauma and victims and the amount of training all influence the therapist's response. Early studies in nursing and medicine evaluating the impact of caring for very ill patients and the relationship of these experiences to burnout demonstrate that the youngest professionals experience the most emotional distress, and both young and old experience difficulties in clinical judgment and make errors (Hinshaw and Atwood, 1984; Jacobson and McGrath, 1983; Norbeck, 1986; Stanton and Schwartz, 1954; Vachon, 1987).

It is humanly impossible for the therapist not to react to the trauma story. Patterns of engagement with the patient will also challenge an empathic and objective stance. The therapist is moved toward either involvement or disengagement (Wilson and Lindy, 1994).

The non-neutral effect of the patterns of interpersonal engagement used by severely traumatized individuals, as well as the vividness of their stories, has been noted by a variety of clinicians supervising the work of therapists (Danieli 1985; Kluft, 1994: Mollica, 1988). Munroe (1991), identified symptoms in therapists that parallel symptoms of post-traumatic stress disorder. Wilson and Lindy (1994) and Figley (1995) have focused on these issues because of the threat to the mental health of providers working with traumatized populations. Ursano and associates (1994) have explored the impact of traumatic events on crisis workers while with victims and after.

A basic premise in the modification of the concepts of transference and countertransference is an acknowledgment of the biological impact of information that is highly arousing emotionally, whether the actual detailing of the trauma stories or in the complexity of the interpersonal engagement patterns associated with victims of trauma. Symptoms of cognitive confusion, anxiety, anger, sleeplessness, disturbing imagery, numbing, altered belief patterns, hyperarousal, loss of perspective, altered sense of self and self-esteem are all assumed to be induced by prolonged emotional arousal that is not dissipated through adequate coping mechanisms. Instead, there is an overriding of the therapist's own alarm system, with a corresponding biological disruption of emotional regulatory and cognitive processes (Figley, 1995; Hartman and Jackson, 1994; McCann and Pearlman, 1990; Munroe et al., 1994; Wilson and Lindy, 1994). Characteristic symptoms seen in victims can be grouped into the following categories (Buie, 1994; Friedman, 1993; Herman, 1992; Horowitz, 1976):

- *Intrusive symptoms:* Flashbacks, vivid nightmares of traumatic events, preoccupation with traumatic events, thoughts of the events when faced with reminders of the environment in which the events took place.
- *Avoidance symptoms:* Purposeful avoidance of reminders of the events, avoiding thinking about the events.
- *Hyperautonomic arousal symptoms:* Heightened startle reflex, constant vigilance, startling response to neutral stimuli, sleep disruption, alterations in pain response, increased heart rate.

- *Numbing symptoms:* Detachment from emotions, memory lapses, lapses in sense of time, detachment from surroundings when either internal or external reminders of the events occur.
- *Distortions of the self-system:* Alterations in the ability to soothe self, self-consistency, self-cohesion, self-monitoring, sustaining self-esteem, and a sense of oneself as part of a social community.

Again, these symptoms in victims are best understood as basic disruptions of biological systems and neural networks and as emerging behavioral and psychological systems to cope with trauma and biological upheaval (Friedman, et al, 1995; van der Kolk and Saporta, 1993; van der Kolk et al., 1996).

Corresponding to the symptoms found in the victim population are those found among health care providers, including the following.

- *Increased physiological and physical reactions:* Rapid heart rate at resting, somatic reactions, sleep disturbances (particularly REM abnormalities), agitation, inattention, drowsiness, and uncontrolled and unintended emotional displays. These reactions are noted to occur in patients and carry over into the private life of the caregiver.
- *Emotional reactions:* Irritability; annoyance or disdain; anxiety and fear reactions; depression and sadness; anger, rage, and hostility; detachment, denial, and avoidance of patients and others; sadistic/masochistic reactions; voyeuristic and sexualized reactions; confusion, psychic overload, overwhelmed reactions, and guilt. As these reactions are manifested in interactions with patients, co-workers, and families, providers often respond to them with shame and embarrassment. Providers, although they admit they need a place to talk about their reactions, also admit they avoid doing so and do not trust their supervisors, to whom they might turn. The erosion of self-esteem and the positive sense of therapeutic efficacy is further challenged when these reactions parallel the disruption of the self-system seen in victims.

• *Psychologic Reactions:* Detachment, overuse of intellectualization, rationalization, isolation, denial, minimization, and fantasy. These reactions provide further evidence of emotional dysregulation.

Other complex responses associated with defensive positions by the therapist are usually out of the awareness of the therapist; they constitute the interpersonal acting out patterns of transference and countertransference. These responses include overidentification with the patient, with increased use of psychological defenses such as projection, interjection, and denial or disengagement from the patient (and others). Denial and disengagement are marked by forgetting appointments, lapse of attention, parapraxes (distorted perceptions of the patient), loss of empathy, hostility and anger toward the patient, relief when the patient misses an appointment or a wish that the patient not show up for appointments, denial of feelings, or denial of the need for supervision or consultations regarding the patient. Often there is a self-centered belief that one has a special "gift" for working with a certain group of victims of violence. Self-medication or numbing by increased use of drugs or alcohol may also occur.

There may be a loss of professional boundaries during work with the patient and reactions in which the professional takes on the total experience of the patient, as can be seen when the therapist takes over as the rescuer of the patient or as the patient's defender against others. There may be excessive preoccupation with the patient, or the therapist may take on aggressor roles, such as the perpetrator, exploiter, or angry/withholding nonprotective parent. These reactions on the part of the provider take on the dimensions of the victim's preoccupation with the traumatic events. The therapist may take on the exploitative relationship of the aggressor or the passive relationship of the hapless and helpless observer who witnessed the event but did nothing to help the victim. These interactive symptoms are the acting out patterns of countertransference and ultimately result in the abandonment of a therapeutic stance and relationship. Countertransference reactions become symptoms of the overriding stress experienced by the provider (Caplan 1970; Danieli, 1980, 1985, 1988; Haley, 1974; Hartman and Jackson, 1994; Kluft, 1989, 1994; McCann and Pearlman, 1990; Munroe, 1991; Wilson and Lindy, 1994).

In summary, in-depth interviews and self-reported measurements and studies have established that there is a parallel process of excessive emotional arousal in both victim and therapist. The factors that influence this arousal are the nature of the stressors confronted by the victim and communicated in the trauma story; specific factors in the victim related to the traumatic event (particularly engagement patterns and symptoms) and personal characteristics of the victim prior to the traumatic events themselves; personal characteristics and background of the therapists; and organizational factors that either support and provide resources for both the victim and therapist or increase the emotional strain on the victim and therapist. These four factors have led students of traumatology and treatment of trauma victims to construct paradigms in an attempt to better understand transference and countertransference.

TWO MODELS OF COUNTERTRANSFERENCE

Thus far two models have evolved that are useful to therapists for helping themselves and helping other providers as well as patients. One model proposed by Wilson and Lindy (1994), focuses on the rupture of empathy and loss of therapeutic role with a negative impact on recovery, the other model, proposed by Valent (1995), focuses on survival strategies as a framework for understanding coping in helpers and vicarious traumatization. The first model details the numerous points to be considered in the four factors that effect the unfolding therapeutic relationship, clueing the therapist to avoidant or counterphobic and detachment reactions, known as *type I countertransference reactions (type I CTRs)*, and overidentification reactions known as *type II countertransference reactions (type II CTRs)*. The second model focuses on the survival strategies that develop around role-engaging patterns as a form of interpersonal response with the potential of being successful and adaptive or unsuccessful and maladaptive. A brief schematic summary of the major points of each model will be presented, as they form the basis of discussion of a variety of countertransference issues confronted by therapists.

INTERACTIVE PROCESSES

Wilson and Lindy (1994) outline three interactive processes that influence countertransference and its potential pathological outcomes.

The first process is the interplay of the *determinants of countertransference reactions (CTRs):* nature of the stressors in the traumatic event and story, personal factors in the therapist, specific factors in the patient, and institutional or organizational factors.

The second process is the *recovery process.* Focusing on the traumatic events themselves, five phases of the recovery process can be identified. They are influenced by the interactions of the determinants of CTRs. The phases of recovery are as follows.

- *Phase 1:* Trauma story and recall immediately after event.
- *Phase 2:* Trauma story as remembered and reconstructed.
- *Phase 3:* Trauma story "unfolds," elaborates, and develops; new affect and imagery.
- *Phase 4:* Trauma story as reappraised and reconstructed; affect and imagery placed in newer meaning system.
- *Phase 5:* Trauma story as integrated; assimilation within changed self-structure.

The third process is *empathic break.* The recovery process follows a time line. At each phase of recovery, there is empathic stress. When the stress results in an empathic break, the fourth

process occurs, which is an outcome. There are a variety of potential pathological outcomes that can be caused by CTRs.

Example of outcomes associated with each phase of recovery follow. When there is empathic break at phase 1, the immediate recounting of the traumatic event and story leads to cessation of the recovery process by a break in beginning therapy. In phase 2, reconstructing and remembering the trauma is encumbered by empathic breaks with a fixation within the phase. There is no movement away from the affective arousal associated with the trauma story and its remembrance. In phases 3 and 4, where there is an elaboration of the trauma story and how it has been organized within the individual and is manifested in the shifting patterns of engagement, empathic stress and loss of the therapeutic role results in the intensification of transference issues pertaining to the patient's self-esteem, safety, affect regulation, fear of abandonment, trust level, fear of betrayal, sense of control, and loss of self-object. And in phase 5, rather than integration of the trauma material, a break in empathy results in acting out on the part of the patient and therapist.

Empathic stress and strains with defensive shifts in both patient and therapist influence the cognitive attributional processes and formulation of affective responses at each phase of recovery. Broadly speaking, two types of CTRs have been identified. The summary of type I and type II CTRs provides markers for a therapist to use in assessing his or her response to a trauma patient.

A continuum of type I countertransference that results in avoidance is as follows. In the beginning there is *denial* of post-traumatic stress disorder (PTSD). Underlying the denial is fear of the trauma story and the patient, as well as fear of contagion. Next is *minimization* of the trauma impact, with a failure to identify PTSD symptoms and to seek quick recovery. Next in the continuum is *distortion*. Here there is a type of engagement of the patient, but there is a shift to pretrauma events, with an overemphasis on childhood dynamics and a failure to appreciate CTRs emerging in the relationship. Next is *avoidance*, with an overreliance on conventional treatments. There is an emergence of strong affective responses to the patient such as dread, guilt, disgust, loathing, numbing shame, horror with counterphobic responses (excessive efforts to re-engage, disregarding boundaries, and resulting in an intensification of the overwhelming feelings pushing the therapist away from the patient). The therapist begins missing appointments and the patient responds with canceled appointments. Next is *detachment*, with rejection, blame, moral judgments, anger, and disdain towards the patient (usually justified on the basis of the behavior of the patient towards the therapist). Numbing increases. Finally, there is *withdrawal*, marked by a referral of the patient elsewhere, or resisting of treatment by the patient, with a treatment standstill marked by acting out. Overmedicating and focusing on medicines is another possibility, distancing the patient and therapist, with premature termination.

A continuum of type II countertransference (overidentification) is summarized here. The first stage is *dependency*. It can be reciprocal or may consist of pathological bonding by the patient, which may be very subtle. Beginning therapists are often subject to pathological bonding, without fully understanding what is occurring. They misinterpret the patient's idealization of the therapist as the patient's being cooperative and functional.

The next response is *enmeshment*, in which there are role and boundary problems that are either partially addressed or unrecognized. Distorted dynamics are set up in the reciprocal role-taking of patient and therapist. There are distorted dynamics, such as believing the patient is making progress while the patient is accommodating the therapist to maintain the dependent attachment. The therapist has a hard time responding in a manner that fosters the client in containing his or her feelings. Often there is a sense of "me too," where the therapist resonates with the patient's positions without inquiry.

Next is *overcommitment/idealization*, which is often reciprocal, but is marked by the therapist's view of the patient. There is excessive advocacy and assumption of responsibility for the patient, as well as a voyeuristic idealization of the patient, with the patient seen as a hero.

Next, the therapist becomes at all costs the *rescuer/healer*. There is a narcissistic belief that the therapist is a specialist in PTSD who very few other therapists can equal. This belief often cuts the therapist off from supervision. Behind this belief is guilt and shame, either a longstanding problem for the therapist or emerging as the burden of overidentification with the patient increases. Finally, there is an overemphasis on the traumatic event or some aspect of the patient's trauma response. For example, there may be an overemphasis without adequate evaluation of the dissociative states of the patient. There can be an overemphasis and focus on the trauma story itself without reduction in its impact on the patient. With this comes a failure to put the trauma story in full lifespan perspective.

SURVIVAL STRATEGIES

Valent's (1995) perspective on survival strategies provides markers for understanding the complex role shifts that occur when working with trauma victims and complements the Wilson and Lindy model.

Munroe and associates (1995) discussed what Parson (1993) and others such as Herman (1992) and van der Kolk and colleagues (1993) regard as the most damaging aspects of victimization—alterations in the self system. In trauma, the alterations are manifested in role assumption and ascription of both patient and therapist. The various roles of the therapist include a failed protector, collaborator, rescuer, comforter, judge, conspirator, perpetrator, fellow survivor, victim, and authority figure.

Valent has proposed to evaluate these roles in terms of survival value. The basic premise is that these roles are a means to successfully survive via an adaptation both physiologically and psychosocially. The adoption of the role can be successful and be manifested in a successful biological, psychological, and social sense; or it can be unsuccessful and be marked by maladaptive responses in biological, psychological, and social spheres.

He identifies eight survival strategies. Table 11–1 summarizes them. These strategies have been arrived at following the empirical and theoretical propositions of MacLean (1990) regarding the triune brain. Through the evolution of species, there are built-in survival responses that have both physiological and psychosocial payoffs. These responses result in patterned interpersonal engagement schema. Overdetermined or misused, they become the province of empathic breaks as both patient and therapist attempt to extricate themselves from maladaptive patterns.

For example, the survival responses of seeking a rescuer and rescuing and protecting are absolutely essential for the survival of the young and the endangered. Care and empathy with devotion lead to socially positive outcomes of responsible, nurturing and altruistic patterns. These activities are supported physiologically with a sense of well-being. However, in the face of sympathetic and parasympathetic arousal associated with maladaptive roles, such as rescuing and protecting, there is a sense of depletion and self-concern where the social experience becomes one of obligation or a turning away with ensuing neglect and rejection.

The recasting of the patient's and therapist's behavior within this framework shifts the interpretive framework of the therapist in viewing his or her own behavior and that of the patient. Furthermore, it assists in understanding more fully the role of defensive identification in transference experiences and the therapist's potential to respond in an "as if" manner by becoming in some manner the feared projection of the patient. More often than not, the rescuer becomes the failed protector by virtue of the impossible expectation that, no matter what, one can "always" rescue the patient.

In an effort to consolidate the use of these two models in understanding CTRs, we will return to the opening case and others to demonstrate the usefulness of these revised concepts to an understanding of transference and countertransference.

APPLICATION OF THE MODELS

The opening example of the student and the clinic system demonstrates clearly the interaction of the four dimensions that interact to create CTRs. The clinic was under stress as to whether it would continue to exist and operate. Further, the case load of providers and those supervising students was extremely heavy, with very complex problems and limited resources. This burden is evident in the assignment of the patient to the student. Part of the rationale for the assignment was that the student was to have supervision. Everyone ignored the supervisor's pregnancy and its disruption of the student's supervision.

The student initially developed a type I CTR marked by a counterphobic response. Mr. M. became her favorite patient because he kept his appointments and she needed to feel that patients accepted her and to feel that she had a patient to refer to as a success at the end of the year. What sustained her was her view of Mr. M. as a child about 9 years old; which was, interestingly enough, the age group she taught for years before deciding to become a therapist. She had no way of understanding this 9-year-old boy because she never discussed him or explored her response to him. Rather, she was attempting to assist him by having him grieve the loss of his wife. He felt responsible for his wife, although they had been separated. He was guilty, feeling he had not done enough to help her. He himself was a counselor in a clinic treating recovering alcoholics, and it was in this clinic that he met his wife. His wife had been a patient at the clinic and, a year after her discharge, they dated and then married. He was 15 years older than his

TABLE 11–1. SURVIVAL STRATEGY COMPONENTS

Appraisal of Means of Survival	Survival Strategies	Successful/Adaptive Responses			Unsuccessful/Maladaptive Responses			
		Biological	Psychological	Social	Biological	Psychological	Social	Trauma Responses
Must save others	Rescuing Protect Provide	↑Estrogen ↑Oxytocin ↑Opioids	Care Empathy *Devotion*	Responsibility Nurture *Altruism*	Sympathetic & parasymp. arousal	Resentment Depletion *Self-concern*	Burden Neglect *Rejection*	Anguished Survivor guilt Caused death
Must be saved by others	Attaching Protected Provided	?↑Opioids	Yearning Need *Contentment*	Reaching out Crying out *Union*	↓Opioids	Abandondment Deprivation *Aloneness*	Clinging Demanding *Separation*	Dread Cast out Left to die
Must achieve goal	Asserting Combat Work	↑E, NE ↓Cortisol ↑Immunocomp.	Strength High morale *Potency*	Will Success *Control*	↑↑E, NE Depletion E, NE ↑BP, ?CHD	Frustration Low morale *Powerlessness*	Willfulness Failure *Lost Control*	Burnout Learned helplessness
Must surrender goal	Adapting Accept Grieve	Parasymp. Arousal Cortisol	Acceptance Mourning *Hope*	Yielding Loss *Turn to new*	↑Cortisol ↓Immunocomp. ↑Infection, ↑CA	Helplessness Depression *Despair*	Overwhelmed Withdrawal *Given in*	Vulnerability Given up Succumbing
Must remove danger	Fighting Defend Rid	Sympathetic arousal ↑NE, E ↑BP	Threat Revenge *Frighten*	Deterrence Wounding *Riddance*	↑↑Sympathetic arousal ↓Cortisol	Hatred Persecution *Killing*	Attack Eradication *Destruction*	Horror Evil Murder
Must remove oneself from danger	Fleeing Retreat Save oneself	Sympathetic & parasymp. arousal	Fear Terror *Deliverance*	Hiding Flight *Escape*	NE depletion ↑E & Cortisol	Phobia Paranoia *Engulfment*	Avoidance Panic *Annihilation*	"Inescapable shock," being hunted, killed
Must obtain scarce essentials	Competing Struggle Acquire	↑Testosterone Sympathetic arousal	Winning Possession *Power*	Dominance Privilege *Take*	↓Testosterone ↓Female hormones ↑Cortisol	Defeat Greed, envy *Crushed*	Submission Plundered *Emptied*	Terrorization Marginalization Elimination
Must create more essentials	Cooperating Trust Mutual gain	↑Opiates ↓BP, E, NE	Mutuality Generosity *Creativity*	Reciprocity Sharing *Synthesis*	↓Opiates ?↑Parasymp. arousal	Ident w aggr Exploited *Stagnation*	Appeasement Robbed *Disintegration*	Alienation Fragmentation Decay

BP, blood pressure; CHD, chronic heart disease; E, epinephrine; NE, norepinephrine.
Reproduced with permission from Valent (1995, p. 32).

wife. Theirs was a stormy relationship, with a variety of suicidal gestures on her part with hospitalization and ultimately a decision to separate. He did continue to have contact with her and gave her money.

The young therapist believed she was addressing this information by being sympathetic to Mr. M. and becoming concerned, as he was, with his fear that he was going to resume drinking and break his sobriety. Although the focus of this work may have been timely, the countertransference responses were not attended to. Rather, the student interpreted her work as supportive. When she found herself becoming angry with Mr. M. over the Christmas holidays and his choice to spend them with a staff member from his agency, she was unaware of what this implied. He had stabilized from his initial depressed state and indicated he wanted to get on with his life. He became involved with a co-worker, who was also a recovering alcoholic. She indicated she wanted nothing but a platonic relationship. He asked her to go to Florida with him to visit with his parents. She agreed, but only on the condition that he realized the relationship was limited. When they came back he was furious with her and felt betrayed and exploited.

The student therapist was angry with him because "she had warned him, told him not to ask her and take her." She felt that something had shifted in their otherwise good working relationship. She had identified his self-defeating behaviors as the focus for the first conference.

These were the issues that she brought to her first consultation, only to have the focus switched to issues surrounding suspicions of the nature of his wife's death. This conference forced her to think of him as a man, not a boy. With the view of him as a man, and a possible abuser and murderer, all of the counterphobic responses dissipated and she found herself angry and withdrawn from him, yet desperate to find someone to work with him.

The second consultation was constructed to accomplish several goals. First, to preserve for the patient and the student the positive aspects of their relationship. Second, to reframe the therapeutic issues to be addressed with Mr. M. so that the staff would be more encouraged in their efforts to work with him. Third, to underscore, with all concerned, how an understanding of early victimization impacts on the therapeutic relationship.

The initial part of the consultation dealt with the 9-year-old boy and the man—a possible perpetrator but also a rescuer. This provided an opportunity to discuss the context in which the clinic initially received the information about Mr. M., as well as the student's context for working with him. This opened up an exploration of the comfort zones established in the initial roles we set up to have a sense of rapport with one another and with patients. It is a very important question to ask whether rapport can be broken in a relationship, yet the relationship maintained. When there is fear that the relationship will end, these early interpersonal and intrapersonal rapport strategies to survive without losing the relationship are taken as a committed relationship, ignoring the defensive nature of the roles and manners being adopted. Here was a caretaker, possibly responsible for the death of a woman he had rescued. For the staff, it was an aversive situation. The possibility of working with a perpetrator and one who had difficulty with boundaries, which were not addressed or explored, resulted in Mr. M. being assigned to a student, who overrode her aversion through a complex processes of identifying him as a 9-year-old boy, for whom she had both positive and personal experiences in teaching. He responded and kept coming, and there are few therapists who do not remember training experiences and the feelings of failure and humiliation when patients did not establish relationships with them and attend meetings. The context for this student was fraught with circumstances that did not allow her counterphobic response to the patient to be identified. She mistook her strategies for survival and the ongoing relationship for a therapeutic one. Thus, a state of disengagement from the patient persisted for the aspiring therapist, which was being gradually revealed when Mr. M. did not heed her advice to refrain from involvement with another woman at his center and was pushed by the prior conference in which less favorable dimensions of his personality were pointed out.

From this, it was easy to open up the whole area of trauma and its impact on patients and therapists and help both staff and student identify with the natural patterns of engaging and disengaging that go on between traumatized patients and therapists. Murder is an overwhelming subject.

Combining the insights of types I and II, with survival strategies and dynamic roles assumed, provided general themes to which many personal examples could be given by the consultant and identified by the group as well as the student. With this background, the next step was to move to the consideration of working with someone who might be a perpetrator. The session refocused on the need for further evaluation of Mr. M. in terms of strengths and vulnerabilities, with the goal of reviewing and reformulating work with him. At the end of the consultation, there again was a review of transference and countertransference issues and how they can be used to understand and clarify treatment involvement.

A poll had been taken before the discussion of Mr. M. as to how many of the staff would want to work with him. At the end of the session, the initial unanimous "no" had changed, with some members of the staff possibly being interested in working with him and others having a different perspective on Mr. M. Further, all had some positive ideas of how to introduce the subject of the ongoing investigation of his wife's death and its impact on him.

► CASE EXAMPLE: SELF-SUFFICIENT OR DEPENDENT? AN IMPORTANT EARLY QUESTION

Dr. K. had finished medical school and a residency in primary care. She was an active athlete, but of late found herself overly involved in dieting to maintain her weight for sports competitions, which were adjusted by weight divisions. She decided to consult a therapist who worked with eating disorders. Approximately 6 months into therapy, she became depressed and realized that her life was most unhappy. She had earlier denied problems with her parents. She began to reflect on a rather bizarre childhood where she and her parents and brothers moved from one religious cult to another. She also felt she was sexually abused by her mother and possibly by her father. The therapist, feeling inadequate to deal with this new information, referred her to another therapist. Work went well for 3 years, at which point the therapist had to terminate with the patient because the therapist planned to marry and leave the state. The therapist was looking for another therapist to take over the therapy. She remarked on how resourceful the patient was, and how much they had accomplished together in therapy. In the process of therapy the patient had renounced her involvement in the last cult that she and her family had joined and thus severed relationships with her parents.

Another therapist agreed to interview the patient, providing that the patient's current therapist also gave her other therapists to see, so that the patient had a sense that she had options when she did select someone to work with. At the initial evaluation, the patient revealed an idolized dependent relationship with her current therapist. She was both sad and angry that she was leaving. The patient also revealed that approximately two times a month she was consumed with suicidal ideation and was unclear what precipitated it. Her terminating therapist had worked closely with her during these times, giving her tapes to see her through when alone. In addition, she had set the patient up with a group therapist who also made herself available. A variety of safety plans had been established. When asked what she wanted in a therapist, the patient responded that it was a woman, who was or had been married, had children and raised them. Although she considered therapy in terms of time frame, she actually imagined an ongoing relationship that she could turn to for the rest of her life; she wanted a therapist who would see her through marriage, and pregnancy, and the rearing of children.

People subjected to early and extensive psychological and physical or sexual abuse present complex pictures. On one hand they can be brilliant and resourceful; on the other, the loss and damage to the self-system, with the resultant alterations in attachment and interpersonal processing of affective exchanges, can be extremely primitive and basic. Thus, a therapist is balancing strengths and weaknesses of patients. The amount of empathic strain is tremendous in the effort to balance the conflicting dimensions of the patient's wants and needs. Anticipating this, the prospective therapist wanted to make sure the patient began to recognize that there could be more than one therapist in the world and that she had choices. The request that she see other therapists was important.

The burden of dependency that the patient expressed in her idealized personification of the therapist was beginning to take its toll. When the therapist revealed that closing her practice and finding someone for her patient afforded her a sense of relief, she found herself trying to pick a replacement for herself—someone who could continue the dependent relationship until the patient was strong enough to leave on her own accord.

Good therapists willing to work with difficult patients are hard to find. Too often they are prevailed upon by others to take on complex cases, only to be overloaded. Such was the case of the referring therapist. She was asking the potential therapist how much time she took for vacations and explained her views on just how much time she believed the patient could tolerate separated from the therapist.

As difficult as it might seem, complex cases such as this should best be referred to a team, so that no one person bears the total burden of very traumatized individuals who are deeply in need. It is important to keep the team healthy. When this is done, the splitting that occurs in the malfunctioning survival strategies of the patient can be addressed in nonpunitive and therapeutic ways (Munroe et al., 1994).

The referring therapist and patient had set up a network for the patient by having her in a group setting as well as in an individual setting; a psychpharmacologist was also available. A level of stability had been achieved; however, it was now falling apart. It had emerged in the process of the patient breaking with her community, the cult, and her family. Naturally, the patient is angry and looking for a replacement. However, her level of distrust of others and of herself has increased.

The therapist who interviewed the patient took all of this dynamic into account and in part used to the interview to (1) frame the termination as a chance for growth; (2) reframe the patient's beliefs and concepts of therapy so she could see multiple therapeutic options; (3) reinforce the positive work done and the courage and determination it had taken; and (4) gently acknowledge with the patient that there were many positive people in her past as well as present life, such as her grandparents and friends she liked within the cult, and how she would eventually (she has a plan and conditions) break totally with the cult yet have a level of contact with her parents and family if she wants. Although this does not necessarily reduce the intensity of transference should the therapist and patient decide to work together, it does lay down important aspects of a therapeutic alliance that can serve as a basis for challenges to disruptive experiences within the therapeutic relationship.

In this second example one therapist distanced herself from the patient and the other became enmeshed in being the protector and rescuer of the patient, and with the break from the parents and family, a substitute for them.

SUMMARY

These two cases underscore the need for therapists to understand that when there is severe trauma in patients' backgrounds, underlying distrust of self and others is perpetuated by an inability to regulate affect and discern interpersonal transactions with a degree of self-observation. Survival strategies, although initially adaptive, become maladaptive, and there are transitions between the two poles of adaptation. As therapists, it is difficult to always divine where the patient is in adaptation. An appreciation of this, as well as of the therapist's own response to the nature of the events that have inflicted harm on the patient, provides a basis for working with and evaluating work with these patients. Mr. M. presents with his passivity and his patterns of being a caretaker and rescuer; Dr. K. makes a break with her family and attempts to substitute not only what she has lost, but what she has ideally sought. These cases underscore some basic principles that must be employed in therapeutic efforts.

First, it is necessary to be aware of the context in which one accepts working with patients and the pathway of referral to services. Second, one must take the time to evaluate and build a therapeutic alliance based on the most realistic expectations of the patient and therapist involved. The limits of this alliance have to be appraised and the alliance has to be renegotiated as therapy progresses. The alliance is the safety zone for the patient and the therapist as the consequences of transference and countertransference issues are addressed in the therapy, whether with groups or individuals. Third, collaboration, consultation, and evaluation of therapy relationships must be a continuous process. Fourth, the therapist has to adopt self-enhancing experiences for herself or himself outside of the role of therapist and caretaker. Basic good mental hygiene—which includes adequate rest, diet, and recreation—are a must. Other self-maintaining activities need to be reviewed and adopted, such as meditation and positive social experiences.

Dr. Figley (1995) has devised a tool to assess participation as therapists and to evaluate whether one is experiencing compassion fatigue (Fig. 11–1). The reader of this chapter is encouraged to take it and then reflect on the principles set forth in the conclusions.

Name _____ Institution _____ Date _____

Please describe yourself: ___ *Male* ___ *Female* _____ *years as practitioner. Consider each of the following characteristics about you and your current situation. Write in the number for the best response. Use one of the following answers:*

> *1=Rarely/Never   2=At Times   3=Not Sure   4=Often   5=Very Often*

Answer all items, even if not applicable. Then read the instructions to get your score.

Items About You:

1. ___ *I force myself to avoid certain thoughts or feelings that remind me of a frightening experience.*
2. ___ *I find myself avoiding certain activities or situations because they remind me of a frightening experience.*
3. ___ *I have gaps in my memory about frightening events.*
4. ___ *I feel estranged from others.*
5. ___ *I have difficulty falling or staying asleep.*
6. ___ *I have outbursts of anger or irritability with little provocation.*
7. ___ *I startle easily.*
8. ___ *While working with a victim I thought about violence against the perpetrator.*
9. ___ *I am a sensitive person.*
10. ___ *I have had flashbacks connected to my clients.*
11. ___ *I have had first-hand experience with traumatic events in my adult life.*
12. ___ *I have had first-hand experience with traumatic events in my childhood.*
13. ___ *I have thought that I need to "work through" a traumatic experience in my life.*
14. ___ *I have thought that I need more close friends.*
15. ___ *I have thought that there is no one to talk with about highly stressful experiences.*
16. ___ *I have concluded that I work too hard for my own good.*
17. ___ *I am frightened of things a client has said or done to me.*
18. ___ *I experience troubling dreams similar to those of a client of mine.*
19. ___ *I have experienced intrusive thoughts of sessions with especially difficult clients.*
20. ___ *I have suddenly and involuntarily recalled a frightening experience while working with a client.*
21. ___ *I am preoccupied with more than one client.*
22. ___ *I am losing sleep over a client's traumatic experience.*
23. ___ *I have thought that I might have been "infected" by the traumatic stress of my clients.*
24. ___ *I remind myself to be less concerned about the well-being of my clients.*
25. ___ *I have felt trapped by my work as a therapist.*

Continued

Figure 11–1. Compassion fatigue self-test for psychotherapists. *(Reproduced with permission from Figley, 1995.)*

26.___ I have felt a sense of hopelessness associated with working with clients.

27.___ I have felt "on edge" about various things and I attribute this to working with certain clients.

28.___ I have wished that I could avoid working with some therapy clients.

29.___ I have been in danger working with therapy clients.

30.___ I have felt that my clients dislike me personally.

Items About Being a Psychotherapist and Your Work Environment:

31.___ I have felt weak, tired, rundown as a result of my work as a therapist.

32.___ I have felt depressed as a result of my work as a therapist.

33.___ I am unsuccessful at separating work from personal life.

34.___ I feel little compassion toward most of my co-workers.

35.___ I feel I am working more for the money than for personal fulfillment.

36.___ I find it difficult separating my personal life from my work life.

37.___ I have a sense of worthlessness/disillusionment/resentment associated with my work.

38.___ I have thoughts that I am a "failure" as a psychotherapist.

39.___ I have thoughts that I am not succeeding at achieving my life goals.

40.___ I have to deal with bureaucratic, unimportant tasks in my work life.

Scoring Instructions: (a) Be certain you responded to all items. (b) Circle the following 23 items: 1–8, 10–13, 17–26, and 29. (c) Add the numbers you wrote next to the items. (d) Note your risk of Compassion Fatigue: 26 or less = Extremely low risk; 27 to 30 = Low risk; 31 to 35 = Moderate risk; 36 to 40 = High risk; 41 or more = Extremely high risk.

Then, (e) Add the numbers you write next to the items not circled. (f) Note your risk of burnout: 17–36 or less = Extremely low risk; 37–50 = Moderate risk; 51–75 = High risk; 76–85 = Extremely high risk.

Scores for this instrument emerged using a sample of 142 psychotherapy practitioners attending workshops on the topic during 1992 and 1993. Psychometric properties of the scale are reported by Stamm and Vara (1993). Alpha reliability scores ranged from 94 to 86; structural analysis yielded at least one stable factor which is characterized by depressed mood in relationship to work accompanied by feelings of fatigue, disillusionment, and worthlessness. Structural Reliability (stability) of this factor, as indicated by Tucker's Coefficient of Congruence (cc), is .91.

Figure 11–1. *(Continued)*

REFERENCES

Buie D. The hateful patient. Paper presented at Bridgewater State Hospital Conference on Violence, Bridgewater, MA, June 1994.

Caplan G. *The Theory and Practice of Mental Health Consultation*. New York: Basic Books; 1970.

Danieli Y. The use of mutual support approaches in the treatment of victims. In: Chigier E, ed. *Grief and Bereavement in Contemporary Society*. 1988;3: 116–123.

Danieli Y. The treatment and prevention of long-term effects and intergenerational transmission of victimization: A lesson from Holocaust survivors and their children. In: Figley CR, ed. *Trauma and Its Wake*. New York: Brunner/Mazel; 1985: 15–35.

Danieli Y. Countertransference in the treatment and study of Nazi Holocaust survivors and their children. *Victimology*. 1980;5:355–367.

Eth S, Pynoos RS. Post-traumatic stress disorder in children. Washington, DC: American Psychiatric Press; 1985.

Figley CR. Compassion Fatigue: Coping With Secondary Traumatic Stress Disorder in Those Who Treat the Traumatized. New York: Brunner/Mazel; 1995.

Figley CR, ed. *Compassion Fatigue: Secondary Traumatic Stress Disorder from Treating the Traumatized*. New York: Brunner/Mazel; 1995.

Friedman MJ. Psychobiological and pharmacological approaches to treatment. In: Wilson JP, Raphael B, eds. *International Handbook of Traumatic Stress Syndrome*. New York: Plenum, 1993.

Friedman MJ, Charney DS, Deutch AU. *Neurobiological and Clinical Consequences of Stress: From Normal Adaptation to Post-traumatic Stress Disorder.* New York: Lippincott-Raven; 1995.

Giller E, ed. *Biological Assessment and Treatment of Posttraumatic Stress Disorder.* Progress in Psychiatry series. Washington, DC: American Psychiatric Press; 1990.

Gleser GC, Green BL, Winget C. *Prolonged Psychological Effects of Disaster: A Study of Buffalo Creek.* New York: Academic Press; 1981.

Haley SA. When a patient reports atrocities: Specific treatment considerations in the Vietnam veteran. *Arch Gen Psychiatry,* 1974;30:191–196.

Hartman CR, Jackson H. Rape and the phenomena of countertransference. In: Wilson JP, Lindy JD, eds. *Countertransference in the Treatment of PTSD.* New York: Guilford Press; 1994:206–244.

Herman JW. *Trauma and Recovery.* New York: Basic Books; 1992.

Hinshaw AS, Atwood JR. Nursing staff turnover, stress, and satisfaction: Models, measures, and management. In: Weley HH, Fitzpatrick JJ, eds. *Annual Review of Nursing Research.* New York: Springer; 1984:133–153.

Horowitz M. Intrusive and repetitive thoughts after experimental stress. *Arch Gen Psychiatry.* 1976;32:1457–1463.

Jacobson SF, McGrath HM. *Nurses Under Stress.* New York: Wiley;1983.

Kluft RP. Countertransference in the treatment of multiple personality disorder. In: Wilson JP, Lindy JD, eds. *Countertransference in the Treatment of PTSD.* New York: Guilford Press;1994:122–150.

Kluft RP. The rehabilitation of therapists overwhelmed by their work with multiple personality disorder patients. *Dissociation.* 1989;2:244–250.

MacLean PD. *The Triune Brain in Evolution.* New York: Plenum; 1990.

McCann IL, Pearlman LA. *Psychological Trauma and the Adult Survivor.* New York: Brunner/Mazel; 1990.

Mollica RF. The trauma story: The psychiatric care of refugee survivors of violence and torture. In: Ochberg FM, ed. *Post-traumatic Therapy and Victims of Violence.* New York: Brunner/Mazel; 1988:295–314.

Munroe JF. Therapist traumatization from exposure to clients with combat related post-traumatic stress disorder: Implications for administration and supervision. Unpublished doctoral dissertation, 1991. Available from Dissertation Abstracts, Ann Arbor.

Munroe JF, Shay J, Fisher L, et al. Presentation of research and team work in the management of stress in the provider. Trauma Group meeting, June 1994.

Norbeck JS. Perceived job stress, job satisfaction, and psychological symptoms in critical care nursing. *Res Nurs Health.* 1986;34:225–230.

Parson ER. Posttraumatic narcissism: Healing traumatic alterations in the self through curvilinear group psychotherapy. In: Wilson JP, Raphael B, eds. *International Handbook of Traumatic Stress Syndromes.* New York: Plenum; 1993:821–840.

Pynoos RS, Nader K. Psychological first aid and treatment approach to children exposed to community violence: Research implications. *J Traumatic Stress.* 1988;1:445–474.

Racker H. *Transference and Countertransference.* New York: International Universities Press; 1968.

Slatker E. *Countertransference.* New York: Aronson; 1987.

Solomon Z. From front line to home front: Wives of PTSD veterans. Paper presented at the sixth annual meeting of the Society for Traumatic Stress Studies, New Orleans, 1990.

Stanton AH, Schwartz MS. *The Mental Hospital.* New York: Basic Books; 1954.

Sullivan HS. *The Interpersonal Theory of Psychiatry.* New York: Norton; 1953.

Ursano RJ, McCaughey BG, Fullerton CS. *Individual and Community Responses to Trauma and Disaster: The Structure of Human Chaos.* New York: Cambridge University Press; 1994.

Vachon MLS. *Occupational Stress in the Care of the Critically Ill, the Dying and the Bereaved.* New York: Hemisphere; 1987.

Valent P. Survival strategies: A framework for understanding secondary traumatic stress and coping in helpers. In: Figley CR, ed. *Compassion Fatigue: Coping With Secondary Traumatic Stress Disorder in Those Who Treat the Traumatized.* New York: Brunner/Mazel; 1995.

Van der Kolk BA, McFarlane AC, Weisaeth L. eds. *Traumatic Stress: The effects of overwhelming experience on mind, body and society.* New York: Guilford Press; 1996.

Van der Kolk BA, Saporta J. Biological response to psychic trauma. In: Wilson JP, Raphael B, eds. *International Handbook of Traumatic Stress Syndromes.* New York: Plenum; 1993:25–33.

Wilson JP, Lindy JD. *Countertransference in the Treatment of PTSD.* New York: Guilford Press; 1994.

CHAPTER 12

TRAUMA AND MEMORY: CLINICAL AND LEGAL UNDERSTANDING OF TRAUMATIC AMNESIA

Charles L. Whitfield

It is neither the job nor the goal of the therapist to be a legal investigator. The therapist's task is to assist the survivor in accomplishing the goals of recovery.

Chapter Overview

► INTRODUCTION

Trauma is any event, usually a non-ordinary one, that harms the body, self, or spirit. It covers a broad range of hurtful experiences, including traumas that involve the physical, sexual, mental, or emotional realms of our being.

The field of trauma psychology has been developing for the past century. We first learned of it from Janet, Brauer, and Freud, and later from numerous observers of combat trauma. More recently, we have begun to fine-tune our knowledge by observing different kinds of trauma, from physical violence to child sexual abuse to growing up in an alcoholic or other dysfunctional family.

If the trauma is accepted as real and the victim or survivor's experience is validated and its expression supported, as happened in the Oklahoma City bombing incident, its short-term effects, which are also known as acute traumatic stress, can be expressed, processed, ameliorated, or "metabolized" in a healthy way so that eventually few or no lasting detrimental effects remain. However, if the reality of the traumatic experience is denied or invalidated by the victim—or by close or important others, such as family, friends, or helping professionals—then the person may not be able to heal completely from the trauma. If the trauma continues, with still no validation and support in expressing its associated pain, it may develop into post-traumatic stress disorder.

To heal from trauma, the experiencer has to be able to grieve the associated pain. To grieve, the individual must remember the trauma well enough to name it accurately (for example, "I was mugged or beaten up on the street last night."). Thus, remembering is a key to resolving the effects of the trauma.

People may accurately remember the essence or core of the trauma, such as a serious auto accident, and some of its details, but they usually misremember one or more of the details. The less they are focused on certain details, and the more time that has elapsed since the trauma, the less they tend to remember accurately about some of those details.

People may accurately remember most of a traumatic experience in any of three ways: completely (or fairly so), partially or not at all. The latter two may be referred to as *traumatic amnesia*, and it is this clinical observation that will be the focus of this chapter. Although traumatic amnesia may occur in most kinds of traumas, it commonly occurs in child sexual abuse.

Accused Child Sexual Abusers

A characteristic of child molesters is that most deny their abusive behavior. That observation, plus the fact that in rare instances a person may be falsely accused of child sexual abuse, has prompted a strong reaction from some of those who have been accused. In 1984, people accused of child molestation formed a group and called themselves Victims of Child Abuse Laws (VOCAL).

THE FALSE MEMORY DEFENSE

In early 1992 the False Memory Syndrome Foundation (FMSF) was formed. It was claimed that persons accusing parents or others of having molested them when children had a "false memory syndrome" and that their false memories were implanted by outside sources, such as their therapists, self-help groups, books, and other suggestive influences (*FMSF newsletter*, 1992–1997).

But prior to and since the FMSF was founded, not a single case report of any clinical condition known as false memory syndrome has been published in any of the peer-reviewed clinical or scientific literature. It is not in any of the diagnostic code books and is not recognized as a bona-fide clinical disorder by any of the mental health professional associations or societies. It is not included or even mentioned in any of the five editions of the *Diagnostic and Statistical Manual of Mental Disorders* (DSM) of the American Psychiatric Association.

Brown and colleagues (in press) argue that there is no convincing evidence in the clinical and scientific literature that anyone can "suggest" or "implant" enduring false memories of childhood sexual abuse or induce the long-term effects of child sexual abuse into individuals or groups of people without actually abusing them.

Some forensic psychologists and sociologists affiliated with the FMSF have coined another term as part of the false memory defense: recovered memory therapy (RMT). Like FMS, RMT is not recognized by the DSM-IV or any similar authoritative source, yet some defense attorneys and their expert witnesses continue to use the term.

BASIS OF THE FALSE MEMORY SYNDROME HYPOTHESIS

The false memory syndrome hypothesis is based on three observations: (1) denial by the person accused of child sexual abuse, (2) the stories of 200 or more retractors (to date not reported in peer-reviewed publications), and (3) a few research studies, most of them concerned with or-dinary memory. The first base is the weakest, as many convicted criminals, especially child molesters, deny that they committed the crime of which they have been accused. It would be useful to study voice inflection and other aspects of expression and behavior to explore exactly how people who are truly innocent say "I didn't do it" and contrast that with how those who are guilty say the same thing. This kind of study would be a useful research project for a team of an attorney and a trauma clinician, for example.

Likewise, it would be useful to study in depth and over time a group of retractors. Retractors are people who subsequently take back their disclosure or accusation of abuse. Some observers suspect that a large but as yet unknown percentage of retractors *were* sexually abused, but may have named the wrong perpetrator. Others probably were abused and named the right perpetrator, but for some reason, perhaps family pressure or fear of losing one or more family relationships, retracted their original and accurate story. From the clinical and scientific literature it is clear that retraction or recantation is a common part of the natural history of the effects of child sexual abuse (Briere, 1992a; Salter, 1995; Summit, 1983; Whitfield, 1995). Some clues that may help differentiate retractors' true memories from untrue ones are described in Table 12–1 (Whitfield, 1995c).

CLINICAL OBSERVATIONS AND UNDERSTANDING

Over the past 100 years we have accumulated a sizable amount of information about the frequency and dynamics of traumatic amnesia (traumatic forgetting, also called dissociative amnesia), and our clinical understanding of it has sharpened during the past 15 years.

POST-TRAUMATIC STRESS DISORDER

Examining the current diagnostic criteria for post-traumatic stress disorder (PTSD) helps in understanding traumatic amnesia. One hundred

TABLE 12–1. OBSERVATIONS AND FINDINGS SUGGESTIVE OF TRUE AND UNTRUE TRAUMATIC MEMORY

Observation	True Memory	Untrue Memory
High risk disorder(s) present	Yes	No
Attractions, fears or avoidances unexplained by known history	May be present	Absent
Indications of emerging memories (e.g., dreams, images, flashbacks, or somatic sensations)	May be present	Absent
Evidence of dissociation	Often present	Absent
Time loss	Often present	Absent to slight
Supplying inconsequential detail in abuse history	May be present	Absent
Story matches depth of pain and symptoms throughout life	Usual	May be present
Tends to avoid sympathy and support	May be present	May be absent
Knows or senses how a perpetrator will act	May be present	Absent
Corroborating data present (e.g., medical, witness, photos)	Usually absent, but helpful if present	Absent
High ambivalence about abuse, memories	May be present	Absent to present
Evidence of florid imagination, psychosis, or pathological lying (but dissociation may resemble and person may be misdiagnosed)	Usually absent	May be present
Duration and evolution of memory	Evolving (once remembered); May evolve to being more real and integrated	Usually degenerates, with or without evolution and integration

Modified with permission from Fredrickson (1992) and Whitfield (1995c)

years ago we called PTSD by the misleading term "hysteria," and in war we have somewhat more accurately called it "shell shock" and "combat neurosis." We have seen it develop following trauma of all sorts, from physical attack, rape, combat, concentration camp experiences, and natural disasters. It is a common result of the battered child syndrome, the battered women syndrome, the rape trauma syndrome, and the child sexual abuse accommodation syndrome (Davidson, 1993; Summit, 1983).

Traumatic stress, which leads to damaging sequelae, occurs when a person is seriously harmed physically or psychologically, especially where there is no supportive human environment in which to process the experience and heal. Its effects are usually more severe when the trauma is of human origin, and are even more severe when it comes from primary caregivers, such as parents or parent figures. The specific trauma of child sexual abuse is harmful in most of these regards.

Traumatic amnesia or forgetting is common in PTSD. Some sort of memory disturbance accounts for about half of the official clinical criteria for making the correct diagnosis of PTSD, as described in the DSM-IV. These disturbances of memory include a range of clinical manifestations of traumatic amnesia, which may be summarized as intrusive memories, unconscious memories, abreactions (dramatic reexperiencing of the trauma), flashbacks, psychological memories, somatic (physical) memories, avoidance of the experience of the memories, and partial or total amnesia for the event or events, as shown in Table 12–2 (DSM-IV, 1994; Whitfield, 1995c, p. 233).

The mental health professions of psychiatry, psychology, social work, and counseling all accept traumatic amnesia as being a valid and integral part of the natural history of the disorder of PTSD, as is reflected in the DSM-IV diagnostic criteria and in the vast body of literature on PTSD and related dissociative disorders (Davidson,

TABLE 12–2. POST-TRAUMATIC STRESS DISORDER (309.81) AND MEMORY (FROM DSM-IV)

A. The person has been exposed to a traumatic event (or events) in which both of the following have been present:
  (1) The person has experienced, witnessed, or been confronted with an event or events that involve actual or threatened death or serious injury, or a threat to the physical integrity of oneself or others.
  (2) The person's response involved intense fear, helplessness, or horror.

B. The traumatic event is persistently **re-experienced** in at least one of the following ways:
  (1) Recurrent and **intrusive** distressing **recollections** of the event, including images, thoughts, or perceptions.
  (2) Recurrent distressing **dreams** of the event.
  (3) **Acting or feeling as if the traumatic event were recurring** (includes a sense of reliving the experience, illusions, hallucinations, and dissociative flashback episodes, including those that occur upon awakening or when intoxicated).
  (4) **Intense psychological distress** at exposure to internal or external cues that symbolize or resemble an aspect of the traumatic event.
  (5) **Physiologic reactivity** upon exposure to internal or external cues that symbolize or resemble an aspect of the traumatic event.

C. **Persistent avoidance of stimuli associated with the trauma** and numbing of general responsiveness (not present before the trauma), as indicated by at least three of the following:
  (1) **Efforts to avoid** thoughts, feelings, or conversations associated with the trauma.
  (2) **Efforts to avoid** activities, places, or people that arouse recollections of the trauma.
  (3) **Inability to recall** an important aspect of the trauma.
  (4) Markedly diminished interest or participation in significant activities.
  (5) Feeling of **detachment** or **estrangement** from others.
  (6) **Restricted** range of **affect** (e.g., unable to have loving feelings).
  (7) Sense of a foreshortened future (e.g., does not expect to have a career, marriage, children, or a normal life span).

D. **Persistent symptoms** of increased arousal (not present before the trauma), as indicated by at least two of the following:
  (1) Difficulty falling or staying asleep.
  (2) Irritability or outbursts of anger.
  (3) Difficulty concentrating.
  (4) Hypervigilance.
  (5) **Exaggerated startle** response.

E. Duration of the disturbance (symptoms in B, C, and D) is more than 1 month.

F. The disturbance causes clinically significant distress or impairment in social, occupational, or other important areas of functioning.

Specify if:
  Acute: if duration of symptoms is less than 3 months.
  Chronic: if duration of symptoms is 3 months or more.

Specify if:
  With delayed onset: onset of symptoms at least 6 months after the stressor

Reproduced with permission from Whitfield (1995c).

1993; Herman, 1992; McCann and Pearlman, 1991; Putnam and Trickett, 1993; Pynoos, 1993; van der Kolk, 1987, 1994). These diagnostic criteria and the diagnosis of PTSD are used by the American Medical Association (AMA) and all health-related regulatory and insurance agencies.

From a thorough review of the clinical and scientific literature, Rowan and Foy (1993) found that PTSD appears to describe the core features of the psychological difficulties of many people who were specifically sexually abused as children. The authors also found a wide array of psychiatric and psychological problems associated with PTSD. These problems include depression; increased fears; sexual problems; feelings of isolation, guilt, distrust, and anger; low self-esteem; self-destructive behaviors; nightmares; sleep difficulties; phobias; substance abuse; a tendency to reenact the trauma and to be revictimized; and aggressive behavior. These psychiatric and psychological symptoms appear in most cases to be the after-effects of the trauma, and do not reflect defects of character or the personality of the victims (Rowan and Foy, 1993).

Likewise, from a detailed analysis of 38 clinical studies (on 2774 child sexual abuse survivors compared to 8388 controls who were not sexually abused) meeting rigorous research criteria, Neumann and colleagues (1996) found that there was a significant association between a sexual abuse history and adult symptoms. These symptoms included anxiety, anger, depression, revictimization, self-mutilation, sexual problems, substance abuse, suicidality, low self-esteem, interpersonal problems, obsessions and compulsions, dissociation, post-traumatic stress responses, and somatization (physical problems). Another review of 45 studies on 1919 sexually abused children (age range 2 to 18 years) versus 1194 controls has shown similar results (Kendall-Tackett et al., 1993).

From the findings of these recent extensive reviews of the clinical research literature, it is clear that child sexual abuse harms most of the victims in numerous ways, and that these symptoms are usually the direct result of the sexual abuse itself and are not likely to be due to other causes (Neumann et al., 1996; Rowan and Foy, 1993). Whether these people always remembered the abuse or had partial or total amnesia for it, the study results were consistent in their findings.

INCIDENCE AND PREVALENCE OF TRAUMATIC AMNESIA

To date there have been 36 studies on more than 6000 children and adults who were abused as children. The studies have shown that from 16 to 78 percent experienced partial to total amnesia for the traumatic event(s) for substantial periods of time. Most of these adults had been sexually abused as children. Some were physically and sexually abused, and a few had been only physically abused. A smaller number had witnessed

severe violence. Clinical researchers commonly observe that mental and emotional abuse nearly always accompanies physical or sexual abuse. Eight of these studies are described in some detail in *Memory and Abuse* (Whitfield, 1995). They are summarized in Table 12–3, with four additional studies.

A survey of 100 self-identified adult survivors of child sexual abuse was done, and it was found that about one third had always remembered the abuse, another third had partial amnesia, and the final third had total amnesia for the abuse (Whitfield and Stock, 1996). I have also conducted a separate ongoing survey of survivors of childhood trauma, most having been sexually abused as children. Of 171 people surveyed, 121 (71 percent) reported experiencing amnesia for significant durations (usually from a few years to decades) for the traumatic events (Whitfield, 1995b).

The consistency of the presence of traumatic amnesia in such high numbers and percentages of case samples among 36 separate studies by independent researchers increases the likelihood that the traumatic amnesia is real, as opposed to an artifact of methodology (e.g., retrospective versus prospective), sample variation, or measurement error that might occur in single studies (Briere, 1992b).

From these studies it is clear, and it is accepted in the body of the clinical scientific literature, that traumatic amnesia is a common result of child sexual abuse experiences. Traumatic amnesia is also clearly and commonly found in PTSD, a disorder often found among survivors of child sexual abuse and physical abuse. Other dissociative disorders may also be found among these populations (DSM-IV, 1994; Kluft, 1988; Lowenstein, 1993).

DISSOCIATIVE AMNESIA

DSM-IV also refers to traumatic amnesia by the alternate term of dissociative amnesia and lists it in a separate diagnostic category (pp. 478–481).

TABLE 12-3. 12 STUDIES OF MEMORY IN CHILDHOOD SEXUAL ABUSE

Number Studied	Study	Delayed Memories
129 women	17 years before all had documented child sexual abuse, and were now re-interviewed. 80/129 (62%) remembered, although 16% (13/80 women, 10% of total) had forgotten at some time in past (Williams, 1994).	49 of them had forgotten the abuse. Add the 10% of the total of 129 who forgot having been abused at some time in the past, and the total with delayed memories is 48%.
450 (93% women)	Briere & Conte (1993) asked 450 people who had been sexually abused, "Between your first forced sexual experience and age 18, did you ever forget the experience?"	59% answered yes. Found more likely to forget if abused at younger age, repeated abuse, fear of death if told others of abuse, associated physical injury, multiple abusers, and greater current symptoms.
60 women	Cameron (1994) surveyed, interviewed, and followed up 60 women over 6 years who were in therapy for various reasons, including having been sexually abused as children.	42% had completely forgotten and another 23% had partially forgotten having been sexually abused decades earlier.
228 women	Roessler and Wind (1994) surveyed 228 women who were survivors of childhood sexual abuse.	28% had repressed memories of the abuse.
53 women	Herman and Schatzow (1987) observed 53 women in weekly therapy groups for incest survivors for 3 months.	64% had partial to severe amnesia and 28% had severe amnesia for having been sexually abused; 2 of 3 had corroborating evidence of their abuse from other sources.
19 (11 girls, 8 boys)	Burgess et al. (1995) prospectively followed 19 children sexually abused by day care staff. Mean age (2½). Follow-up into teens.	Even with extrafamilial abusers only, 16% (3) totally forgot on follow-up and 26% (5) partially forgot, for a total of 42%.
52 women	Roe et al. (1995) studied 52 women with a history of adult inpatient treatment for the effects of child sexual abuse.	Forty (78%) had experienced amnesia for the abuse for from 3.5 to 45 years, with a mean of 23 years.
100 women	Loftus et al. (1994) studied 100 women in outpatient treatment for substance abuse in NYC.	19% had delayed memories of having been sexually abused as children. Authors state that there could have been more who were abused but repressed the memory and had not yet regained it.
79 (31 men, 66 women)	Of 330 psychologists surveyed, 79 (24%) had been sexually (78%) and/or physically (22%) abused as children.	32 (40.5%) had completely or partially forgotten the abuse; 47% found external corroboration (Feldman-Summers & Pope, 1994).
171 (34 men, 137 women)	171 attendees at workshops self-identified as having been sexually abused as children.	121 (71%) had completely forgotten the abuse for long durations (Whitfield 1995b, 1996a).
36 men and women	Van der Kolk & Fisler (1995) studied 36 adults (average age 42) experiencing childhood trauma (29 CSA, 11 physical abuse, 4 other trauma).	15 (42%) had experienced significant or total amnesia for their traumas; 27 (75%) had direct (external) corroboration of the trauma.
113 men and women	Elliott & Briere (1995) studied 498 adults from the general population randomly and found 113 (23%) with a history of child sexual abuse.	49 (42%) had experienced traumatic amnesia, including 23 (20%) with total amnesia for the trauma.
TOTAL 1490	By interviews, surveys and clinical observations 20 authors studied 1,490 people, mostly women, regarding their memories of having been sexually abused in childhood.	16% to 78% were found to have delayed memories (traumatic amnesia or forgetting) of having been sexually abused or traumatized in other ways.

Compiled in part from Whitfield (1995c).

The diagnostic criteria for dissociative amnesia include the following:

- The predominant disturbance is one or more episodes of inability to recall important personal information, usually of a traumatic or stressful nature, that is too extensive to be explained by ordinary forgetfulness.
- The disturbance does not occur exclusively during the course of dissociative identity disorder, dissociative fugue, post-traumatic stress disorder, acute stress disorder, or somatization disorder (see below) and is not due to the direct physiologic effects of a substance (e.g., a drug of abuse, a medication) or a neurologic or other general medical condition (e.g., amnestic disorder due to head trauma).
- The symptoms cause clinically significant distress or impairment in social, occupational, or other important areas of functioning.

According to DSM-IV, the amnesia may last for minutes to years, and there may be one or more episodes of it in a person's history (p. 479). DSM-IV also includes the statement that, "Some individuals with chronic amnesia may gradually begin to recall dissociated memories. Other individuals may develop a chronic form of amnesia" (p. 479). Amnestic disorders due to other general medical conditions, such as epilepsy or stroke, are usually identified by a complete medical evaluation (pp. 158–160).

As documented in DSM-IV, the four mental health professions of psychiatric nursing, psychiatry, psychology, and social work accept dissociative amnesia as a valid and integral part of the natural history of traumatic experience and of several disorders in which trauma plays or appears to play a causal role. These disorders include acute stress disorder, dissociative identity disorder (pp. 484–487), somatization disorder (pp. 446–450), dissociative fugue (pp. 481–484), dissociative disorder not otherwise specified (p. 490), as well as PTSD. The diagnostic criteria for dissociative amnesia and these other disorders are used by the AMA and all health-related regulatory and insurance agencies.

THE NATURAL HISTORY OF TRAUMATIC AMNESIA

ASSOCIATIONS

According to our current understanding of the natural history of traumatic experience, based primarily on our knowledge of the effects of child sexual abuse, about one half to two thirds of the victims will always remember all or parts of the experience. In most of these cases, the trauma occurred as (1) a single episode by one offender, the traumatized person was (2) validated, and (3) grieving of the trauma was supported by important others in the person's life.

Conversely, about one third to one half of people traumatized by child sexual abuse experience traumatic amnesia for these events. Factors that tend to precede or be associated with traumatic amnesia include (1) multiple or repeated episodes of the trauma, (2) multiple offenders, (3) young age when traumatized, (4) the person's experience was invalidated, (5) grieving was not supported, (6) the offender was a primary caregiver, (7) force or violence or the threat of violence was used during or around the abuse, (8) there was perceived distress at the time of the abuse, and (9) more current symptoms than average were present (Briere and Conte, 1993; Elliot and Briere, 1995; Terr, 1991; Whitfield, 1996). These people suffered more abuse and were not supported in the aftermath.

In summary, about one third of the reported survivors of childhood sexual assault always cognitively remembered their experience, one third had full traumatic amnesia for the event(s), and one third had only partial memory for the abuse (van der Kolk, 1996; Whitfield and Stock, 1996). Traumatic or dissociative amnesia has been accepted in numerous courts as a valid theory and as a scientifically verified clinical observation, as it fulfills all five of the *Daubert* legal criteria:

- The theory has been tested (in numerous published reports of clinical cases).
- The theory has been peer reviewed and published (described above).

- Standards control the theory's operation (shown in the literature on traumatic amnesia).
- There is a known or potential rate of error (see range of results described in Table 12–3).
- The theory is generally accepted within the relevant scientific (psychiatric and psychological) community (published in DSM-IV and numerous other places) (Holmgren, 1996).[1,2]

DEFENSES AGAINST PAIN

For the past 100 years clinical scientists have used three terms to describe how traumatic amnesia develops. These terms include dissociation, repression, and denial. *Dissociation* means to separate from something, in this case, from the extreme pain of the trauma. *Repression* means to separate completely from the awareness of the pain. *Denial* is a complex psychological defense against the pain (Whitfield 1995c pp. 93–126). These three terms, along with others such as splitting, displacement, and projection, are theoretical concepts of defenses against psychological pain based on countless cases of trauma that help us explain how and why the fact of traumatic amnesia develops.

TRIGGERS AND PATTERNS OF TRAUMATIC MEMORY RECOVERY

A sexual abuse survivor's initial recovered memories are often triggered by one or more external stimuli, such as hearing of someone else's abuse or being touched in a certain way. Being in a safe or close or intimate relationship may also trigger memories. These relationships may include being in psychotherapy or counseling, as closeness reminds the survivor of prior times when he or she was close and was abused (Terr, 1994; Whitfield, 1995c, pp. 46–47).

---

[1] *Shahzade v. Gregory*, no. 921213 9 EFH, U.S. District Court, MA. Memorandum and Order by Judge D.J. Harrington. May 8, 1996.

[2] *Daubert v. Merrell Dow Pharmaceuticals*, 113 S. CT at 2796-97, 1993.

Some expert witnesses for defendants in child abuse cases have claimed that the presence of such external triggers indicates a false memory that was "implanted" in some way, but the ability of even highly suggestive external influences to actually cause false memories of trauma is unproven and purely speculative. Even if it were possible in some circumstances, this does not by any means indicate that all or even a significant number of such later recalled memories are false.

In traumatic amnesia, the process of memory return, when it occurs, usually takes place in a fragmented manner, in bits and pieces, as it evolves over time into a more complete recollection of the traumatic event and experience. When it follows a period of partial or total traumatic amnesia, this piecemeal pattern of memory return and evolution is also part of the natural history of the *effects* of trauma. This pattern does not in itself invalidate the authenticity and essential accuracy of the person's memory of the trauma.

Sexual abuse survivors tend to have more psychological and physical symptoms during the early stages of memory retrieval. The patient may describe symptoms or even appear to be mentally ill, when the patient is not (Elliott and Briere, 1995; Rowan and Foy, 1993; Whitfield, 1995). The cognitive symptoms represent the intrusive, repetitive phenomenon of PTSD necessary in reconstruction of the trauma memory.

DIFFERENTIATING ESSENCE FROM DETAILS

Finally, it may at times be important to differentiate the essence or core of the memory from the details. In traumatic experiences such as child sexual abuse—whether always remembered or previously forgotten—the essence of the memory is nearly always accurate, while one or more of the details may be inaccurate (Terr, 1994; Whitfield, 1995c). Thus, a person may accurately remember the event(s) and the actual abuser, but misremember exactly where or how the abuse occurred. Finding one or more errors in the details does not by itself invalidate the veracity of a traumatic memory.

LEGAL OBSERVATIONS

Since the late 1980s legal scholars and some therapists have been accumulating observations of traumatic amnesia in numerous legal cases in which adults who were molested as children sue their alleged offenders. Some cases are described in Whitfield (1995c) and Lazo (1995). In Lazo's comprehensive survey, she covers some of our current legal understandings of traumatic amnesia (as of early 1995).

It is difficult to determine the outcome of legal cases. A problem in compiling an accurate picture of how cases involving traumatic amnesia have fared in our legal system is that cases that go to trial but are not appealed are not generally published or reported. Most cases are settled before they get to trial.

EVIDENCE OF CHILD SEXUAL ABUSE

Child molesters nearly always commit their crimes in private and threaten their victims into keeping them a secret. When their behavior is exposed, they deny it. Lack of witnesses or manifestations of physical injury, forced secrecy, and denial usually make it difficult to prove that the sexual abuse happened. Thus, victims and some of their advocates usually have to search for direct and/or circumstantial evidence of the abuse.

Most child molesters do not fit the stereotype of a sleazy stranger lurking in a trenchcoat by the schoolyard fence. Those who sexually abuse children are usually men and women who already know the children and are close to them in some way. They may be a parent or parent figure, older sibling or other family member, a teacher, member of the clergy, scout leader, babysitter, or a friend of the family.

Nor do they offend suddenly. Rather, the offender usually gradually warms up to the child and follows a pattern that extends as a slow process over a fairly lengthy and painful period of time. The process of sexually offending a child has been described as including four stages or phases: engagement, grooming, assault, and concealment (Emrick, 1994, 1996; Whitfield, 1995c, pp. 307–310).

DEFINING THE SEXUAL ABUSE OF CHILDREN

Sexual abuse may be defined as any sexualized behavior that harms or traumatizes a child. It may be overt or covert. Overt sexual abuse includes any inappropriate touching of a child's genitals or breasts and intercourse or penetration—or touching—with adult genitals, a finger or fingers, or another object. In covert sexual abuse there is often a lack of physical contact. Covert sexual abuse has its own traumatic and stressful features. It may include telling a child sexual jokes, inappropriate nudity, preoccupation with a child's genitals or with one's own genitals with the child, preoccupation with a child or adolescent's sexuality, telling a child or adolescent of one's own sexual escapades, preoccupation with talking about sexual behaviors, taking nude photographs of the child, showing a child explicit sexual pictures, or flirting with the child. Covert sexual abuse nearly always accompanies the overt (Briere, 1992a; Courtois, 1989; Salter, 1995; Whitfield, 1995c).

In a survey of 39 adults (33 women and 6 men) who self-identified as having been sexually abused as children, 32 (82 percent) gave a history of having been overtly sexually abused, and all had also been covertly abused. These 39 adults named their type of covert abuse in the following frequency: 21 (54 percent) had been told sexual jokes as a child by their offender(s), 25 (64 percent) had been exposed to inappropriate nudity, 14 (36 percent) had experienced offender preoccupation with their own or the child's genitals, and 24 (62 percent) experienced the offender as being preoccupied with talking about sexual behaviors or showing them explicit sexual pictures. Fourteen (36 percent) experienced their offender(s) telling them about their sexual escapades, and 28 (72 percent) experienced their offender(s) flirting with them (Whitfield, 1996b).

EVIDENCE

In the discovery and disclosure of evidence in abuse cases it may thus be useful to explore and examine the statements and behavior of the accused offender and close others in the family, such as a spouse who may support the offender's denial. We know that nearly all (about 97 percent) of sex offenders deny having committed any overt or covert offense on first confrontation (Bowen, personal communication, 1994; Whitfield, 1995c). Of those offenders who undergo long-term (that is, years of) treatment, only about half will eventually admit that they offended, and then only to their therapist or to one or two others whom they may trust (Bowen, personal communication, 1994). The problem is in trying to determine who is innocent. It is of course up to the accuser, who sometimes may be assisted by the state, to prove that the accused committed the offense or crime.

In trying to arrive at the truth, as a practical matter most courts tend to accept only direct ("hard" or external) evidence for a sexual offense on a child, such as probative information from witnesses, others who were abused by the same defendant, photographs, letters, diaries, clinical records (rare), scars (still rarer), or confessions by the abuser. Because of the traumatic and secretive nature of the crime and its effects on the victim, this kind of information is hard to uncover shortly after the offense. Because of the mind-altering effects of the trauma on the trusting, vulnerable young victim, it is usually even harder to uncover decades later.

CIRCUMSTANTIAL EVIDENCE FROM CLINICAL OBSERVATION

Some courts, such as in the State of Washington in 1994 in the case of *Crook v Murphy*

(Whitfield, 1995c), have allowed circumstantial or indirect evidence that, taken as a whole, helps prove that the plaintiff was sexually abused as a child. This may be a different kind of circumstantial evidence than some courts are used to considering and admitting. It includes appropriate clinical findings that a therapist may have observed, recorded, and accumulated during evaluation and therapy. Clinical circumstantial evidence may include finding at least four of the following (Whitfield, 1995c):

- A high-risk disorder.
- Post-traumatic stress disorder.
- Frequent age-regressions, flashbacks, or abreactions (sudden, dramatic expressing of a past trauma).
- Reenactments of the trauma; repetitions or repetition compulsions.
- Characteristics of the memories themselves.
- Other patterns, dynamics, and connections.

These six observations are based upon and synthesized from the clinical findings reported in numerous studies, some of which are exemplified in the conclusions of Rowan and Foy (1993) and Neumann and associates (1996). They are also based on the vast experience of countless mental health clinicians, some of which has been documented in the writings and testimony of experts in the evaluation and treatment of traumatic disorders and conditions, such as child sexual abuse (Terr, 1994).

A high-risk disorder may be one or more of a number of medical and psychiatric diseases, disorders, or conditions, nearly all of which are listed in the medical and psychiatric diagnostic codebooks, that have been found to occur frequently in association with a history of childhood trauma, including especially sexual abuse. These are listed in Table 12–4, with comments and references that verify their high-risk or high-association nature.

These kinds of clinical findings are important to consider because they rarely occur spontaneously in nontraumatized people. These abnormal findings occur frequently in those who

TABLE 12–4. HIGH-RISK DISORDERS ASSOCIATED WITH CHILD ABUSE

Disorder or Situation	Frequency Found
Psychiatric inpatients	50 to 60% abused as children; 20 to 50% with a dissociative disorder.
Psychiatric outpatients	40 to 70% abused as children.
Dissociative identity disorder ("MPD")	Nearly all have severe, chronic child abuse.
Eating disorders	Likelihood of higher abuse history than general population.
Chemical dependence (Alcoholism and other drug dependence)	Likelihood of higher abuse history than general population.
Depression, major depression, and suicide attempts	High incidence among those with these disorders and a history of child abuse.
Somatization disorder	Likely abused as children.
Borderline personality disorder	Majority have severe, chronic child abuse.
Psychosis	44% self-admit child abuse history.
Abused and neglected children	
General disorders	
Sexual dysfunction	Common.
Self-destructive behaviors	
Violent behaviors (including sadomasochistic behaviors)	
Prostitution	About 80% sexually abused as children.
Pedophilia; child sex offenders	About 65% sexually abused as children, nearly 100% traumatized in some way.

Reproduced with permission from Whitfield (1995a).

have been significantly traumatized. These common observations are generally the results and effects of childhood trauma. Except in rare circumstances (such as in some combat veterans who try to claim that they have PTSD to receive benefits, when in fact they do not), they generally cannot be feigned.

As an example, in the *Crook v Murphy* case, the characteristics of Lynn Crook's delayed memories, combined with the diagnosis of PTSD due to no other cause than the alleged child sexual abuse and the fact that one of her sisters testified that she had also been sexually abused by their father, led the superior court judge to rule in Crook's favor.

This kind of circumstantial evidence may or may not be sufficient to prove that the defendant(s) committed the offense. Nonetheless, it is circumstantial evidence, which is accepted in most states as being equal to or as strong as direct evidence in proving the fact that a crime such as child abuse happened. Specifically, regarding

circumstantial evidence in California (see *California Jury Instructions, Civil*, 8th ed, pages 18–23), the jury is instructed that:

- Evidence means testimony, writings, material objects, or other things presented to the senses and offered to prove the existence or non-existence of a fact.
- Evidence is either direct or circumstantial. Direct evidence proves a fact without an inference, and if true, conclusively establishes that fact. Circumstantial evidence proves a fact from which an inference of the existence of another fact may be drawn.
- An inference is a deduction of fact that may logically and reasonably be drawn from another fact or group of facts established by the evidence.
- The law makes no distinction between direct and circumstantial evidence as to the degree of proof. Each is respected for such convincing force as it may carry.

The childhood amnesia defense is a myth

Some defense lawyers hire "false-memory" advocating expert witnesses to try to support a childhood amnesia defense (also called infantile amnesia). By this hypothesis, false memory syndrome advocates say that a person cannot remember any event before age three or four. The reason, they claim, is that the very young child's brain is insufficiently developed to be able to remember anything. Once again, they cite experiments and studies on normal memory and try to transfer them, inappropriately, to traumatic memory. But the available data from published case reports, based upon careful clinical observation, indicates that this defense is doubtful at best and clearly untrue in many cases.

Psychiatric nurse Ann Burgess and her colleagues evaluated and monitored 19 children who had been sexually abused (corroborated in court) by day care staff (Burgess, et al., 1995). The children's ages at the time of the abuse ranged from 3 months to 4½ years, with a mean age of 2½ years. Three independent clinicians evaluated each child just after the abuse became evident and then every 5 years thereafter. At each evaluation they checked for four kinds of memory: cognitive (or verbal), behavioral, visual, and somatic. The most common kind of nonverbal memory manifested was somatic (100 percent), followed by behavioral (82 percent) and visual (59 percent). Eleven (58 percent) of the children always verbally (cognitively) remembered the abuse, 5 (26 percent) partially remembered, and 3 (16 percent) totally forgot experiencing any abuse.

In Linda Williams' follow-up study of 129 women who had experienced childhood sexual abuse, as documented in emergency room medical records (the first study listed in Table 12–3), 5 of 11 women (45 percent) who were under 4 years old at the time of being sexually abused remembered the abuse (Williams, 1994). If we combine Williams' figures with those of the Burgess study, we find that of a total of 30 very young children (below age 4 to 4½), 16 (53 percent) later remembered the sexual abuse that was also proven by direct evidence (Burgess et al., 1995; Williams, 1994).

Other studies have found similar results (Bauer, 1996; Bruhn, 1990; Hewitt, 1994; Terr, 1988, 1991). In fact, after extensive research, Bauer (1996) concludes that many very young children (ages 2 years and under) remember certain events for long durations. What *is* true is that because language skills are not fully developed by these very young ages, abused children are not usually able to talk about their traumatic experiences in the way that an older person would. For example, in the Oklahoma City bombing, most of the traumatized child survivors were supported by their family and peers when they reported what happened to them and how the experience affected them. They were able to more effectively consolidate their traumatic memories into memory storage through a process that memory researchers call rehearsal. Trauma clinicians explain that talking about (or rehearsing) a traumatic event or experience is the best way to help anyone remember the event. This sequence is shown in the following diagram.

Young children who are traumatized at a preverbal stage of development are at a significant disadvantage because they are not able to

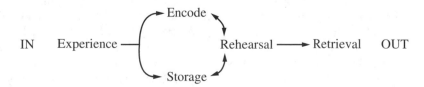

TABLE 12–5. STAGES OF RECOVERY FROM PTSD

Condition	Stage		
	One (Herman's stages)	Two	Three
Hysteria	Stabilization, symptom-oriented treatment	Exploration of traumatic memories	Personality reintegration and rehabilitation
Combat trauma	Trust, stress-management, education	Reexperiencing trauma	Integration of trauma
Complicated post-traumatic stress disorder	Stabilization	Integration of memories	Development of self, drive integration
Dissociative identity disorder (MPD)	Diagnosis, stabilization, communication, cooperation	Metabolism of trauma	Resolution, integration, development of post-resolution coping skills
Adult child syndrome	Stabilization and treatment of stage zero disorder	Awakening, remembering, naming, grieving, core issues,transformations, integration. Stage 3 continues as spirituality (Whitfield, 1995c)	
Traumatic disorders	Safety	Remembrance and mourning	Reconnection

Expanded from Herman, 1992; Whitfield, 1995c.

process the experience by talking about it. This disadvantage is compounded by the fact that, in most cases of child sexual abuse, the offender threatened the child with serious harm if he or she were to disclose the abuse.

Differentiating True from Untrue Traumatic Memory

Differentiating true from untrue traumatic memory can be a complex process. From a clinical perspective, it often takes courage and persistence on the part of the survivor and skill and experience on the part of the therapist to sort these out, and both usually require time and patience. Although therapists do have some guidelines (Table 12–1), it is neither the job nor the goal of the therapist to be a legal investigator (Herman, 1992; Whitfield, 1995a). The therapist's task is to assist the survivor in accomplishing the goals of recovery through the stages of recovery (Table 12–5). (Whitfield, 1990, 1992).

Using Memory in Healing the Effects of Trauma

Remembering and accurately naming what happened in any traumatic experience is crucial to healing. We can estimate that somewhat more than half (with a range of 22 to 84 percent) of survivors have always remembered on one level or another their abusive or traumatic experience of having been sexually abused, and that a little under half (with a range of from 16 to 78 percent) have had prolonged periods when they experienced traumatic amnesia for what happened. There are also those in a gray zone, who remember parts but not all of their experience that would be important in their process of healing.

But simple remembering is not always associated with accurately naming what happened. People are abused or mistreated, or experience other traumas, and for a number of reasons they frequently are not fully aware of the nature of their experience. To heal the detrimental effects usually requires a series of several actions, including stabilizing, awakening, remembering, naming what happened, grieving, working through core issues, making transformations, and finally integrating all of these into our psyche and daily life. Although these actions are described in more detail elsewhere (Whitfield, 1995), it may be useful here to look at an overview of recovery from trauma that Herman (1992) compiled in *Trauma and Recovery*. Over the last century these stages and tasks of recovery have been described for various guises of PTSD, yet there are enough similarities for us to discern a pattern that has become progressively clearer over time, as is shown in Table 12–5.

In four out of these six descriptions, remembering the traumatic experiences is an integral part of the recovery process, and in the other two remembering is implied as being a part of reexperiencing and "metabolizing" the trauma. The process of recovery is described in more detail in *Memory and Abuse* (Whitfield, 1995c).

Summary

Child sexual abuse is widespread and traumatic amnesia for it is common. Looking back on the 1990s, it is to be hoped that historians will view this as the time when our legal and criminal justice system began to deal appropriately with the many forms of family violence, including the sexual and physical abuse of children. Important aspects of this change should include the ability to differentiate ordinary memories from traumatic memories and an understanding of the relationship between traumatic memory and amnesia.

REFERENCES

Bauer PJ. What do infants recall of their lives? *Am Psychologist.* 1996;51:29–41.

Briere JN, Conte J. Self-reported amnesia for abuse in adults molested as children. *J Traumatic Stress.* 1993;6:21–31.

Briere JN. *Child Abuse Trauma*: Theory and Treatment of the Lasting Effects. Thousand Oaks, CA: Sage; 1992a; second edition, 1996.

Briere JN. Methodological issues in the study of sexual abuse effects. *J Consult Clin Psychol.* 1992b; 60:196–203.

Brown D, Scheflen A, Hammonds C. *Memory, Trauma Treatment, and Law* (in press).

Bruhn AR. *Earliest Childhood Memories*. NY: Praeger; 1990.

Burgess A, et al. Memory presentations of childhood sexual abuse. *J Psychosoc Nurs.* 1995;33:9–16.

Cameron C. Women survivors confronting their abusers: Issues, decisions and outcomes. *J Child Sex Abuse.* 1994;3:7–35.

Cheit RE. *Moving Forward.* Fall 1995;3:8–10.

Courtois CA. *Healing the Incest Wound: Adult Survivors in Therapy.* New York: Norton; 1989.

Davidson J. Issues in the diagnosis of post-traumatic stress disorder. In: Pynoos RS, ed. *PTSD: A Clinical Review.* Luterville, MD: Sidran Press; 1993.

Elliot DM, Briere J. Posttraumatic stress associated with the delayed recall of sexual abuse: A general population study. *J Traumatic Stress.* 1995;8: 629–647.

Emrick RL. *Sexual Offenders: A Provider's Handbook.* Thousand Oaks, CA: Sage; 1996.

Emrick RL. Child sexual abuse: A closer look at offenders, offense cycle, process of abuse and victim trauma. Unpublished, Phoenix, 1994.

False Memory Syndrome Foundation. *Newsletter.* 1992–1997.

Feldman-Summers S, Pope KS. The experience of "forgetting" childhood abuse: A national survey of psychologists. *J Consult Clin Psychol.* 1994;62: 636–639.

Fredrickson R. *Repressed Memories: A journey to recovery from sexual abuse.* NY: Simon & Schuster Fireside/Parkside; 1992.

Herman J. *Trauma and Recovery.* NY: Basic Books; 1992.

Herman J, Schatzow E. Recovery and verification of memories of childhood sexual trauma. *Psychoanalytic Psychol.* 1987;4:1–14.

Hewitt SK. Preverbal sexual abuse. *Child Abuse Neglect.* 1994;18:819–824.

Holmgren B. Limitations on forensic application of children's memory and suggestibility research—a criminal justice perspective. Talk given at the

Trauma and Memory conference, University of New Hampshire, July 27, 1996.

Kendall-Tackett KA, et al. Impact of sexual abuse on children: A review and synthesis of recent empirical studies. *Psychol Bull.* 1993;113:164–180.

Kluft RP. *The Dissociative Disorders.* Washington, DC: American Psychiatric Press; 1988.

Lazo J. True or false: Expert testimony on repressed memory. *Loyola of Los Angeles Law Rev.* 1995;28: 1345–1414.

Loftus EL, et al. Memories of childhood sexual abuse: Remembering and repressing. *Psychol Women Q.* 1994;18:67–84.

Lowenstein RJ. Psychogenic amnesia and psychogenic fugue: A comprehensive review. In: Pynoos RS, ed. *PTSD: A Clinical Review.* Lutherville, MD: Sidran Press; 1993.

McCann E, Pearlman L. *Psychological Trauma in the Adult Survivor.* NY: Bruner/Mazel; 1991.

Neumann DA, et al. The long-term sequelae of childhood sexual abuse in women: A meta-analytic review. *Child Maltreatment.* 1996;1:6–16.

Putnam FW, Trickett PK. Child sexual abuse: A model of chronic trauma. *Psychiatry—Interpersonal Biol Processes.* 1993;56:82–95.

Pynoos RS, ed. *Post-Traumatic Stress Disorder: A Clinical Review.* Lutherville, MD: Sidran Press; 1993.

Roe CM, et al. Memories of previously forgotten childhood sexual abuse: A descriptive study. St Louis, MO: Masters and Johnson Sexual Trauma and Compulsivity Programs; 1995.

Roessler TA, Wind TW. Telling the secret: Adult women describe their disclosures of incest. *Interpersonal Violence.* 1994;9:327–338.

Rowan AB, Foy DW. PTSD in child sexual abuse survivors: A literature review. *J Traumatic Stress.* 1993; 6:3–20.

Salter AC. *Transforming Trauma: A Guide to Understanding and Treating Adult Survivors of Child Sexual Abuse.* Thousand Oaks, CA: Sage; 1995.

Summit R. The child sexual abuse accommodation syndrome. *Child Abuse Neglect.* 1983;7:177–193.

Terr L. *Unchained Memories.* NY: Basic Books; 1994.

Terr L. Childhood traumas: An outline and overview. *Am J Psychiatry.* 1991;148:10–20.

Terr L. What happens to the memories of early childhood? *J Am Acad Child Adolesc Psychiatry.* 1988; 27: 96–104.

Van der Kolk BA. Testimony in *Shahzade v Gregory*, 1996.

Van der Kolk BA. The body keeps the score: Memory and the evolving psychobiology of post traumatic stress. *Harvard Rev Psychiatry.* 1994;1:253–265.

Van der Kolk BA, Fisler R. Dissociation and the fragmentary nature of traumatic memories: Overview and exploratory study. *J Traumatic Stress.* 1995;8: 505–525.

Van der Kolk BA, et al. *Psychological Trauma.* Washington, DC: American Psychiatric Press; 1987.

Whitfield CL. Survey of 171 adults who self-identified as having been sexually abused as a child. Unpublished, Atlanta, January 1996a.

Whitfield CL. Survey of 39 adults who self-identified as having been sexually abused as a child. Unpublished, Atlanta, March 1996b.

Whitfield CL. Traumatic amnesia: The evolution of our clinical and legal understanding. Unpublished paper presented at the Fairfax Co. Judicial Continuing Education conference, Fairfax, VA, March 1996c.

Whitfield CL, The forgotten difference: Ordinary memory vs. traumatic memory. *Consciousness Cognition.* 1995a;4:88–94.

Whitfield CL. How common is traumatic forgetting? *J Psychohistory.* 1995b;23:119–130.

Whitfield CL. *Memory and Abuse: Remembering and Healing the Effects of Trauma.* Deerfield Beach, FL: Health Communications; 1995c.

Whitfield CL. *My Recovery Plan for Stage 2 Recovery* (booklet). Deerfield Beach, FL: Health Communications; 1992.

Whitfield CL. *A Gift to Myself: A Personal Workbook and Guide to Healing the Child Within.* Deerfield Beach, FL: Health Communications; 1990.

Whitfield CL, Stock WE. Traumatic memories in 100 survivors of child sexual abuse. Paper presented at Trauma and Memory: An International Research Conference, University of New Hampshire, Durham, July 27, 1996. (submitted for publication).

Williams LM. Recall of childhood trauma: A prospective study of women's memories of child sexual abuse. *J Consult Clin Psychol.* 1994;62: 1167–1176.

Williams MR. Statutes of limitations. In: Rix R, ed. *Sexual Abuse Litigation: A Practical Resource for Attorneys.* Washington, DC: One Voice; 1996.

CHAPTER 13

BRIEF INDIVIDUAL PSYCHOTHERAPIES

Susan H. McCrone

Recently, focus has shifted from brief therapy to single-session therapy. Single-session therapy is probably the oldest form of therapy and now appears to be the newest as well.

Chapter Overview

► INTRODUCTION

In the social, political, and economic context of the 1990s, the length of therapy (termed brief, short term, or time limited) has become a national focus. Indeed, the necessary and desirable length of psychotherapy has been a matter of discussion and controversy since the beginning of psychotherapy. In the early days of psychoanalytic psychotherapy, it was thought that for therapy to be effective, it had to be intensive, reconstructive, and lengthy. Brief therapy was identified as "supportive or directive," less effective, and only palliative (Garfield, 1989). Yet as early as the turn of the century, accounts were written about the efficacy of brief therapy. A symphonic conductor with psychogenic pain in his conducting arm described a significant session in his brief therapy:

> His advice was to conduct. "But I can't move my arm." "Try it at any rate." "And what if I should have to stop?" "You won't have to stop." "Can I take upon myself the responsibility of possibly upsetting the performance." "I'll take the responsibility." And so the conductor did a little conducting with his right arm, then with his left, and occasionally with his head. . . . So by dint of much effort and confidence, by learning and forgetting, I finally succeeded in finding my way back to my profession (Walter, 1946, pp. 167–168).

This passage is a description by Bruno Walter of one of his six sessions with Sigmund Freud. This account directly or indirectly highlights the critical elements of brief psychotherapy, as presented in Table 13–1.

The question has been raised as to how many sessions constitute brief therapy. Although there is a range in the literature, short-term or brief therapy is often arbitrarily defined as 20 sessions or less (Hoyt, 1995, p. 76). There is, however, a growing body of literature on single-session psychotherapy, which is also considered brief therapy. Authors support the idea that brief therapy is determined more by the critical elements than the length.

> When a therapist and patient endeavor to get from Point A (the problem that led to therapy) to Point B (the resolution that ends therapy) via a direct, effective and efficient route, we say that they are deliberately engaging in brief therapy (Hoyt, 1995, p. 281).

TABLE 13–1. CRITICAL ELEMENTS OF BRIEF PSYCHOTHERAPY

Focus	Therapist and client focus on a key area of personal or interpersonal concern.
Role of therapist	Active and direct in promoting client function. Positive belief in client's capacity to change.
Role of client	Therapist encourages client activity rather than passivity by assigning tasks outside of the therapeutic session.
Role of time	Therapist and client work within a time-limited context, usually explicitly conveyed, emphasizing the immediacy of the change process.
Nature of relationship	Collaboration with mutual goal setting.

Adapted with permission from Hoyt (1995).

A HISTORY OF BRIEF PSYCHOTHERAPY

Although with selected patients Freud practiced brief therapy, in most cases he advocated analysis lasting 6 months to 1 year. Other psychoanalysts, such as Rank and Ferenczi experimented with attempts at reducing the time of psychoanalysis, but were viewed as aberrants and heretics by their fellow analysts (Garfield, 1989).

By the mid-1940s, brief therapy had gained enough impetus and followers to warrant a council at a meeting on psychosomatic medicine. Alexander (1944, p. 3) described his work with brief therapy, stating "occasionally, one or two psychotherapeutic interviews, rich in emotional experience and insight, may have a more revelatory effect upon certain patients than months of analysis on others." Later, in their book on psychoanalytic therapy, Alexander and French (1946) explained their success with briefer therapy. Herzberg (1946) practiced "active psychotherapy," in which the therapist prescribed tasks for the patient to perform and fostered the patient's independence. Frohman (1948) described his form of brief psychotherapy of 20 to 30 sessions in which an eclectic approach was adapted to fit the requirements of individual cases.

Despite these isolated explorers in the realm of brief psychotherapy, prior to World War II most psychiatric treatment in the United States had become the long-term luxury of the privileged and was under the purview of psychoanalysts (Garfield, 1989). World War II created a situation in which many GI's were in need of treatment. Attempts were made to streamline and modify the system for provision of psychiatric care. Psychologists and clinical social workers attained recognition as psychotherapy providers. Group therapy became more common as the treatment of choice and necessity. Veterans Administration Medical Centers emerged as a training ground for mental health professionals, and there arose an increased interest in crisis intervention (Hoyt, 1995). Brief psychotherapies did not, however, emerge as legitimate therapeutic methods until the 1950s, when several changes in practice were taking place. Two important developments were the emergence of behavioral and family therapy and the accumulation of a substantial body of research on the process and outcome of psychotherapy (Wells and Giannetti, 1990).

The emphasis on shorter forms of therapy was given further impetus by a report by the Joint Commission on Mental Illness and Health (1961). In it, psychoanalysis was singled out for the lengthy preparation of its practitioners and length of treatment. "It is principally effective for a limited number of carefully selected patients who are not incapacitated by their illness and do not require hospitalization" (p. 80). The Joint Commission advocated a model of crisis intervention with 24-hour emergency coverage for patients. Bellak and Small (1965) described the role of the therapist in brief therapy in the context of emergency services:

> In brief psychotherapy, the therapist does not have time for insight to develop; he must foster insight. He does not have time to wait for working through, he must stimulate working through. And where these basic aspects of the therapeutic process are not forthcoming, he must invent alternatives (p. 6).

Another impetus to the development of brief therapies was the Avnet Report published in 1965. This document described the results of a project cosponsored by Group Health Insurance, the American Psychiatric Association, and the National Association for Mental Health in which short-term outpatient psychiatric care (15 individual sessions) was offered to 76,000 people who were already insured for other medical services. Seven hundred and forty of the participating patients were queried 2½ years after the completion of treatment. Eighty-one percent of those completing the sessions saw some improvement in their condition, and 17 percent felt that they were completely recovered. Although skeptical about the efficacy of short-term treatment, the psychiatrists rated 76 percent of the patients as improved and 10.5 percent of them as recovered.

Since the 1960s, there has been a proliferation of types of brief psychotherapies (Table 13–2). Behavioral therapy gained acceptance in the late 1960s, and with it came controlled studies to measure symptomatic improvement. Published studies began to indicate that a large number of patients dropped out of therapy, with an actual average number of sessions attended of 6 to 8 (Garfield, 1989).

The Collaborative Study of the Treatment of Depression, sponsored and coordinated by the National Institute of Mental Health, was an important study on the efficacy of brief psychotherapy. In this study depressed patients were assigned to one of four treatment groups. Two of the treatments were the cognitive therapy developed by Beck and associates (1979) and the interpersonal therapy developed by Klerman and colleagues (1984). Training manuals were used by the therapists to insure strength and comparability of treatments among therapists. The two therapies were compared to imipramine and with a placebo plus clinical management. No significant differences in reduction of depressive symptoms or overall functioning were found either between the two psychotherapies or between the psychotherapies and imipramine. Patients improved but no single treatment was more effective than another. Many other studies have continued to document the equal efficacy of short-term psychotherapy with long-term treatment (Koss and Butcher, 1986).

> Virtually without exception, these empirical studies of short-term outpatient psychotherapy or inpatient care . . . have found that planned short-term psychotherapies are essentially equally effective and are, in

general, as effective as time-unlimited psychotherapy virtually regardless of diagnosis or duration of treatment (Bloom, 1992, p. 9).

TABLE 13–2. TIMELINE FOR THE DEVELOPMENT OF BRIEF PSYCHOTHERAPY

1900s	Freud
1925	Rank and Ferenczi
1946	Alexander and French, Herzberg
1940s	World War II
1948	Frohman
1951	Perls, Hefferline, and Goodman 　　Theory and technique of gestalt therapy
1952	Bateson communication project 　　Weakland 　　Haley 　　Fry 　　Jackson
1956	*Toward a Theory of Schizophrenia* 　　(Bateson et al.)
1958	Jackson founded Mental Research Institute 　　Weakland 　　Haley 　　Riskin 　　Satir 　　Watzlawick
1961	Joint Commission on Mental Illness and 　　Health, Berne (1972), transactional 　　analysis
1962	Ellis (1992), rational-emotive therapy
1963	Haley published *Strategies of* 　　*Psychotherapy* 　　Strategic therapy 　　Malan, Short-term dynamic psychotherapy
1966	Fisch started brief therapy project in MRI 　　Wolpe, Wolpe and Lazarus, behavior 　　therapy
1972	Sifneos, short-term anxiety-provoking 　　psychotherapy (STAPP)
1973	Mann, time-limited (Mann and Goldman, 　　1982)
1976	Horowitz, stress response therapy (1979)
1978	Davanloo (1980, 1991), short-term 　　intensive-dynamic
1980	Milton Erickson, Ericksonian hypnotherapy
1981	Madanes, strategic
1982	de Shazar, Brief Therapy Center of 　　Milwaukee
1984	Strupp and Binder, time-limited dynamic 　　psychotherapy

In the 1990s, the practice of psychotherapy has been influenced and shaped by a number of sociocultural forces, including economic pressures to decrease the cost of health care, the rapidity of the pace of life, the information explosion fueled by advances in technology, and the expansion of managed care. No longer are many consumers, covered under managed care, determining the site and cost of services or the nature and length of treatment (Hoyt, 1995). "The successful therapist will need to define his or her market, and once this is done, develop explicit strategies for capturing a fair share of it" (Wells and Giannetti, 1990, p. 23). To remain competitive in today's health care market, it would seem that these strategies would, by necessity, need to be brief.

PATIENT SELECTION CRITERIA

Although each model of brief psychotherapy has its own selection criteria, there appear to be some common characteristics that make particular patients well suited for brief therapy (Hoyt, 1995). The first criterion is that the patient comes to therapy to solve some focal problem for which the solution is in his or her control. Depending upon the model, this could be called circumscribed chief complaint, or focus, or core conflict; but it always involves some identifiable problem. The second criterion is that the patient is motivated to change. The third is that the patient is psychologically minded, and has the ability to actively use the ideas of the therapist (flexible interaction). The last criterion is that the patient has had a history of beneficial relatedness in some interpersonal relationships. In a factor analysis of the criteria for selection, Hoglend and colleagues (1992) found that these criteria were more significant predictors of long-term dynamic change than patient background and DSM-III variables. Brief therapy is not, however, limited to patients with mild symptoms or symptoms of recent onset. "The best strategy, in my opinion, is to assume that every patient, irrespective of diagnosis, will respond to short-term treatment unless he proves himself refractory to it" (Garfield, 1989, p. 140).

PHASES OF THERAPY

Time is essential in brief therapy. The message, by definition, is brevity. At the core, brief therapy is defined more by an attitude of the patient and therapist than by the number of sessions. The therapist believes and expects that change can occur *in the moment*, and that the patient has within himself or herself the power to be different or to remain the same (Goulding and Goulding, 1978, 1979). In keeping with the concept of time, brief therapy can be conceptualized to have a structure of sequenced phases. In practice, these phases may blend into one another rather than remain discretely organized (Hoyt, 1995). The structure builds upon the previous phase so that successful work in one phase becomes a precondition for the next. For example, if the patient has thought about the goals in the pretreatment phase, the identification of the focus or central issue in the beginning phase is facilitated. Table 13–3 describes the key phases in brief therapy.

MODELS OF BRIEF THERAPY

Various models or "schools" of brief therapy have emerged in the last 30 years. Although the application of any of these models to the treatment of an individual patient may be influenced by the style of the practitioner, there are general guidelines in theory and practice that distinguish different forms of brief therapy. Although review of all of the models of brief therapy is beyond the scope of this chapter, several of the more clearly articulated models will be briefly reviewed with references provided for a more in-depth investigation by the reader. Clearly the

TABLE 13–3. KEY PHASES OF BRIEF THERAPY

Pretreatment
Potential patient gives thought to what he or she
wants to accomplish
Identifies how he/she expects therapy to help
Thinks about how long it will take

Beginning
Develop rapport and therapeutic alliance
Confront resistance and negative transference
Identify focus, central issue
Set therapeutic limits
Contract for number of sessions/payment
Homework assignments

Middle
Working through, increasing awareness
Clarification/redefinition of focus
Confrontation (if compatible with model)
Interpretation of resistance (if compatible)
Application of lessons outside of office
Monitor progress

End Phase/Termination
Extract therapist from successful equation

Follow-through
(Determined by philosophy of the model)
Check in for booster

Adapted with permission from Garfield (1989).

words of Milton Erickson in 1980 remain relevant to the practice of brief psychotherapy today. "Each person is a unique individual. Hence, psychotherapy should be formulated to meet the uniqueness of the individual's needs rather than tailoring the person to fit the Procrustean bed of a hypothetical theory of human behavior" (quoted in Zeig and Gilligan, 1990, p. xix).

SHORT-TERM DYNAMIC PSYCHOTHERAPY

In the past few decades, clinical researchers have conducted systematic studies into short-term dynamic psychotherapy. This research has been enhanced by audiovisual technology that documents the psychotherapeutic process and increases replicability. Additionally, three in-

ternational congresses on short-term dynamic psychotherapy (Montreal in 1975 and 1976, and Los Angeles in 1977) documented the efficacy of several different models with regard to selection criteria, techniques, and outcome evaluation.

Beginning with Freud, numerous theoreticians and clinicians have applied the psychoanalytic concepts of the unconscious, resistance, and transference to brief forms of treatment. Unlike traditional psychoanalytic psychotherapy, the emphasis in all of the various short-term dynamic psychotherapies has been on increased therapist activity within a limited (central) focus. Brief dynamic therapists strive to promote change within a focalized area of conflict through a mixture of de-repression and affective release, corrective emotional experience, relearning, and application of the patient's will.

Presentation of all of the forms of short-term dynamic psychotherapy is beyond the scope of this chapter, but Table 13–4 highlights the central characteristics, techniques, and length of treatment for six of these forms.

Research data has supported the efficacy of short-term dynamic psychotherapy in treating patients with varied disorders. Svartbery and associates (1995) found a clinically significant improvement in anxiety in 3 of 4 patients treated with short-term anxiety-provoking psychotherapy (STAPP). Weiss and Marmar (1993) described the effectiveness of time-limited dynamic psychotherapy for PTSD, pathological grief, and other stress response syndromes in the treatment of over 200 patients. The comparative efficacy of two psychodynamically based therapies—short-term dynamic psychotherapy and brief adaptive psychotherapy—were evaluated in a sample of 81 patients with personality disorders. The authors found that patients in the two therapy conditions improved significantly on all measures in comparison with the patients on the waiting list, with no significant differences between the two treatments.

TABLE 13–4. SELECTED SHORT-TERM DYNAMIC PSYCHOTHERAPIES

Approach	Central Characteristic	Techniques	Length
Short-term anxiety provoking psychotherapy (STAPP) (Sifneos, 1972, 1987, 1992)	carefully selected patient with oedipal conflict	anxiety-provoking confrontation transference interpretation emotional relearning	6–15
Short-term dynamic (STD) (Malan, 1963, 1976)	oedipal conflict or loss	interpretative links between past and present issues	30–40
Time-limited (Mann, 1973; Mann & Goldman, 1982)	focus on patient's self present and chronically endured pain themes: unresolved mourning, activity vs. passivity, independence vs. dependence, adequacy vs. diminished self-esteem	therapist help pt. master underlying separation issues	12
Stress-response and microanalysis (Horowitz, 1976, 1979; Horowitz et. al., 1984)	focus on pt.'s state of mind (images of self and others and information processing style)	help pt. rework and emotionally master recent stress event	12
Short-term intensive dynamic (Davanloo, 1978, 1980, 1991; Worchel, 1990)	emphasis on characterological defenses basic analytic "triangle of unconscious" (impulse-feeling/anxiety/defense) "triangle of feeling" (transference/current significant person/past significant person)	confrontation interpretation of defenses "unlocking the unconscious"	5–40
Time limited dynamic (Strupp & Binder, 1984; Butler, Strupp & Binder, 1992)	cyclical maladaptive pattern identified and interpreted: acts of self, expectations of others, acts of others, self-introjects	empathic uses countertransference to provide corrective emotional experience	25

Adapted with permission from Hoyt (1995).

COGNITIVE-BEHAVIORAL APPROACHES

Cognitive-behavioral therapy has its roots in the resurgent interest in cognition that affected the field of psychology in the late 1960s and early 1970s (Wells and Giannetti, 1990). From the perspective of this model, human behavior originates from the processing of both internal and external information (Ingram and Kendall, 1986). Of central importance to the clinician is the interrelationship of cognitions, affect, and behavior in the etiology and treatment of psychopathology. Because psychopathology is believed to result from and be maintained by dysfunctional cognition and emotion, cognitive-behavioral therapy attempts to alter the meaning a client attaches to events (Meichenbaum and Butler, 1980). Cognitive-behavioral approaches by nature are almost always brief. They are highly goal directed, offering clear and specific remedies for distinct problems. Goals of cognitive-behavioral therapy include cost-effective treatment for a wide range of client problems; altering interpretations of self and environment by change in behavior, environment, or cognition; increasing coping skills; and increasing likelihood that gains will be maintained after termination (Lehman and Salovey, 1990, p. 245).

Cognitive approaches (typically with behavioral aspects) have been categorized by Mahoney and Arnkoff (1978) into three main groups:

- Cognitive restructuring, including the rational-emotive therapy of Ellis (1962, 1992) and Beck's cognitive therapy (1976, 1988).
- Coping skills, including Wolpe's systematic desensitization (1958) and Meichenbaum's stress inoculation training (1977, 1985, 1992).
- Problem-solving, including D'Zurilla and Goldfried's behavioral problem-solving therapy (1973) and Mahoney's personal science approach (1974, 1977).

"Faulty learning is revised as distortions in cognitive schemata are corrected, relaxation skills and relapse prevention methods are taught, and constructive decision making is increased" (Hoyt, 1995, p. 306).

In addition to the research supporting the effectiveness of cognitive-behavioral therapy in the treatment of depression, recent research data have supported the efficacy of cognitive-behavioral therapy with substance abuse patients. In a review of brief interventions for alcohol problems, Bien and colleagues (1993) found that relatively brief interventions have consistently been found to be more effective in reducing alcohol consumption or achieving treatment referral of problem drinkers than no counseling, and have often been as effective as more extensive treatment. Although Richmond and associates (1995) did not find a significantly greater reduction in consumption of alcohol at follow-up after a general practitioner-based brief intervention, patients did report a significantly greater reduction in alcohol-related problems. Minicucci (1994) challenges nurses to reconceptualize their ideas about alcohol abuse and dependence as progressive diseases that are managed but never cured, and to incorporate research data that support the concept that the disease is a learned habit that is treatable with cognitive-behavioral interventions.

Saunders and colleagues (1994) found brief motivational interventions to be a useful adjunct to methadone programs. Although there was no difference between the educational and motivational group in terms of severity of reported opiate dependence,

> over the 6-month follow-up period the motivational subjects demonstrated a greater, immediate commitment to abstention, reported more positive expected outcomes of abstention, reported fewer opiate related problems, . . . complied with the methadone programme longer and relapsed less quickly (p. 415).

Clearly, more research is needed to identify the types of patients for whom cognitive-behavioral therapy is most effective.

INTERPERSONAL PSYCHOTHERAPY (IPT)

Among the forms of short-term psychotherapy, interpersonal psychotherapy (IPT) is a relative newcomer. It has evolved over the last half of the 20th century and has been used in carefully controlled studies. Several American psychiatrists have been important in the development of the interpersonal approach to psychotherapy. Adolph Meyer's work (1957) at John's Hopkins University began the Baltimore-Washington group of interpersonal therapists. In his approach, called psychobiology, he focused on details of the patient's life history, experiences during each stage of development, and the impact of these life events on feelings and behavior (Cornes, 1990). Harry Stack Sullivan, a student of Meyer, and Freida Fromm-Reichman continued to apply an interpersonal approach to the treatment of patients.

The emergence of short-term IPT of depression occurred in the early 1970s in the New Haven-Boston Collaborative Depression Research Project. "It is a focused, short-term, time-limited therapy that emphasizes the current interpersonal relations of the depressed patient while recognizing the role of genetic, biochemical, developmental, and personality factors in the causation of and vulnerability to depression"

(Klerman et al., 1984, p. 6). The rationale and techniques of IPT were originally described in a training manual developed for research and then published as a textbook. When IPT was initially developed, 12 to 20 weekly sessions were found to be effective in achieving the therapeutic goals. IPT is not associated with a specific etiologic theory of depression but is based on the belief that the psychopathology is manifest in the interpersonal sphere. A major focus is the determination of how problems in interpersonal relations contribute to the symptoms and how psychosocial events are correlated in time with the onset of depressive symptoms.

IPT treatment has several goals. The first, reduction in depressive symptoms, is achieved by helping patients understand that their experiences are part of a depressive syndrome. The second goal is to help patients develop more successful patterns for dealing with current social and interpersonal problems that are linked to the onset of depression. The four major problem areas associated with depression are delayed or distorted grief reactions, interpersonal role disputes, role transitions, and interpersonal deficits (Klerman et al., 1984).

There are three phases in IPT treatment. The initial three sessions are used to obtain a history of the illness, explain the rationale and intent of IPT, complete an interpersonal inventory, identify the major problem areas, and agree on a focus and plan for treatment. The middle phase (sessions 4 to 13) focuses on one or two identified problem areas using goals and strategies appropriate to each problem area. During this phase, the therapist uses the therapeutic relationship to further the goals of treatment. During the termination phase (sessions 14 to 16), the course of therapy is reviewed and progress reinforced. There is increased recognition of the patient's competence, ability to function independently, and new capacities to decrease vulnerability to future episodes of depression (Cornes, 1990).

This psychotherapeutic approach relies on the techniques of exploration for information gathering, reassurance, clarification of emotional states, improvement in interpersonal communication, and reality testing of perceptions and performance. The emphasis is on current problems and feelings experienced in the interpersonal context (Cornes, 1990).

IPT has been modified for use with depressed adolescents (IPT-A) (Moreau et al., 1991). The authors describe the beginning of clinical trials to test the modification on adolescents with a range of depressive disorders and to incorporate these findings into a manual.

Recently, IPT has been used to treat HIV-positive, depressed adults (Markowitz et al., 1992). Of 23 depressed subjects, 20 recovered from the depression, after a mean of 16 sessions. Six aspects of interpersonal therapy make it especially well suited for the treatment of HIV-positive outpatients. These include "a here-and-now framework, formulation of problems from an interpersonal perspective, exploration of options for changing dysfunctional behavior patterns, identification of focused interpersonal problem areas, and the confidence that therapists gain from a systematic approach to problem formulation and treatment" (p. 885).

Klerman and colleagues (1984) view interpersonal psychotherapy as a set of skills built upon prior training in the mental health clinical disciplines. Training requires mastery of the training manual, participation in didactic seminars, and case supervision (Bloom, 1992).

STRATEGIC THERAPY

Strategic therapy was derived from the work of Milton Erickson. In addition to its roots in hypnotherapy, strategic therapy has rich interconnections with systems thinking and the family therapy movement. The Mental Research Institute in Palo Alto, California, was developed in 1958 from the work of Bateson, Jackson, Haley, and Weakland on a theory of schizophrenia that brought systems thinking to the attention of clinicians.

The Mental Research Institute group developed a theory of change based upon communications and systems concepts and coupled it with a symptom-focused, brief treatment approach. At the same time, strategic and problem-solving approaches were being developed by Haley (1973, 1976) and Madanes (1981), and further developed by de Shazar (1985) and others. Jay Haley (1973) described strategic therapy as follows:

> Therapy can be called strategic if the clinician initiates what happens during the therapy and designs a particular approach for each problem. . . . He must identify solvable problems, set goals, design interventions to achieve these goals, examine the responses he receives to correct his approach and ultimately examine the outcome. . . . (p. 17).

Lankton (1990) identifies seven features that characterize Erickson's work and that form the basis for strategic therapy. This is a nonpathology-based model. Problems are seen as part of, and a result of, attempts at adaptation. Symptoms are seen as natural responses of unique individuals. The techniques used are often indirect, allowing the individual and family members resources and options, seemingly without the aid of the therapist. The therapist utilizes whatever the patient brings to the office (understandings, behaviors, and motivations) as part of the treatment. Clients are expected and encouraged to quickly get into actions related to desired goals. The strategy of the therapist is to take responsibility for influencing the patient and to be active in setting or initiating the stages of therapy. The focus is on action and experience in the present and future, not the past. The therapist enchants the patient by engaging his or her mind, appealing to the patient for collaboration, and capturing the ear of the listener (Hoyt, 1995).

The procedure has five steps that are carried out more simultaneously than sequentially.

1. Decide what to communicate to the patient.
2. Decide how to communicate it (usually indirectly).
3. Determine the patient's values.
4. Divide the solution into manageable steps.
5. Present the intervention within a therapeutic sequence, tailoring the intervention to fit the patient's values (Zeig and Gilligan, 1990, p. 373).

For Erickson, the basic problem was not one of pathology but of people getting "stuck" by being unable to use their range of skills, competencies, and learning. From this basic ideology came a wide range of techniques employed to help the patient get "unstuck." These include indirection; imagery; hypnosis; teaching stories; metaphoric communication; provocation to challenge and motivate patients; prescribing ordeals, symptoms, and other paradoxical maneuvers; assigning ambiguous tasks; and providing directives to alter conflict-generating rules. The basic premise underlying all of these techniques is utilizing whatever patients brings with them. The essential shift in strategic therapy is from deficits to strength, problems to solutions, the past to the future.

> The paradox of strategic therapy is that, after mastering its techniques, ultimately we employ them almost playfully, in an effort to just be with our patients as they find the changes inherent in what they brought with them with their "problems." In this way the strategic therapist is not a "doctor" but rather a midwife. The pleasures of strategic therapy are the pleasures of aiding in a birth and wondering at what emerges inevitably. . . . The completion of the birth is not an end, but yet another beginning (Rosenbaum, 1990, p. 401).

SOLUTION-FOCUSED THERAPY

An aspect of strategic treatment that has recently received a great deal of attention is called solution-focused (de Shazar, 1985, 1988, 1991) or solution-oriented therapy (O'Hanlon and Martin, 1992; O'Hanlon and Weiner-Davis, 1989; O'Hanlon and Wilk, 1987). The focal areas of this therapy are to increase that which works and decrease that which doesn't; to identify the "exceptions" to the problem, and what the patient is doing differently at those times; to determine what has worked before, so that those strengths can be applied to the current situation; and to identify a useful solution and how to construct it. The shift is from dysfunction to competency, with an orientation toward the future utilization of human abilities. Budman and Gurman (1988) describe the assumptions of solution-oriented therapy:

• Change is not just possible but inevitable.
• Problems dealt with in therapy are those defined by the client.
• The real world outside of therapy is the most important part of a client's life, one where supportive relationships need to be fostered and positive change practiced.

The assessment becomes the intervention as solution-oriented questions are posed to help clients set personal goals to find solutions to their problems. See Table 13–5 for solution-oriented questions.

Webster (1990) and Tuyn (1992) have examined the benefits for psychiatric nurses of using brief solution-focused approaches. These include mobilizing hope, using existing support systems, and supporting a client's strengths. Montgomery and Webster (1994) believe that the use of brief solution-focused therapy may be more congruent with the values of nursing's metaparadigm and role as advocates for patients. Webster and associates (1994) describe several approaches to introducing solution-focused ideas to inpatient psychiatric nursing staff and nursing students. Baker and Geise (1992) found that an inpatient psychiatric unit that implemented brief therapy techniques reported decreased conflict and more support and consistency in relationships between nursing, medicine, and managed care organizations. They

TABLE 13–5. SOLUTION-ORIENTED QUESTIONS

Pre-session Change Questions
   Many times in between the call for an appointment and the first session, people notice that already things seem different. What have you noticed about your situation?

Miracle Question
   Suppose one night there is a miracle while you are sleeping and the problems that brought you to therapy are solved. Because you were sleeping, you don't know that a miracle has happened. What do you suppose you will notice is different the next morning that will tell you that there has been a miracle?
   Who will be the first person to notice the next day that something is different after the miracle?
   What will be different between you and your (mother, boss, husband) after the miracle happens?

Exception Questions
   Are there times now that some of this miracle happens even just a little bit?
   Tell me about those times when this problem doesn't occur. How do you get that to happen?

Scaling Questions
   On a scale of 1 to 10, where 10 is the problem solved and 1 is the worst it's ever been, where are you today?
   On a scale of 1 to 10, with 10 being that you have every confidence this problem can be solved and 1 being no confidence at all, where would you put yourself today?
   What would it take for you to go (e.g.) from a 3 to a 3.5 or a 4?

Coping Questions
   How have you prevented things from getting worse?
   How did you manage to get yourself up this morning?
   What keeps you going?

also found a decrease in length of stay, and no increase in recidivism.

SINGLE-SESSION THERAPY (SST)

Recently, focus has shifted from brief therapy to single-session therapy (SST). Single-session therapy is the most frequent form of psychological treatment. SST is probably the oldest form of therapy and now appears to be the newest as well (Hoyt, 1995). Accounts of significant changes occurring after one session have existed at least since Freud's cure of Gustav Mahler's sexual problem on a single long walk (Breuer and Freud, 1955). Studies have indicated that in most outpatient settings, single-session therapy, whether planned or not, is very common (Bloom, 1992; Cummings and Follette, 1976).

Certain ideologies on the part of the therapist promote the efficacy of SST. The therapist's attitude is that not only is change inevitable, but it is already happening. Therapy focuses and amplifies the ongoing change process. At the end of the session, the therapist leaves the client with the idea that change will continue to occur.

The therapist views each encounter as a whole, complete in itself. The problem must be elicited and its resolution developed in one meeting. "Treatment begins when the client first telephones in and continues through the final words of the leave taking" (Hoyt, 1995, p. 120).

Therapists avoid rushing or trying to be brilliant. If a therapist enters a session thinking he or she must develop something extraordinary or brilliant to create a change in the client, it decreases the chance that this will occur by denying the client's autonomy. The therapist need only facilitate the client's natural change process.

Like other types of brief therapists, SST therapists emphasize the client's abilities and strengths, rather than the client's pathology. The therapist believes that ultimately the client knows himself or herself better than the therapist does. The task of the therapist is to facilitate the client's finding the solution.

SST therapists believe that what happens in therapy can provide the impetus for the client to make significant changes outside of the session. They recognize that life, not therapy, is the great teacher.

One important task of the single-session therapist is to identify the client's difficulty in such a way that it can function as a pivotal focus for change. The therapist helps the client put the symptom into a larger pattern from which new directions can be developed. The client is directed by the therapist to use the ambiguity of the problem as a bridge to new behaviors and experiences.

To make SST complete, it must contain an appropriate ending. When concluding SST, the therapist asks the client if he or she feels that enough has been accomplished in the session for the client to move on. If an affirmative response is obtained, the therapist asks the client to review the progress. This then serves as a resource for further utilization with other problems. In most cases, the therapist lets the client know that he or she will remain available on an as-needed basis after the client has taken some time on his or her own. Often a follow-up phone call is arranged by the therapist.

Single-session therapy is not wedded to one model. SST generally is successful by mirroring within therapy the problems encountered by the clients in their lives.

> Our effort in SST is to create awakenings, a sense that there need be "no more hesitating or lingering." We see "beginnings [in which] dwells a magic force," whose magic is intrinsic to the very brevity of the intense, mutative moment, in which dwells the experience that the time for change is now. . . . (Hoyt, 1995, p. 138)

Research data support the effectiveness of SST both individually and with families. De Johgh and associates (1995) described the efficacy of a single session of cognitive restructuring in a sample of phobic dental patients. Significant gains were made in frequency and believability of negative cognitions and dental trait anxiety. Talmon (1990) reported that more than three quarters of 200 patients seen only once reported that they were improved or much improved. If the research data continue to support the utilization of this much briefer form of brief therapy, it would have a significant impact on the delivery of mental health care in the future.

THE FUTURE OF BRIEF PSYCHOTHERAPY

Brief therapy has had a long history, starting with the work of Freud, and appears to have a long future as well. Factors contributing to the ongoing success of this treatment include market forces, the desire of most people for rapid relief from psychological distress, and the development of new treatment technologies that increase the possibility of greater diagnostic and treatment specificity. The burgeoning of health maintenance organizations, the acceleration of managed care, and the continuing emphasis on some form of universal health care as responses to the continuing escalation of health care costs all point to the further expansion of brief therapy (Hoyt, 1995). Research data supporting efficacy equal to that with long-term therapy and the development of training manuals for the education of new mental health practitioners also supports the continuing emphasis on brief therapy as the treatment of choice for many patients.

> Combining the fiscal imperative of the managed care movement with the fact that brief therapy is the treatment of choice for many patients, serving the needs as well as providing the socioeconomic advantage of allowing patients who would otherwise go without to receive the benefits of professional mental health care, we can expect increasing attention to the practice and study of brief psychotherapy in the years ahead (Hoyt, 1995, p. 326).

REFERENCES

Alexander F. The brief psychotherapy council and its outlook. *Psychosomatic Medicine, Proceedings of the Second Brief Psychotherapy Council*. Chicago: Institute of Psychoanalysis; 1944.

Alexander F, French TM. *Psychoanalytic Therapy: Principles and Applications*. New York: Ronald Press; 1946.

Baker N, Geise A. Reorganization of a private psychiatric unit to promote collaboration with managed care. *Hosp Commun Psychiatry*. 1992;43: 1126–1129.

Beck AT, Rush AJ, Shaw BF, Emery G. *Cognitive Therapy of Depression*. New York: Guilford Press; 1979.

Bellak L, Small L. *Emergency Psychotherapy and Brief Psychotherapy*. New York: Grune & Stratton; 1965.

Bloom BL. *Planned Short-term Psychotherapy*. Boston: Alyn Bacon; 1992.

Breuer J, Freud S. Studies in hysteria. In: Strachey J, ed. *The Standard Edition of the Complete Works of Sigmund Freud*. London: Hogarth Press; 1955;2.

Budman SH, Gurman AS. *Theory and Practice of Brief Therapy*. New York: Guilford Press; 1988.

Butler SF, Strupp HH, Binder JL. Time-limited dynamic psychotherapy. In: Budman SH, Hoyt MF, Friedman S, eds. *The First Session in Brief Therapy*. New York: Guilford Press; 1992.

Cornes C. Interpersonal therapy of depression (IPT). In: Wells R, Giannetti V, eds. *Handbook of the Brief Psychotherapies*. New York: Plenum; 1990.

Cummings NA, Follete WT. Brief psychotherapy and medical utilization. In: Horken H, et al. *The Professional Psychologist Today*. San Francisco: Jossey-Bass; 1976.

Davanloo H. *Unlocking the Unconscious: Selected Papers*. London: Wiley; 1991.

Davanloo H, ed. *Basic Principles and Techniques in Short-term Dynamic Psychotherapy*. New York: Spectrum; 1978.

Davanloo H, ed. *Short-term Dynamic Psychotherapy*. New York: Jason Aronson, 1980.

De Johgh AD, Muris P, Horst GT, et al. Case histories and shorter communications. *Behav Res Ther*. 1995;33:944–954.

De Shazar S. *Putting Differences to Work*. New York: Norton; 1991.

De Shazar S. *Clues: Investigating Solutions in Brief Therapy*. New York: Norton; 1988.

De Shazar S. *Keys to Solution in Brief Therapy*. New York: Norton; 1985.

D'Zurilla TJ, Goldfreid MR. Cognitive processes, problem solving, and effective behavior. In: Goldfried MR, Merbaum M, eds. *Behavior Change*

Through Self-control. Troy, MO: Holt, Rinehart & Winston; 1973.

Ellis A. Brief therapy: The rational-emotive method. In: Budman SH, Hoyt MF, Friedman S, eds. *The First Session in Brief Therapy*. New York: Guilford Press; 1992.

Ellis A. *Reason and Emotion in Psychotherapy*. New York: Stuart; 1962.

Follette WT, Cummings NA. Psychiatric services and medical utilization in prepaid health plan setting. *Med Care*. 1967;5:25–34.

Frohman BS. *Brief Psychotherapy*. Philadelphia: Lea & Febiger; 1948.

Garfield SL. *The Practice of Brief Psychotherapy*. New York: Pergamon Press; 1989.

Gustafson JP. *The Complex Secret of Brief Psychotherapy*. New York: Norton; 1986.

Goulding RL, Goulding MM. *Changing Lives Through Redecision Therapy*. New York: Brunner/Mazel; 1979.

Goulding RL, Goulding MM. *The Power is in the Patient*. San Francisco: Transactional Analysis Press; 1978.

Haley J. *Problem-solving Therapy*. San Francisco: Jossey-Bass; 1976.

Haley J. *Uncommon Therapy: The Psychiatric Techniques of Milton Erickson, MD*. New York: Norton; 1973.

Herzberg A. *Active Psychotherapy*. New York: Grune & Stratton; 1946.

Hoglend P, Sorbye O, Sorlie T, et al. Selection Criteria for Brief Dynamic Psychotherapy: Reliability, Factor Structure and Long-term Predictive Validity. *Psychother Psychosomat*. 1992;57:67–74.

Horowitz MJ. *States of Mind*. New York: Plenum; 1979.

Horowitz, MJ. *Stress response syndrome*. New York: Jason Aronson; 1976.

Horowitz MJ. *Personality Styles and Brief Psychotherapy*. New York: Basic Books; 1984.

Howard KI, Kopta AM, Krause MS, et al. The dose-effect relationship in psychotherapy. *Am Psychol*. 1986;41:159–164.

Hoyt MF. *Brief Therapy and Managed Care*. San Francisco: Jossey-Bass, 1995.

Ingram RE, Kendall PC. Cognitive-clinical psychology: A paradigm shift without a paradigm. In: Ingram RE, ed. *Information Processing Approaches to Psychopathology and Clinical Psychology*. Orlando: Academic Press; 1986.

Joint Commission on Mental Illness and Mental Health. *Action of Mental Health*. New York: Basic Books; 1961.

Klerman GL, Weissman MM, Rounsaville B, Chevron ES. *Interpersonal Psychotherapy of Depression*. New York: Basic Books; 1984.

Koss MP, Butcher JN. Research on brief psychotherapy. In: Garfield SL, Bergin AE, eds. *Handbook of Psychotherapy and Behavior Change: An Empirical Analysis*. 3rd ed. New York: Wiley; 1986.

Lankton SR. Erickson strategic therapy. In: Zeig JK, Munson WM, eds. *What is Psychotherapy: Contemporary Perspectives*. San Francisco: Jossey-Bass; 1990.

Lehman A, Salovey P. An introduction to cognitive-behavior therapy. In: Wells R, Giannetti V, eds. *Handbook of the Brief Psychotherapies*. New York: Basic Books; 1990.

Luborsky L. *Principles of Psychoanalytic Psychotherapy*. New York: Basic Books; 1984.

Madanes C. *Strategic Family Therapy*. San Francisco: Jossey-Bass; 1981.

Mahoney MJ. Personal science: A cognitive learning therapy. In: Ellis A, Grieger R, eds. *Handbook of Rational-Emotive Therapy*. New York: Springer; 1977.

Mahoney MJ. *Cognition and Behavior Modification*. New York: Ballinger; 1974.

Mahoney MJ, Arnkoff D. Cognitive and self-control therapies. In: Garfield SL, Bergin AE, eds. *Handbook of Psychotherapy and Behavior Change*. 2nd ed. New York: Wiley; 1978.

Malan DH. *The Frontier of Brief Psychotherapy*. New York: Plenum; 1976.

Malan DH. *A Study of Brief Psychotherapy*. London: Tavistock; 1963.

Mann J. *Time-limited Psychotherapy*. Cambridge, MA: Harvard University Press; 1973.

Mann J, Goldman R. *A Casebook in Time-limited Psychotherapy*. New York: McGraw-Hill; 1982.

Markowitz JC, Klerman GL, Perry SW. Interpersonal psychotherapy of depressed HIV-positive outpatients. *Hosp Commun Psychiatry*. 1992;43:885–890.

Meichenbaum D. Stress inoculation training: A twenty-year update. In: Woofold RL, Lehrer PM, eds. *Principles and Practices of Stress Management*. New York: Guilford Press; 1992.

Meichenbaum D. *Stress Inoculation Training*. New York: Pergamon; 1985.

Meichenbaum D. *Cognitive Behavior Modification*. New York: Plenum; 1977.

Meichenbaum D, Butler L. Cognitive ethology: Assessing the streams of consciousness and emotion. In: Blankstein KR, Pliner P, Polivy J, eds. *Advances in the Study of Communication and Affect: Assessment and Modification of Emotional Behavior*. New York: Plenum; 1980.

Meyer A. *Psychobiology: A Science of Man*. Springfield, IL: Thomas; 1957.

Minicucci DS. The challenge of change: Rethinking alcohol abuse. *Arch Psychiatr Nurs*. 1994;8:373–380.

Montgomery CL, Webster D. Caring, curing and brief therapy: A model for nurse psychotherapy. *Arch Psychiatr Nurs*. 1994;8:291–297.

Moreau D, Mufson L, Weissman M, Klerman G. Interpersonal psychotherapy for adolescent depression: Description of modification and preliminary application. *J Am Acad Child Adolesc Psychiatr*. 1991;30:642–651.

O'Hanlon WH, Martin M. *Solution-oriented Hypnosis: An Ericksonian Approach*. New York: Norton; 1992.

O'Hanlon WH, Weiner-Davis M. *In Search of Solutions: A New Direction in Psychotherapy*. New York: Norton; 1989.

O'Hanlon WH, Wilk J. *Shifting Contexts: The Generation of Effective Psychotherapy*. New York: Guilford Press; 1987.

Richmond R, Heather N, Wodak A, et al. Controlled evaluation of a general practice-based brief intervention for excessive drinking. *Addiction*. 1995;90:119–132.

Rosenbaum R. Strategic psychotherapy In: Wells RA, Giannetti VJ, eds. *Handbook of Brief Psychotherapies*. New York: Plenum; 1990.

Saunders B, Wilkinson C, Phillips M. The impact of brief motivational intervention with opiate users attending a methadone programme. *Addiction*. 1994;90:415–424.

Shires B, Tappan T. The clinical nurse specialist as brief psychotherapist. *Perspect Psychiatr Care*. 1992;28:15–18.

Sifneos PE. *Short-term Anxiety-provoking Psychotherapy: A Treatment Manual*. New York: Plenum; 1992.

Sifneos PE. *Short-term Dynamic Psychotherapy: Evaluation and Technique*. Rev. ed. New York: Plenum; 1987.

Sifneos PE. *Short-term Psychotherapy and Emotional Crisis*. Cambridge, MA: Harvard University Press; 1972.

Stern S. Managed care, brief therapy and therapeutic integrity. *Psychotherapy*. 1993;30:162–174.

Strupp HH, Binder JL. *Psychotherapy in a New Key: A Guide to Time-limited Dynamic Psychotherapy*. New York: Basic Books; 1984.

Svartbery M, Seltzer MH, Stiles TC, Khoo S. Symptom improvement and its temporal course in short-term dynamic psychotherapy. *J Nerv Ment Dis*. 1995;183:242–248.

Talmon M. *Single Session Therapy: Maximizing the Effect of the First (and Only) Therapeutic Encounter*. San Francisco: Jossey-Bass; 1990.

Tuyn LK. Solution-oriented therapy and Rogerian nursing science: An integrative approach. *Arch Psychiatr Nurs*. 1992;6:83–89.

Walter B. *Theme and Variation: An Autobiography*. New York: Knopf; 1946.

Webster DC. Solution-focused approaches in psychiatric/mental health nursing. *Perspect Psychiatr Care*. 1990;26:17–21.

Webster DC, Vaughn K, Martinez R. Introducing solution-focused approaches to staff in inpatient psychiatric settings. *Arch Psychiatr Nurs*. 1994;8:254–261.

Weiss DS, Marmar CR. Teaching time-limited dynamic psychotherapy for post-traumatic stress disorder and pathological grief. *Psychotherapy*. 1993;30:587–591.

Wells R, Giannetti V, eds. *Handbook of the Brief Psychotherapies*. New York: Plenum; 1990.

Wolpe J. *Psychotherapy by Reciprocal Inhibition*. Palo Alto: Stanford University Press; 1958.

Worchel J. Short-term dynamic psychotherapy. In Wells R, Giannetti V, eds. *Handbook of the Brief Psychotherapies*. New York: Plenum; 1990.

Zeig JK, Gilligan SG, eds. *Brief Therapy: Myths, Methods, and Metaphors*. New York: Brunner/Mazel; 1990.

CHAPTER 14

TREATING SUBSTANCE ABUSE IN FAMILY THERAPY

Linda S. Cook

Family systems theory is a growth-centered modality; one is encouraged to explore self and others in the family and to move beyond eliminating symptoms. Indeed, many psychiatric and physical symptoms are viewed as the behavioral expression of increased anxiety within the family. Addiction to any chemical substance is viewed as a response to anxiety.

Chapter Overview

► INTRODUCTION

Advanced psychiatric nursing practice is facilitated with the use of a theoretical framework to guide patient assessment and practice, particularly when caring for a chronically ill and frequently resistant population. Bowen's family systems theory (FST) is an established framework within which mental health professionals define and treat psychiatric dysfunction. Bowen's FST is especially useful in dealing with addicted patients, because the family, its history, and its support (or lack thereof) is addressed as a key issue in treatment. This chapter describes elements of Bowen's family systems theory and discusses its application to the assessment and treatment of addicted patients.

BOWEN'S FAMILY SYSTEMS THEORY

Family systems theory was developed by Murray Bowen (1978) in the 1940s as a result of his work with schizophrenic adolescent girls at the Menninger Clinic and Georgetown University. In the course of his work with the girls, he noticed the emotional reactivity and increased symptoms that accompanied their rising anxiety resulting from maternal interactions. He progressed quickly from working with the mother-daughter dyads to working with the entire family in an attempt to decrease anxiety and reduce symptoms.

From this work evolved a complex theory of eight interlocking concepts that described human interaction in terms of differentiation and emotional reactivity. These concepts include differentiation of self, family emotional system, family projection process, sibling position, triangles, cut-offs, multigenerational transmission, and societal regression.

DIFFERENTIATION OF SELF

The cornerstone concept of the theory is differentiation of self. Differentiation of self refers to the individual's ability to separate intellectual and emotional systems. Differentiation is marked by a perception of personal boundaries. The well-differentiated person is able to separate thinking and feeling and is able to act, rather than react, on an emotional level. Because the individual thinks before acting, responses are based on problem solving rather than a rigid, predictable pattern.

The poorly differentiated individual blends intellect and emotional response to the point of being unable to separate them. Responses to problems are reactive in nature and dependent upon those around him or her. As little actual problem solving is done, fewer options are available, and the person is easily stressed into decompensation.

FAMILY EMOTIONAL SYSTEM

The family emotional system is the emotional climate in which the child is raised. A poorly differentiated family will be unable to escape the "stuck together" emotional fusion of the family. This fusion of feelings of family members raises anxiety and makes individual rational function difficult, if not impossible. Family members use to excess three mechanisms to deal with the anxiety: marital conflict, dysfunction of a spouse, and projection of undifferentiation onto a child. Children reared in this environment generally will not have the skills to differentiate a self and may well become symptomatic.

A well-differentiated family rears children able to separate thinking from feeling. Subjective feeling states are not allowed to interfere with decision making. Children reared in this environment do not bear symptoms for the family.

FAMILY PROJECTION PROCESS

Family projection process describes the transmission of undifferentiation and anxiety from parents onto a specific child or children. The most common example is that of the mother who resolves her anxiety by focusing her attention on a child. The selection of the particular child usually occurs as a result of significant, or nodal, events occurring during the pregnancy or birth of that child or as a result of "special" needs of the child such as occur through illness or physical challenge. This focus of anxiety occurs in all families, but does not become potentially pathological unless a particular child is singled out for attention consistently.

SIBLING POSITION

Sibling position describes position in the family by sex and birth order. In family systems theory, the genders are considered mutually interdependent, but certain clusters of behaviors are learned as a result of sex and birth order. For example, first-borns tend to be caretakers. As differentiation levels drop across families, learned sex roles tend to become more rigid.

TRIANGLES

Triangles refer to the most stable emotional system. A two-person system is inherently unstable: as emotional intensity and anxiety rise, a third person is sought to diffuse the anxiety so that the couple may remain stable. This triangling and diffusion of anxiety is considered normal unless the triangles become fixed and rigid. Again, the rigidity is seen as symptomatic of fusion and reactivity.

CUT-OFFS

A cut-off is the process of achieving distance from the family of origin when emotional intensity has become unbearable. The cut-off may involve establishing geographic distance from the family of origin. It may also be emotional, such as is seen when an individual behaves in such a way as to guarantee ejection from the family. Cut-offs are problematic in that the isolated individual must use later relationships to resolve issues from the family of origin.

MULTIGENERATIONAL TRANSMISSION

Multigenerational transmission involves the transference of levels of differentiation down generations within a family. In addition to levels of differentiation, other patterns of behavior may also be passed along. In his early work with schizophrenia (predating neurotransmitter discovery), Bowen saw multigenerational transmission as the process that resulted in schizophrenia in a poorly differentiated family with a downward spiraling of differentiation over seven generations.

SOCIETAL REGRESSION

The final concept, societal regression, applies family systems theory to society at large. Stressors to the society, such as overpopulation and pollution, are viewed as increasing the anxiety level of the society. As stressors become chronic, the society tends to behave in more emotionally reactive and less thoughtful ways. Persons or groups of persons behaving in antisocial ways are seen as acting out the system's anxiety.

ASSUMPTIONS OF FAMILY SYSTEMS THEORY

As with other natural systems theories, FST carries with it some basic assumptions—the most basic being interdependence within the system. Family members interact in predictable patterns. A change in one person's behavior of necessity affects the entire system and how the family members relate to each other. Although work with the family is facilitated with the entire family present in therapy, systemic change is still possible by working with only one family member.

Even though FST moved away from linear, cause-and-effect thinking, it is assumed that families operate in a rule-driven, hierarchical model. The 1950s patriarchal assumption of a two-parent nuclear family with the father firmly in charge of the financial life and the mother in charge of the emotional life of the family is apparent. Parenting done by mothers and fathers is viewed as qualitatively different. Although the two-parent family does not comprise the majority of families four decades later, the emotional roles filled by adult role models remain unchanged (Firestone, 1970).

Everyone in the family system is assumed to have power and agency to change within FST. This power, however, does not exist equally throughout the family and is different qualitatively for different family members. Physical power has traditionally centered on the father. Walters and associates (1988) state that the basis for power in the family is economic; the person with the largest paycheck has the most power. Again, this person has historically been the adult male. The emotional power held by the adult female within the family provides little access to resources, but may promote or inhibit the growth of the family. The power possessed by children within the family is of the same emotional quality, but of lesser quantity, as that possessed by the adult female. Agency for changing behavior is related to physical, emotional, and financial power.

Power gradients are seldom discussed in Bowen's family systems theory. FST views behaviors as interactional, rather than causal: phenomena as behavioral interactions to be described rather than explained. Viewing an abuse of power, such as domestic violence, as behavioral interaction is useful in demonstrating the way in which violence in perpetuated in the family. It also, however, has the unfortunate potential for blaming the victim for the abuse. To avoid blaming the victim, power gradients must be clearly understood. The identified patient is usually the least powerful family member and the individual who is demonstrating the effects of anxiety for the family.

Anxiety refers to the subjective feeling of distress provoked by a perceived threat. Although it may vary in intensity and degree, anxiety is perceived by Bowen to be present at all times. Behavior is motivated by a desire to reduce anxiety. Substance abuse, in Bowen's FST, is a maladaptive response to increased anxiety. This maladaptive response may progress to addiction, a life-consuming process of obtaining and using drugs to the detriment of personal relationships and employment, and a cause of legal entanglement.

In summary, FST is a growth-centered modality; one is encouraged to explore self and others in the family and to move beyond eliminating symptoms. Indeed, many psychiatric and physical symptoms are viewed as the behavioral expression of increased anxiety within the family. Addiction to any chemical substance is viewed as a response to anxiety.

BOWEN'S THERAPY WITH THE ADDICTED PATIENT

Prior to any psychiatric intervention it is critical that the addicted patient first be assessed for physiological stability. Therefore, information to be gathered first is data concerning the substance used, the amount used and the time interval since the last use. This information will allow the nurse to determine the likelihood of impending withdrawal symptoms, some of which are potentially lethal.

PSYCHIATRIC ASSESSMENT

After physical stability is assured, psychiatric assessment may be started. Within Bowen's FST, assessment involves appraising individual and family function and coaching to improve the level of function, that is, to behave in a more differentiated way. In the typical initial interview, the nurse is usually dealing only with the addicted person rather than with the entire family. How then does the nurse assess family function?

One of the techniques of Bowen's therapy involves avoidance of emotional "hotspots." Dwelling on the individual's recent (and perhaps ongoing) use of drugs is likely to increase resistance. Thus, after assessing the potential for withdrawal symptoms, the interview shifts to less threatening topics. A beginning genogram of family members frequently serves this function. It is important not to delve into family dynamics as they may provoke as much anxiety as the issues around addiction. Rather, one should at this point simply identify members of families of origin (two or more generations, if possible) and procreation. The patient will ask the purpose of this genogram; a useful rationale is that of looking for potential sources of support during the recovery process.

The genogram is not only a diagnostic tool but also a wonderful way to focus therapy. As patients begin to work on the roster of family members, the possibilities of and degree of support become apparent. Even with the listing of family members, there will usually be high levels of emotion present. Patients may experience feelings of guilt, anger, or remorse as they talk about each person. It is not uncommon for the addicted person to be so removed from these feelings as to experience alexithymia, or the inability to identify specific feeling states. What is instead felt is a feeling of vague discomfort that has been masked by alcohol or drugs. The first task of the therapist may then be to help the patient identify feelings in the safe context of the therapeutic environment. It is frequently a new discovery for the addict that one may "feel the feeling" without acting on it with drugs or alcohol.

Completing the baseline genogram provides the therapist with an enormous amount of information. The first piece of useful information is that of birth order. As noted earlier, gender and birth order roles tend to be somewhat rigid in less differentiated families. Thus, if the patient is an oldest sister of sisters, she is likely to be a caretaker within the family and is also likely (regardless of the degree to which she is addicted) to feel responsible for younger family members. This responsibility will be compounded with guilt over perceived failures to take care of these siblings. A younger brother of sisters, on the other hand, may feel little guilt related to his lack of caretaking behaviors, as they were never expected of him. Regardless of birth order and gender, the genogram will provide the therapist with clues as to possible patient behavior patterns.

A second piece of information readily available will be the presence of cut-offs in the family. Sometimes the addict has been ejected from the family for such things as repetitive lying or thefts from family members to support a drug or alcohol habit. The ejected family member will be able to report little current information and may, in fact, state that he or she has been thrown out by the family. The addict may also have voluntarily have cut himself or herself off. It is not unusual for an addict to report that "I don't want them to see me this way." Patients are encouraged to gradually begin reconnecting with members of their families of origin. The patient is coached to first approach family members who provoke less anxiety—a patient who has had a highly conflictual relationship with her mother might instead contact a sibling first. This reconnection with the family of origin is key. Success in new relationships is difficult to reach if conflicts in the family of origin have never been resolved.

Other key family members may also be cut off or absent. Stanton and Todd have reported an unusually high number of deaths of first-degree relatives in addicts' families. As information is gathered, dates of deaths, births, and departures should be attached to the genogram for each member whenever possible. These nodal events are typically the cause of an increase of anxiety in families, and thus may mark periods of increased substance use in the addict's life.

As therapy progresses and trust is established, the family therapist continues to examine the patient in relation to the family. As the patient talks about issues in maintaining sobriety, the family emotional system will become more clear. In addicted families, it is likely that high levels of marital conflict (between the patient's parents and between the patient and his or her significant other) will be present. These conflictual relationships may be explored in the light of drug and alcohol use. Does the conflict spark an increase in the use of the drug of choice? If so, then the patient may benefit from coaching in conflict management to provide an alternative to drug use.

The patient may present as the dysfunctional spouse or partner. The dysfunctional spouse or partner faces a difficult challenge in recovery. The family is likely to have a difficult time in accepting feedback or information from "the family drunk." It may be difficult for the family to accept that the addict in recovery has opinions worth hearing. These are the families that convey subtle hints to the patient that life was easier when he or she was intoxicated and not functioning as an adult. The patient perceives a lack of support and becomes angry. Patients may be helped enormously, and freed from anger and frustration, if the situation is reframed for them. A family that is learning how to behave with a sober individual is very different from a family that doesn't want that person sober.

The patient may also present as the "projected child" on whom most of the anxiety fell in the family of origin. These patients are, with some degree of regularity, named after addicted or alcoholic family members in previous generations. Multigenerational transmission of anxiety and dysfunction is clearly seen in such families. These patients are usually astounded to look at their genogram and see the degree to which addiction or alcoholism pervades their families. Drug and alcohol use can be reframed for these people as "family traditions" that can be altered or stopped.

Nodal events (deaths, births, marriages, children leaving home), which are defined as times of high anxiety, are assessed. Dates of these events are recorded on the genogram. Outbursts of aberrant behavior frequently accompany nodal events.

Triangles are identified in the family as some members prove to be more or less supportive. These triangles tend to be rigid in that the same people act as "family hero," "scapegoat," "lost child," "clown," and so forth, in successive conflicts and crises. The therapist's goal is not to eradicate triangles; triangling is a normal human behavior. Rather, the addict should be coached to expand the number of triangles and lessen the rigidity surrounding the use of the triangled person. In this way, the patient will be altering communication patterns within the system, as well as increasing his or her support system.

Most of the individual concepts of Bowen's FST are not typically addressed directly. Differentiation of self is indirectly assessed through the process of therapy by seeing how the patient deals with anxiety and decision-making. Is the patient able to think rationally when anxious, or does he or she have an automatic "knee-jerk" reaction to anxiety? For the addict or alcoholic, the response to anxiety has typically been use of the drug of choice to decrease anxiety as a primary response. For those therapists wishing a more empirical approach, Haber's Level of Differentiation of Self Scale (1990) provides scaled information on the patient's level of emotional maturity. This tool has been used in a variety of populations, but probably needs further use in addicted populations before making generalizations.

Assumptions made about behavior patterns associated with gender role and birth order must be validated with the patient. If, indeed, the assumptions have a basis in reality, the patient must be guided to an understanding of learned and shaped behavior. It is usually helpful for the patient to gain the understanding of expected behavior within a family system (e.g., the family drunk). If the patient understands that the family has certain expectations of his or her behavior based on a lifetime of responses to anxiety, it will be less surprising to the addict that the family does not immediately trust him or her or that subtle "change-back" messages are sent. Patients in recovery are frequently frustrated by a lack of family enthusiasm for their sobriety and sometimes feel (and are) sabotaged by family members who have not had to deal with a sober adult in the past.

GROUP THERAPY AND RECOVERY GROUPS

The FST work done by the patient and therapist is tremendously aided with attendance at a group. In group therapy, the patient learns that his or her feelings, frustrations, and temptations are shared by others in recovery. They may learn from the coping skills of others and may be in the new position of providing support for others. Although 12-step meetings are not therapy groups, many patients benefit from this kind of assistance.

Most people in recovery benefit from a psychoeducational group that teaches about short-and long-term drug effects as well as what to expect in terms of physical, cognitive, emotional, and spiritual symptoms in recovery. Although patients clearly understand how the drugs made them feel, many do not understand the mechanisms, nor the long-term implications, of use. It is important, for example, for a cocaine addict to realize that craving for the drug may still be strong 9 to 12 months after ceasing drug use. Without this information, it is easy for the patient to conclude that the treatment has not helped, and relapse.

These groups add much to the recovery of addicted persons. It is critical, however, that the therapeutic process include treatment of issues likely to provoke a relapse. Family systems theory provides a framework and the therapy provides a mechanism to treat those issues.

► CASE EXAMPLE

Patrice was a 26-year-old mother of three. She came to the clinic for treatment of a 5 year addiction to crack cocaine. She had attempted several times to stop using cocaine, but had relapsed each time. During her intake interview, it was found that she was also experiencing physical withdrawal symptoms from alcohol that she used to "take the edge off" the cocaine high. Patrice was spending $250 to $500 per week on cocaine and consuming approximately a fifth of alcohol per week. She was diagnosed with concurrent dependencies on cocaine and alcohol. After receiving medical intervention during a period of detoxification, Patrice reported to the clinic for therapy.

► FAMILY OF PROCREATION

A brief history of Patrice's use of drugs and alcohol was done. As with many women, Patrice began using drugs and alcohol with the father of her children. They had never married; he and Patrice had separated after having a fight about her ongoing use of drugs. She discussed having a male friend whom she was dating. This man did not and had never used drugs or alcohol. The relationship was important to her, and Patrice overtly stated that she wanted to get clean to maintain the relationship.

Patrice had three children. Her oldest child, Evelyn, was 7 years old. Patrice said she depended heavily on her to help with the other two children "when I'm not home." This child had been drug-free when born and Patrice said "you can tell because she's really smart and grown-up for her age." Her son Michael, age 4, was "a crack baby." Patrice said he had problems sitting still and paying attention; she had strong concerns about his future ability to do well in school. Her youngest child, Theresa, had been conceived while Patrice was drug-free and was born within days of the death of Patrice's mother. Theresa was named for her grandmother.

▶ FAMILY OF ORIGIN

In the next several sessions, Patrice and her therapist talked about her family of origin (Fig. 14–1). Patrice was the youngest of six siblings. Her parents had separated before her birth; she said she had met her father "a few times" but did not have a close relationship with him. Her parents had apparently split up due to her mother's inability to stop drinking. Her mother had died of complications due to alcoholism one year before Patrice began therapy; Patrice reported being "devastated" by her mother's death, as the two of them had been very close. As the youngest child, Patrice had been the last to leave home and had had much time alone with her mother. It was, in fact, her mother's death that had sparked the most recent episode of drinking and drugging.

Of her siblings, only two (Renee and William) had never had problems with drugs or alcohol. Her oldest sister, Martha, her oldest brother, Marcus, and her third sister, Sandra, had each had significant, life-altering difficulties with cocaine, heroin, or alcohol. Until this attempt at sobriety, Patrice and her sister Sandra had frequently used cocaine together.

When asked about her home life while she was growing up, Patrice said that while the family loved each other, the house was "always full of fighting." With her father's departure, the oldest children had had to get jobs to help support the family. Martha and Marcus had trouble holding down steady jobs because they were already drinking regularly as teenagers. Renee resented these two because she was consistently working and giving her paycheck to her mother, who then supported the drinking habits of Martha and Marcus. Martha moved out of the home when she was 17 and went to live with her aunt Virginia, who also drank. Marcus remained in the family home; he and Renee continued to fight. Patrice reports idolizing her brother Marcus and took his side against Renee while growing up. Renee married at the age of 18 and left Marcus and William to support the family. William soon took Renee's place as the family hero/martyr, working long hours and paying bills run up by his mother and Marcus. Patrice had a close relationship with her sister Sandra. Sandra had assumed care of Patrice shortly after her birth, bathing and dressing her as other little girls did with their dolls. This relationship remains close, but became strained whenever Patrice attempted to stop using drugs and alcohol.

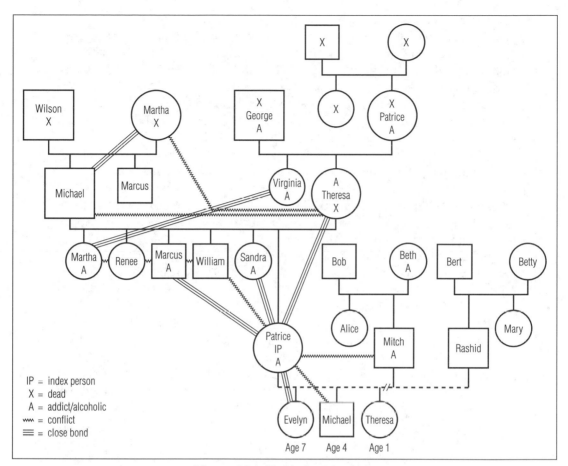

Figure 14-1. Patrice's genogram.

Moving back two generations, Patrice knew her mother's family very well but had only heard about her paternal relatives. Her mother's family had all had problems with alcohol. Her mother was the youngest of two daughters. Her older sister, Virginia, drank heavily and had been diagnosed with liver cancer. Patrice was named after her maternal grandmother, who had died with her husband, George, in an alcohol-related motor vehicle accident when Theresa was a young woman. Patrice had been told that these grandparents were "partying people."

Patrice had never met her father's parents, but had been told about them by her mother. Her father, Michael, had been the oldest of two sons. Michael's father, Wilson, had been a minister in a Protestant church, and the whole family had grown up very involved in church activities. Both parents had died of natural causes as "very old people."

Patrice's mother reported strong conflicts with Michael's mother, Martha. Her husband had divided loyalties and frequently took his mother's side against her. She had told Patrice repeatedly that her mother-in-law's "holier-than-thou attitude" had been responsible for a lot of her drinking. Patrice's mother had, over the years, begun to bestow upon her parents saintly qualities—they never fought, everyone loved them, they were the perfect couple. Patrice cannot remember ever hearing anything negative about her maternal grandparents.

Over the course of therapy, Patrice was able to identify strong patterns of drug and alcohol use in her families of origin and procreation. She was able to see the high risk the youngest siblings were at for addiction. She was also able to see the pattern of naming children for older addicted persons and the patterns that these children then followed.

She was able to identify rigid triangles in both her families of origin and procreation. She made efforts to communicate with other people outside her usual triangles. She was able to see the fused relationship she shared with her sister Sandra and began to make moves towards differentiation by identifying her values as compared to Sandra's values.

She was able to identify roles played in her family of origin—hero, martyr, scapegoat, and so on. She also saw the danger her own children were in based on birth order, sex, and perception of illness versus health. She was able to identify a wish to support her children to achieve.

She recognized that her failed relationship with her children's father was a relationship between two people who were accustomed to being cared for rather than being caretakers. She had more confidence in her new relationship based on sibling placement.

Patrice was able to identify strengths in her families and in herself. She was able to identify ways in which she used problem solving in her quest for drugs, and was able to find new ways to apply her skills at problem solving to maintain sobriety. These skills were reinforced by attending groups in which experiences were shared and education provided (Kaschak, 1992).

At the end of 2 years, Patrice was still clean and sober. She had married her friend, Rashid. She had had a fourth child and was attending classes on a part-time basis. Her dream had become to eventually finish college and work with other recovering addicts. She had regained her health and her life, and had developed a new sense of self.

REFERENCES

Bowen M. *Family Therapy in Clinical Practice*. New York: Jason Aronson; 1978.

Haber J. The Haber Level of Differentiation of Self Scale. In: Strickland O, Waltz C, eds. *Measurement of Nursing Outcome*, vol. 4. New York: Springer; 1990.

Firestone S. *The Dialectic of Sex: The Case for Feminist Revolution*. New York: Quill; 1970.

Kaschak E. *Engendered Lives: A New Psychology of Women's Experience*. New York: Basic Books; 1992.

Walters M, Carter B, Papp P, Silverstein O. *The Invisible Web: Gender Patterns in Family*. Guilford Family Therapy Series. New York: Guilford Press; 1988.

CHAPTER 15

COGNITIVE THERAPY IN ADVANCED NURSING PRACTICE

Arthur Freeman • M. Jane Yates

*B*y learning to un-
derstand the idio-
syncratic way in which
he or she perceives self,
world and experience,
and the prospects for
the future, the patient
can be helped to alter
negative affect, change
his or her view of life
experience, and behave
more adaptively.

Chapter Overview

► INTRODUCTION

In the last several years, cognitive therapy (CT) has become a meeting ground for mental health professionals from different theoretical orientations, professions, and cultures. For example, psychodynamic therapists find in cognitive therapy a dynamic core that involves working to alter basic schemas. The behavioral therapists find in CT a short term, active, directive, collaborative, psychoeducational model of psychotherapy that has as its goal direct behavioral change. Cognitive behavioral interventions have been written about in the psychiatric, medical, nursing, social work, and psychological literature. Cognitive therapy is consistent and imbedded in the basic tenets of nursing. Bowler and associates (1993) state that "the cognitive model of treatment conforms with many widely held beliefs and assumptions of psychiatric nursing regarding the etiology and treatment of mental disorders" (p. 248). Moreover, the nurse's role as educator, leader, resourceperson, therapist, and caretaker fits well with the conceptual, theoretical, philosophical, and therapeutic model of CT.

The literature on CT has grown in an almost exponential fashion. Rooted in the early work of Beck on the treatment of depression (Beck, 1967, 1977; Beck et al., 1979), contemporary CT has become a broad-spectrum model of therapy that is being applied to virtually every treatment problem, patient type, and therapeutic context. As a general model of psychotherapy, CT has been applied to anxiety (Beck et al., 1985; Costello and Borkavec, 1992; Freeman & Simon, 1989); eating disorders (Fairburn, 1985; Garner and Bemis, 1985); personality disorders (Beck et al., 1990; Freeman, 1988; Freeman and Leaf, 1989); suicide (Freeman and Reinecke, 1993; Free-

man and Simon, 1989); sexual disorders (McCarthy, 1989); and schizophrenia (Eimer and Freeman, 1992; Perris et al., 1992). The model has been successfully applied to the treatment of women (Davis and Padesky, 1989); the elderly (Gallagher-Thompson and Thompson, 1992; Glantz, 1989); gay men (Kuhlwein, 1992); gay women (Wolfe, 1992); and children (DiGiuseppe, 1989; Kendall, 1991). CT has been applied in individual therapy (Freeman et al., 1990); groups (Wright et al., 1993); couples (Baucom and Epstein, 1989; Epstein and Baucom 1989); with families (Epstein et al., 1988); and with inpatients (Freeman and Greenwood, 1987; Wright et al., 1993).

The basic model has been adapted to a variety of cultures rather easily because it is *process focused* rather than being *content focused*. Helping individuals to develop the process to examine their beliefs (whatever those beliefs might be) appears to be far more helpful cross-culturally than focusing on some point of culturally related content (e.g., the oedipal conflict).

The historical and theoretical bases of CT are quite broad and encompass the early work of Beck (1967, 1976, 1989); Beck, Rush, Shaw, and Emery (1979); Ellis (1962, 1973, 1977, 1985, 1989); Lazarus (1976, 1981); and Meichenbaum (1977). Contemporary cognitive therapy is rooted in the earlier work of Adler (1927), Arieti (1980), Bandura (1977a, 1977b, 1985), Bowlby (1985), Frankl (1985), Freud (1892), Horney (1936), and Sullivan (1953).

The common element in the different cognitive-behavioral models is helping the patient to examine the manner in which he or she construes and understands the world (cognitions), and to experiment with new ways of responding (behaviors). By learning to understand the idiosyncratic way in which he or she perceives self, world and experience, and the prospects for the future, the patient can be helped to alter negative affect, change his or her view of life experience, and behave more adaptively.

Cognitive therapy does not focus on cure, but is a psychoeducational or coping model of therapy. This teaching focus is inherent in nursing theory care models. A major reason that individuals have difficulty dealing or coping with internal or external stimuli is a lack of basic skills. Skill deficits might include difficulty or inability to respond to depressogenic or anxiogenic thoughts; social skills deficits, making it difficult to cope in social situations; or difficulty in recognizing the beginnings of a panic attack and then taking the appropriate action. The major goal of cognitive therapy is to increase the patient's skills so that he or she can more effectively deal with the exigencies of life, and thereby have a greater sense of control and self-efficacy.

The directive nature of the model involves the therapist working to enhance therapeutic collaboration. The therapist works, through the technique of Socratic questioning, to develop greater awareness in the patient. Further, the therapist can offer hypotheses for consideration, act as a resourceperson, or directly point out areas of difficulty. The therapist's ability to develop hypotheses and to then translate them into workable therapeutic goals is essential.

CT requires that the patient be an active participant in the therapeutic process. One of the most important elements for a positive therapeutic outcome is a strong working alliance. This implies that the patient has made a decision and commitment to change. Without that motivation and commitment, therapy will be difficult if not impossible.

The therapist must be able to generate a collaborative set so that the patient sees himself or herself as a partner in the process, not merely coming to be "therapized" or "worked on." The collaboration may not always be equally shared, but may be divided 30–70, or 70–30, with the therapist providing most of the energy or work within a particular session or in the therapy more generally. The vegetatively depressed patient may be able to muster the strength to sit up in bed and talk to the therapist. Later, the patient may get out of bed and sit in the chair in the room. When the patient can leave his or her room and walk down the hall for a therapy session, major changes have occurred. As the therapy progresses successfully, the proportion of patient to therapist work would shift. In some cases, the patient's problems may preclude taking a more active part in the therapy. This would be true with dependent personality disorders. In these cases, the therapeutic goal may be to help the patient work to the limit of his or her ability.

Perhaps the strongest elements in CT are the structure, focus, and goal orientation of the model. By avoiding the casual, free-associative meandering that has been typical of most dynamic therapies, CT can move quickly and directly into those areas that create the most difficulty.

The time-limited nature of CT is not measured in the number of sessions, but rather in the manner in which the therapy is conducted. The CT therapist sees therapy as having a beginning, middle, and an end. By setting near-point, midpoint and far-point goals, the patient's problem list can be dealt with in an ordered and reasonable fashion.

THE BASIC COGNITIVE THERAPY MODEL

The CT model posits three issues in the formation and maintenance of the common psychological disorders: the cognitive triad, cognitive distortions, and the schema (Beck et al., 1979; Freeman et al, 1990).

THE COGNITIVE TRIAD

The construct of the cognitive triad was first developed to better understand depression (Beck et al., 1979). In depression, the triad helps to understand the interaction of the patient's negative views of self, world or experience, and of the future. In anxiety, the triad represents the patient's concern about threat to self, from the world or experience, and oriented toward the future. Virtually all patient problems can be subsumed under one of these three areas, or some combination of the three. The therapist can start to focus and structure the therapy from the onset of treatment by paying special attention to the triad. Personal issues relating to self, world, and future differ for each patient. Each constituent of the triad does not necessarily contribute equally to the depression. By assessing the degree of contribution of each of the three factors, the therapist can begin to develop a conceptualization of the patient's problem(s).

COGNITIVE DISTORTIONS

An individual can distort in a variety of positive or negative ways. The patient who distorts in a positive direction may view life in an unrealistically positive way and take chances that most people would avoid (e.g., starting a new business or investing in a risky new stock). If successful, the positive distorter is vindicated and may be envied for courage. If unsuccessful, the positive distorter may see the failure as a consequence of taking a low-yield chance. The positive distorter can, however, take chances that may eventuate in being in situations of great danger (e.g., experiencing massive chest pains and not consulting a physician). The positive distortion in this case might be, "I'm too young and healthy for a heart attack." The manic individual might be seen as the extreme example of the positive distorter.

It is, however, the negative distortions or maladaptive thoughts (also called automatic thoughts) that generally become the focus of therapy. One job of the therapist is to make the distortions manifest in content, degree of patient belief, and style, and to help identify the impact of the distortions on the patient's life. The distortions are the thematic directional signs that point to, or suggest, the underlying schema. The distortions occur in many combinations and permutations, and are essentially "normal." It is when these distortions become exaggerated and a source of discomfort or dysfunction that the patient will generally seek help. Often these distortions are parenthetic statements to what the patient is saying. For example, when the patient says, "I'll be embarrassed" and then has a strong emotional reaction to the notion of embarrassment, the parenthetic or unspoken part of the statement might be, "and that would be terrible/awful" or "I won't survive the embarrassment," or "and it will serve me right for thinking I could do that." Certain types or combinations of distortions have become emblematic of particular styles of behaving or of certain clinical syndromes.

The distortions and patient styles are presented here in isolation for the sake of discussion. This is not meant to be a comprehensive list, but is rather presented for illustrative purposes. Typical distortions and examples of the common clinical correlates follow.

- *All or nothing thinking.* "I'm either a success or a failure." "The world is either black or white." (At the extreme, this is common in borderline and obsessive-compulsive disorders.)
- *Mind reading.* "They probably think that I'm incompetent." "I just know that he disapproves." (At the extreme, this is common in avoidant and paranoid personality disorders.)

- *Emotional reasoning*. "Because I feel inadequate I am inadequate." "Because I feel uncomfortable, the world is dangerous." (At the extreme, this is common in anxiety and panic disorders.)
- *Personalization*. "That comment wasn't just random, it must have been directed toward me." "Problems always emerge when I'm in a hurry." (At the extreme, this is common in avoidant or paranoid personality disorders.)
- *Overgeneralization*. "Everything I do turns out wrong." "It doesn't matter what my choices are, they always fall flat." (At the extreme, this is common in depression.)
- *Catastrophizing*. "If I go to the party, there will be terrible consequences." "I'd better not try because I might fail, and that would be awful." (At the extreme, this is common in anxiety disorders, especially social anxiety, social phobia, or panic.)
- *Should statements*. "I should visit my family every time they want me to." "They should do what I say because it is right." (At the extreme, this is common in obsessive-compulsive disorders.)
- *Control fallacies*. "If I'm not in complete control all the time, I will go out of control." "I must be able to control all of the contingencies in my life." (At the extreme, this is common in anxiety disorders, especially obsessive-compulsive disorders.)
- *Comparing*. "I am not as competent as my co-workers or supervisors." "Compared to others, there is clearly something flawed about me." (At the extreme, this is common in depression.)
- *Heaven's reward fallacy*. "If I do everything perfectly here, I will be rewarded later." "I have to muddle through this life, maybe things will be better later." (At the extreme, this is common in obsessive-compulsive disorders or depression.)
- *Disqualifying the positive*. "This success experience was only a fluke." "The compliment was unwarranted." (At the extreme, this is common in depression.)
- *Perfectionism*. "I must do everything perfectly or I will be criticized and a failure." "A merely adequate job is akin to failure." (At the extreme, this is common in anxiety.)
- *Selective abstraction*. "The rest of the information doesn't matter. This is the salient point." "I must focus on the negative details while I ignore and filter out all the positive aspects of a situation." (At the extreme, this is common in depression.)
- *Externalization of self-worth*. "My worth is dependent on what others think of me." "They think, therefore I am." (At the extreme, this is common in depression and low self-esteem.)
- *Fallacy of change*. "You should change your behavior because I want you to." "They should act differently because I expect it." (At the extreme, this is common in narcissism.)
- *Fallacy of worrying*. "If I worry about it enough, it will be resolved." "One cannot be too concerned." (At the extreme, this is common in anxiety disorders.)
- *Fallacy of ignoring*. "If I ignore it maybe it will go away." "If I don't pay attention I will not be held responsible." (At the extreme, this is common in depression and anxiety.)
- *Fallacy of fairness*. "Life should be fair." "People should all be fair." (At the extreme, this is common in avoidant and socially anxious patients.)
- *Being right*. "I must prove that I am right, as being wrong is unthinkable." "To be wrong is to be a bad person." (At the extreme, this is common in obsessive-compulsive disorders and in narcissistic disorders.)
- *Fallacy of attachment*. "I can't live without a man." "If I was in a relationship, all of my problems would be solved." (At the extreme, this is common in depression and anxiety.)

Although all of the above distortions are stated in the first person, they can also apply to expectations of others, including family, social, religious, and gender groups.

SCHEMA

The dynamic element of cognitive therapy is understanding and making manifest the underlying rules/assumptions/beliefs/schema. Beck (1967, 1976, 1976) and Freeman (1986, 1993) have suggested that schemas generate the various cognitive distortions seen in patients. Although there have been attempts to differentiate between rules, assumptions, underlying rules, beliefs, and schema, Beck and co-workers (1990) have used the term "schema" to denote this dynamic substrate, a convention that will be followed here. These schemas or basic rules of life begin to be established as a force in cognition and behavior from the earliest points in life, and are well fixed by the middle childhood years. They are the accumulation of the individual's learning and experience within the family, religious, ethnic, gender, or regional subgroups, and the broader society. A schema that is strongly held and is seen to be essential for the person's safety, well-being, or existence will be more powerful as a directing force within the person's life. If the schema was adopted and internalized early in life and was powerfully reinforced by significant others, it will similarly be more apparent in the personality style (Beck et al., 1990). If the schema was acquired prior to the acquisition of language, during the sensorimotor stage, the schema will be very powerful and direct behavior, although the individual may not be able to identify the source of the schema. It appears to come from out of a "fog" (Layden et al., 1993).

The schema are very rarely isolated and separate but, like the distortions, occur in complex combinations and permutations. The schema become, in effect, how one defines oneself, both individually and as part of the group. The schema can be active or dormant, with the more active schema being the rules that govern day-to-day behavior while the dormant schema are called into play to control behavior in times of stress. An active schema might be "Thou shalt not kill," although the individual might eat meat (killed by others) or kill an attacker of one's children (protect one's family). Schema may be either compelling or noncompelling. The more compelling the schema, the more likely it is that the individual or family will respond to it. The more strongly held the schema, the less likely it is to be surrendered. Individuals who would rather die than surrender their beliefs are termed martyrs. Similarly, some schema are seen to be essential for survival and will not yield to therapeutic interventions.

Schema are in a constant state of change and evolution. From the child's earliest years there is a need to alter old schema and develop new ones to meet the different and increasingly complex demands of the world (adaptation). The infant's conception of reality is governed by the limited interaction with the world, so the infant may initially perceive the crib and the few caretakers that care for and comfort it as the entire world. As the infant develops additional skills of mobility and interaction, the schema are altered by the new data. Infants then perceive their worlds as significantly larger. Environmental data and experience are only taken in by the individual as the individual can use this data in terms of his or her own subjective experiences. The schema are self-selective in that the individual may ignore certain environmental stimuli that he or she is not able to integrate or synthesize. There is an active and evolutionary process where all perceptions and cognitive structures are applied to new functions (assimilation), while new cognitive structures are developed to serve old functions in new situations (accommodation) (Rosen, 1985, 1989). Some individuals may persist in using old structures without fitting them to the new circumstances in which they are involved. They may further fail to accommodate or build new structures.

A particular schema may engender a great deal of emotion and be emotionally bound by the individual's past experience, by the sheer weight of the time in which that schema has been held, or by the relative importance and meaning of the individuals from whom the schema were acquired. There is a cognitive element to the schema that pervades the individual's thoughts and images. The patient can, with the proper training, describe schema in great detail. The therapist can also deduce them from behavior or automatic thoughts. In some cases, however, the schema that govern behavior were acquired very early in the developmental process. Schema that are acquired through sensorimotor channels may be powerful for the individual and have a profound effect on the person's life. These early schema may be among the hardest to change in that the therapist is attempting to change sensorimotor learning using abstract formal operations techniques (Layden et al., 1993).

Finally, there is a behavioral component that involves the way the belief system governs the individual's responses to a particular stimulus or set of stimuli. In seeking to alter a particular schema that has endured for a long period of time, it would be necessary to help the individual deal with the belief from as many different perspectives as possible (i.e., cognitive, behavioral, and affective). There is no "pure" strategy; for example, a behavioral intervention will have cognitive and affective elements. A change in behavior, therefore, will also often bring about changes in cognition and affect. In many cases we find that an individual's particular schema are consensually validated. Significant others not only help to form but also maintain the particular schema, be they negative or positive.

Patients will often describe themselves as displaying particular characteristics "as far back as I can remember." Objective observations may support the patients' views that they have behaved in a certain way as far back as early childhood. What then differentiates the child who develops a schema that is held with moderate strength and is amenable to change later on from the individual who develops a core belief that is powerful and apparently immutable? There are several possibilities:

- In addition to the core belief, the individual maintains a powerful associated belief that no matter what he or she might do, he or she cannot change.

- The belief system is powerfully (and continually) reinforced by parents or significant others.
- Although the dysfunctional belief system may not be especially reinforced, any attempt to believe the contrary may not be reinforced or may even be punished (e.g., any attempt to assert a sense of worth would be ignored).
- The parents or significant others may offer direct instruction contrary to developing a positive image (e.g., "It's not nice to brag" or "It's not nice to toot your own horn because people will think less of you").

GENERAL TREATMENT APPROACH

Cognitive therapy requires all of the characteristics of any effective therapy, including rapport building, trust, empathy, active listening, and the maintenance of the therapeutic alliance. A full developmental, family, social, occupational, educational, medical, and psychiatric history is taken. The data are essential in helping to turn patient complaints into a working problem list and in developing the treatment conceptualization. The establishment of a discrete problem list helps both patient and therapist have an idea of where the therapy is going, to agree on a general time/energy framework, and to be able to assess the therapeutic progress. Having established and agreed upon a problem list and focus for therapy, the individual sessions are then structured through agenda setting.

Rather than having the therapy session meander, the therapist can work with the patient to focus the therapy work and to make better use of time, energy, and available skills. Agenda setting at the beginning of the session allows both patient and therapist to put issues of concern on the agenda for the day. It also allows the therapist to structure the time by working to set an agenda that is broad enough to use the available time without being so broad as to leave much of the agenda work incomplete. The agenda setting allows for a continuity between sessions so that sessions are not individual events, but rather part of a whole. A typical agenda might include:

1. Rapport building to reestablish the personal connection with the patient.
2. Review of any self-report scales filled out by the patient prior to the session. Any items or questions from those scales can be put on the agenda.
3. Setting the agenda. This is the opportunity for the therapist to maintain the continuity of the sessions by placing on the agenda items from the previous session.
4. Overview of the week. The patient can fill the therapist in on events of importance during the week, including the patient's response to the last therapy session.
5. Review of homework. Success or problems in doing the homework and the results or learning consequent from the homework.
6. Particular problems are put on the agenda. This might involve teaching a particular skill (social or assertiveness skills) or the questioning of particular dysfunctional thoughts.
7. Three to five minutes prior to the ending of the session, the patient can be asked to review the session and outline what he or she has gotten from it. This gives the therapist an opportunity to help the patient clarify the goals and accomplishments of the session. The homework for the next session can be emphasized and the session given a closure. Finally, the patient can be asked for his or her response to the session.

ASSESSMENT METHODS

When depression is the primary problem, the Beck Depression Inventory (BDI) is among the most useful tools available to the therapist. The Beck Depression Inventory (Beck et al., 1961) is one of the most widely used self-report measures for depression in the world. Translations have been made into virtually every major language. It consists of 21 items designed to reflect the various factors in the depression, and yields a score that offers an overall level of depression. Weekly administration of the BDI, prior to each session, can serve to provide objective data regarding therapeutic progress, and as an aid in helping validate or challenge the patient's assumptions about self, world, and the future. The BDI can be used as a homework form when patients report diurnal mood fluctuations. The patient is given a supply of the forms and is asked to fill them out at regular intervals each day (waking, noon, 4:00 PM, time of sleep). The therapist can then evaluate high and low points during the day and the change in specific items. By doing a weekly item analysis, the specific content of the depression can be elicited and then used in the agenda. For example, if a patient who is a chronic "1" on the suicide item (9) endorses either a "0" or a "3," it would be important for the therapist to elicit information about the reason(s) for the change.

When anxiety is a target symptom, the therapist can use the Beck Anxiety Inventory (BAI), a 21-item self-report symptom checklist designed to measure the severity of anxiety-related symptoms (Beck et al., 1983). The BAI is a useful, objective measure of the overall level of anxiety, and is diagnostic both quantitatively and qualitatively in a fashion similar to the BDI.

For patients who report suicidal thinking, the Hopelessness Scale (HS) was developed as a measure of the negative view of the future and the intensity of that view (Beck et al., 1974). The HS is frequently used in conjunction with the BDI as a measure of potential for suicide. This measure may also be used as an index of change. As the patient learns new ways of coping, experiences greater self-efficacy, and perceives change, the level of hopelessness decreases.

DIAGNOSIS AND TREATMENT PLAN

The initial step in establishing a treatment plan for the patient involves the therapist developing a working conceptualization of the problem(s). This conceptualization will, of necessity, be based on family and developmental histories, test data, interview material, and reports of previous therapists or other professionals. This conceptualization must meet several criteria. It must be useful, simple, theoretically coherent, explain past behavior, make sense of present behavior, and be able to predict future behavior. Part of the conceptualization process involves the compilation of a problem list, which is then prioritized to identify a sequence of problems to be dealt with in therapy. A particular problem may be the primary focus of therapy because of its debilitating effect on the individual. In another case, there may be no debilitating problems, thereby placing the focus on the simplest problem, giving the patient practice in problem-solving and some measure of success. In a third case, the choice of a therapy focus might be on a "keystone" problem, that is, a problem whose solution will cause a ripple effect in solving other problems. Having set out the treatment goals with the patient, the therapist can begin to develop strategies and the interventions that will help effect the strategies.

CT is proactive, and so the therapist must plan and develop hypotheses as to what reinforces and maintains dysfunctional thinking and behavior. If a particular belief is only partially believed by the individual, it is much easier for the individual to give it up because he or she is giving up a small piece of a belief system as opposed to being asked to challenge what is seen and regarded as "self." The more chronic patients who seek treatment, including those who exhibit the chronic "neurotic" behaviors and character disorders, often see their symptoms as "me." They will readily verbalize, "This is who I/we are and this is the way I/we have always been." When the challenge to self is perceived, the individual usually responds with anxiety. Any challenge to the self needs to be the result of a careful, guided discovery based on collaboration, as opposed to a direct, confrontational, and disputational stance.

TREATMENT INTERVENTIONS

Several cognitive and behavioral techniques can be used by the therapist to identify and to then question both the distortions and the schema that underlie them. These techniques are taught to the patients to help them respond in more functional ways. The precise mix of cognitive and behavioral techniques will depend on the patient's skills, the therapist's skills, the level of pathology, and the treatment goals. For the severely debilitated patient, the initial goals of treatment would be focused on the patient doing self-help tasks. Graded task assignments can be used with great success. Starting at the bottom of a hierarchy of difficulty and moving through successively more difficult tasks can help the patient achieve a greater sense of personal efficacy. This personal efficacy can then be used as evidence for the cognitive work in therapy. Pharmacotherapy may be an essential ingredient in the therapy program developed for different patients. Contrary to popular myth, CT and pharmacotherapy are not mutually exclusive, but can be integrated into effective treatment (Wright et al., 1993).

COGNITIVE TECHNIQUES

The goal of CT is for the therapist to become skilled in the broad therapy "menu." By skillfully moving between various interventions, the therapist can teach the patient specific intervention skills so that the patient can be his or her own therapist. Intervention skills are as follows.

- *Idiosyncratic meaning*. It is essential to question the patient directly on the meanings of the patient's words and thoughts. This also models the need for active listening skills, increased communication, and a means for checking out assumptions.
- *Questioning the evidence*. It is essential to teach the individual to question the evidence that is being used to maintain and strengthen an idea or belief. Questioning the evidence also requires examining the source of data and recognizing that the individual may ignore major pieces of data and focus on the few pieces of data that support the dysfunctional view.
- *Reattribution*. The patient often takes responsibility for events and situations that are only

minimally attributable to the patient. The therapist can help the patient distribute responsibility among all relevant parties.

- *Examining options and alternatives*. This cognitive strategy involves working with the patient to generate additional options. The prime example of this appears in the suicidal patient. These patients see their options and alternatives as so limited that among their few choices, death might be the easiest or simplest choice.

- *De-catastrophizing*. This involves helping the patient to evaluate if he or she is overestimating the catastrophic nature of a situation. The patient can be helped to see that the consequence of life actions are not "all or nothing" and thereby are less catastrophic. It is important that this technique be used with great gentleness and care so that the patient does not feel ridiculed or made fun of by the therapist. Questions that might be asked of the patient include, "What is the worst thing that can happen," or "And if it does occur, what would be so terrible?"

- *Fantasized consequences*. The individual is asked to describe a fantasy about a feared situation and to describe their images and the attendant concerns. In the verbalization, patients can often see the irrationality of their ideas. If the fantasized consequences are realistic, the therapist can work with the patient to realistically assess the danger and develop coping strategies. This technique allows the patients to bring imaged events, situations, or interactions that have happened previously into the consulting room. The explication and investigation of the style, format, and content of the fantasy can yield material for the therapy work.

- *Advantages and disadvantages*. By asking the patient to examine both the advantages and the disadvantages of both sides of an issue, a broader perspective can be achieved. This basic problem solving technique is useful in gaining a perspective and in then plotting a reasonable course of action.

- *Turning adversity to advantage*. There are times that a seeming disaster can be used to ad-

vantage. Losing one's job can be a disaster but may, in some cases, be the entry point to a new job or even a new career. Having a deadline imposed may be seen as oppressive and unfair, but may be used as a motivator. There is a balancing that puts experience into a perspective.

- *Guided association/discovery*. This therapist-guided technique stands in opposition to the technique of free association basic to the psychoanalytic process. The use of what is called the chained or guided association technique involves the therapist working with the patient to connect ideas, thoughts, and images using Socratic questioning. The therapist provides the conjunctions to the patient's verbalizations. The use of statements such as, "And then what?" "What evidence do we have that is true?" allows the therapist to guide the patient along various therapeutic paths, depending on the conceptualization and therapeutic goals.

- *Use of exaggeration or paradox*. There seems to be room at the extremes for only one person. By taking an idea to its extreme, the therapist can often help to move the family to a more central position regarding a particular belief. Given a hypersensitivity to criticism and ridicule, some patients may experience the paradoxical strategies as making light of their problems. The therapist who chooses to use the paradoxical or exaggeration techniques must have a strong working relationship with the patient, good timing, and the good sense to know when to back away from the technique.

- *Scaling*. For those patients who see things as "all or nothing," the technique of scaling or seeing things as existing on a life-referenced continuum is very important. The scaling of a feeling can force patients to use the strategy of gaining distance and perspective. Because patients may be at a point of extreme thoughts and extreme behaviors, any movement towards a midpoint is helpful. A patient is first asked to rate their response to a particular experience from 0 to 10. They can then establish anchor points for that experience from the greatest response (10) to the least response (0).

- *Externalization of voices.* Patients "hear" the dysfunctional voices in their head. When they externalize the voices, both patient and therapist are in a better position to deal with the voices or messages in a variety of ways. By having the therapist take the part of the dysfunctional voice, the patient can get practice in adaptive responding. The therapist can first model being adaptive to the patient's verbalization of the dysfunctional thoughts. After modeling the functional voice, the therapist can, via a graded manner, become an increasingly more difficult dysfunctional voice for the patient to respond to. The patient can recognize the dysfunctional nature of the voice. The therapist can hear the tone, content, and general context of the suicidal thoughts and generate strategies for intervention.
- *Self-instruction.* Meichenbaum (1977) has developed an extensive model for using self-instruction. Patients can be taught to offer direct self-instructions for more adaptive behavior or, in some cases, counterinstructions to avoid dysfunctional behavior. In this technique, the therapist is not introducing anything new. Rather, the patient is being helped to use and strengthen a technique that we all use at various times. The patient can start with direct verbalizations that will, with practice, become part of the behavioral repertoire.
- *Thought stopping.* Dysfunctional thoughts often have a snowball effect for the individual. What may start as a small and insignificant problem can, if left to roll along, gather weight, speed, and momentum. Thought stopping is best used when the thoughts are about to start or have just started not in the middle of the process. The patient can picture a stop sign, "hear" a bell, picture a wall. Any of these can be helpful to stop the progression and growth of the thoughts.
- *Distraction.* This technique is especially helpful for patients with anxiety problems. Because it is almost impossible to maintain two thoughts at the same strength simultaneously, anxiogenic thoughts generally pre-

clude more adaptive thinking. Conversely, a focused thought distracts from the anxiogenic thoughts. By having patients focus on complex counting, addition, or subtraction, they are rather easily distracted from other thoughts. Having the patient count to 200 by 13s is very effective (having the patient count by 2, 5, 10, or 11 is not as effective because these number sequences are overlearned). When out of doors, counting cars or people wearing the color red, or any cognitively engaging task, will work. Distraction or refocusing of attention may be achieved by focusing on some aspect of the environment, engaging in mental exercise or imagery, or initiating physical activity. Although this technique is a short-term technique, it is very useful to allow patients the time to establish some degree of control over their thinking. This time can then be used to use other cognitive techniques.
- *Direct disputation.* There are times when direct disputation is helpful. A major guideline as to when direct disputation is necessary is the imminence of a suicide attempt. When it seems clear to the clinician that a patient is going to make an attempt, the therapist must directly and quickly work to challenge the patient's hopelessness. Although it might appear to be the treatment technique of choice, the therapist risks becoming embroiled in a power struggle or argument with the patient. Disputation coming from outside the patient may, in fact, engender passive resistance and a passive-aggressive response that might include suicide. Disputation, argument, or debate are potentially dangerous tools. They must be used carefully, judiciously, and with skill.
- *Labeling of distortions.* The fear of the unknown is a frequent issue for anxiety patients. The more that the therapist can do to identify the nature and content of the dysfunctional thinking, and to help label the types of distortions that patients use, the less frightening the entire process becomes.
- *Developing replacement imagery.* Inasmuch as the anxiety is constantly being generated by

imagery, patients can be helped to develop coping images. For example, rather than imaging failure, or recalling defeat or embarrassment, the therapist can practice with the patient new and effective coping images. Once well practiced, patients can do image substitution.

BEHAVIORAL TECHNIQUES

The goals in using behavioral techniques within the context of cognitive therapy are manifold. The first goal is to use direct behavioral strategies and techniques to test dysfunctional thoughts and behaviors. By having the patient try feared or avoided behaviors, old ideas can be directly challenged. A second use of behavioral techniques is to practice new behaviors as homework. Certain behaviors can be practiced in the office, and then practiced at home. Homework can range from acting differently, practicing active listening, being verbally or physically affectionate, or doing things in a new way.

1. *Activity scheduling.* The activity schedule is perhaps the most ubiquitous technique in the therapist's armamentarium. For patients who are feeling overwhelmed, the activity schedule can be used to plan more effective time use. The activity schedule is both a retrospective tool to assess past time use and a prospective tool to help plan better time use.

2. *Mastery and pleasure ratings.* The activity schedule can also be used to assess and plan activities that offer patients both a sense of personal efficacy (mastery, 1 to 10) and pleasure (1 to 10). The greater the mastery and pleasure, the lower the rates of anxiety and depression. By discovering the low or high anxiety activities, plans can be made to increase the former and decrease the latter.

3. *Social skills or assertiveness training.* If patients lack specific social skills, it is incumbent upon the therapist to either help them to gain the skills or to make a referral for skills training. The skill acquisition may involve anything from teaching patients how to properly shake hands to practicing conversational skills.

4. *Bibliotherapy.* Several excellent books can be assigned as readings for homework. These books can be used to socialize or educate patients to the basic CT model, emphasize specific points made in the session, or introduce new ideas for discussion at future sessions. Some helpful books include *Love Is Never Enough* (Beck, 1989), *Feeling Good* (Burns, 1980), *Woulda, Coulda, Shoulda* (Freeman and DeWolfe, 1990), and *The 10 Dumbest Mistakes that Smart People Make* (Freeman and DeWolfe, 1992).

5. *Graded tasks assignments.* GTAs involve a series of small, sequential steps that lead to the desired goal. By setting out a task and then arranging the necessary steps in a hierarchy, patients can be helped to make reasonable progress with a minimum of stress. As patients attempt each step, the therapist can be available for support and guidance.

6. *Behavioral rehearsal/role-playing.* The therapy session is the ideal place to practice many behaviors. The therapist can serve as teacher and guide offering direct feedback on performance. The therapist can monitor the patient's performance, offer suggestions for improvement, and model new behaviors. In addition, anticipated and actual road blocks can be identified and worked on in the session. There can be extensive rehearsal before the patient attempts the behavior in vivo.

7. *In vivo exposure.* There are times when the practice in the consulting room needs to be expanded. Although very time intensive, the therapist can go with a patient into feared situations. The therapist can drive with a patient across a feared bridge, go to a feared shopping mall, or travel on a feared bus. The in vivo exposure can be part of the office-based therapy along with the patient-generated homework.

8. *Relaxation training.* The anxious patient can profit from relaxation training inasmuch as the anxiety response and the quieting relaxation response are mutually exclusive. The relaxation training can be taught in the office and then practiced by the patient for homework. Ready-

made relaxation tapes can be purchased, or the therapist may easily tailor a tape for a patient. The therapist-made tape can include the patient's name and can focus on particular symptoms. The tape can be modified, as needed.

CHALLENGING DYSFUNCTIONAL THINKING

One of the most powerful techniques in CT involves helping the patient to challenge dysfunctional thinking. The CT model posits an interaction between the individual's thoughts and the emotions. The model does *not* posit a direct linear relationship of thoughts causing feelings.

The daily record of dysfunctional thoughts (DTR) is an ideal format for testing the dysfunctional thoughts. Whether the patient's problems are depression, anxiety, phobia, or whatever, the therapeutic approach would be substantially the same. The process begins with the patient identifying the thought, emotion, or situation that causes them difficulty. If the patient presents with an emotional issue ("I'm very sad"), the therapist needs to inquire as to the situations that might engender the emotion, and the attendant thoughts. If the patient presents with a thought ("I'm a loser"), the therapist needs to ascertain the feelings and the situation. Finally, the patient may present a situation ("My husband left me"). The therapist needs to determine the thoughts and the emotions. Statements such as, "I feel like a loser" need to be reframed as thoughts, and the emotions that are a concomitant of the thought elicited. The following examples demonstrate the use of the DTR.

Often, patients phrase their thoughts as questions. "Why does this always happen to me?" "Why can't I maintain a relationship?" "Why doesn't my life turn out better?" A heuristic view is that questions are generally functional. It is important to ask questions, and then to answer them. The dysfunctional thoughts are more generally declarative rather than interrogatory. "This always happens to me," "I can't maintain a relationship," and "my life is less than I had hoped for." The cognitive techniques can be used to question the patient's conclusions. For example, if the patient has the dysfunctional thought, "There's something terribly wrong with me," sample adaptive responses are as follows.

What do you mean by something WRONG with you? (Idiosyncratic meaning.)

What evidence are you using that there's something wrong with you? (Questioning the evidence.)

Has it always been you who has been wrong or bad? (Reattribution.)

Are you saying that there is something so terribly wrong with you that you have never been right about anything? (Exaggeration.)

On a scale from 1 to 10, where would you place your having something wrong? (Scaling.)

One possibility is that there is something terribly wrong with you. Are there any other possible conclusions? (Alternatives and options.)

As can be seen, use of the techniques is limited only by the creativity of the therapist. The techniques need to be learned so that the therapist can move quickly and easily among the appropriate ones.

HOMEWORK

No therapy takes place solely within the confines of the consulting room. It is important for the patient to understand that extension of the therapy work to the nontherapy hours allows for a greater therapeutic focus. Burns and Auerbach (1992, p. 464) have found that "differences in homework compliance are significantly correlated with recovery from depression." The homework can be either cognitive or behavioral. It might involve having the patient complete an activity schedule (an excellent homework for the first session), complete several DTRs, or try new behaviors. The homework needs to flow from the session material, rather than being tacked onto the end of the session simply because CT should include homework. The more meaningful and collaborative the homework, the greater the likelihood of patient compliance with the therapeutic regimen. If the homework is not reviewed as part of the session agenda, the patient will quickly stop doing the homework.

VULNERABILITY FACTORS

Vulnerability factors are circumstances, situations, or deficits that have the effect of decreasing the patient's ability to effectively cope with life stressors by losing options, or failing to see available options. These factors work to lower the patient's threshold or tolerance for life stress situations and, alone or in combination, may serve to increase the patient's suicidal thinking or actions, lower the threshold for anxiety stimuli, or increase the patient's vulnerability to depressogenic thoughts and situations (Freeman and Simon, 1989). These factors include the following.

1. *Acute illness*. This may run the range from a severe and debilitating illness to more transient illnesses such as headaches and virus infections.
2. *Chronic illness*. In situations where the health problem is chronic, there can be an acute exacerbation of the suicidal thinking.
3. *Deterioration of health*. In aging, there may a loss of activity due to the body's inability to perform up to the expectations that were appropriate at other times in the patient's life.
4. *Hunger*. During times of food deprivation, the individual is often more vulnerable to a variety of stimuli. In literature, Jean Valjean was willing to break the conventions of society. Studies have indicated that in times of hunger, individuals should not attempt to shop for food because of the probability of overpurchasing food.
5. *Anger*. When individuals are angry, there appears to be a loss of appropriate problem-solving ability. There may be a loss of impulse control or overresponding to stimuli that may more usually be ignored.
6. *Fatigue*. In a similar fashion, fatigue decreases both problem-solving strategies and impulse control.
7. *Loneliness*. When individuals see themselves as isolated and apart from others, leaving this unhappy world may seem to be a reasonable option.
8. *Major life loss*. With the death of a significant other through death or through divorce or separation, individuals often see themselves as having reduced options, or do not care what happens to them.
9. *Poor problem-solving ability*. Certain individuals may have impaired problem-solving ability. This deficit may not be obvious until the individual is placed in situations of great stress. Being able to deal with minor problems may never test the individual's ability.
10. *Substance abuse*. The abuse of many substances can increase suicidality. This may be of two types: acute problems, where the patient's judgment is compromised during periods of intoxication, and more chronic problems, where judgment may be impaired more generally.
11. *Chronic pain*. Chronic pain may have the effect of causing the individual to see suicide as one method for achieving surcease from the pain.
12. *Poor impulse control*. There are certain patients who have poor impulse control because of organic (hyperactivity) or functional problems. Patients with bipolar illness or borderline, antisocial, or histrionic personality disorders may have impulse control deficits.
13. *New life circumstance*. Changing jobs, marital status, homes, or family status all are stressors that are vulnerability factors.

The therapist's work will often involve helping the patient avoid the vulnerability factors.

TERMINATION

Termination of CT begins in the first session. Because the goal of CT is not cure, but more effective coping, the cognitive therapist does not plan for therapy indefinitely. As a skill-building model of psychotherapy, the therapist's goal is to assist patients in acquiring the skills to deal with the internal and external stressors. When the depression inventory, patient report, therapist observation, and feedback from significant others confirm decreased depression, greater activity, and a higher level of adaptive abilities, the therapy can move towards termination. The termination is accomplished gradually to allow time for ongoing modifications and corrections. Sessions are tapered off from once weekly to biweekly. From that point sessions can be set on a monthly basis, with follow-up sessions at 3 and 6 months until therapy is ended. Patients can, of course, still call and set an appointment in the event of an emergency. Sometimes patients will call simply to get some information, a reinforcement of a particular behavior, or to report a success. With the cognitive therapist in the role of a consultant/collaborator, this continued contact is appropriate and important.

NONCOMPLIANCE

Noncompliance, sometimes called resistance, often carries the implication that the patient doesn't want to change or "get well," for either conscious or unconscious reasons. The resistance may be manifested directly (e.g., tardiness or missing of appointments) or more subtly through omissions in the material reported in the sessions. Clinically, we can identify several reasons for noncompliance. They can appear in any combination or permutation, and the relative strength of any non-compliant action may change with the patient's life circumstances, progress in therapy, or relationship with the therapist. Several reasons for noncompliance or resistance are as follows.

- Lack of patient skill to change behavior.
- Lack of therapist skill to help the patient change.
- Environmental stressors precluding changing.

- Patient cognitions regarding the possibility of failure.
- Patient cognitions regarding consequences of changing.
- Congruent patient and therapist distortions.
- Poor socialization to the CT model.
- Secondary gain from maintaining the dysfunctional behavior.
- Lack of collaboration of therapeutic alliance.
- Poor timing of interventions.
- Patient fear of changing.
- Lack of patient motivation.
- Patient rigidity.

CLINICAL APPLICATIONS OF COGNITIVE THERAPY

In this section, brief applications of CT to problems typical to nursing practice will be discussed. These include the treatments for anxiety and personality disorders, and the applications of the CT model to crisis intervention, group therapy, and family therapy.

ANXIETY

Complaints of anxiety, nervousness, and tension are among the most common problems presented to mental health professionals. It is also apparent that clinical anxiety often presents as a concomitant to a number of other physiological and psychological disorders, including psychosomatic disorders, that may in fact mask the anxiety. In still other cases, the presenting symptoms are physiological, and may or may not have been anxiety related. Therefore, the incidence and prevalence of anxiety are most likely underestimated in medical, nursing, and psychotherapeutic practice.

The basic theme of anxiety is a perception of threat and danger. The threat may cause psychological or physical symptoms, all labeled as "anxiety." Anxiety can affect virtually all response systems—respiratory, muscular, circulatory, dermal, or gastrointestinal, singly or in combination. The manifestations of debilitating anxiety usually include behavioral responses, either by commission (fight/flight or paralysis) or omission (avoidant behavior). There are the physiological sensations that signal the presence of the anxiety, the affective experience of the anxiety, and the cognitive events and processes that stimulate and maintain the anxiety. All of these may be disabling in personal, occupational, and social functioning.

The basic cognitive therapy model of anxiety (Beck et al., 1985; Freeman and Ludgate, 1988; Freeman and Simon, 1989; Freeman et al., 1990) involves several elements. The process of anxiety formation starts with a situation. The individual has a perception of that situation that is based on that individual's schema. The individual then must make an assessment of the perceived threat or perceived self-efficacy (resources). In perceiving a situation as very threatening, it is seen as dangerous. If a mild threat is perceived, the individual will respond as to a challenge, and may very well feel excitement and enthusiasm. When the individual starts feeling anxious, he or she is likely to become even more vigilant to perceived threats and begin to see threat where none existed before. This escalates so that as the individual becomes hypervigilant, virtually everything becomes a threat.

The course of CT for anxiety is similar to the basic model discussed. An important difference is the explanation and the de-catastrophizing of the anxiety symptoms.

The first area to be assessed is the patient's anxiety threshold. Each person has a general anxiety threshold and thresholds for specific situations and experiences. These thresholds may shift. In times of stress, thresholds may lower and the individual becomes sensitive to experiences that in ordinary circumstances have little or no effect. The therapist must ask what events, situations, or interactions trigger the individual to become anxious.

A second assessment issue is the cognitive content of the anxiety. This content may reflect the broad themes of a syndrome, and the more specific and idiosyncratic content of the problem. For example, generalized anxiety involves a fear or threat of physical or psychological danger; panic disorders involve a catastrophic misinterpretation of both external and internal proprioceptive cues (more than, "I'm really worried about that," rather "I'm going to die"). In phobias the cognitive content involves danger or threat in a situation, fear of an object, or fear of a specific circumstance.

A third issue is the risk to resources ratio. When anyone enters a situation they make two evaluations. The first is, "What risk do I perceive for myself in this situation?" Second is an assessment of the personal or environmental resources the individual perceives to have available. If the individual perceives his or her resources as adequate to cope with the risk, typically the individual does not experience anxiety. This is not a single evaluation, but an ongoing series of evaluations. An essential differentiation is whether there is a perception of skill deficit or an actual skill deficit, a perception of high or low resources or a reality of high or low resources. If there is a skill deficit, behavioral interventions would be appropriate. If it is a perception of low resources when the individual is, in fact, socially skilled, more cognitive interventions would be used to help challenge the negative view.

The fourth area to be evaluated is the personality factors of autonomy and dependence. These two factors are highly relevant to the anxiety response (Beck et al., 1983). Autonomy and dependence are usually thought of as anchor points on a linear continuum. At one end is the person who is very dependent and at the other end is a person who is autonomous. Autonomy and dependence are not on a linear continuum, but can be seen as orthogonally related. When people are predominantly dependent or autonomous, their responses to stress are quite different one from the other.

The usual responses to stress are fight, flight, or freeze. The more autonomous individual, when stressed, will rarely seek help, and does not come into therapy willingly. The style of these individuals is to run or fight. They often report their anxiety in terms of vague physiological symptoms, such as "I kinda just feel this lump in my chest" (or "in my throat" or "a little bit of nausea"). The autonomous individual tends to feel trapped and encroached upon (in an almost claustrophobic manner). The therapist who tries to engender a warm, close rapport with the autonomous patient may find the patient becoming more anxious and possibly leaving therapy.

Dependent individuals enter therapy willingly, again and again. Their more frequent response is to freeze or become paralyzed. They may ask how often they can come for therapy. Dependent patients are concerned that if they don't tell the therapist everything, the therapist's ability to help will be impaired. When stressed, dependent patients become very vulnerable to feelings of abandonment (agoraphobic-like). Being late for a single appointment with a dependent patient may engender anxiety for this reason.

Not all anxiety reactions are the same in terms of the symptom picture. By assessing the particular symptoms the patient is experiencing, or has experienced, the therapist can begin to structure the therapy to deal with the symptoms. One person may have predominantly physical symptoms, such as difficulty breathing, indigestion, wobbliness, hot flashes, necessitating the structuring of one sort of intervention. If, however, the patient experiences fear of the worst happening and is terrified and frightened of losing control, the therapist is dealing with a very different set of symptoms. Anxiety must be broken up into its component symptoms, with each weighted by the patient.

The environmental stressors that the individual experiences are identified on axis IV of DSM-IV. Both the type and degree of stress should be assessed. It should be noted that what may be a very severe stressor for one person may be a relief for someone else. It is clear that perception, expectation, and other cognitive factors play a major role in the individual's assessment of what constitutes a stressor and how severe the stressor is perceived to be.

Other factors for assessment are the vulnerability factors discussed earlier. The therapist's task is to help patients recognize and respond to such factors.

It is important to note that when a patient reports a long personal or family history of anxiety, panic, or phobic or avoidant behavior, the argument over whether the anxiety is biological or psychological becomes academic. The patient has habituated to an anxiety response. Does the patient experience single episodes of anxiety, or are we dealing with chronic anxiety? A full anxiety response history needs to be elicited. If data can be collected from a family member, it may be used to verify or question the patient's perception.

The patient's personal rules or schema will dictate the anxiety experience and responses. These rules will then govern or influence much of the manner, style, frequency, and content of the anxiety response.

An assessment of medical history, both individual and family, and examination by a physician are important prior to making a diagnosis of anxiety.

The use of caffeine, cocaine, and amphetamines has been related to the organic anxiety syndrome. Further, withdrawal from CNS-depressing substances such as alcohol or sedatives may cause anxiety syndrome response (DSM-IV).

In developing the conceptualization, the following questions must be answered to generate the most complete clinical picture of why this individual feels/thinks/behaves as he or she does.

- Is the patient in real danger?
- What attribution does the patient make as to the responsibility and causation of the anxiety?
- Has the patient made an accurate self-assessment?
- What are the expectations that the patient has governing his or her behavior and the behavior of others?
- Are the expectations for self (or therapist) within the bounds of probability (for example, "they must change").

- What are the dysfunctional/distorted/auto-matic thoughts that are part of the day-to-day life of the patient?
- What are the schema that are represented by the distortions, and how do the schema affect the behaviors?
- What skills are needed to cope more effectively?
- What behavioral responses need to be modified to allow more effective coping?

Consideration of these areas should help to guide the therapist toward a more systematic and effective intervention.

PERSONALITY DISORDERS

Personality-disordered patients often take more of the therapist's time and more of the therapist's energy, and cause greater difficulty both on the unit and in outpatient settings. They typically present for therapy with issues other than their axis II problems, most often with complaints of depression and anxiety. The duration of treatment, frequency of treatment sessions, goals and expectations for both therapist and patient, and the techniques and available strategies need to be altered in the treatment of personality disorders.

Although some personality disorders may not be obvious early in therapy, other axis II problems are clear within the first therapeutic contact. These tend to be those patients whose social functioning is poor.

It is important to remember that the patient's goals, and not those of others (including the therapist), are the focus of treatment. If an externally referred patient is not willing to work on "core" issues, the therapeutic work may include helping the patient to be trusting, and to understand the therapist's suggestion for work on the more core issues. This can be set up as a series of therapeutic experiments. Although clearly taking longer, the gradual uncovering and guided discovery will be far more fruitful than a direct confrontation.

Diagnostic signs that may point to the possibility of axis II problems might include the following.

- The patient or significant other may report, "Oh, he has always done that, since he was a little boy," or the patient may report, "I've always been this way."
- The patient is not compliant with the therapeutic regimen.
- Therapy seems to have come to a sudden stop, with no apparent reason.
- The patient seems entirely unaware of the effect of his or her behavior on others.
- There is a question as to the motivation of the patient to change.
- The patient may give lip service to the therapy and to the importance of change, but seems to manage to avoid changing.
- The patient's problems appear to be self-consonant. For example, a depressed patient without an axis II diagnosis may say, "I just want to get rid of this depression. I know what it is like to feel good, and I want to feel that way again." The axis II patient has no previous point of reference and sees the problems as them.
- The axis II patient sees the problems as "out there."

Axis II patients manifest behavior that has been reinforced by parents and other caregivers. They maintain early developmental rules and do not seem to have developed more adaptive alternative schema or have not adapted the schema to the changing demands and circumstances of the world.

Axis II patients do not see the problem, or they may externalize and see the problem as outside of themselves. They see others as too demanding or picking on them. "It's not me, it's them." The very "me-ness" of the problem must be addressed.

Following the assessment, the therapist must make sure that there is socialization or education of the patient to the CT model. The initial therapeutic focus may be on relieving the presenting symptoms, (anxiety or depression). In helping the patient to deal with anxiety or depression the therapist can teach the patient the basic cognitive therapy skills that are going to be necessary in working with the more difficult personality disorder. If the therapist can help the patient become less depressed or less anxious, the patient may accept that this therapy may have some value after all, and it may be worthwhile continuing to work in therapy. Some axis II patients, having brought the anxiety and depression under control with fairly standard techniques, may choose to leave therapy. One technique that may be helpful with these patients is to differentiate between "symptom therapy" and "schema therapy." By explaining the importance of working on the schema, the patient may choose to stay in therapy.

The therapeutic relationship will be one of the key ingredients in the therapy of the personality disorder. The therapeutic relationship will be a microcosm of the patient's responses to others in his or her environment. The sensitive nature of the relationship means that the therapist must exercise great care in working with this patient group. Being even two minutes late for a session with the dependent personality may signal anxiety about abandonment. The same two minute lateness will raise the specter of being taken advantage of by the paranoid personality. Given the imperative nature of trust and a relationship, few patients test the patience and mettle of a therapist more than the axis II group. The therapy of the personality disorder must include a strong supportive/expressive component. Without the therapist's active support, the patient may quickly become frightened and disillusioned and leave therapy. The collaborative set involves setting mutually acceptable goals for therapy. These goals must be reasonable and proximal. The patient who expects to become a totally different person as a result of therapy will, invariably, be disappointed. By making small steps towards the desired goals, therapy can move ahead slowly but effectively.

The patient's significant others can be invaluable allies in the therapeutic endeavor by helping the patient to do homework, do reality testing, and offering support in making changes.

The significant others can also be important sources of data about the patient's past behaviors. In a negative vein, meeting with the significant others may enable the therapist to piece together a family history of problems, and what keeps the patient behaving in the same dysfunctional way. Finally, the significant others might be involved in marital or family therapy with the patient.

CRISIS INTERVENTION

A crisis may be defined as a temporary state of upset and disorganization, characterized chiefly by an individual's inability to cope with a particular situation using customary methods of problem solving, and by the potential for a radically positive or negative outcome. The first part of the definition addresses the transient nature of crises. For some individuals, crises are immediate, transient, and temporary. For other individuals, however, life crises may be more long-term and chronic and in fact, become a way of life.

The individual's ability to cope, the focus of the second and third parts of the definition, revolves around the issue of problem-solving ability. By using the common or traditional techniques for personal coping, suicidal individuals find themselves overwhelmed. The traditional techniques are simply not adequate to the present task requirements. The final part of the definition involves the potential for rather weighty consequences.

Normally, when individuals are in a crisis situation and their present resources are not adequate to the task, they may call upon little-used reserves of personal fortitude and spirit or upon the resources of their social network. In addition, they may search for, or create, systems of support to assist them through the crisis. For individuals with few resources (internal or external) that can be called upon to assist them in dealing with crisis, life may be overwhelming. If one has a supportive family system, good friends, or a therapist to call upon, various life crises can be more easily weathered.

As discussed earlier, the CT approach involves the internal focus on the automatic thoughts and schema, and the external focus of changing behaviors, trying new behaviors, and developing and using available resources.

Although crisis is often thought of as a response to a specific and identifiable event or circumstance, the personal perceptions of the event and the beliefs of the individual cannot be overlooked. Short-term, time-limited therapy is a treatment option in crisis situations. In this respect, cognitive therapy is the ideal treatment model. The immediate goals of the cognitive therapy crisis intervention are threefold. First, the evaluation and assessment of the immediacy of the crisis situation. Second, an assessment of the individual's coping repertoire to deal with the crisis. Third, the generation of options of thought, perception, and behavior in addition to the suicide option.

The crisis intervention may come in the form of immediate crisis counseling and problem solving with the acutely suicidal individual, or a more supportive role with active listening being the major tool in dealing with a lonely person. Of course, the lonely person seeking human contact needs more than a listening ear, and more long-term problem solving (and appropriate skill development) may be necessary.

The focused cognitive therapy approach for crisis intervention involves five stages: the first stage involves building rapport. Instrumental in developing this rapport is the therapist's behavior, both on the phone and in person. The therapist has to be able to convey an interest and concern in the person's problem and a nonjudgmental attitude towards the person.

The second stage involves making an initial evaluation regarding the severity of the crisis situation. By doing this, the therapist must be able to develop some idea of the immediate physical danger to the person, the society, or to a significant other. It might also offer some idea as to the type of person with whom the therapist is dealing. There must be a determination as to the course of action that should be taken by the therapist, whether continued therapy is needed or some more drastic action, such as hospitalization or contact with the police or some state agency. Finally, the therapist must work to assist the person in identifying the specific problem he or she is experiencing (establishing a problem focus). The patient is often confused and disorganized and unable to define his or her problem. The therapist must make every effort to help the individual focus on the specific areas creating problems, as opposed to attempting to deal with the vagaries of "depression," "anxiety" or "communication problems." It is important, however, to avoid focusing on one specific problem too early in the contact, because there is a chance that by doing that the therapist could be overlooking other significant problems.

Once the problem has been established the third stage involves helping the patient assess and mobilize strengths and resources. This may be in the form of helping him or her to identify friends in the immediate vicinity who could be capable of helping, as well as identifying various internal strengths and resources that the person in crisis is very likely to overlook.

In the fourth stage the therapist and patient must work jointly to develop a positive plan of action (collaboration and problem solving). An essential aspect of this stage includes eliciting the patient's commitment to this plan of action. At this point, the technique of problem solving is especially applicable. If the nature of the crisis is such that problem solving is not an appropriate mechanism, the last stage becomes necessary.

Stage five involves ongoing collaboration and monitoring of the patient's behavior regarding the crisis issue.

GROUP COGNITIVE THERAPY

In the last 20 years the literature on behavioral and cognitive-behavioral approaches to group psychotherapy has grown enormously, with applications to specific disorders such as borderline personality disorder (Linehan, 1984) and schizophrenia (Perris et al., 1992), or to specific populations such as couples (Abrahms, 1983; Baucom and Epstein, 1988) or inpatients (Bowers, 1989; Freeman and Reinecke, 1993). There are several facets to cognitive group therapy.

UNIVERSALITY

One of the resistances that often surfaces in individual therapy may be framed as "You [the therapist] don't understand what I am going through." One patient continually used the statement, "You don't know a person unless you have walked a mile in their shoes" as a way of disregarding the therapist's viewpoint. It is, however, far more difficult to ignore other patients who share many of the same experiences. Sharing perceptions and reactions in the group allows patients to see that they are not alone in their suffering and that other people have problems of a similar nature. The ultimate effect is that the patient does not feel so isolated in his or her problems.

SUPPORT AND RELATEDNESS

The group can help to foster relatedness for the chronically isolated patient. The group can operate as a support for the patient who is faced with having to work toward modifying external life stressors. By group members sharing of their personal experience in similar situations, and by a sharing of coping strategies and techniques that were used in those situations, the patients can be mutually supportive.

The group can also "dilute" therapy for isolated patients who are overwhelmed by the requirement of the sharing and intimacy of the one-to-one therapy experience. These patients can be participant-observers in the group and can gain from the opportunity to listen to the thoughts, ideas, interactions, and experiences of others. The group may, in fact, serve as a motivator for individual therapy as group members speak of the help they get in their individual therapy. By offering an opportunity for the patient to discuss and process the group experience, the individual therapist may be able to work more

effectively with isolated patients. The patient can use material from the group experience as the vehicle for therapy rather than having to resurrect old memories and experiences.

DIAGNOSTIC FUNCTION

The group can also serve a diagnostic function. The group experience allows the therapist to directly observe the patient's behavioral interactions with other patients. The contained interactions allow for a here-and-now experience that offers the therapist a window into the patient's repertoire of interpersonal skills, threshold for responding, and range of responses to others. The therapist does not have to depend on the patients' reports of how others react to them or how they react to others, as the scenario unfolds before the therapist's eyes. Patients who can appear quite intact in the one-to-one interview may have more trouble maintaining their stability when they are faced with added stimuli of the group setting.

PSYCHOEDUCATION

The basic psychoeducational nature of cognitive therapy is very apparent in the group. The basic principles of the cognitive approach are taught and reinforced in a variety of experiments and group exercises. A blackboard is used in many settings to allow a visual display of therapy concepts. For many patients, reading materials are used as a helpful adjunct to the therapy. Through the use of social skills practice, assertiveness training and other skills can be introduced, practiced, and assigned as homework. Many group therapy programs develop standard written materials for the patients that help the patients learn the cognitive therapy skills in an orderly sequence. These are often combined in a folder or notebook and serve as a place for keeping homework.

PEER FEEDBACK

Involvement in the group allows patients to experience peer feedback. For many patients whose social functioning in the world has been limited, the group provides the only opportunity for constructive peer responses to their behavior. Patients who are more reactively isolated because of their problems can get feedback about how others perceive and react to them. It is not only feedback about problems that is helpful, but also feedback about progress. When a patient makes therapeutic gains, the group can reinforce the progress.

MODELING

The sharing of ideas in the group allows for a great deal of imitative behavior. Patients often model the behaviors of other group members. In the process, the patient can learn effective coping strategies (e.g., assertiveness, empathic responses, goal setting, and problem solving). However, negative behaviors can also be modeled (e.g., withdrawal, passive aggression, rebellion and hostility). The therapist needs to reinforce positive modeling and steer the group away from regressive and destructive behaviors.

SOCIAL SKILL BUILDING

The very nature of the social interaction inherent in the group meeting, format, and procedures fosters a high level of social awareness or interest. Basic social skills can be taught, modeled, discussed, and role-played in the group. The opportunity for feedback and practice is important for all patients. But for those with severe social skills deficits, there is a greater need for the group to assist with building the level of social competence.

LABORATORY EXPERIENCE

The group is a laboratory where patients can test out their automatic thoughts and experiment with different behaviors in a safe, and highly structured, environment. It is important to point out that although the group can provide opportunities for a broad range of cognitive and behavioral experiments, it also has the potential to be an arena

for acting out. This problem can best be dealt with by maintaining a highly structured therapeutic approach. Group cognitive therapy adheres to the highly focused and structured model of individual cognitive therapy.

REALITY TESTING

The group can also offer a vehicle for reality testing and increasing patient responsibility.

TRANSITION

By participating in the group, the patient can try out certain new behaviors or approaches to interpersonal situations that will be encountered in the outside world.

FAMILY THERAPY

The role of significant others cannot be underestimated. The patient on the unit or in an outpatient setting may be living within a family system or group. The family is often asked to come in when problems have become severe or traumatic, rather than at the start of a crisis or conflict. Problems might include physical or emotional abuse of elderly parents by children, abuse of children by parents, issues of child management, demonstrated needs for proper and appropriate parenting, or general relationship issues. Because of the general crisis nature of the presenting problems, the therapist attempts to intervene in the family dynamics in a direct manner.

By involving the family members in the therapeutic process, the interventions can be implemented more quickly, collaboration strengthened, and stigmatization mediated. Frequently, certain members of a family system need treatment or information. In other situations, an entire family requires treatment. When a family is having difficulty adjusting to a next phase in the family life cycle, or when a family crisis has disrupted the normal progression through the family life cycle, it would be appropriate to engage the family in the therapeutic endeavor.

The personal and/or family distortions become the thematic directional signs that point to the underlying family schema.

A major focus of family-centered therapy is on understanding and explicating the underlying rules, beliefs, and schema held by families and family members. The CT approach to family therapy, therefore, promotes self-disclosure of individual cognitions in order to increase mutual understanding through enhanced knowledge and an understanding of the thoughts, beliefs, and attitudes of the different family members. As early schema develop and are modified within the family group, cognitive therapy with families provides a context for observing these schema in operation, and for testing and modifying family member's distorted perceptions and cognitions.

Family schema are often difficult to alter because they are generally reinforced by the other family members. If, for example, a particular family schema is "Family secrets must not be shared with outsiders," the therapist can expect that any family member who speaks up will be censured, either overtly or covertly, by the other family members. McGoldrick and co-workers (1982) stress that families view the world through their own cultural filters so that the particular belief systems may be familial or more broadly cultural. Family systems theorists have described the phenomenon of the entire "system" working toward maintaining a balance. If an individual within a family system attempts to change that system or alter his or her strength of belief in the system, the system may be mobilized into action to close ranks against the "heretic" or to work toward keeping the individual within the system. This is a situation often seen in working with adolescents. Adolescents are most often referred by school, family, or court. As the adolescent begins to make changes toward a more functional style of behaving, which may involve an alteration in belief system, it is not unusual for the family to be unhappy or even disgruntled about the results of therapy, and threaten to or actually remove the child from therapy, claiming that the adolescent is now "worse." By "worse" these families often mean that the adolescent is at greater variance with the family schema. Although the adolescent's pre-therapy behavior was undesirable and destructive to both self and others, it appears that in developing a new belief system or modifying a belief system, the individual may run afoul of the family schema and be seen as destructive.

Examples of a family schema based on the culture in which the family is immersed might be basic rules regarding sexual behavior; reaction to other racial, ethnic, or religious groups; or particular religious beliefs. Related, and very much a part of the family or cultural belief system, are those belief systems that may be rooted in a religion's theology or its tradition. A family belief about heaven and hell may be part of the dogma of a religion; however, much of the "religious" response that individuals have is to the tradition of the religion that has been developed over a number of years within small cultural groups.

The beginning of the therapy is the establishment of a problem list. Each of the presenting problems is investigated with the family as a group to get an overview of the problem. Subsequent to that initial interview, each participating member is interviewed. There are often issues that will not come up within the family interview but that need to be stated and understood by the therapist. Further, certain issues that may affect the family difficulty are not appropriate for family discussion (e.g., sexual performance difficulties of mother or father). Although the therapist may learn of family secrets, the possible keeping of secrets is a worthwhile risk in exchange for the additional information and insight into the dynamic workings of the family. Once the problem list is developed, it can then be prioritized within a family session. Issues of greatest dysfunction or possible threats to health and well-being would be placed higher in the hierarchy.

A full developmental, family, social, occupational/educational, medical, and psychiatric history is taken for each family member.

The therapist is not limited to meeting with the family as a group. There are many different treatment configurations that can be used in working with the family. In working with a family, the therapist could meet with the mother alone, each of the children individually, the children together, or the entire family. The frequency of the meetings is also negotiable, based on family need.

Having established and agreed upon a problem list and focus, the individual sessions are then structured through agenda setting and homework. The therapist, working with the family, can set an agenda for each session.

TRAINING

It is noteworthy that the Medical School at the University of Pennsylvania, where Aaron T. Beck worked for 40 years, and where he developed cognitive therapy, has never offered an academic course in cognitive therapy. Similarly, the University of Pennsylvania graduate programs in social work, clinical psychology, and counseling psychology have never offered a course in cognitive therapy. The only graduate course in CT has been offered as part of the graduate program in the University's School of Nursing. The course is presently being taught as a series of one-day workshops covering basic theory, philosophy, and technique, which are followed by the clinical applications of CT with depression, suicide, anxiety, personality disorders, substance abuse, eating disorders, couples, families, children and adolescents, groups, and psychotic patients. The final workshop sessions involve in-class practice in using CT. The teaching format is didactic, observation via videotape, and role-play. This training format is an excellent beginning. It prepares the graduate psychiatric nurse.

Full training must involve ongoing case supervision on a one-to-one or small group basis. It is this supervised practice that allows for the applications of the workshop material to the real world.

SUMMARY

The points listed here have been adapted from several key assumptions pertaining to the applications of cognitive therapy in nursing practice (Bowler et al., 1993).

1. Psychiatric nursing is concerned with understanding psychopathological relationships between a patient's thoughts, feelings, and behavior, as well as what has happened in a person's life and environment.
2. The nurse works with the patient as part of a multidisciplinary team.
3. Patient problems are addressed in a collaborative and empirical manner.
4. The patient's thoughts and feelings represent responses to both internal and external stimuli. These cognitive, affective, and behavioral responses tend to occur in repetitive patterns that are schema driven, and shape what we see as the person's overt behavior.
5. The nurse's evaluation of the patient's mood and behavior, whether on the ward or in follow-up treatment, must include exploring, discussing, and recording the patient's thoughts, precepts, and attributions.
6. Helping the patient to concretize the cognitions relative to beliefs about self, world, and the future helps to organize the patient's thinking.
7. Cognitive therapy is an effective tool with a broad range of patient populations, contexts, and problems.
8. The focus in the therapy is on helping patients to understand the process of their thinking and the sequelae of that process rather than on identifying specific theoretically driven content.
9. Cognitive therapy can be used in many contexts including individual, group, and family therapy.
10. Psychiatric nurses must receive special training in order to use this therapy effectively.

REFERENCES

Adler A. *Understanding Human Nature*. New York: Fawcett; 1927.

Arieti S. Cognition in psychoanalysis. *J Am Acad Psychoanalysis*. 1980;8:3–23.

Bandura A. Model of causality in social learning theory. In: Mahoney M, Freeman A, (eds.) *Cognition and Psychotherapy*. New York: Plenum; 1985.

Bandura A. Self-efficacy: Towards a unifying theory of behavior change. *Psychol Rev.* 1977a;84:191–215.

Bandura A. *Social Learning Theory*. Englewood Cliffs, NJ: Prentice-Hall; 1977b.

Baucom DH, Epstein N. *Cognitive Behavioral Marital Therapy*. New York: Brunner/Mazel; 1988.

Beck AT. *Love Is Never Enough*. New York: HarperCollins; 1989.

Beck AT. *Cognitive Therapy and the Emotional Disorders*. New York: International Universities Press; 1976.

Beck AT. Cognitive therapy: Nature and relation to behavior therapy. *Behav Ther.* 1970;1:184–200.

Beck AT. *Depression: Causes and Treatment*. Philadelphia:University of Pennsylvania Press; 1967.

Beck AT. Thinking and depression: I. Idiosyncratic content and cognitive distortions. *Arch Gen Psychiatry*. 1963;9:324–333.

Beck AT. Epstein N, Brown G, Steer RA. An inventory for measuring clinical anxiety: Psychometric properties. *J Consult Clin Psychol*. In press.

Beck AT, Freeman A, et al. *Cognitive Therapy of Personality Disorders*. New York: Guilford Press; 1990.

Beck AT, Emery G, Greenberg RL. *Anxiety Disorders and Phobias: A Cognitive Perspective*. New York: Basic Books; 1985.

Beck AT, Epstein N, Harrison R. Cognitions, attitudes and personality dimensions in depression. *Br J Cognitive Psychother*. 1983;1:1–16.

Beck AT, Rush AJ, Shaw BF, Emery G. *Cognitive Therapy of Depression*. New York: Guilford Press; 1979.

Beck AT, Weissman S, Lester D, Trexler L. The measurement of pessimism: The hopelessness scale. *J Consult Clin Psychol*. 1979;42:861–865.

Beck AT, Ward CH, Mendelson M, et al. An inventory for measuring depression, *Arch Gen Psychiatry*. 1961;4:561–571.

Bowers W. Cognitive therapy with inpatients. In: Freeman A, Simon KM, Beutler L, Arkowitz H, eds. *Comprehensive Handbook of Cognitive Therapy*. New York: Plenum; 1989.

Bowlby J. The role of childhood experience in cognitive disturbance. In: Mahoney M, Freeman A, eds. *Cognition and Psychotherapy*. New York: Plenum; 1985.

Bowler KA, Moonis LJ, Thase ME. The role of the nurse in the cognitive milieu. In: Wright JH, Thase ME, Beck AT, Ludgate JW, eds. *Cognitive Therapy With Inpatients: Developing a Cognitive Milieu*. New York: Guilford Press; 1992.

Burns DD. *Feeling Good*. New York: Morrow; 1980.

Burns DD, Auerbach AH. Does homework compliance enhance recovery from depression? *Psychiatr Ann*. 1992;22:464–469.

Costello E, Borkovec TD. Generalized anxiety disorder. In: Freeman A, Dattilio FM, eds. *Comprehensive Casebook of Cognitive Therapy*. New York: Plenum; 1992.

Davis DD, Padesky C. Enhancing cognitive therapy with women. In: Freeman A, Simon, KM, Beutler L, Arkowitz H, eds. *Comprehensive Handbook of Cognitive Therapy*. New York: Plenum; 1990.

DiGiuseppe R. Cognitive therapy with children. In: Freeman A, Simon KM, Beutler L, Arkowitz H, eds. *Comprehensive Handbook of Cognitive Therapy*. New York: Plenum; 1989.

Eimer BN, Freeman A. The schizophrenic patient. In: Freeman A, Dattilio FM, eds. *Comprehensive Casebook of Cognitive Therapy*. New York: Plenum; 1992.

Ellis A. *The history of cognition in psychotherapy*. In: Freeman A, Simon KM, Beutler L, Arkowitz H, eds. *Comprehensive Handbook of Cognitive Therapy*. New York: Plenum; 1989.

Ellis A. Expanding the ABC's of RET. In: Mahoney M, Freeman A, eds. *Cognition and Psychotherapy*. New York: Plenum; 1985.

Ellis A. The basic clinical theory of rational-emotive therapy. In: Ellis A, Grieger R, eds. *Comprehensive Handbook of Rational-Emotive Therapy*. New York: Springer; 1977.

Ellis A. *Humanistic Psychotherapy: The Rational-Emotive Approach*. New York: Julian Press; 1973.

Ellis A. *Reason and Emotion in Psychotherapy*. New York: Lyle Stuart; 1962.

Epstein N, Baucom DH. Cognitive-behavioral marital therapy. In: Freeman A, Simon, KM, Beutler L, Arkowitz H, eds. *Comprehensive Handbook of Cognitive Therapy*. New York: Plenum; 1989.

Epstein N, Schlesinger SE, Dryden W. *Cognitive-Behavioral Therapy With Families*. New York: Brunner/Mazel; 1988.

Fairburn CG. Cognitive-behavioral treatment for bulimia. In: Garner DM, Garfinkel PE, eds. *Handbook of Psychotherapy for Anorexia Nervosa and Bulimia*. New York: Guilford Press; 1985.

Frankl V. Cognition and logotherapy. In: Mahoney M, Freeman A, eds. *Cognition and Psychotherapy*. New York: Plenum; 1985.

Freeman A. Understanding schema. In: Kuhlwein KT, Rosen H, eds. *The Practice of Cognitive Therapy*. San Francisco: Jossey-Bass; 1993.

Freeman A. Cognitive therapy of personality disorders. In: Perris C, Eienmann M, eds. *Cognitive Psychotherapy*. Umea, Sweden: Dopuu Press; 1988.

Freeman A. Understanding personal, cultural, and family schema in psychotherapy. In: Freeman A, Epstein N, Simon KM, eds. *Depression in the Family*. New York: Haworth Press; 1986.

Freeman A, DeWolfe R. *The 10 Dumbest Mistakes That Smart People Make*. New York: HarperCollins; 1992.

Freeman A, DeWolfe R. *Woulda, Coulda, Shoulda*. New York: HarperCollins; 1990.

Freeman A, Leaf R. Cognitive therapy of personality disorders. In: Freeman A, Simon KM, Beutler L, Arkowitz H, eds. *Comprehensive Handbook of Cognitive Therapy*. New York: Plenum; 1989.

Freeman A, Ludgate J. Cognitive therapy of anxiety. In: Keller PA, Heyman SR, eds. *Innovations in Clinical Practice*. Sarasota, FL: Professional Resource Exchange; 1988;7.

Freeman A, Reinecke M. *Cognitive Therapy of Suicidal Behavior*. New York: Springer; 1993.

Freeman A, Simon KM. Cognitive therapy of anxiety. In: Freeman A, Simon KM, Beutler L, Arkowitz H, eds. *Comprehensive Handbook of Cognitive Therapy*. New York: Plenum; 1989.

Freeman A, Simon KM, Pretzer J, Fleming B. *Clinical Applications of Cognitive Therapy*. New York: Plenum; 1990.

Freud S. Treatment by hypnosis. In: Freud S. *Collected Works*. London: Hogarth Press; 1892.

Gallagher-Thompson D, Thompson LW. The older adult. In: Freeman A, Dattilio FM, eds. *Comprehensive Casebook of Cognitive Therapy*. New York: Plenum; 1992.

Garner DM, Bemis KM. Cognitive therapy for anorexia nervosa. In: Garner DM, Garfinkel PE, eds. *Comprehensive Handbook for Psychotherapy for Anorexia Nervosa and Bulimia*. New York: Guilford Press; 1985.

Glantz MD. Cognitive therapy with the elderly. In: Freeman A, Simon KM, Beutler L, Arkowitz H, eds. *Comprehensive Handbook of Cognitive Therapy*. New York: Plenum; 1989.

Horney K. *The Neurotic Personality*. New York: Norton; 1936.

Jakubowski P, Lange AJ. *The Assertive Option*. Champaign, IL: Research Press; 1978.

Kendall PC, ed. *Child and Adolescent Therapy*. New York: Guilford Press; 1991.

Kuhlwein KT. Working with gay men. In: Freeman A, Dattilio FM, eds. *Comprehensive Casebook of Cognitive Therapy*. New York: Plenum; 1992.

Layden MA, Newman C, Freeman A, Byers S. *Cognitive Therapy of the Borderline Patient*. Boston: Allyn & Bacon; 1993.

Lazarus AA. *The Practice of Multimodal Therapy*. New York: McGraw-Hill; 1981.

Lazarus AA, *Multimodal Behavior Therapy*. New York: Springer; 1976.

McCarthy B. A cognitive-behavioral approach to sex therapy. In: Freeman A, Simon KM, Beutler L, Arkowitz H, eds. *Comprehensive Handbook of Cognitive Therapy*. New York: Plenum; 1989.

McGoldrick M, Pearce JK, Giordano J, eds. *Ethnicity and Family Therapy*. New York: Guilford Press; 1982.

Meichenbaum D. *Cognitive-Behavior Modification*. New York: Plenum; 1977.

Perris C, Nordstrom G, Troeng L. Schizophrenic disorders. In: Freeman A, Dattilio FM, eds. *Comprehensive Casebook of Cognitive Therapy*, New York: Plenum; 1992.

Rosen H. Piagetian theory and cognitive therapy. In: Freeman A, Simon KM, Beutler L, Arkowitz H, eds. *Comprehensive Handbook of Cognitive Therapy*. New York: Plenum; 1989.

Rosen H. *Piagetian concepts of Clinical Relevance*. New York: Columbia University Press; 1985.

Sullivan HS. *The Interpersonal Theory of Psychiatry*. New York: Norton; 1953.

Wolfe JL. Working with gay women. In: Freeman A, Dattilio FM, eds. *Comprehensive Casebook of Cognitive Therapy*. New York: Plenum; 1992.

Wright J, Beck AT, Thase M, eds. *Cognitive Therapy With Inpatients: Establishing the Cognitive Milieu*. New York: Guilford Press; 1993.

CHAPTER 16

PSYCHIATRIC CONSULTATION-LIAISON NURSING

Lenore H. Kurlowicz

*P*sychiatric consul-
tation-liaison
nursing has evolved
in response to an in-
creased awareness and
recognition of the im-
portance of psycho-
physiological inter-
relationships and their
impact on physical ill-
ness and recovery.

Chapter Overview

- Psychiatric Consultation-Liaison Nursing Practice
    Consultation
    Liaison
    Additional PCLN Roles
- Preparation for Practice
    Situational Needs
- Historical Perspective
- Organizational Placement and Models of PCLN Practice
- Types of Consultation
    Client Centered
    Consultee Centered
    Program Centered
    Consultee-centered Administrative
    Diagnosis of the Total Consultation: A Holistic
        Theoretical Model
- Four Phases of Consultation
- PCLN Consultative Dilemmas
- PCLN Evaluation and Research
    Future Research Needs
- Trends and Future Issues
- Summary
- References
- Appendix

► INTRODUCTION

Psychiatric Consultation-Liaison Nursing (PCLN) is a subspecialty of advanced nursing practice within the specialty of psychiatric nursing. The scope of PCLN practice is multifaceted and includes direct and indirect practice roles ranging from primary prevention through intervention and rehabilitation (American Nurses Association, 1990). The focus of PCLN practice is on the emotional, behavioral, cognitive, developmental, and spiritual responses of clients and families who enter the health care system with actual or potential physical dysfunction. This specialty area of advanced psychiatric nursing practice is based on the synthesis and application of theoretical models in nursing, psychiatry, psychology, and sociology and includes systems theory, stress theory, crisis intervention, change theory, adult learning theory, as well as principles of the consultation process. PCLNs are knowledgeable in the interaction of biological, psychological, and sociocultural factors in health and illness and the range of normal to pathological psychological responses to physical conditions (Lewis and Levy, 1982).

PCLN practice is distinctive in its emphasis on three interlocking characteristics:

- Consideration of the interaction between physical, psychological, spiritual, developmental, and sociocultural phenomena and their behavioral manifestations in the specific environmental context.
- Promotion of health and prevention of dysfunction.
- The interaction of clients and families, caregivers, and health care delivery systems.

The PCLN is also involved in the care of individuals who present with physical symptoms or dysfunctions in the absence of organic pathology for which a psychodynamic formulation is critical in understanding these processes (ANA, 1990). In general, the goals of PCLN practice are to facilitate the integration and application of mental health concepts into clinical nursing practice, to enhance psychiatric nursing intervention, to promote quality nursing practice and professional self-esteem within nursing, and to encourage tolerance among the members of the health care team of those situations in which effective intervention or resolution is not immediately attainable (Lewis and Levy, 1982).

PSYCHIATRIC CONSULTATION-LIAISON NURSING PRACTICE

PCLN practice includes both consultation and liaison activities (ANA, 1990). The goals of consultation and liaison activities are complementary and interdependent and become inseparable areas of clinical practice. The PCLN uses both processes in conjunction with specific theoretical knowledge, clinical expertise, and an ability to synthesize and integrate information to influence health care delivery systems.

CONSULTATION

Consultation is an interactive process between a consultant, who has expertise in a specific area(s), and a consultee, who is seeking help or advice, usually about a patient-related problem, which the consultee has identified as within the realm of expertise of the consultant (Caplan, 1970). Mental health consultation implies a process of interaction between two professionals about a specific patient or organizational problem (Caplan, 1970). The mental health consultant is a professional "problem-solver" requested by or "invited in" by a colleague or organization to assist persons, groups, or systems to resolve mental health issues. The mental health consultant functions in an objective and independent manner. The consultees are usually individuals or groups who influence or participate in health care delivery (nurses, physicians, administrators). Although remaining available to other members of the health care team and working within a collaborative model, PCLNs provide consultation primarily to nursing staff and are specifically concerned with psychological issues that relate to nursing care and nursing management. Within the consultation process, the PCLN provides psychiatric nursing consultation relevant to a particular piece of the client's or family's life presented to them. Most often, clinical expertise is provided by the PCLN regarding the delivery of psychological care in response to a request from a health care provider. Consultation is a supportive, interpersonal process in which the consultant collaborates with the consultee who has requested assistance with problem solving. Furthermore, the nature of the consultant-consultee relationship is usually collaborative rather than hierarchical, and the consultant typically has no direct authority or evaluative responsibilities over the consultee. Intervention is left in the domain of the consultee, and thus allows freedom for the PCLN to work with individuals at any level (Caplan, 1970). The consultant's authority is based on "expert knowledge" where the consultee perceives that the consultant has expertise that is useful (Smith, 1987). The PCLN, in general, has "informal" authority that is based on the qualities of the PCLN. The primary responsibility remains within the jurisdiction of the consultee, who may accept or reject the offerings of the

PCLN. The consultation process is not psychotherapy but it can be therapeutic. It frequently yields positive benefits for the individuals, groups, or organizations that have requested the service, and it results in an overall sense of accomplishment and self-worth for those involved (Caplan, 1970).

LIAISON

Liaison describes the linkage of the knowledge base of psychiatric nursing and the care of patients with actual or potential physical dysfunction in a variety of health care settings (ANA, 1990). It is also a process that facilitates the relationship that exists among the patient, the adjustment to the illness, the consultee(s), and the hospital, ward, or unit milieu (Lewis and Levy, 1982; Robinson, 1987). Within the liaison process, there is a linkage of health care professionals to facilitate communication between clients, families, and specific health care professionals. The liaison process usually occurs in conjunction with each individual consultation. Furthermore, additional liaison activities include unit-based nursing education programs, patient education programs, participation in discharge planning, nursing care planning (or health care team rounds), patient care conferences, and facilitation of patient, family, or staff nurse support groups (Krupnick, 1995).

ADDITIONAL PCLN ROLES

PCLNs frequently have additional roles in a health care organization. They include, but are not limited to psychotherapist, educator, support group facilitator, clinical supervisor, participant in policy development and program planning, consultant to administrative systems and other groups, and researcher (ANA, 1990). Referrals for PCLN services are generated by networks of professionals who recognize their availability and value. When a liaison nurse is established in a health care agency, much of the initial work consists of developing a referral network by educating staff members about the liaison service and its potential value to themselves and their patients. As a network develops, referrals will originate from various health care providers. For example, a staff nurse may request PCLN services to assist with the nursing plan of care for a depressed, psychologically regressed patient. A physician may request PCLN consultation for assistance with treatment interference issues in an older acutely confused, delirious surgical patient. A physical therapist may request assistance from the PCLN for a patient with angry and hostile interactions affecting their ability to maintain an exercise program. A nurse manager may request PCLN assistance regarding a unit-based nursing care approach for nursing home residents with verbally disruptive behaviors. Depending on the setting, the PCLN report will be included in the nurses' notes, integrated progress notes, or a separate consultant's report. Initiation of a referral to a PCLN is often made independently by the consultee and, for nurses, without a physician's order. In some settings, the request must be made in writing.

PREPARATION FOR PRACTICE

The PCLN is an advanced practice nurse who has attained at least a master's degree in psychiatric nursing and has successfully completed a supervised graduate level clinical program (ANA, 1990; Robinette, 1996). The PCLN's education includes classroom and supervised clinical experiences in individual, group, and family therapy, models that are all used in practice. Most graduate programs also include courses in organizational theory in which the principles of power and influence and planned change are emphasized. Generally, prior combined clinical experience in both and psychiatric and medical-surgical nursing is recommended and can help to demystify the role, to assist in its development within the general hospital, and to provide those in the role with an increased sense of professional gratification (Lewis and Levy, 1982). Administrative experience as a head nurse or nurse manager can also enhance the PCLN's knowledge of the consultee

and the health care organizations. Because a hospital is an incredibly complex organization, a successful PCLN needs a solid theoretic and experiential base, along with competence, confidence, and concern (Lewis and Levy, 1982).

Although ANA certification in the subspecialty of PCLN practice does not currently exist, certification as a clinical nurse specialist in psychiatric nursing is recommended (ANA, 1990). PCLNs may also choose a subspecialty such as oncology or critical care nursing for which they may have additional certification (Moschler and Fincannon, 1992; Robinette, 1996).

PCLNs possess leadership ability and generally function independently in a staff rather than a line position. They have skill at enabling others to learn and carry out specific tasks and possess patience and high-level interpersonal skills. Ideally, they possess expert and referent power evolving from expertise and pleasant personality characteristics (Smith, 1987). Moreover, the personal and professional attributes that are necessary for successful PCLN practice include accessibility, flexibility, objectivity, creativity, resilience, and behavior reflective of a personal and professional maturity (Lewis and Levy, 1982). Central characteristics helpful in the PCLN role are acceptance of ambiguous situations, tolerance of personal rejections, and the capacity and willingness to tolerate consistently stressful and often unpredictable, "difficult" situations with clients, families, and health care providers (Krupnick, 1995).

SITUATIONAL NEEDS

Because the PCLN responds to the immediate issue or problem as it is presented by the consultee, the PCLN does enter the process with predetermined information and must be able to respond with information as it is uniquely relevant to the needs manifested by the consultee and the goals of the consultation. The content and processes of PCLN work vary in response to each request and situation. In this manner, the PCLN role is different from other advanced practice roles in the organization such as staff development nurses or nurse educators, whose relationships with staff are more hierarchical, like teacher and student where predetermined content is brought to the situation. PCLNs must be able to practice in an independent, autonomous manner while making linkages and coalitions with other professionals and systems. The ability to manage their own emotional wellness and professional collaborative relationships is essential in a role in which isolation often accompanies autonomous, albeit stressful and sensitive, practice situations with a high potential for compassion fatigue (Frigley, 1995; Krupnick, 1995). Many PCLNs obtain clinical supervision, often on a fee-for-service basis, on an ongoing or periodic basis from more experienced PCLNs or other advanced practice psychiatric nurses (Platt-Koch, 1986). Peer networking is also available through the International Society of Psychiatric Consultation-Liaison Nurses (ISPCLN).[1]

HISTORICAL PERSPECTIVE

Psychiatric consultation-liaison nursing has its origins in both nursing and psychiatry. Physicians were the first to practice consultation-liaison psychiatry, providing psychiatric consultation to clients in the general hospital, based on the concepts of psychophysiologic medicine and preventive psychiatry. Liaison psychiatry originated in the 1950s. Paralleling this trend, psychiatric nurses began to act as consultants to their colleagues in medical and surgical settings. At first, liaison nurses remained based on their psychiatric units, providing indirect assistance when it was requested. Later, they began to work directly with clients and their families. Johnson (1963) at Duke University Medical Center was the first to describe psychiatric nursing consultation to nurses in the general hospital. Psychiatric nursing consultation was carried out within a

hospital-wide nurse-to-nurse consultation program that attempted to maximize the use of available nursing resources. The psychiatric nurses who participated assisted medical-surgical nurses in problem solving and comprehending the emotional impact of illness, suffering, and recovery on the client (Johnson, 1963). The need for a theoretical and clinical framework to guide their practice gradually became evident throughout the early experiences of psychiatric nurses attempting to provide consultation without formal education. Subsequently, graduate schools began to respond by offering specialized programs geared to liaison nursing. The University of Maryland in 1972 and Yale University in 1979 were the first two graduate programs to provide a specialized program in liaison nursing. Since then, PCLN education has been integrated into graduate psychiatric nursing curriculums throughout the country, and many provide clinical experiences in a general hospital setting. With the formation of the ISPCLN in 1994, a graduate core curriculum is now being developed by the organization that will propose a core liaison curriculum that will adequately prepare advanced practice nursing students to meet the complex, multidimensional needs of medically ill patients and families as well as changing health care organizations.

The first national meeting of PCLNs was held in 1986. Since that time, annual PCLN conferences have expanded to include PCLNs from other countries. As stated previously, the ISPCLN was formally established in 1994 and continues to support membership for nurses internationally who are practicing or interested in psychiatric consultation-liaison nursing.

ORGANIZATIONAL PLACEMENT AND MODELS OF PCLN PRACTICE

The practice arenas for PCLNs continue to expand and the role has evolved from being primarily acute care or general hospital based to practice

---

[1] 437 Twin Bay Drive, Pensacola, FL 32534-1350; telephone 904-474-4147.

in a variety of settings such as home care, rehabilitation settings, and managed care organizations (Hellwig, 1993; Millar, 1993). Furthermore,
throughout the past 5 years, the visibility of
PCLNs in long-term care, nursing homes in particular, has increased considerably (Santmyer and
Roca, 1991). Traditional organizational placement for the PCLN has been either in the department of nursing, usually psychiatric nursing, or
within the department of psychiatry. Within nursing, however, PCLNs may be positioned in such
departments as medical or surgical nursing, or
in departments of nursing education. Historically, it has been proposed that successful clinical relationships and alliances are best facilitated when the PCLN is in a nonhierarchical
position within the organization with no direct
evaluation responsibilities for staff performance.
As a great deal of the actual work is based on
the liaison nurse's ability to establish consultative alliances, these responsibilities would prove
counterproductive to clinical practice (Lewis
and Levy, 1982).

In many instances, psychiatrists and PCLNs
have worked together on liaison teams, either informally or formally, to broaden the focus of each
discipline in addressing the needs of patients and
staff in the various settings, and in some settings,
as a financial necessity (Krupnick, 1995). The
"shared domain" of the PCLN and the liaison
psychiatrist lies in the assessment and treatment
of patients and their families. In general, PCLNs
recommend to a consultee a referral to a psychiatrist for patients who are suicidal or homicidal,
those who require or who may benefit from psychotropic medication, and those who require
complex differential diagnosis (Platt-Koch et al.,
1990). Conversely, psychiatrists often refer to the
PCLN patients whom they believe would relate
better to a nurse than a psychiatrist, family members who require support or follow-up, nursing
staff who need assistance with countertransference feelings stimulated by certain patients, or patients for whom there are issues particular to the
staff nurse role, which the psychiatrist may feel
unable to adequately address.

Lewis and Levy (1982) have described three
variations on psychiatric liaison teams. In the first,
the entire, usually multidisciplinary, team operates
out of the department of psychiatry and is usually
headed by a psychiatrist. In this model, the PCLN
is administratively as well as clinically responsible to the psychiatrist and has no formal tie to the
department of nursing. The second model is one in
which a medical liaison psychiatric service is
based in the department of psychiatry while a parallel service is based in the department of nursing.
In this model, each discipline reports to its professional department, and there are no formal ties between the two services. Ideally, in this system,
there is good communication between the two services, with many cross-referrals as one service
recognizes the need for input from the other. Table
16–1 displays one example of a preliminary PCLN
classification system or descriptor of PCLN services (complexity/intensity plus time) that depicts
the potential areas of crossover and cross-referral
by PCLNs to liaison psychiatry. This classification was inductively created by a content analysis
of a PCLN's consultations over a 10-year period
(Kurlowicz, 1996). As depicted, the PCLN may
maintain an independent clinical practice in many
situations; and, at certain levels, PCLNs and liaison psychiatrists would collaborate regarding the
psychosocial needs of the patient and health care
provider's management of the problem.

A third model is one in which the departments of psychiatry and nursing each hire their
own psychiatric personnel for liaison work, but
the psychiatrist and liaison nurse collaborate in
providing a psychiatric consultation-liaison service. In this model, each discipline is administratively accountable to its own professional department, but there is an officially sanctioned
combined liaison service. They both may respond to requests for formal psychiatric consultations, but an attempt is made to divide clinical
responsibilities according to their particular area
of expertise. This model differs from the first primarily in that the relationship is collaborative
and neither one is administratively accountable
to the other. It differs from the second in that

TABLE 16–1. DIRECT PCLN LEVELS OF CARE

Level I	—	Least complex Example: reaction to diagnosis, prognosis; concerns/questions about coping; patient and/or family assessment Initial assessment: 30 minutes to 1 hour F/U: 0–1
Level II	—	Least complex but more complicating factors Example: adjustment reaction (to sudden/traumatic loss; crisis of diagnosis or complicated medical course requiring further testing, hospitalization) with beginning treatment interference issues (anorexia, impaired health care interactions); patient and/or family assessment Initial assessment: 1 hour F/U: 1–2
Level III	—	Mild complexity Example: adjustment disorder (to illness/loss) with recent psychiatric history, treatment including dementia; identified treatment interference; patient or family Initial assessment: 1 hour + possible psychiatric evaluation F/U: 1–3
Level IV	—	Very complex; moderate to high index of medical/psychiatric interplay but factors more readily identifiable Example: alcohol, drug withdrawal, metabolic disturbance with associated behavioral disturbance interfering with Rx; moderate to severe depression/anxiety; potential for suicide; possible factitious disorder Initial assessment: 30 minutes to 1 hour + psychiatry evaluation F/U: 1–2
Level V	—	Most complex; severe medical/psychiatric interplay requiring additional medical/psychiatric evaluation Example: brain tumor/injury with severe emotional/behavioral disturbance and threat to self or others (aggression interfering with Rx); severe, unresolving acute mental status change (hallucinations, catatonia); severe depression with active SI/HI Initial assessment: 30 minutes to 1 hour + psychiatry evaluation F/U: 1–4

there is more visible interrelationship and working together.

Much overlapping of roles as well as role confusion occurs in the field of psychiatry because all the disciplines share a related body of theoretical knowledge. Although there is differentiation among disciplines in terms of medical and clinical training and the depth of knowledge acquired, it is the educational process unique to each discipline and the primary focus of professional attention that distinguishes the clinical focus of one discipline from the other (Robinson, 1987). Successful teams, regardless of the model, can occur if there is administrative support for a practice that involves a physician and nurse functioning in a collaborative rather than a supervisor–subordinate relationship, with each team member understanding and respecting the needs of the other, and neither discipline feeling that it is subservient to the other. As each team works to identify its particular contribution to the team, anxiety or conflict may develop with regard to the other members' contributions and can lead to issues of territoriality and sharing of responsibility.

TYPES OF CONSULTATION

Caplan (1970) defined four types of mental health consultation: client centered, consultee centered, program centered administrative, and consultee centered administrative. Although

Caplan described the four categories for use in community mental health settings, they can be applied readily to the hospital consultation process as well as consultation in other practice settings for the PCLN. Which type of consultation is to be provided by the PCLN remains flexible and a firm commitment to one type of consultation rarely occurs. Most often in clinical situations, client-centered and consultee-centered consultations are employed by the PCLN. Examples of the combined use of the various types of consultation in clinical practice were described by Grant (1988) and Kurlowicz (1991) in their analyses of PCLN consultation activities with nurses of hospitalized AIDS patients. The ultimate goals of all consultations are the welfare of the patient and the continued growth of the consultee's supportive skills.

CLIENT-CENTERED

Client-centered consultation, the most common type of PCLN consultation, focuses on helping the consultee find the most effective management approach for a particular patient problem. The primary goal of client-centered or "direct" consultation is on how the patient can be helped. A secondary goal is improving the consultee's knowledge and skills to enhance their handling of similar problems in the future. An example of this type of consultation is the surgical staff nurse who requests PCLN consultation for a patient who she suspects is psychotic. The PCLN interviews the patient, validates the nurse's perception that the patient is indeed hallucinating and delusional, and identifies the need for an evaluation by the liaison psychiatrist for further diagnostic and medication evaluation. The PCLN then assists the staff nurse in planning a formal treatment plan for the patient that includes specific nursing interventions regarding maintenance of patient safety and therapeutic nursing communication strategies. Robinette's (1996) description of PCLN consultation with emergency department and oncology nusing staff are additional examples of client-centered PCLN consultation.

CONSULTEE-CENTERED

Another common type of consultation employed by PCLNs is consultee-centered consultation. The PCLN's main attention in this type is focused on trying to understand the nature of the consultee's difficulties with a patient and helping the consultee remedy the shortcomings. The nature of the consultee's problem is central to this type of consultation. An example of this type of consultation is the medical staff nurse who requests to meet with the PCLN upon the suggestion of her nurse manager because of difficulty maintaining professional objectivity and a professional demeanor with a patient with a substance abuse problem. In this "indirect" consultation, the PCLN helps the nurse recognize this problem and its effects on her health care interactions with the patient, explores possible origins of the problem, and facilitates the formation of a more effective plan of care. The client or patient is generally not interviewed in consultee-centered consultation.

PROGRAM-CENTERED

In program-centered administrative consultation, the focus of the consultation is on the development of a new program or the improvement of an existing one. The goal of this type of consultation is to prescribe an effective course of action in program planning. One example is a PCLN who is consulted by a newly formed pre-heart transplant team to assist with the development a psychosocial support program for patients and their significant others who are awaiting heart transplantation. In this consultation type, the PCLN meets with the team to further discuss their requests and identified needs, analyzes any existing data describing specific psychosocial issues with this specific population, and selectively meets with members of the nursing and medical staff, as well as patients and family members. The PCLN then provides recommendations for a multilevel program that would enhance the mental health care of these patients during the pre-heart transplant waiting period, including a patient support group. Additional examples of program-centered administrative consultation by PCLNs in the general hospital setting described in the literature are Baldwin's (1978) work in a critical care unit, Minarik's (1984) consultation for families in acute care, and Davidson and Noyes' (1973) consultation to a burn service.

CONSULTEE-CENTERED ADMINISTRATIVE

Lastly, PCLNs can engage in consultee-centered administrative consultation. The focus of this type of consultation is on an organizational or administrative problem and is generally requested by administrative or managerial personnel. The goal of the consultation is the elucidation and resolution of consultee's difficulties or shortcomings that interfere with the tasks of program development and organization and to help the consultees accomplish the mission of the organization. An example of this type of consultation is an assistant director of nursing who requests PCLN consultation to facilitate the communication patterns of his nurse manager group who are not functioning optimally within the specific nursing department, and thus not accomplishing specific administrative objectives. Through a series of meetings with the nurse manager group that includes education and exercises to enhance communication competencies, the PCLN improves the group's communication skills, enhances their cohesiveness and subsequent functioning as a group, and ultimately facilitates their accomplishment of departmental and organizational objectives.

DIAGNOSIS OF THE TOTAL CONSULTATION: A HOLISTIC THEORETICAL MODEL

An additional framework for operationalizing the PCLN consultation process has been proposed and described by Lewis and Levy (1982). Within this process, PCLNs consider the identified patient, nurse, milieu, and all other aspects of the consultation. Lewis and Levy have termed this process "diagnosis of the total consultation." Within this holistic theoretical model, a series of identifiable steps are systematically performed in the consultation process by the PCLN and the assessment of the patient becomes only one, albeit an important, aspect of the evaluation. Johnson (1963), in writing about psychiatric nursing consultation in the general hospital, emphasized that the request for the consultation was related to more than just the degree of the patient's disturbance. Since that time, reports have also described that consultations can be requested for many, often not clearly explicated, reasons beyond a patient problem (Kucharski and Groves, 1977; Strain and Grossman, 1975). The PCLN is often consulted when the problem is unclear and much skill is required to recognize this phenomenon. Through the use of a holistic model, the meaning of the "total" consultation can be explicated and effective intervention determined.

The specific parameters of diagnosing the total consultation are the specific consultation request, the consultee, the physician or health care team, the unit environment, the family system, the medical illness, and evaluation of the patient's chart. These parameters aid in identifying and understanding overt and covert consultation questions, defining the scope of the problem, clarifying expectations, determining the need for direct and indirect services, and planning nursing interventions. Interventions and recommendations are based on the total consultation and should be practical suggestions. Interventions should begin simply and progress as needed. Many times the involvement of the PCLN aids in clarifying the problem, and subsequently all parties are able to interact more productively. Interventions should not be static and should be evaluated and changed when needed.

FOUR PHASES OF CONSULTATION

The consultation process is time limited and in general involves four phases: entry (beginning with the consultation request), diagnosis, response or intervention, and closure and evaluation. A collaborative process is maintained throughout the various phases. The goals of the consultation are to enhance the consultee's skill in managing a work-related problem and to facilitate the consultee's ability to master similar problems in the future (Caplan, 1970).

PCLN CONSULTATIVE DILEMMAS

Certain stresses are inherent in the nature of consultation for the PCLN. Furthermore, many of these stresses cannot be removed without destroying the consultant–consultee relationship. The existence of the various stresses amidst a delicately balanced and intricate system of human relationships can contribute to uncertainty, suspiciousness, resentment, frustration, and conflict and create interpersonal barriers to effective PCLN practice. Awareness of these stresses and their implications, for the neophyte PCLN in particular, can reduce the ill effects of these difficulties. Specific consultative dilemmas include the authority factor (expert versus position), intrusion of an outsider, threat of an expert, resistance to change, dependency, compulsive (quick action) solutions, client insecurity, lack of consultant objectivity, conflict in roles, unclear consultee motivation, and interference with disengagement from the consultation (Beckhard, 1982).

PCLN EVALUATION AND RESEARCH

Evaluation of PCLN activities is important, though often difficult. Factors that contribute to evaluation difficulties include the multifaceted nature of the role (direct care, indirect care, education, administrative support), the lack of agreement on specific evaluation or performance criteria, and overlap of activities with other psychosocial services. Similar to other advanced practice roles, the PCLN frequently shifts emphasis among the various role components in order to meet the changing needs of patients, providers, and health care institutions (Gurka, 1991). Caplan (1970) recommended that evaluation of professional mental health consultation be focused on three major areas: changes in the mental health condition of the client; changes in consultee performance, perceptions, and/or attitudes; and consultee satisfaction.

The greatest difficulty is that the effects of PCLN activities may be indirect and not readily visible. PCLNs may influence or contribute to patient or provider outcomes through consultation, education, or direct service, but may not be credited with achieving the positive outcome. Bloch (1975) reported that evaluation must encompass a delineation of specific processes to which an outcome can be attributed and that only an evaluation that encompasses both process and outcome has the potential for great impact on the quality of care. PCLNs should continue to explicate their unique activities within their clinical practice while attempting to link PCLN-specific activities with patient, provider, and institutional or system-related outcomes. In addition, PCLNs must continue to examine which outcomes are most sensitive to PCLN activities (Brooten and Naylor, 1995). The timing, length, and intensity of services provided by PCLNs to different patient groups is also warranted (Naylor and Brooten, 1993). The current availability of intervention classification systems for advanced practice nurses can facilitate the explication of PCLN process activities.

Similar to other advanced practice psychiatric nursing roles, PCLNs contribute to nursing and the psychiatric field through innovations in theory and practice and utilization of and participation in research, and communication about these contributions (ANA, 1990). PCLNs participate in research in a variety of ways. PCLNs apply and incorporate available and relevant research to practice, conduct research as appropriate, promote "research consumership" in the specific health care institution, and collaborate with colleagues in research activities (LoBiondo-

Wood and Haber, 1986). Affiliations with university schools of nursing provide the opportunity for many PCLNs to collaboration with doctorally prepared nurse researchers on specific research projects (Krupnick, 1995). PCLNs with a doctoral preparation can also foster a spirit of inquiry, critical thinking, and research, as well as provide research mentorship for PCLN colleagues in the practice setting. PCLNs also use research utilization models to integrate research into their practice. For example, a research utilization project by Kane and Kurlowicz (1994) employed the Iowa Model of Research in Practice (Titler et al., 1994) to guide the development of a research-based standard of practice protocol for nursing management of postoperative delirium.

PCLN and PCLN-related research occurs at many levels of inquiry. At the most basic level, PCLNs who maintain accurate daily records, descriptions, and statistics of clinical consultations and liaison activities build a database upon which to generate clinical investigation and validation of clinical practice (Krupnick, 1995; Wu et al., 1994). An example of published research by PCLNs at this level of inquiry includes a report by Davis and Nelson (1980) that described referral patterns and reasons for PCLN consultation. PCLNs must continue to develop databases and infrastructures that will describe and quantify their multifaceted activities and, in particular, the linkage of various PCLN activities with patient, provider, and institutional outcomes (Robinette, 1996). Descriptive reports of PCLN processes and activities will continue to be important to examine how health care delivery trends, such as shortened hospital stays, and system reorganization and redesign operations, have influenced PCLN practice. In several reports, PCLNs have also described the specific activities or processes implemented during their consultations. Hart's (1990) description of PCLN activities on a hospital ethics committee, Kurlowicz's (1991) retrospective analysis of PCLN interventions with nurses of hospitalized AIDS patients, and Santmyer and Roca's (1991) analysis of PCLN consultation activities with nursing home residents and staff are a few examples.

PCLNs have also examined and described outcomes associated with various aspects of their practice. Important PCLN research at this level of inquiry includes a report on the effects of PCLN interventions on the care of patients with sitters (Talley et al., 1990), consultee satisfaction with PCLN services (Newton and Wilson, 1990), the impact of a PCLN-facilitated staff support group on the work environment of a specialty unit (Tommasini, 1992), and a study of nursing care hours of clients receiving varying amounts and types of psychiatric consultation-liaison services (Mallory et al., 1993).

FUTURE RESEARCH NEEDS

Future PCLN research will require a focus on outcomes analysis in three major domains: (1) patient related, such as a decrease in psychological symptom distress, a decrease in treatment interference, and maintenance of patient safety, (2) provider related, such as consultee satisfaction, learning, and/or improved health care interactions; and (3) institutional or system related, such as decreased length of stay, prevention of medical complications associated with psychiatric comorbidity, a decline in number of re-admissions, or an increase in referrals to other hospital support services such as psychiatry, pastoral care, or psychiatric nursing home care services. Donabedian's (1966) framework has been proposed as a model that can be used to guide evaluation research for advance practice nurses and may be applicable to PCLNs (Gurka, 1991). Within this model, key aspects of PCLN structure, process activities, and outcomes would be evaluated that together that may ultimately affect the quality of care for various patient populations, their providers, and the health care institution (Donabedian, 1966). Appendix 16–1 contains an example of one PCLN's quality improvement and evaluation initiatives guided by Donabedian's (1966) framework that encompass the structure, process, and outcome components suggested for PCLN practice evaluation. For PCLNs, outcomes research should not be an end in itself.

TRENDS AND FUTURE ISSUES

PCLN practice continues to evolve and be influenced by changes within the profession of nursing. Furthermore, changes in psychiatry and reforms in the delivery of health care, such as costs of service delivery and an emphasis on quality of care issues, will significantly influence PCLN practice (Krupnick, 1995). The "downsizing" of acute care hospitals will further necessitate a strong emphasis on PCLN practice evaluation, in particular the impact of specific PCLN activities on various multilevel outcomes within the organization. A greater emphasis on objective, data-based information regarding PCLN practice that includes the routine use of standardized measurements of various psychological states and other quality of care outcomes will be needed to further explicate the practice. Peer review models will become especially important to ensure quality PCLN practice (Titlebaum et al., 1992). As today's health care environments explore creative ways to increase and develop new sources of revenue, all positions will be scrutinized for their value to the institution. The ability to generate revenue, therefore, will be an important issue for PCLNs. Platt-Koch and associates (1990) stated that "Bringing in the dollars is an important and obvious way for PCLNs to improve their chance of survival in today's health care institutions" (p. 208).

Furthermore, PCLNs will need to continue to make themselves visible, accessible, and marketable in a variety of health care delivery systems such as community-based settings and long-term care. PCLNs must also publicize and document their contributions to as well as their demonstrated effects on patient outcomes and cost of care to further legitimize the role. Krupnick (1995) proposed specific elements that will be integral to the future viability of the PCLN role. They include ongoing PCLN outcome research, marketing of PCLN services in both traditional and nontraditional health care settings, ongoing education of nurse colleagues,

nurse administrators in particular, as well as consumers and lawmakers regarding the PCLN role and potential contributions to the current health care environment, and continued political activity for the expansion of prescriptive authority.

SUMMARY

Psychiatric consultation-liaison nursing has emerged as an advanced practice subspecialty within psychiatric nursing. This subspecialty has evolved in response to an increased awareness and recognition of the importance of psychophysiological interrelationships and their impact on physical illness and recovery (Krupnick, 1995). Psychiatric consultation is defined as the provision of clinical expertise regarding the provision of psychological care in response to a specific request from health care providers (Lewis and Levy, 1982). The liaison process is the linkage of health care professionals to facilitate communication, collaboration, and building of partnerships between clients and health care providers (Robinson, 1987).

PCLN practice has expanded from the traditional indirect model of assisting with psychological interventions to direct care and organizational consultations. Furthermore, PCLN practice has also expanded beyond the general hospital setting to more diverse health care settings including home care and long-term care. PCLNs must continue to evaluate the structure, process, and outcomes of their practice as well as educate colleagues and consumers about their unique contributions and expertise.

REFERENCES

American Nurses' Association. *Standards of Practice: Psychiatric Consultation-Liaison Nursing*. Washington, DC: ANA; 1990.

Baldwin CA. Mental health consultation in the intensive care unit: Toward a greater balance and precision of attribution. *J Psychosoc Nurs Ment Health Serv*. 1978;161:17–21.

Beckhard R. *The Leader Looks at the Consultative Process*. Washington: Leadership Resources; 1982.

Bloch D. Evaluation of nursing care in terms of process and outcome: Issues in research and quality assurance. *Nurs Res*. 1975;24:256–263.

Brooten D, Naylor MD. Nurses' effects on changing patient outcomes. *IMAGE J Nurs Sch*. 1995;27: 95–99.

Caplan G. *The Theory and Practice of Mental Health Consultation*. New York: Basic Books; 1970.

Davidson S, Noyes R. Psychiatric nursing consultation on a burn unit. *Am J Nurs*. 1973;73:1715–1718.

Davis DS, Nelson JK. Referrals to psychiatric liaison nurses: Changes in characteristics over a limited time period. *Gen Hosp Psychiatry*. 1980;2:41–45.

Donabedian A. Evaluating the quality of medical care. *Milbank Memorial Fund Q*. 1966;44:166–196.

Frigley R. *Compassion Fatigue: Coping With Secondary Traumatic Stress Disorder in Those Who Treat the Traumatized*. New York: Brunner/Mazel; 1995.

Grant SM. The hospitalized AIDS patient and the psychiatric liaison nurse. *Arch Psychiatr Nurs*. 1988;5: 370–377.

Gurka AM. Process and outcome components of clinical nurse specialist consultation. *Dimensions Crit Care Nurs*. 1991;10:169–175.

Hart CA. The role of the PCLN in the ethical decisions to remove life-sustaining treatments. *Arch Psychiatr Nurs*. 1990;5:370–377.

Hellwig K. Psychiatric home care nursing: Managing patients in the community setting. *J Psychosoc Nurs Ment Health Serv*. 1993;31:21–24.

Johnson BS. Psychiatric nurse consultant in a general hospital. *Nurs Outlook*. 1963;2:728–729.

Kane AM, Kurlowicz LH. Improving the postoperative care of acutely confused older adults, *Med/Surg Nursing*. 1994;3:453–458.

Krupnick SW. Psychiatric consultation-liaison nursing. In: Antai-Otong D, ed. *Psychiatric Nursing: Biological and Behavioral Concepts*. Philadelphia: Saunders; 1995.

Kucharski A, Groves J. The so-called "inappropriate" psychiatric consultation request in a medical-surgical ward. *Int J Psychiatr Med*. 1976–77;13: 209–220.

Kurlowicz LH. Psychiatric consultation-liaison nursing interventions with nurses of hospitalized AIDS patients. *Clin Nurse Specialist*. 1991;5:124–129.

LoBiondo-Wood G, Haber J. *Nursing Research: Critical Appraisal and Utilization*. St. Louis: Mosby; 1986.

Lewis A, Levy JS. *Psychiatric Liaison Nursing: The Theory and Practice*. Reston, VA: Reston Publishing; 1982.

Mallory GA, Lyons JS, Scherubel JP, Reichelt PA. Nursing care hours of patients receiving varying amounts and types of C/L services. *Arch Psychiatr Nurs*. 1993;7:353–360.

Millar MP. Planning and program development for psychiatric home care. *J Nurs Admin*. 1993;23: 35–41.

Minarik PA. The psychiatric liaison nurse's role with families in acute care. *Nurs Clin North Am*. 1984; 19:161–171.

Moschler LB, Fincannon J. Subspecialization in psychiatric consultation-liaison nursing. *Arch Psychiatr Nurs*. 1992;6:234–238.

Naylor MD, Brooten D. The roles and functions of clinical nurse specialists. *Image J Nurs Sch*. 1993; 25:73–78.

Nelson J, Davis D. Educating the psychiatric liaison nurse. *J Nurs Ed*. 1979;18:14–20.

Newton L, Wilson KL. Consultee satisfaction with a psychiatric consultation liaison service. *Arch Psych Nurs*, 1990; 4:207–208.

Platt-Koch LM. Clinical supervision for psychiatric nurses. *J Psychosoc Nurs Ment Health Serv*. 1986; 4:7–15.

Platt-Koch LM, Gold A, Jacobsma B. Setting up a fee for service program for psychiatric liaison nurses. *Clin Nurse Specialist*. 1990;4:207–210.

Robinette AL. PCLNs: Who are they? How can they help? *Am J Nurs*. 1996;96:48–50.

Robinson L. Psychiatric consultation liaison nursing and psychiatric consultation liaison doctoring: Similarities and differences. *Arch Psychiatr Nurs*. 1987;1:73–80.

Robinson L. A psychiatric nursing liaison program. *Nurs Outlook*. 1972;20:454–457.

Santmeyer KS, Roca RP. Geropsychiatry in long term care: A nurse-centered approach. *J Am Geriatr Soc*. 1991;14:156–159.

Smith MC. Group and Organizational Theory. In TP Hoskins, AM Leach and BS Sideleau. *Comprehensive Psychiatric Nursing* 3 ed., New York: McGraw Hill; 1987:410–411.

Strain J, Grossman S. *Psychological Care of the Medically Ill*. New York: Appleton-Century-Crofts; 1975.

Talley S, Davis DS, Goicoechea N, et al. Effect of psychiatric liaison nurse specialist consultation on the care of medical-surgical patients with sitters. *Arch Psychiatr Nurs.* 1990;4:114–123.

Titlebaum H, Hart CA, Roamano-Egan J. Interagency psychiatric consultation liaison nursing peer review and peer board: Quality assurance and empowerment. *Arch Psychiatr Nurs.* 1992;6: 125–131.

Titler MG, Kleiber C, Steelman V, et al. Infusing research into practice to promote quality care. *Nurs Res.* 1994;43:307–313.

Tommasini NR. The impact of a staff support group on the work environment of a specialty unit. *Arch Psychiatr Nurs.* 1992;6:40–47.

Wu YWB, Crosby F, Ventura M, Finnick M. In a changing world: Database to keep the pace. *Clin Nurse Specialist.* 1994;8:104–108.

Psychiatric Consultation-Liaison Nursing Quality Improvement Initiatives

A. Finding the opportunity/"triggers" to improve practice
   1. Clinical problems and practices (recurrent, high volume, high risk, and revenue-depleting) identified from clinical practice and quality improvement/risk management data.
   2. Scientific evidence that specific mental health problems lead to delayed recovery from medical illness or surgery, amplification of pain and disability, prolonged hospitalization, and suicide and nonsuicide mortality (especially in older patients).
   3. Service/departmental initiative to enhance quality improvement program, provide efficient psychiatric nursing (and medical) consultations, and enhance professional practice environment—through infusion of research into nursing practice.
   4. Concurrent institutional imperative to enhance quality of care, reduction of costs, improve patient/family satisfaction, and enhance professional practice environment.
B. Scope
   1. Medical/surgical units
C. Targeted populations
   1. Patients on 1:1 nursing observation
   2. Elderly surgical patients with acute postoperative confusion and related behavior(s)
   3. Elderly patients with depressive symptoms

OVERVIEW OF PROJECTS

1. Patients on 1:1 Nursing Observation

   Phase I.   Collect preliminary data on approx. 30 to 50 patients housewide (not ER) to develop a profile of these patients and current process.
   Phase II. Analyze data from Phase I and present to NMC with plan for PCLN intervention process: intervention process to be developed based on analysis of preliminary data.
   Phase III. Evaluate PCLN interventions and outcomes of interventions. Proposed outcomes (will depend on Phases I and II).

   Examples
   Patient
      1. Patient safety maintained
      2. Improved interactions with care providers
   Nurse/provider
      1. Improved health care interactions
      2. Increased confidence and clinical competence in working with these patients
      3. Decrease in behavioral symptoms
      4. Standard of care for suicidal patients maintained

Institutional
1. Decrease in duration of 1:1 observation
2. Decrease in lag time for Med/psych evaluations/referral to inpatient psychiatry units
3. Policy for suicidal patients followed

Time frame: To continue throughout this fiscal year

2. Geriatric Surgery Patients (65 and Older) With Delirium (Acute Confusion) and Related Behavior(s) Postoperatively

PCLN intervention process: To be further outlined

Examples: Review of Clinical Practice Guidelines (CPG) with nurse and other providers
Formal education of nurses on a designated unit
Review of meds/lab data
Patient/nurse interview with standardized delirium/confusion assessment method (CAM)
Referrals to Med/Psych for medication evaluation/adjustment, diagnostic evaluation (complex interplay of medical/psychiatric factors), psychosis, suicide, homicide, transfer to inpatient psychiatry
Referral to other disciplines as relevant
Individualized care plan suggestions based on patient needs
Cross-referral to other CPGs as relevant (e.g., aggression toward others)

Proposed outcomes
Patient
1. Delirium resolved/mental status improved (change in CAM score)

2. Patient safety maintained (no attempts at self-harm and other injuries)

Nurse/provider (as measured by a brief nurse survey)
1. Improved health care interactions
2. Decrease in treatment interference
3. Increased confidence and clinical competence in working with delirious patients
4. Decrease in behavioral symptoms
5. Increase in patient cooperation/participation in care

Institutional
1. Decrease in LOS
2. Increase in Med/psych consultations (for medication and/or diagnostic evaluation)
3. Increased referrals to other services (PT, OT, esp. mental health OT)

Time frame: To continue throughout one fiscal year

3. Geriatric Patients (65 and Older) With Depressive Symptoms

PCLN intervention activities: To be developed

Examples: Administration of Geriatric Depression Scale (GDS)
Review of meds/lab data
Referral to Med/Psych for medication evaluation/adjustment, diagnostic evaluation (complex interplay of medical/psychiatric factors), suicide, homicide, transfer to inpatient psychiatry
Referral to other disciplines as relevant
Institution of suicide precautions
Cross referral to suicide or aggression CPG as relevant
Counseling (includes cognitive, IPC, behavioral)
Self-efficacy enhancement
Strengths identification

Stress management/relaxation techniques
Sleep hygiene techniques
Support group referral
Psychoeducation
General PCLN support strategies
Individualized care plan suggestions based on patient needs

Proposed outcomes
Patient
1. Patient safety maintained (no attempts at self-harm)
2. Decrease in depressive symptoms (change in GDS score)

Nurse/provider (as measured by a brief nurse survey)
1. Improved health care interactions
2. Decrease in treatment interference

3. Increased confidence and clinical competence in working with depressed patients
4. Decrease in behavioral symptoms
5. Improved participation in care

Institutional
1. Decrease in LOS and/or readmissions within 48 hours.
2. Increase in Med/psych consults (for medication and/or diagnostic evaluation)
3. Increased referrals to other services (PT, OT, esp mental health OT)
4. Evidence of referral to outpatient mental health care delivery system

Time frame: To continue throughout one fiscal year

CHAPTER 17

ASSESSMENT MEASURES FOR BATTERED WOMEN

Albert R. Roberts • Patricia Petretic-Jackson

---

*I*f intervention ser-
vices for battered
women are to achieve
their stated objectives,
they must be based on a
systematic plan and
evaluation of the pro-
gram's stated goals.

Chapter Overview

COMMON MYTHS

A number of myths and stereotypes hinder both an accurate knowledge of the nature, extent, and intensity of woman battering and effective intervention. Enormous progress has been made in the past few years in regard to major policy reforms, assessment measures, and new treatment strategies for battered women. Recent legislation, more sensitive police and court responses, empirically based assessment measures and short-term intervention strategies offer much promise to lessening the battering of women in the United States (Roberts, 1996b). But in order for agency policies and clinical practices to be implemented effectively, our attention needs to be directed toward the realities of domestic violence against women, other than the myths. This article was written to debunk the traditional myths and replace them with new knowledge, research, public policy, and intervention strategies.

Although considerable progress has been made in funding domestic violence programs in the past ten years, much still remains to be done. There is disproportionately less funding for victim assistance programs when compared with programs and institutions for convicted felons. For example, the Violent Crime Control and Law Enforcement Act of 1994 authorizes nearly $9.9 billion for prisons and an additional $1.7 billion for alternative detention programs, whereas the Violence Against Women Act of the 1994 crime bill authorizes a total of only $1.2 billion over five years for criminal justice programs and social services to aid battered women and victims of sexual assault.

Myth 1
Woman battering is a problem in only the lower socioeconomic class.

Reality. Woman battering takes place in all social classes, religions, races, and ethnic groups. Although violence against women seems to be more visible in the lower class because it is more frequently reported to the police and hospital emergency rooms in inner-city poor neighborhoods, it is increasingly being recognized as a pervasive problem in middle- and upper-class homes as well. For example, the murder of Nicole Brown Simpson in 1994 received intensive media scrutiny because of reports that she had been beaten by her exhusband, former football legend O.J. Simpson. In her new book, Georgette Mosbacher, former wife of the CEO of Fabergé, describes the battering she endured during her marriage.

Although woman battering occurs in all socioeconomic classes, it is reported to be more prevalent in the lowest economic groups. The U.S. Department of Justice's 1994 *National Crime Victimization Survey Report* states that women with a family income under $9999 were more than five times as likely to be a victim of a violent incident perpetrated by an "intimate" than were women with a family income over $30,000 (BJS, 1994).

Myth 2
Woman battering is not a significant problem because most incidents are in the form of a slap or a punch that do not cause serious injury.

Reality. Woman battering is a very serious problem. *National Crime Survey* data estimate the number of visits each year for medical care resulting from domestic violence: 28,700 visits to a hospital emergency room, 39,900 visits to a physician's office, 21,000 inpatient hospitalizations, and 99,800 days of hospitalization. The total health-care costs per year are approximately $44 million (McLeer and Anwar, 1989; National Crime Surveys, 1981).

For example, Dolores, 42 years old, described her injuries from years of battering: "Two broken ribs, scars on my elbows and thighs, bruises on my back and neck. Broke my bridge in five places. All of my top teeth are loose. My glasses were broken." In addition, "He threatened to kill me. If he was drunk enough, I thought he would. He always said, 'If I ever catch you with another man, I'll kill you' and 'If you leave me, I'll blow your brains out.'"

Myth 3

Elder abuse (abuse of one's elderly parent or other relative) is not much of a problem.

Reality. According to the 1990 report of the House of Representatives Select Committee on Aging, *Elder Abuse: A Decade of Shame and Inaction*, more than 1.5 million older persons may be victims of abuse by their adult children. This figure is only an estimate because there is no accurate reporting system for elder-abuse incidents. Brownell (1996) discusses battered elderly women, police complaint reports as a source of early case findings, the need for statutory or mandatory reporting of elder abuse, financial exploitation, and a model case-management strategy.

Myth 4

The police do not want to arrest the batterer because they view domestic violence calls as a private matter.

Reality. Before 1985, the police often did not want to arrest the batterer when they were called to the scene in a domestic violence case. However, the court decision in the case of *Thurman* v *The City of Torrington* (1985) served notice to police departments across the country to treat domestic violence reports as they would a crime in which the perpetrator and victim do not know each other.

In this Torrington, Connecticut, case, Tracey Thurman had repeatedly begged the police for protection from her former husband, Charles "Buck" Thurman. In one instance, the police were called to Ms. Thurman's residence because her former husband was beating and stabbing her just outside her home. When the police officer finally arrived (his arrival was delayed for approximately 20 minutes while he went to the station to "relieve himself"), he asked Buck for the knife but did not handcuff or attempt to arrest him. Buck then continued to brutalize Tracey, kicking and stomping on her. Tracey suffered very serious injuries, including partial paralysis. She won her lawsuit against the Torrington police department for its negligence in not arresting Buck and for violating her constitutional rights to equal protection. Ms. Thurman was awarded $2.3 million in compensatory damages, which was later reduced to $1.9 million. The large settlement in the Thurman case is credited as being the catalyst for the development of mandatory arrest laws in a growing number of states.

By 1989, 13 states had enacted mandatory arrest policies for the perpetrators of domestic violence, although in several of the states, arrest is mandatory only when the batterer violates a restraining order. Frisch and Caruso (1996) discuss the far-reaching changes in New York's Family Court Protection and Domestic Violence Intervention Act of 1994, which requires police to make arrests in cases in which there is reasonable cause to believe that a felony or misdemeanor was committed by one family or household member against another or if an order of protection was violated. As of 1994, in New Jersey, arrest became mandatory if a woman suffers an injury or complains of an injury by her husband or boyfriend. New Jersey law states that arrest is mandatory for violating a restraining order if it involves a new act of domestic violence.

For example, Beth stated: "I had black eyes from his hitting and punching me. I called 911 and the police came, and I said to arrest him. He told them I was nuts because I was on pills from the doctor. The house was a mess, and I had the baby. The police officer believed me, and they arrested him. One officer asked me if I had anywhere to go, so I said I was from New Jersey and my mother was there. He advised me to go back to New Jersey with the money I had. The police said otherwise it would happen again. So I called my mother, bought a ticket, and left the next morning. He [the batterer] called and told me to drop the charges while I was packing to leave. I told him no." (Roberts, 1996b).

Myth 5

All batterers are psychotic, and no treatment can change their violent habits.

Reality. The majority of men who assault women can be helped. Two main types of intervention for men who assault women are arrest and counseling. Studies have shown that mandatory arrest has worked for some type of batterers, but not others. In their 1992 study of 1200 cases in Milwaukee, Sherman (1992) and associates found that arrest seemed to result in an escalation of battering among unemployed minorities, whereas arrest had a deterrent effect among abusers who were employed, white, and married at the time of the study. Roberts (1996c) details recent studies of the deterrent effect of arrest on different subgroups of batterers.

The Duluth, Minnesota, Domestic Abuse Intervention Project (DAIP) conducted a 12-month follow-up study in which battered women were asked their opinion of the intervention that the project had used in an effort to make the batterer change his violent habits. Of the women studied, 60 percent said they felt there was improvement when the batterer took part in education and group counseling, whereas 80 percent of the women stated that the improvement had resulted from a combination of involvement by the police and the courts, group counseling, and the shelter (Pence and Paymar, 1993).

Myth 6
Although many battered women suffer severe beatings for years, only a small percentage experience symptoms of post-traumatic stress disorder (PTSD).

Reality. Three clinical studies of battered women living in shelters or women attending community-based self-help groups found PTSD rates ranging from 45 to 84 percent (Astin et al., 1990; Houskamp and Foy, 1991; Kemp et al., 1991). These studies revealed a significant association between the extent and intensity of battering experiences by abused women and the severity of their PTSD symptoms. Jackson and Jackson (1996) provide a detailed discussion of PTSD symptoms and mental health interventions with battered women.

Mechanic (1996) provides a detailed review of the admissibility of expert testimony on the battered woman syndrome and PTSD to support self-defense claims made by battered women charged with homicide for killing their abusers. In some cases the expert testimony and the distortions of it by the press lead to a more severe sentence (e.g., 15 to 20 years or a life sentence).

Tina, 25 years old, recounted her suicide attempt and intrusive thoughts about the traumatic abusive incidents:

> I tried to kill myself because of depression over life in general. I was fed up—sick and tired of being beaten, and miserable, and taken advantage of. I kept having recurring nightmares about the battering and death threats. Thoughts of the beatings kept popping into my mind almost every morning. My body took the drugs. I couldn't O-D [overdose]. I tried to hang myself in my backyard, but someone pulled into my driveway and rescued me. I found recently I have a lot to live for. (Roberts, 1996b).

Myth 7
Battered women who remain in a violent relationship do so because they are masochistic.

Reality. Most battered women who remain in an abusive relationship do so for the following reasons.

- Economic need (financial dependency).
- Intermittent reinforcement and traumatic bonding (e.g., the development of strong emotional attachments between intimate partners when the abusive partner is intermittently kind, loving, and apologetic for the past violent episodes and promises that it will never happen again, interspersed with beatings and degrading insults).
- Learned helplessness (e.g., when someone learns from repeated, unpleasant, and painful experiences that he or she is unable to control the aversive environment or escape, that person will gradually lose the motivation to change the situation).
- The fear that the abuser will hunt down the victim and kill her if she leaves.
- Concern that leaving the relationship and moving to a new location will be a major disruption for the children (Roberts, 1996b).

Dwyer and associates (1996) have thoroughly reviewed the theories and causal explanations of woman battering.

Myth 8

Children who have witnessed repeated acts of violence by their father against their mother do not need to participate in a specialized counseling program.

Reality.

> We had been arguing; I can't remember what about. He became violent and ripped the phone wire off because I tried to call the police. He tied me up with the wire and burned me with an iron. He ran outside and ripped some kind of plug from my car so that it wouldn't work. Both my children were there. My daughter was 6, and she was screaming. My son was 5, and he just stayed away and hid under his bed. (Roberts, 1996b).

A report from the American Bar Association (1994) entitled *The Impact of Domestic Violence on Children* urges lawyers and judges to try more actively to protect children from the devastating impact (both physical and psychological) of domestic violence. The report provides the following revealing statistics about children and youth who have witnessed domestic violence: 75 percent of the boys who were present when their mothers were beaten were later identified as having demonstrable behavior problems; between 20 and 40 percent of chronically violent teens lived in homes in which their mother was beaten; 63 percent of the males in the 11 to 20 age group incarcerated on homicide charges had killed the man who battered their mother.

Jaffe and associates (1990) found that although group counseling was helpful for children with mild to moderate behavior problems, more extensive individual counseling was required for children who had witnessed ongoing and severe violent episodes. Jaffe and associates reported on a 4-year study of 371 children who had lived in violent homes. They found that group counseling had helped the children "improve their self-

concept, understand that violence in the home was not their fault, become more aware of protection planning, and learn new ways of resolving conflict without resorting to violence" (p. 90).

Carlson (1996) provided a detailed discussion of shelter-based programs and group therapy for children of battered women, as well as a review of the evaluations and outcome studies of these programs.

Myth 9

Alcohol abuse and/or alcoholism causes men to batter their partners.

Reality. Although research indicates that a higher rate of domestic violence seems to occur among heavy drinkers than among nondrinkers, the majority of batterers are not alcoholics and the overwhelming majority of men classified as high-level or binge drinkers do not abuse their partners (Straus and Gelles, 1990).

In many cases, alcohol is used as an excuse for battering, not a cause. Disinhibition theory suggests that the physiological effects of heavy drinking include a state of lowered inhibitions or control over the drinker's behavior. Marlatt and Rohsenow (1980) found that the most significant determinant of behavior right after drinking is not the physiological effect of the alcohol itself, but the expectations the individuals place on the drinking experience. Removing the alcohol does not cure the abusive personality.

Traditional substance abuse treatment programs are unable to meet the critical needs of abused women, whether those with abusive partners who are addicts or those women who themselves have a substance abuse or polydrug problem. Two independent forms of treatment are needed by chemically dependent battered women as well as chemically dependent batterers. A well-coordinated and effective working relationship between the two service-delivery systems—domestic violence and addictions treatment—needs to be developed in every city, county, and state or province throughout the United States and Canada. Domestic violence treatment providers need training on assessment protocols and treatment strategies with chemically dependent women, and addiction treatment specialists need training on the mental health needs and therapeutic programs available to traumatized battered women.

ASSESSMENT

Assessment must focus on the nature of the woman's battering experiences and the consequences of the battering as reflected in the woman's current psychological functioning. In part, the clinician's choice of methods and measures is determined by the purpose of the assessment: court evaluation, determination of trauma, or program evaluation.

For practical reasons, the use of multiple, brief, problem-specific standardized measures is advisable. If the battered woman has a history of psychopathology or of multiple traumas, a more comprehensive assessment of global functioning may be warranted. The goal for most clients is to select those instruments or methods that will provide relevant information without taking too much time to be completed.

Clinicians must also be sensitive to the stress inherent in the assessment process. Often they forget that the battered woman is a survivor, as well as a victim. The focus on her experience during the assessment may thus intensify the woman's distress, and the clinician may forget to identify her existing skills and strengths. The assessment process should identify client strengths, which can be used to formulate strategies for intervention and to promote change. Thus, examination of the woman's coping and survival skills is a crucial area which must not be omitted in the assessment process.

ASSESSING THE VIOLENCE

To assess the dimensions of the traumatic event or battering episode and obtain a history of battering, clinicians have a choice of several methods. A multimodal assessment of battering can be quite successful, using a combination of structured interviews, open-ended interviews, and a standardized scale or questionnaire. For a comprehensive review of clinical issues and methods of assessing family violence among children and adults, see Ammerman and Hersen's (1992) outstanding sourcebook.

Interviews

Most psychiatric nurses and social workers begin with an open-ended interview, allowing the woman to "tell her story." This format makes it easier for the clinician to build rapport with the woman and to establish the woman's prioritization of issues. A second option is to use a structured interview instead of the open-ended format. The structured interview permits contextual issues to be examined in more detail. A third option, which we recommend, is to begin with an open-ended interview and follow it with a structured interview.

The clinician must obtain information about the last few battering incidents, about the first incident of abuse, and about a representative incident. This will help determine the pattern of the abusive cycle and the potential for escalation over time. The clinician should ascertain the sequence of events, but without phrasing the questions to appear to blame the victim.

One structured interview that clinicians may want to consider, primarily for use in forensic evaluations, is the Battered Woman Syndrome Questionnaire (BWSQ) (Walker, 1984). Used in a major research study by Walker, the highly comprehensive interview requires 8 hours of face-to-face interviewing by a trained interviewer. Although its length makes the routine administration of this measure impractical, clinicians may consider this measure a model from which to derive their own clinical interview protocol.

Standardized Measures and Questionnaires

Originally, self-report questionnaires assessing battering experiences were designed to identify the nature of abusive incidents to which the battered woman was exposed in a battering relationship. The earliest measures (e.g., Conflict Tactics Scales; Straus, 1979) concentrated on physically abusive acts, with a minimal focus on sexually and psychologically abusive acts. Later questionnaires incorporated more information regarding these other forms of abuse. Most recently, attention has shifted to more detailed assessment of psychological abuse in the battering relationship.

The clinician has several measures from which to choose when assessing psychological abuse. The need for a detailed analysis of psychological maltreatment will guide the selection of the most appropriate questionnaire for a particular client. If a highly detailed measure of psychological abuse is desired, the Psychological Maltreatment of Women Inventory (PMWI) (Tolman, 1989) is recommended. The 30-item Index of Spouse Abuse (ISA) (Hudson and McIntosh, 1981) would also be an appropriate choice if a general assessment of both physical and psychological abuse is desired in a single measure. The ISA has adequate psychometric properties and discriminates between battered and nonbattered women. Its wording is designed for female victims; no version for male self-report is available. Both of these scales are preferable to the Conflict Tactics Scale (CTS) (Straus, 1979) if the clinician wants a comprehensive assessment of the dimension of psychological abuse. Only six items are used to measure verbal and symbolic aggression in the original version of the CTS, although recent variations of it (Brekke, 1987) have expanded the questions on psychological abuse. A final measure still being developed is the Severity of (Physical) Violence Against Women Scales (Marshall, 1992), in which 46 events involving threats and actual violent acts are rated according to seriousness, aggressiveness, and physical and emotional harm. Marshall suggests both clinical and research applications for the scale, and community and student norms are available.

Thus, in order to determine the nature of the abuse, a clinician may select from several measures. When selecting a measure, the clinician should decide whether it provides specific information regarding the forms of abuse experienced by a particular client. Possible options are the Conflict Tactics Scale, the Abusive Behavior Observation Checklist, and the Psychological Maltreatment of Women Inventory.

Conflict Tactics Scale. In its original form, the Conflict Tactics Scale (CTS) (Straus, 1979) is not generally recommended if a comprehensive assessment of sexual and psychological abuse is desired, although the measure does sample a wide range of physically abusive acts and a number of verbal abuse items. There have been several modifications of the original CTS (Brekke, 1987) that have added questions regarding psychological and sexual abuse. Straus (1979) has developed several methods of combining items into different indices of family violence.

If the clinician is interested in a brief screening measure of psychological and physical abuse that can be used to supplement information from the primary interview, the CTS can be found in Schumm and Bagarozzi (1989).

Abusive Behavior Observation Checklist. The Abusive Behavior Observation Checklist (Dutton et al., 1988) assesses the frequency of specific acts of physical, sexual, and psychological abuse.

Psychological Maltreatment of Women Inventory. The Psychological Maltreatment of Women Inventory (PMWI) (Tolman, 1989) is a 58-item scale that samples a wide range of behaviors. Parallel forms for men and women determine the relative frequency of abusive behaviors. The PMWI yields two subscales, measuring dominance-isolation and verbal-emotional abuse. Preliminary validation research indicates that the scale does discriminate between battered and nonbattered women based on the number of acts endorsed and the two factor sum scores (Tolman, 1989).

ASSESSING DANGER

Danger Assessment Scale

The Danger Assessment Scale (Campbell, 1989) was designed for use in the initial screening of battered women to determine their danger of homicide. The most recently revised version includes 15 yes-no items. Either the woman herself or a health or mental health professional can administer the scale. The total assessment takes approximately 10 minutes, and the follow-up with the woman to discuss her risk takes approximately 5 minutes. The scale is based on a match with demographic factors associated with increased risk of homicide, such as the presence of firearms in the home, sexual abuse, use of drugs or alcohol by the batterer, high level of control, violent jealousy, abuse during pregnancy, violence toward children, and attempts or threats of suicide by the woman. This measure is recommended for its short administration time, empirical underpinnings, and ability to give the woman a concrete measure of her risk of danger. Because informed decision-making is an important goal in working with battered women, this quick measure will permit her to make an informed decision about her safety or risk of danger. (For an examination of the latest study of battered women who kill and the causal links of homicide to being a high school dropout, being on welfare, cohabiting with the abusive partner, and suicide attempts, see Roberts, 1996a.)

ASSESSING PRIOR ATTEMPTS AT AVOIDANCE, ESCAPE, OR PROTECTION FROM ABUSE

Most clinicians assess the battered woman's prior use of specific coping strategies in response to the abuse in the context of the clinical interview. However, Dutton developed a written questionnaire to measure this dimension: the Response to Violence Inventory (Dutton et al., 1989). The measure assesses the nature and frequency of use of specific strategies in the past, perceived effectiveness with regard to protection from danger, and rationale for not using particular strategies. The measure is designed to be followed by an interview with the clinician to provide clarification and greater detail. A copy of this inventory can be found in Dutton (1992b). Dutton also stresses the importance of giving an opportunity to the battered woman, using an unstructured interview format, to describe the means she has employed in the past to protect herself and others.

ASSESSING PTSD SYMPTOMS

Literature seldom reports on the use of psychometric measures to look at symptoms of intrusion, avoidance, and arousal in battered women (Dutton, 1992a). Administering the Structured Clinical Interview (SCID) used for determining DSM-IV diagnosis is one option (Spitzer and Williams, 1986), but some level of training is required for its administration. Another measure that assesses intrusion and avoidance symptoms is the Impact of Events Scale (IES) (Horowitz et al., 1979). This 15-item scale has the advantage of being used in several empirical studies of battered women. Scores on the measure are correlated with the PTSD subscale of Keane and associates (1984), which was derived from the Minnesota Multiphasic Personality Inventory (MMPI), and the Crime-related Post-traumatic Stress Disorder Scale (CR-PTSD) (Saunders et al., 1990), which is a modification of the SCL-90-R (Dutton et al., 1990). We believe that if the IES is used to determine PTSD symptomatology, it should be supplemented by a measure that assesses arousal symptoms, such as the SCL-90-R.

In addition, assessing PTSD symptoms is complicated by the difficulty of differentiating between post-traumatic responses to trauma and the traumatic responses by which the woman copes with battering. For example, if a woman is abusing substances in an attempt to cope with the stresses of battering, although substance use may be considered a form of avoidance, other intrusion or avoidance symptoms may not be evident in the assessment. Therefore, any assessment of trauma symptoms must consider the moderating effects of both threats of abuse and actual substance abuse, both of which may mask signs of

PTSD (Dutton, 1992a). As with the assessment of pre-existing personality disorders, an accurate assessment of PTSD symptoms may not be possible until the woman has been in a safe environment for a period of time (Horowitz, 1986).

ASSESSING OTHER PSYCHOLOGICAL SYMPTOMS

Depression

Beck Depression Inventory. The Beck Depression Inventory (BDI) (Beck et al., 1979) is a 21-item scale that examines cognitive and somatic components of depression. Once question specifically assesses level of suicidal risk. BDI scores of 11 to 20 indicate mild to moderate depression, and scores over 20 point to severe depression.

For a number of reasons, the BDI is recommended as a means of monitoring depression in battered women. First, the BDI has been used widely in both research and clinical practice with battered women, which gives the clinician a normative standard of comparison. The measure is also highly sensitive to change in mood, which enables monitoring of fluctuations in self-reported depression levels over time. Its brief administration time makes it less intrusive and provides a consistent, standardized, objective measure of depressive symptomatology over the course of intervention. Research with battered women suggests considerable variability in levels of reported depression, although women in shelter samples appear to have greater elevations on the BDI than comparison groups do.

Trauma Symptoms

Derogatis Symptom Checklist-90-Revised. The Derogatis Symptom Checklist-90-Revised (SCL-90-R) (Derogatis, 1977) is a 90-item scale in which symptoms are rated for the severity of discomfort that they have caused in the past week. The test yields separate scores for somatization, obsessive-compulsiveness, interpersonal sensitivity, depression, anxiety, hostility, phobic anxiety, paranoid ideation, and psychoticism.

Advantages include the correspondence between item content and common trauma sequelae and the scale's utility as a screening device for more severe problems associated with compounded trauma response.

Saunders and co-workers (1990) derived the Crime-related Post-traumatic Stress Disorder Scale (CR-PTSD) from the SCL-90-R. Although data on the clinical use of the CR-PTSD are limited, the normative information provided for crime victims may provide a useful standard of comparison of trauma effects.

Trauma Symptom Checklist-33, Trauma Symptom Checklist-40, and Trauma Symptom Inventory. Particularly relevant to battered women who report a history of early childhood assault, the Trauma Symptom Checklist (TSC) (Briere et al., 1994; Elliot and Briere, 1992) assesses current emotional, behavioral, and somatic symptoms associated with childhood assault history. Although scores are not yet available for women whose assault experience is limited to adult violence, norms for both abused and nonabused clinical, community, and college samples have been published. Given the multiple trauma history of many battering victims, the scale may be appropriate, and the overlap of its items with the SCL-90-R permits the multiple assessment of such common sequelae as depression and anxiety. The 40-item version is particularly useful in assessing current sexual problems. The scales yield both a total trauma score and scores on five symptom subscales that measure depression, anxiety, dissociation, sleep disturbance, and post-sexual abuse trauma. Briere (1995) has published a 117-item version of this trauma scale, renamed the Trauma Symptom Inventory (TSI; Available from Psychological Assessment Resources). The TSI expands the clinical symptom list, includes nine clinical scales, and provides norms on various trauma groups, including victims of adult interpersonal victimization (Briere et al., 1994). However, the TSI was not designed to confirm a diagnosis of PTSD.

ASSESSING ATTITUDES

Domestic Violence Blame Scale and Modified Domestic Violence Blame Scale

The Domestic Violence Blame Scale (DVBS) (Sandberg et al., 1985) and the modified version developed for administration to clinicians (MDVBS) (White and Petretic-Jackson, 1992) are clinical research scales designed to assess multidimension blame attribution concerning domestic violence in professional, public, and clinical groups. The DVBS provides four blame scores, consisting of offender, societal, situational, and victim blame attribution. The MDVBS provides five blame scores, assessing victim, internal disposition (personality) of both victim and offender, societal, situational, and relationship blame. Norms are available for physicians, psychologists, lawyers, shelter workers, mental health professionals, and college students. The scale can be used to examine attitude change following educational programming or training. It also can be a means of clinician self-assessment, as patterns of blame scores have been found to be related to clinicians, as well as a theoretical orientation and a source of recommendations for treatment. Although clinical norms for battered women using the DVBS are now being developed, the scale can be used to identify salient attributional issues that would be a focus of treatment with battered women, such as the degree of self-blame versus perpetrator blame. In the clinical administration, the woman is asked to complete the scale twice, first as it applies to battered women in general and then as it applies to her own situation.

Inventory of Beliefs About Wife Beating

The Inventory of Beliefs About Wife Beating (Saunders et al., 1987) contains the norm-based responses of 675 students, 94 community respondents, 71 batterers, and 70 advocates for battered women. The measure yields five reliable subscales. Sympathetic attitudes toward battered women are correlated with liberal views of women's roles and sympathetic attitudes toward rape victims. Abusers and advocates differ the most in their attitudes, and male and female students also obtain significantly different scores.

ASSESSING GLOBAL PERSONALITY FUNCTIONING

Given the varied emotional and behavioral sequelae associated with battering, serious consideration should be given to routinely administering a global measure of personality functioning.

Minnesota Multiphasic Personality Inventory-2

Clinicians are strongly encouraged to consider the routine use of the Minnesota Multiphasic Personality Inventory-2 (MMPI-2) (Butcher et al., 1989) with battered women, particularly those with a suspected or confirmed compounded rape reaction or history of psychiatric care. Its clinical utility makes it a worthwhile assessment tool, despite its lengthy administration time (1 to 1½ hours). The test is also particularly useful in detecting underlying anxiety and depression in women whose behavioral coping style may mask such problems.

Variability in profiles may reflect differences in premorbid adjustment, time since assault, type of assault, and overall level of posttraumatic stress. Rosewater's (1982, 1985, 1987, 1988) study of MMPI profiles of battered women suggested that clinical scales on the MMPI are often highly elevated, indicating high levels of distress. The profiles of women still in a battering relationship, or those only recently removed from one, differ from the profiles of women who have been out of the battering relationship for a year. Analysis of the Harris-Lingoes subscales (Harris and Lingoes, 1968) is recommended to interpret any clinical scale elevations more accurately. The MMPI-2 also has two PTSD subscales.

Millon Clinical Multiaxial Inventory

The Millon Clinical Multiaxial Inventory (MCMI) (Millon, 1983) is designed to differentiate between acute psychopathology (e.g., DSM-IV axis I disorders) and chronic, pervasive, interpersonal personality dysfunction (e.g.,

DSM-IV axis II disorders). The 175-item measure consists of 20 clinical scales, and its administration time is approximately 15 to 25 minutes. The original MCMI (now referred to as the MCMI-I) has been revised (MCMI-II) (Millon, 1987). But because of problems reported with the reliability and validity of the diagnostic profiles obtained when the MCMI was administered to battered women, no empirical research using the MCMI-II with this population has been available to date. Walker (1987) believes that the MCMI cannot accurately differentiate BWS from serious personality disorders. In our clinical work, we have found that a diagnosis of borderline personality disorder is frequently obtained based on MCMI test results for battering victims who have both problems of substance abuse and a history of childhood abuse, although interview information and behavioral observation often do not confirm such a diagnosis. Along similar lines, clinical research has indicated that when the MCMI is used to assess battered women in a crisis situation, axis II personality disorders are often more accurately assessed when the MCMI is administered at least 6 months after a woman has left the battering relationship.

SUMMARY

If intervention services for battered women are to achieve their stated objectives, they must be based on a systematic plan and evaluation of the program's stated goals. Unfortunately, program planning, coordination with other disciplines, and program evaluation have not been given the necessary attention, despite the provision of what appears to be quality care in many programs.

Little research has been done on the impact of the short and long-term adjustment of battered women using mental health services. The clinical literature has suggested that cognitive-behaviorally oriented crisis and time-limited treatment models are the desired approaches in treating battered women. The adequacy of services (program evaluation) and information regarding the woman's adjustment should be obtained at the end of crisis interventions. The client's satisfaction with time-limited intervention should be obtained at the end of the brief treatment course, along with measures of the client's current psychological functioning. Both crisis and time-limited intervention should use client satisfaction questionnaires, in which women are asked to rate the usefulness of specific strategies, the overall perceived utility of the services, the adequacy of the educational information provided, the availability of services, and the clinician's skills. Clients could also make suggestions for program changes and additional services. This form could be provided in a packet along with self-help information. With a telephone follow-up, such information could also be obtained at the end of the contact.

REFERENCES

American Bar Association. *The Impact of Domestic Violence on Children*. Chicago: American Bar Association; 1994.

Ammerman RT, Hersen M, eds. *Assessment of Family Violence: A Clinical and Legal Source Book*. New York: Wiley; 1992.

Astin MC, Lawrence K, Pincus G, Foy D. Moderator variables for PTSD among battered women. Paper presented at the convention of the International Society for Traumatic Stress Studies, New Orleans, October 1990.

Beck A, Rush A, Shaw B, Emery G. *Cognitive Therapy of Depression*. New York: Guilford Press; 1979.

Brekke J. Detecting wife and child abuse in clinical settings. *Social Casework*. 1987;68:332–338.

Briere J. *Trauma Symptom Inventory*, Odessa, FL: Psychological Assessment Resources, Inc. 1995.

Briere J, Elliot D, Smiljanich K. The Trauma Symptom Inventory: Reliability and Validity in Clinical and Nonclinical Groups. Unpublished manuscript, 1994.

Brownell P. Social work and criminal justice responses to elder abuse in New York City. In: Roberts AR, ed. *Helping Battered Women: New Perspectives and Remedies*. New York: Oxford University Press; 1996.

Bureau of Justice Statistics (BJS). *Criminal Victimization in the United States, 1992.* Washington, DC: U.S. Department of Justice; 1994.

Butcher JN, Dahlstrom WG, Graham JR, et al. *MMPI-2: Manual for Administration and Scoring.* Minneapolis: University of Minnesota Press; 1989.

Campbell J. Women's responses to sexual abuse in intimate relationships. *Health Care Women Int.* 1989; 10:335–346.

Carlson B. Children of battered women: Research, programs and services. In: Roberts AR, ed. *Helping Battered Women: New Perspectives and Remedies.* New York: Oxford University Press; 1996.

Derogatis LR. *SCL-90: Administration Scoring and Procedures Manual.* Baltimore: John Hopkins University Press; 1977.

Dutton M. Assessment and treatment of post-traumatic stress disorder among battered women. In: Foy D, ed. *Treating PTSD: Cognitive-Behavioral Strategies.* New York: Guilford Press; 1992a.

Dutton M. *Empowering and Healing the Battered Woman.* New York: Springer; 1992b.

Dutton M, Hass G, Hohnecker L. Response to Violence Inventory. Unpublished manuscript. Nova University, 1989.

Dutton MG, Freeman M, Stumpff A. Abusive behavior observation checklist. 1988, unpublished manuscript, Ft Lauderdale, FL: Nova Univ.

Dutton M, Perrin S, Chrestman K, Halle P. MMPI Trauma Profiles for Battered Women. Paper presented at the annual meeting of the American Psychological Association, Boston, August 1990.

Dwyer DC, Smokowski PR, Bricourt JC, Wodarski JS. Domestic violence and women battering: Theories and practice implications. In: Roberts AR, ed. *Helping Battered Women: New Perspectives and Remedies.* New York: Oxford University Press; 1996.

Elliot DM, Briere J. Sexual abuse trauma among professional women: Validating the trauma symptom checklist-40 (TSC-40). *Child Abuse and Neglect* 1992;16:391–398.

Frisch LA, Caruso JM. The criminalization of woman battering. In: Roberts AR, ed. *Helping Battered Women: New Perspectives and Remedies.* New York: Oxford University Press; 1996.

Harris RE, Lingoes JD. Subscales for the Minnesota Multiphasic Personality Inventory. Mimeograph, Langley Porter Clinic, 1968.

Horowitz M. *Stress Response Syndromes,* 2 ed. Northvale, N.J.: Jason Aronson, 1986.

Horowitz M, Wilner N, Alvarez, W. Impact of events scale. A measure of subjective distress. *Psychosomatic Medicine,* 1979;41:209–218.

Houskamp BM, Foy DW. The assessment of posttraumatic stress disorder in battered women. *J Interpersonal Violence.* 1991;6:367–375.

Hudson W, McIntosh S. The assessment of spouse abuse: Two quantifiable dimensions. *J Marriage Family.* 1981;43:873–885.

Jaffe PG, Wolfe DA, Wilson SK. *Children of Battered Women.* Newbury Park, CA: Sage; 1990.

Keane T, Malloy P, Fairbank J. Empirical development of an MMPI subscale for the assessment of combat related post-traumatic stress disorder. *J Consult Clin Psychol.* 1984;52:888–891.

Kemp A, Rawlings EI, Green BL. Post-traumatic stress disorder (PTSD) in battered women: A shelter sample. *J Traumatic Stress.* 1991;4:137–148.

Marlatt GA, Rohsenow DJ. Cognitive process in alcohol use: Expectancy and the balanced placebo design. In: Mellow NK, ed. *Advances in Substance Abuse: Behavioral and Biological Research.* Greenwich, CT: JAI; 1980.

Marshall LL. Development of the Severity of Violence Against Women Scales. *J Family Violence.* 1992;7:103–120.

McLeer SV, Anwar R. A study of battered women presenting in an emergency department. *Am J Public Health.* 1989;79:65–66.

Mechanic MB. Battered women, homicide and the legal system. In: Roberts AR, ed. *Helping Battered Women: New Perspectives and Remedies.* New York: Oxford University Press; 1996.

Millon T. *Millon Clinical Multiaxial Inventory Manual.* 3rd ed. Minneapolis: National Computer Systems; 1983.

Millon T. Millon Clinical Multiaxial Inventory-II Manual. Minneapolis: National Computer Systems; 1987.

National Crime Surveys. National Sample, 1973–1979. Ann Arbor: Inter-University Consortium on Political and Social Research, University of Michigan; 1981.

Pence E, Paymar M. *Education Groups for Men who Batter: The Duluth Model.* New York: Springer; 1993.

Roberts AR. Battered women who kill: A comparative study of incarcerated participants with a community sample of battered women. *J Family Violence.* 1996a;11.

Roberts AR. Introduction: Myths and realities regarding battered women. In: Roberts AR, ed. *Helping Battered Women: New Perspectives and Remedies.* New York: Oxford University Press; 1996b.

Roberts AR. Police responses to battered women: Past, present, and future. In: Roberts AR, ed. *Helping Battered Women: New Perspectives and Remedies.* New York: Oxford University Press; 1996c.

Rosewater LB. Battered or schizophrenic? Psychologists can't tell. In: Yllo K, Bograd C, eds. *Feminist Perspectives on Wife Abuse.* Beverly Hills: Sage; 1988.

Rosewater LB. A critical analysis of the proposed self-defeating personality disorder. *J Personality Disorders.* 1987;1:190–195.

Rosewater LB. Schizophrenic, borderline or battered? In: Rosewater LB, Walker L, eds. *Handbook of Feminist Therapy: Women's Issues in Psychotherapy.* New York: Springer; 1985.

Rosewater LB. The development of an MMPI profile for battered women. Ph.D. dissertation, Union Graduate School, Yellow Springs, Ohio, 1982.

Sandberg GG, Petretic-Jackson P, Jackson TL. Definition and attribution of blame in domestic violence. Paper presented at the Midwestern Psychological Association Convention, Chicago, May 1985.

Saunders D, Lynch A, Grayson M, Linz D. The inventory of beliefs about wife beating: The construction and initial validation of a measure of beliefs and attitudes. *Violence and Victims,* 1987;2:39–57.

Saunders BE, Arata C, Kilpatrick D. Development of a crime-related post-traumatic stress disorder scale for women within the Symptom Checklist-90-Revised. *J Traumatic Stress.* 1990;3:439–448.

Schumm WR, Bagarozzi DA. The Conflict Tactics Scale. *Am J Family Therapy.* 1989;17:165–168.

Sherman LW. *Policing Domestic Violence: Experiments and Dilemmas.* New York: Free Press; 1992.

Spitzer RL, Williams JB. *Structured Clinical Interview for DSM III-R.* New York: New York State Psychiatric Institute; 1986.

Straus M. Measuring intrafamilial conflict and violence: The Conflict Tactics (CT) Scale. *J Marriage and Family.* 1979;45:75–88.

Straus M, Gelles R. *Physical Violence in American Families.* New Brunswick, NJ: Transactions; 1990.

Tolman RM. The development of a measure of psychological maltreatment of women by their male partners. *Violence Victims.* 1989;4:159–177.

Walker L. Assessment and intervention with battered women. In: Ritt L, Keller P, eds. *Innovations in Clinical Practice: A Source Book.* Sarasota, FL: Professional Resource Exchange; 1987;6.

Walker L. *The Battered Woman Syndrome.* New York: Springer; 1984.

White P, Petretic-Jackson P. Psychologists' Patterns of Blame Attribution for Wife Abuse. Paper presented at the annual meeting of the American Psychological Association, Washington, DC, August 1992.

CHAPTER 18

CONSIDERATIONS OF MALTREATMENT IN THE ASSESSMENT OF PEDIATRIC PATIENTS

Joann H. Grayson

Several factors usually separate accidental bruises from those that are inflicted. First, the age of bruises is important. A child's having many bruises in different stages of healing suggests repeated battering. Location is also important. Accidental bruises often include those on the shins, knees, elbows, and hands, as well as forehead, nose, and face. Bruises on the back, buttocks, stomach, backs of legs, and forearms suggest inflicted injury.

Chapter Overview

- Serious and Fatal Neglect
- Physical Abuse
    - Abusive Head Injury
    - Burns
    - Skin and Soft Tissue Injury
    - Fractures
    - Abdominal Injuries
    - Poisoning
- Sexual Abuse
- Intervening for the Child
- References

Adapted with permission from the Virginia Child Protection Newsletter, *1995;45.*

► INTRODUCTION

A multidisciplinary approach must be taken by health care providers in assisting families whose children have been maltreated. Nurses are urged to stay involved with children and adolescent patients, who may be victims of neglect or physical and psychological abuse. In their work, nurses have a duty to attend not only to physical injuries, but also to address the emotional needs of a child and family and to ensure referral and follow-up services.

SERIOUS AND FATAL NEGLECT

Neglect is the most prevalent type of maltreatment. It is a pattern of failing to provide one or more of the essentials for survival: food, fluid, medical care, or supervision. Almost half of all cases of maltreatment are cases of neglect. Neglected children are, for the most part, the most severely impaired with the poorest developmental outcomes (Becker et al., 1995). For example, preschool victims often have severe deficits in peer interaction skills (Gaudin, 1993).

Failure to provide food results in acute starvation if the failure is short-term. The child may not appear malnourished, even if death results. If the nutrition is inadequate, rather than absent, failure to thrive may result. Failure to thrive is a condition in which the child fails to gain the weight or height expected and no organic disease accounts for the growth failure. The child appears profoundly malnourished and emaciated. For both acute starvation and failure to thrive, the medical staff should check carefully for other signs of abuse. A skeletal survey, evaluation for sexual assault, and toxicology screens may be indicated (Rosenberg, 1994).

Failure to provide fluids results in dehydration, which also has many disease-related causes. In cases of child neglect the most common reasons for dehydration are punishment for toileting accidents or other offenses. The child will present with dry eyes, dry mouth, decreased or absent urine output, vascular collapse, and blood vessel clots (Rosenberg, 1994).

Parents or caretakers may fail to access medical care for several reasons, such as religious beliefs, fear of having abuse diagnosed, costs of care, underestimation of the severity of the problem, lack of judgment, or lack of motivation. When failure to provide care results in death, permanent impairment, or other serious consequences for the child, neglect is indicated.

Failure to supervise is a frequent precursor of accidents for children. A caretaker may be inattentive due to substance abuse, mental illness, physical illness, low intelligence, or low motivation. A parent may leave children with a sibling or an inadequate babysitter.

Failure to intervene is also a form of neglect. One parent may witness abuse of children, yet fail to intervene or take the children for medical care. A parent may not intervene for many reasons. A study of 2500 Oregon children who were victims of maltreatment found that neglected children were three times more likely to reside in families with substance-abusing mothers who are seriously dysfunctional (Bolstad et al., undated).

Neglect generally affects all children in the family. Thus, not only the identified child but siblings and all other children within the home need to be evaluated. Because neglect is a repetitive, chronic situation, treatment and intervention need to be long term.

Physical abuse

In the 1940s and 1950s, radiologists began to note suspicious limb and rib fractures associated with head injuries in infants. In 1962, the late C. Henry Kempe and his colleagues wrote an article for the *Journal of the American Medical Association* entitled "The Battered Child Syndrome." Public attention soon focused on the problems of the abused child (Rice et al., 1993).

Over the past 30 years, the medical literature has expanded to include thousands of studies and increasingly sophisticated diagnostic techniques. Several publications summarize voluminous and technical medical literature concerning inflicted injuries. This chapter presents information about maltreatment that should be known by pediatric nurses; however, by necessity, the chapter is incomplete.

ABUSIVE HEAD INJURY

The leading cause of death among abused children is head injury (Annable, 1994; Levitt et al., 1994; Smith, 1994). Severe accidental head trauma is uncommon in children under 2 years of age. Only 20 percent or less of deaths from head trauma in children under 2 are due to accidental trauma (Bruce and Zimmerman, 1989). Death rates from fatal head injury compare to deaths from serious congenital heart disease and deaths due to HIV, while far exceeding the prevalence of childhood cancer deaths (Smith, 1994). Thus, abusive head injury is a major source of mortality for American children.

The incidence of abuse among children with serious head injuries appears high. One study of admissions to a Cincinnati hospital over a 2-year period found a high percentage of abusive injury in infants less than 1 year old presenting with serious head injury. Excluding uncomplicated skull fractures, 64 percent of head injuries and 95 percent of serious intracranial injury were the result of child abuse. In one study (Alexander et al., 1990), over 70 percent of victims of inflicted head trauma had evidence of prior abuse, neglect, or both. This included a quarter of the sample who had experienced multiple intracranial hemorrhages.

Head injury differs from more visible forms of child abuse. It may be a single event. There may be no external signs of injury (Alexander et al., 1990). There may be no intent to harm the child. Not all children die as a result of abusive head trauma. Approximately 88 percent of children diagnosed with abusive head injury live (Smith, 1994). However, the immediate and delayed outcome of abusive head injury is worse than with any other cause of head injuries, in part because of ineffective treatment due to misdiagnosis. Early diagnosis can improve outcome.

An abusive head injury may be inflicted in several ways. Methods include, singularly or in combination, direct impact injuries, strangulation, malnutrition, and shaking. The latter appears to be the most common method (Smith, 1994). Carole Jenny, of the Children's Hospital in Denver, comments, "I think shaken baby syndrome and head trauma is most often missed. These injuries can present like many other conditions."

Direct impact injuries occur when high-speed objects hit a child's head. Direct impact can be due to slapping, hitting with an object, punching, or throwing an object and hitting the child's head. Neglect of auto restraints can also cause head injury. Dropping a child from a great height is another possibility (Levitt et al., 1994).

If an object is irregular or hard enough, it can penetrate the scalp. Often such injuries arise from knives, glass, or a spear-like object. Choking or suffocating children, especially if repeated, can lead to cerebral atrophy, as blood flow and oxygen delivery is compromised. Damage from shaking can also occur during choking.

Diagnosis may be compounded by false history. The most frequent complaint offered by the caretaker is respiratory distress. Other observations by caretakers are lethargy, irritability, seizures, or poor muscle tone ("floppy" or "limp") (Ludwig and Warman, 1984). Infants can also present with seizures, failure to thrive, vomiting, coma, or death (Dykes, 1986; Spaide et al., 1990; Wissow, 1990).

Several clues can alert the nurse to the possibility of abuse. The literature is nearly unanimous that falls of less than 4 feet are unlikely to cause serious brain injury (Smith, 1994). Serious injury requires serious trauma. Any child with serious head injury who has not been involved in an automobile accident or a fall from several stories should be considered a possible victim of child abuse.

In children with head injuries, computed tomography (CT) imaging will often delineate acute injuries not seen with other imaging methods. Magnetic resonance imaging, however, is more effective in dating subdural hematomas and will reveal lesions missed by CT imaging, especially 5 days or more after the initial injury (Jenny and Hay, 1994).

The presence of associated injuries can also support diagnosis. Approximately half the children who suffer an abusive head injury have accompanying long bone fractures. Therefore, all children under age 2 with possible abusive head injury should receive a radiographic long bone study (Smith, 1994). Radiology is limited because significant brain injury can occur without evidence of a fracture (Bruce and Zimmerman, 1989). CT imagery can be helpful; however, CT data underestimate the severity of injury. Fatal cases of abusive head injury with normal CT are documented. Thus, a normal CT does not exclude the possibility of head injury or of abuse. The converse is not true, however. It is rare that an abnormal CT will be associated with no or minimal symptoms (Smith, 1994). It is important to follow cases carefully for weeks as some brain injury develops gradually (Frank et al., 1985; Giangiacomo et al., 1988).

As retinal findings may be the only external clue to serious head injury and child abuse, a careful ophthalmologic evaluation is essential in the diagnosis of suspected abusive head injury (Annable, 1994; Apolo, 1987; Dykes, 1986; Giangiacomo and Barkett, 1985; Levitt et al.,

1994; Riffenburgh and Sathyavagiswaran, 1991; Wissow, 1990). Retinal hemorrhages are common, occurring in as many as 75 percent of cases. In some studies, retinal hemorrhages were seen only in infants with inflicted injuries (Billmire and Myers, 1985). Other ocular problems include detached retina and optic nerve injury (Lambert et al., 1986), tears to the cornea, inflammation of the iris, glaucoma, and dislocation of the lens (Wissow, 1990).

Differential diagnosis of abusive head injury should rule out accidental injuries, metabolic disorders, pre-existing intracranial vascular abnormalities, and sudden infant death syndrome (SIDS). The overall outcome of children with abusive head injury is poor. Only a third emerge without handicapping conditions. Mortality is high, ranging from 12 to 27 percent. The remainder of victims experience conditions such as blindness, seizure disorders, mental retardation, developmental delay, cerebral palsy, quadriplegia, or even coma (Levitt et al., 1994; Ludwig and Warman, 1984). Protecting victims from further abuse is of paramount importance. Siblings also need protection (Alexander et al., 1990), as no effective treatment for perpetrators has been found (Bruce and Zimmerman, 1989; Smith, 1994).

BURNS

Burns are among the most serious manifestations of child abuse. The mortality rate for children who are deliberately burned is as high as 30 percent, compared to a 2 percent death rate for children with accidental burns (Purdue and Hunt, 1992). Between 10 and 25 percent of pediatric burns are deliberately inflicted by adults, accounting for about 10 percent of all physical child abuse cases (Purdue and Hunt, 1992). Furthermore, there is some evidence that perpetrators who burn children are likely to reabuse the children, because of premeditation.

Infants and toddlers are at greatest risk for inflicted burns (Wissow, 1990). Infants younger than 1 year have limited mobility and climbing skills. Although accidental spill scald burns are common, immersion burns that are accidental are rare for this age group. In children ages 5 and older, abuse by burning of any type is rare, but when it does occur, it is generally targeted at children who are neurologically impaired or have developmental deficits (Purdue and Hunt, 1992). Scald burns are the most common (Purdue and Hunt, 1992; Wissow, 1990). Scald burns may be immersion, random splash, or spill injuries.

Immersion burns result from falling into, being placed in, or being forced down into hot liquid. Accidental immersion burns display splash marks, varying depths of burn, indistinct areas between burned and unburned skin, and multiple burn areas caused by the child's struggle. In contrast, immersion burns show uniform depths, little evidence of motion (as the child is held down) and indistinct (although not "perfect") wound borders. In a few cases, areas in contact with the cooler tub bottom will be spared severe burning (Purdue and Hunt, 1992). There may be "stripes" of unburned skin if areas were flexed or bent so that the skin was pressed against other skin and thus not burned (Rice et al., 1993).

Many children with inflicted immersion burns are burned on their buttocks. This is consistent with observations that problems with toilet training or soiling precipitate the abuse. Other likely areas for immersion burns are hands and feet.

Spill or "splash" injuries result when a hot liquid falls or is poured from above onto a child. Pediatric burns caused by deliberate throwing or pouring hot liquid on a child are rare, in contrast to assaults by adults on other adults where throwing or pouring hot liquid is common. Instead, spill injuries to children are generally caused by placing the child under running hot tap water (Purdue and Hunt, 1992). Because children's skin is more sensitive, children can be burned at lower temperatures than adults. Thus some hot tap water that would not cause a burn to an adult will burn a child (Ludwig and Kornberg, 1992; Wissow, 1990). Accidental spill burns are more likely to affect the face or chest. Burns to extremities or buttocks are more likely

to be inflicted. Spill burns are generally not as severe, because the liquid cools as it falls through the air and runs off the skin before severe damage is done (Rice et al., 1993). Usually there are several small, scattered "satellite" burns.

Clothing or diapers may alter the pattern of the burns. Clothing may act to hold the hot liquid closer to the skin for a longer period of time, leading to burns in areas that would ordinarily be spared (Wissow, 1990). Diapers with an outer barrier layer may, on the other hand, offer protection against the scald burn (Purdue and Hunt, 1992).

Chemical burns are often deeper and more severe than scald burns. This is because the burning process continues as long as the substance is in contact with skin (Rice et al., 1993). Flame burns are much less common. Inflicted flame burns are characterized by extreme depth in a fairly circumscribed area. One frequent site for inflicted open flame burns is between fingers or toes. The history given typically is not consistent with the injury.

Burns in the shape of hot solids (such as cigarettes, hair curlers, heating grates, or irons) are highly suggestive of abuse. Accidental burns by such objects generally have a lack of apparent pattern, due to the child's reflex movement as soon as contact is felt. Deliberately inflicted burns, on the other hand, often show a distinct outline of the object. (Very brief accidental contact with a hot object may produce a superficial second-degree burn with the object pattern.) Cigarette burns may be confused with impetigo, although the depth of the lesion is greater with cigarette burns. Healed cigarette burns may appear as either darkened areas or absent of pigment (Rice et al., 1993). Infections, severe diaper rash, and hypersensitivity reactions can sometimes be mistaken for intentional burns.

Suspicious burns include multiple burns of varying ages and types that could not have happened at the same time. Other inflicted injuries are present in about 20 percent of cases. Thus, long bone, chest, and skull X-rays are recommended in cases of suspicious burns (Purdue and

Hunt, 1992). A history of unexplained injuries or prior burns is also suspicious.

The history of the injury should be correlated with the observed pattern, burn depth, and general burn appearance. The precise timing of the injury and its purported cause should be carefully noted. Blistering can take several hours to develop. Electrical or microwave burns transfer energy to deep tissue more than to the surface and internal damage may be greater than the obvious surface injury. Thus, burns need to be observed over time before conclusions are drawn (Wissow, 1990).

Burns incompatible with the child's developmental abilities are suspect. A carefully detailed history should include any prior trauma, developmental milestones, illness, immunization status, and status of routine medical care. The most common cause of death in burn cases is pneumonia. Poor nutritional status compromises healing.

Inflicted burns are more likely to be correlated with a delay in seeking medical treatment. Further inquiry is needed for burns attributed to actions of siblings or cases where someone other than the person present at the time of the injury brings the child for treatment (Wissow, 1990).

Evaluation and documentation of the burn size and pattern should be precise and include careful drawings. Burn size should be expressed as a percentage of total body surface. Charts with correct body proportions by age are helpful in reliable determination of burn size. Photographic documentation is also recommended. No specific laboratory tests distinguish deliberate from accidental burns (Purdue and Hunt, 1992).

Positive outcome in burn cases is especially dependent upon follow-up care. Healing is prolonged, and very active outpatient therapy is required for a period of six to eight times longer than the hospitalization. After this, evaluations are needed at least yearly until growth stops. As abusive parents are often noncompliant with treatment, a burned child can be severely compromised if returned to the abusive household. Adequate supports need to be in place if the abused burn victim is returned home.

SKIN AND SOFT TISSUE INJURY

The skin is the most common site for physical abuse. Skin bleeding has only four causes: trauma (accidental or inflicted), coagulation protein disorders, platelet disorders, and vasculitis (Kornberg, 1992). It is important to note that the presence of a bleeding disorder does not necessarily rule out child abuse. A study of 50 children suspected of having experienced abuse found 8 (16 percent) to have bleeding disorders. Seven of the 8 were ultimately proven to be cases of child abuse (Kornberg, 1992).

A standard clotting screen will detect platelet and coagulation disorders. Vasculitis can be excluded through skin biopsy, but this is rarely necessary as it can also be diagnosed by related findings available by inspection. Therefore, the major diagnostic problem is separating accidental from inflicted injuries.

Several factors usually separate accidental bruises from those that are inflicted. First, the age of bruises is important. A child's having many bruises in different stages of healing suggests repeated battering. Location is also important. Accidental bruises often include those on the shins, knees, elbows, and hands, as well as forehead, nose, and face. Bruises on the back, buttocks, stomach, backs of legs, and forearms suggest inflicted injury (Rice et al., 1993).

Patterned bruising is often a clue to abuse. Bruising in the shape of identifiable objects is typically abuse. Common findings are loop marks (caused by electric cord or rope folded over), handprints (slap marks), stick or hair brushes. Sharp borders between normal and damaged skin generally indicates inflicted injury. Restraint marks from cord or rope are one example.

As is true in other types of physical abuse, the history offered by the caretaker may not match the injury. Delay in seeking treatment is also likely for inflicted injury. The age of the child should also be noted. A toddler might be expected to have bruising whereas an infant who cannot walk is not capable of self-inflicted injury.

The general level of care and presentation of the parents may also be a clue. In a 1982 study in Children's Hospital of Michigan (reported in Commonwealth of Kentucky Protocol, 1989), an "unkempt" child with signs of "abnormal parenting" had a 30 percent chance of being abused. "Unkempt" referred to conditions such as severe diaper rash, dirty body, or odor. "Abnormal parenting" was defined as one or more of the following: aggressive or hostile behavior towards staff, critical or overly demanding behaviors towards the child, lack of bonding, signs of being under the influence of drugs or alcohol, and signs of euphoria or depression.

Hair loss is another manifestation of child abuse. Several conditions such as nutritional deficiencies and fungal infections (e.g., ringworm) need to be considered as causes of hair loss. A fairly rare disorder is trichotillomania, in which the child systematically pulls out patches of his or her own hair.

Some congenital conditions, such as mongolian spots (discoloration, present from birth, often on the buttocks and lower back) can mimic abuse. Cases of hemophilia are also misdiagnosed as abuse, as well as conditions such as connective tissue disorders or photodermatitis, which can be mistaken for abuse.

Finally, certain cultural practices such as coin rolling or cupping may present as inflicted injury. Coin rolling is a Vietnamese and Chinese method to treat fever, headache, and chills. Oil is applied to the chest and back and massaged until warm. Then the edge of a coin is vigorously rubbed into the skin. Cupping is used to treat pain. A heated cup or glass is placed on the skin. According to Kornberg (1992) such bruising is not abuse as it involves minimal discomfort, no scarring, and is "harmless and well intentioned" (p. 103).

Documentation is extremely important as bruises fade rapidly. If bruising appears to be from a recognizable object, child protection and police need to search the home promptly for the weapon. Photographs are vital. Radiological studies of very young children are indicated if bone fractures are a concern.

FRACTURES

It is now estimated that abuse accounts for 20 percent of the skeletal trauma in children (Rice et al., 1993). As early as 1946, Caffey suggested the connection between unexplained fractures and battered children.

Any fracture can be caused by abuse. Certain patterns of fractures are considered pathognomonic for abuse (Jenny and Hay, 1994). Fractures of the ribs and the metaphyses of long bones are felt to be diagnostic of intentional injury (Wissow, 1990). The latter are thought to occur when the limbs are subjected to pulling and tension as the child is shaken or pulled violently. Rib injuries may occur from a direct blow on the back or from squeezing. Although rib fractures represent less than 25 percent of the fractures found in abuse cases (Huyer, 1994), in children younger than 2 an estimated 90 percent of abusive fractures involve ribs (Rice et al., 1993).

Suspicion of abuse should also be considered in any of the following:

- Unsuspected fractures discovered accidentally during examination.
- Skeletal injury out of proportion to history given.
- Multiple fracture, especially if symmetrical.
- Multiple fractures in various stages of healing.
- Skeletal trauma accompanied by burns or injuries to other body parts (Rice et al., 1993).
- Caretaker reports no injury but says there was a change in behavior, abnormality, or seizure (Leventhal et al., 1993).

Abusive fractures most commonly occur in very young children, below age 2 or 3 (Merten et al., 1994; Rice et al., 1993; Wissow, 1990). Only ten percent of abusive fractures occur in children over age 5 (Rice et al., 1993). In contrast, 80 percent of abuse fractures are found in infants less than 18 months while only 2 percent of accidental fractures are found in this age group (Merten et al., 1994). The age range is more variable, however, for children with mental or physical handicaps (Wissow, 1990).

When evaluating a fracture, medical staff should consider the mechanism of trauma and the direction of force required to fracture the bone. This information should be compared with the history offered. Unfortunately, no data are available on the strength of children's bones at various ages, although variability in bone strength and susceptibility to fracture is likely. Individual cases should be compared to other children of similar health and constitution (Jenny and Hay, 1994).

Differential diagnosis includes birthing trauma (especially after a breech birth), "Little League elbow" (epiphyseal separations occurring due to the child continually flexing the elbow while throwing a ball), leukemia, congenital syphilis, infantile cortical hyperostosis, Menke's kinky hair syndrome, osteogenesis imperfecta, osteomyelitis, congenital indifference to pain, Blount's disease, rickets, and scurvy (Jenny and Hay, 1994; Rice et al., 1993). Most of these conditions are uncommon and have characteristic clinical or radiological appearances that help to differentiate them from abuse (Wissow, 1990).

ABDOMINAL INJURIES

Abdominal injuries are second only to head injuries in causing death in child abuse cases. Studies suggest a 40 to 50 percent mortality rate for the 0.5 to 8 percent of physically abused children with abdominal injuries. Such high mortality rates are likely due to delays in seeking treatment and delays in diagnosis caused by inaccurate or misleading information offered by the parents. Also, because children are small, a single blow to the abdomen may injure more than one organ, with greater consequences than a similar blow to an adult (Huyer, 1994).

Serious abdominal injury results from significant force. Most accidental injuries to the abdomen result from falls from great heights or from motor vehicle accidents (generally where the child is a pedestrian). Inflicted abdominal trauma results from direct blows, such as a punch or a kick, or from an indirect shearing force generated from rapid deceleration of the body, as when a child is thrown across a room and hits a wall. Stomach and intestines rupture, spilling their contents into the abdominal cavity (Huyer, 1994; Rice et al., 1993).

Accidents most frequently injure the kidney, spleen, and liver. In contrast, spleen injuries are rare in inflicted trauma, while the liver is frequently injured and the kidney is the second most commonly injured organ. Gastric rupture, intestinal perforations, and intramural hematoma of the intestine are common.

The child will present with vomiting, dehydration, abdominal pain, and tenderness. The abdomen will be distended or swollen and muscles of the abdominal wall will be tense. The child may show labored breathing. External injury, bruising, or abnormality, may or may not be present. Delays of symptom onset can be from 1 hour to more than 2 days. In cases of serious liver injury, the child will be in shock with internal bleeding, abdominal distention, and decreased or absent bowel sounds. Minor liver injuries may remain asymptomatic (Huyer, 1994; Wissow, 1990).

Wissow (1990) suggests that abdominal trauma may be a marker for extremely disturbed families in the late stages of abuse. He cites a study of children from two urban hospitals where over half of those with abdominal injuries were already known to CPS as founded cases.

POISONING

Accidental poisoning of children is common. More than 400,000 poisoning accidents involving children occur annually in the United States (Bays, 1994). Yet fewer than 100 cases of child abuse by poisoning are described in the literature. This may be because only more severe or more unusual cases are reported.

The true incidence of child abuse poisonings is unknown, and it is likely that the majority of cases go undetected and unreported. In fatalities, detection is possible only if an autopsy is performed, and then only if the appropriate tests are also done. In nonfatal cases, detection happens only in those children with severe or bizarre symptoms which lead physicians to test for toxic agents (Bays, 1994).

Four common motivations for poisoning have been suggested: (1) impulsive acts under stress, such as trying to quiet a fussy baby; (2) neglect or not supervising a child's activities; (3) bizarre or overcontrolling child rearing; and (4) Münchhausen syndrome by proxy. Intentional poisoning is thought to be more lethal than accidental poisonings. Accidental poisonings have a death rate of 0.04 percent in contrast to the 17 to 50 percent mortality rate reported in the literature for intentional poisonings.

The peak age for accidental poisonings is 2 to 3 years. Two-year-olds account for about one half of all cases. Accidental poisoning is rare in infants younger than 1 year or for children between the ages of 6 and 10 years. After age 10, the incidence of intentional ingestion and suicide attempts begins to rise (Bays, 1994).

Accidental poisonings of children typically occur at home, during daylight hours peaking at 10 in the morning and 4 to 7 in the evening. Over three-fourths occur while the child is being watched or within earshot of the parent. Drugs are the most common poison for 2 to 3-year-olds, and household products are most common for the 1 to 2-year group. Often, the substance ingested had been used by an adult and moved to a location more accessible to the child. Typically, less than 2 hours of time elapses before seeking medical treatment (Bays, 1994).

When eliciting history from the caretaker, a complete list of drugs and remedies in the household should be made. Inquiry should extend to grandparents, babysitters, or others where the child spends time in their home.

Developmental status is important. To ingest a toxin accidentally, the child must be able to crawl, cruise, or walk to the location of the poison, extract the poison from its container, and get the substance into the month. In evaluating developmental status, it is preferred that the med-

ical personnel test the child's developmental levels, rather than accept the parents' report.

Inquiry should be made concerning adults in the family with a history of mental illness, with a history of abuse as children, drug or alcohol abuse, and frequent or chronic health problems. Marital discord has been cited as a causative agent in child poisonings. If a parent attacks a child, especially a child favored by the other parent, the child's illness may be perceived to "restore balance" in the household (Bays, 1994).

Care should be taken to try to identify prior incidents of poisonings. One study (Litovitz et al., 1989, cited in Bays, 1994) reported that 41 percent of children between ages 3 and 5 who had been accidentally poisoned were "repeaters." Of the 585 "repeaters," 18 percent had had two prior ingestions, and over 4 percent had had three. One child had 9 prior ingestions, one had 12, and one had 15. Twelve percent of the "repeaters" were younger than 1 year.

"Repeaters" apparently occur in families with increased stress, poor emotional support, low coping abilities, and higher levels of adult physical and mental illness. Even if the child poisons himself or herself, the family creates the conditions for the poisoning to happen. Similarly, neglect should at least be considered if a sibling is blamed for the poisoning.

A number of children who are poisoned have been prior victims of physical abuse, with studies suggesting that about 20 percent show evidence of physical abuse. A history of traumatic injury was reported in 40 percent of 147 children presenting with presumed accidental poisonings (reported in Bays, 1994). There may be a strong association between "accidental" poisoning and more classic forms of child abuse.

Drugs sometimes may be administered in an attempt to cover up physical or sexual abuse. Children may be given drugs to make them more pliable to sexual overtures. Drugs may be administered in an attempt to control a child's pain from physical abuse.

Toxicology screens are the major tool for detecting poisonings. Unfortunately, routine toxicology screens are limited. Some common poisons are not detected unless specifically requested. The time elapsed since ingestion also affects results (Bays, 1994).

A commonly used poison is syrup of ipecac, which is available without prescription. Clues to this substance include chronic or recurrent vomiting and diarrhea as well as elevated level of CPK, aldolase, and emetine. Laxative abuse also manifests with chronic or recurrent diarrhea, and can lead to failure to thrive. Stools are voluminous and watery but do not contain blood, pus, or abnormal levels of carbohydrates or fat. Ex-Lax may cause a pink tinge to the diaper.

Common punishments include putting soap, liquid detergent, black or red pepper, or other noxious substances in the mouth. One researcher alone has described 8 children who died after aspiration of pepper (cited in Bays, 1994). A thorough history is important. Many children punished in this manner have had prior instances of abuse. Examination of the pepper container is also suggested.

In addition, fresh or dried hot peppers can cause mucosal injury to the eyes and respiratory and gastrointestinal tracts, and death. Children should be asked whether they have had anything put into their mouths or if they have been made to eat anything as punishment.

Salt poisoning is not as common, but 17 cases (6 of whom died) have been reported in the literature (Bays, 1994). These children present with vomiting, lethargy, dehydration, hypothermia, and seizures. Some salt poisoning is accompanied by water deprivation or restriction. Conversely, water can be forcibly administered as punishment. These children present with apnea, seizures, and hypothermia. Some clinicians suspect that many cases of psychosocial dwarfism with bizarre eating and/or drinking behaviors are directly related to abuse involving food or water (Bays, 1994).

Bays (1994) notes several nonabusive causes of water intoxication. One growing problem is when parents do not have sufficient formula and offer water to the infant instead. The daily allotment of formula provided by the Supplemental Food Program for Women, Infants and Children (WIC) is indeed supplemental and will not provide adequate calories for infants over 4 months of age. If a family does not or cannot buy additional formula and offers water instead, water intoxication can result. Ingestion of insulin or oral hypoglycemic agents will produce lethargy, coma, and unexplained hypoglycemia. Intentional caffeine poisoning leading to death has been reported, although this appears rare. Ingestion of large numbers of caffeine diet pills, diuretic tablets, or "amphetamine look-alike" caffeine capsules can poison children and lead to death. Prescription drugs are frequent choices for nonaccidental poisoning, including barbiturates, phenothiazine, antidepressants, diuretics, and antiepileptic drugs. However, any drug may be used.

Lye, household cleaners, and other industrial compounds can be administered intentionally for punishment. Caustic ingestions may be overlooked by professionals as a potential form of abuse.

Alcohol and illicit drugs damage many children and claim some lives each year. Some are administered or offered by the caretakers. In other cases, addicted caretakers leave the substances where children can access them. A few children receive harmful doses of drugs via breast milk. Passive inhalation can be damaging, especially in cases of PCP or free-base cocaine. There are reports of infants and children's bodies being used to "hide" drugs, such as by placing plastic-wrapped drugs in the rectum.

Drugs may be given to children to sedate them or to amuse their caretakers. A survey of middle-class adolescent girls enrolled in drug treatment revealed that 11 percent had deliberately intoxicated children while babysitting. No parents had discovered the abuse despite some children being exposed as many as 15 times (reported in Bays, 1994).

Symptoms vary, depending on the drug(s) and dosage, and upon the child's age, weight, and condition. Symptoms include cardiac arrest, lethargy, unresponsiveness, seizures, respiratory distress, neurological abnormalities, and intracranial hemorrhage.

Another source of poisoning, intentional or nonintentional, is herbal remedies and vitamins. Accidental poisonings can occur from contaminated well water, deadly home-canned foods, and ingestion of household or outdoor plants. Labeling and dispensing errors are another differential diagnosis as well as errors in medication administration by caregivers.

If a child is found on one occasion to be a victim of intentional poisoning, it is likely that previous episodes of poisoning have occurred and/or that future episodes will occur if the child is left unprotected with the caretaker. Child abuse by intentional poisoning appears resistant to psychotherapeutic intervention and may reflect greater pathology than some other forms of child abuse. A careful history should be taken, not only of the child, but of siblings, parents, and caretakers. Complete medical records should be obtained. A psychological evaluation of the alleged perpetrator is warranted (Bays, 1994).

Sexual Abuse

Medical evaluation for suspected sexual abuse is a relatively recent phenomena. Only in the last decade have studies and commentary begun to address the question of physical findings in sexually abused children. Prior to the child's disclosure or before the caretaker suspects sexual abuse, the nurse may become suspicious in the course of examining a child for some other complaint. "Masked" presentations typically include early pregnancy, depression, suicidal thinking, and psychosomatic complaints (Hunter et al., 1985; Neinstein et al., 1984).

A nurse may be asked to assist in the evaluation of a child suspected of having been abused sexually. The request for a medical evaluation may be from a parent, law enforcement official, or staff member from child protective services. In these cases in particular, a medical evaluation for physical evidence of sexual abuse is only one aspect of the overall assessment. Many, if not most, physical exams will yield normal findings, even if sexual abuse is proven (Adams, 1992; Bays and Chadwick, 1993; Berkowitz, 1992; Meltzer and Kuchuk, 1991). Thus, medical diagnosis is based on a combination of history, physical findings, and when appropriate, laboratory tests (Bays and Chadwick, 1993).

A normal physical examination is expected, as many types of sexual abuse, such as fondling or oral sodomy, leave no physical signs. In addition, treatment following abuse may be delayed. It is known through follow-up studies that sexually abused children who have experienced recent penetration may show physical signs. Within 24 hours to 1 month, however, signs of sexual assault may be gone. Further, onset of puberty can obscure evidence of injury. For example, even if an exam is timely, only about half the cases of acute anal penetration will have visible findings (Berkowitz, 1992). Overall, findings diagnostic of sexual abuse are found in only 3 to 16 percent of child victims (Bays and Chadwick, 1993).

It is important that both professionals and families realize that a normal physical exam does not "rule out" sexual abuse. Otherwise, the physical will only contribute to a family's denial of problems (Vandeven, 1992).

Although some disagreement exists in the literature, certain findings are accepted by most clinicians as diagnostic of sexual abuse, even in the absence of a complaint from the child or history from a caretaker. These findings include the following.

- Presence of semen, sperm, or acid phosphatase.
- Pregnancy.
- Fresh genital or anal injuries including lacerations, abrasions, contusions, transection, avulsions, hematomas, ecchymoses, petechiae, or bite marks in the absence of an adequate explanation.
- Positive test or culture for syphilis or gonorrhea that is not acquired perinatally or through intravenous routes.

- A markedly enlarged hymenal opening for age with associated findings of hymen disruption including absent hymen, hymenal remnants, healed transection, or scars (in absence of an adequate accidental or surgical explanation) (Bays and Chadwick, 1993).

Others argue convincingly for concern and labeling with a broader range of findings. Wissow (1990) notes that only a small proportion of sexually abused children are found to be infected with a STD. Krugman (1991) states, "Any child with a sexually transmitted disease is a child who has a substantial risk of having been sexually abused" (p. 339). He adds that children who have chlamydia, trichornoniasis, venereal warts, or herpes type II should be considered "probably sexually abused." Bays and Chadwick (1993) agree that these STDs should trigger an evaluation for sexual abuse, as transmission of STDs outside the perinatal period by nonsexual means is a rare occurrence (Bays and Chadwick, 1993; Neinstein et al., 1984).

At the time abuse is disclosed or suspected, the identity of the abuser, nature of his or her medical problems, and type of sexual contact are generally not known. Young males, especially, may have been victims of older men who are at risk of carrying STDs. Also, the growing realization that STDs can be acquired by a child from sexual contact with other children has served to explain some cases of STDs that might previously have been attributed to nonsexual contact (Wissow, 1990).

There is disagreement about the need to perform laboratory tests for STDs in cases of suspected abuse. Wissow (1990) notes that gonorrhea is fairly common, citing findings of 10 percent in children enrolled in a sexual abuse treatment program. Wissow suggests that cultures for both gonorrheal and chlamydal infections be obtained from the pharynx, anus, and genitalia of suspected victims.

The medical examinor who checks for genital and anal trauma must be knowledgeable about normal anatomy and the developmental changes that occur in size and appearance of the genitalia as a child progresses from infancy through puberty.

A spectrum of findings—specific and nonspecific—are produced by molestation. The types of physical findings vary according to many variables including types of sexual abuse, objects or body parts used, age of the child, amount of force used, use of lubricants, number of episodes of abuse, and the time elapsed before the exam (Bays and Chadwick, 1993). For particular data, readers are referred to Dejong (1992, in Ludwig and Kornberg, 1992) and to Wissow (1990).

Some conditions may mimic findings of sexual abuse. If genital injuries are present, accidental trauma or conditions that present with bleeding must be ruled out, such as infections, irritation, or inflammation due to nonsexual etiology. A variety of dermatologic and congenital conditions may be confused with findings indicative of sexual assault. Anal findings can be due to poor hygiene, pinworms, infection, gastroenteritis, and inflammatory bowel disease, as well as sexual abuse. It is worth noting, however, that accidents, masturbation, and the use of tampons are very unlikely to cause injury to the hymen or internal genital structures (Bays and Chadwick, 1993).

If the most recent incident of abuse occurred within the previous 72 hours, forensic specimens need to be collected. The overriding consideration is to perform the physical examination in a manner that is nontraumatic. The physical exam should determine whether the child has diseases or injuries relating to the abuse that warrant medical care. It is important that the child emerge from the exam reassured about his or her physical integrity and well-being (Berkowitz, 1992; McHugh, 1991).

The medical evaluation for physical evidence is only one aspect of the overall assessment for sexual abuse. Physical findings, when they exist, are strong evidence. The history and statement of the child are equally important, whether they are gathered by the physician or other team member (Dubowitz et al., 1992).

INTERVENING FOR THE CHILD

Children's reactions to the same type of abusive act vary. Some children show few symptoms; others may model the abusive behaviors and become aggressive. Maltreated children may display a combination of symptoms: they may withdraw, develop somatic complaints, or dissociate. Research indicates that maltreated children suffer behavioral and emotional problems in virtually all areas of development; therefore, no single profile emerges (Graziano and Mills, 1992).

Barriers to medical research on child abuse have been tremendous. There are few well-trained researchers and little funding, as child abuse does not fit into "disease-specific" categories. Clinicians in full-time practice have provided more than 85 percent of the studies (Jenny, 1994). Understanding the medical consequences of actions toward children can be a major step in education and prevention of serious damage and child fatalities.

REFERENCES

Adams JA. Significance of medical findings in suspected sexual abuse: Moving towards consensus. *J Child Sex Abuse*. 1992;1:91–99.

Alexander RC, Crabbe L, Sato Y, et al. Serial abuse in children who are shaken. *Am J Dis Child*. 1990; 144:58–60.

Annable WL. Ocular manifestations of child abuse. In: Reece RM, ed. *Child Abuse: Medical Diagnosis and Management*. Malvern, PA: Lea & Febiger; 1994.

Apolo J. Bloody cerebrospinal fluid: Traumatic tap of child abuse? *Pediatr Emerg Care*. 1987;3:93–95.

Bays J. Child abuse by poisoning. In: Reece RM, ed. *Child Abuse: Medical Diagnosis and Management*. Malvern, PA: Lea & Febiger; 1994.

Bays J, Chadwick D. Medical diagnosis of the sexually abused child. *Child Abuse & Neglect*. 1993;17: 91–110.

Becker JV, Alpert JL, BigFoot DS, et al. Empirical research on child abuse treatment: Report by the child abuse and neglect treatment working group, American Psychological Association. *J Clin Child Psychol*. 1995;24:23–46.

Berkowitz C. Babies, bath water and sexual abuse. *J Child Sex Abuse*. 1992;1:101–103.

Billmire EM, Myers PA. Serious head injury in infants: Accidents or abuse? *Pediatrics*. 1985;75: 340–342.

Bolstad O, Johnson E, Magnuson L. *2500 Families: A Treatment Effectiveness Study of the Morrison Center Child and Family Mental Health Program 1982–88*. Portland, OR: Morrison Center Youth and Family Services; undated.

Bruce D, Zimmerman R. Shaken impact syndrome. *Pediatr Ann*. 1989;18:482–494.

Commonwealth of Kentucky Protocol. Inflicted vs. accidental bruises: How to tell the difference. In: Cowen FJ, ed. *Sexual Assault/Abuse: A Hospital/Community Protocol for Forensic and Medical Examination*. Frankfort, KY: Department of Social Services, Commonwealth of Kentucky; 1989.

Dubowitz H, Black M, Harrington D. The diagnosis of child sexual abuse. *Am J Dis Child*. 1992;6: 688–693.

Dykes L. The whiplash shaken infant syndrome: What has been learned? *Child Abuse Neglect*. 1986;10: 211–221.

Frank Y, Zimmerman R, Leeds N. Neurological manifestations in abused children who have been shaken. *Devel Med Child Neurol*. 1985;27:312–316.

Gaudin JM. Effective intervention with neglectful families. *Criminal Justice Behav*. 1993;20:66–89.

Giangiacomo J, Barkett KJ. Ophthalmoscopic findings in occult child abuse. *J Pediatr Ophthalmol Strabismus*. 1985;22:234–237.

Giangiacomo J, Khan JA, Levine C, et al. Sequential cranial computed tomography in infants with retinal hemorrhages. *Ophthalmology*. 1988;95:295–299.

Graziano A, Mills J. Treatment for abused children: When is a partial solution acceptable? *Child Abuse Neglect*. 1992;16:217–228.

Hunter RS, Kilstrom N, Loda F. Sexually abused children: Identifying masked presentations in a medical setting. *Child Abuse Neglect*. 1985;9:17–25.

Huyer D. Abdominal injuries in child abuse. *APSAC Advisor*. 1994;7:5–8.

Jenny C. The state of child abuse medical research—1993. In: Reece RM, ed. *Child Abuse: Medical Diagnosis and Management*. Malvern, PA: Lea & Febiger; 1994.

Jenny C, Hay TC. *The Visual Diagnosis of Child Physical Abuse*. Elk Grove Village, IL: American Academy of Pediatrics; 1994.

Kornberg AE. Skin and soft tissue injuries. In: Ludwig SL, Kornberg AE, eds. *Child Abuse: Medical Diagnosis and Management*. New York: Churchill Livingston; 1992.

Krugman RD. Physical indicators of child sexual abuse. In: Tasman A, Goldfinger SM, eds. *American Psychiatric Press Review of Psychiatry*. Washington, DC: American Psychiatric Press; 1991;10.

Lambert SR, Johnson TE, Hoyt CS. Optic nerve sheath and retinal hemorrhages associated with shaken baby syndrome. *Arch Opthalmol.* 1986;104: 1509–1512.

Leventhal JM, Thomas SA, Rosenfield NS, Markowitz RI. Fractures in young children distinguishing child abuse from unintentional injuries. *Am J Dis Child.* 1993;147:87–90.

Levitt CJ, Smith WL, Alexander RC. Abusive head trauma. In: Reece RM, ed. *Child Abuse: Medical Diagnosis and Management*. Malvern, PA: Lea & Febiger; 1994.

Ludwig S, Kornberg AE. *Child Abuse: A Medical Reference* 2nd ed. New York: Churchill Livingstone; 1992.

Ludwig S, Warman M. Shaken baby syndrome. A review of 20 cases. *Ann Emerg Med.* 1984;13: 104–107.

McHugh M. Medical assessment of the sexually misused child. In: Lopatto AD, Neely JC, eds. *Sexual Abuse of Children*. New York: Office of Projects Development, Appellate Division, First Department, Supreme Court of the State of New York; 1991.

Meltzer AH, Kuchuk A. Evaluating allegations of child sexual abuse: The "validation" process.

In: Lopatto AD, Neely JC, eds. *Sexual Abuse of Children*. New York: Office of Projects Development, Appellate Division, First Department, Supreme Court of the State of New York; 1991.

Merten DF, Cooperman DR, Thompson GH. Skeletal manifestations of child abuse. In: Reece RM, ed. *Child Abuse: Medical Diagnosis and Management*. Malvern, PA: Lea & Febiger; 1994.

Neinstein LS, Goldenring J, Carpenter S. Nonsexual transmission of sexually transmitted diseases: An infrequent occurrence. *Pediatrics.* 1984; 74: 67–76.

Purdue GF, Hunt JL. Burn injuries. In: Ludwig S, Kornberg AE, eds. *Child Abuse: A Medical Reference*. New York: Churchill Livingston; 1992.

Rice H, Pisapia J, Bar-on ME, *Child Abuse*. Richmond: Children's Medical Center Child Protection Team, Medical College of Virginia; 1993.

Riffenburgh RS, Sathyavagiswaran L. The eyes of child abuse victims: Autopsy findings. *J Forensic Sci.* 1991;36:741–747.

Rosenberg D. Fatal neglect. *APSAC Advisor.* 1994; 7:38–40.

Smith WL. Abusive head injury. *APSAC Advisor.* 1994;7:16–19.

Spaide RF, Swengel RM, Scharre DW, Mein C. Shaken baby syndrome. *AFP.* 1990;41:1145–1152.

Vandeven AM. Commentary on the medical evaluation of suspected sexual abuse revisited: 1992. *J Child Sex Abuse.* 1992;1:105–107.

Wissow LS. *Child Advocacy for the Clinician*. Baltimore: Williams & Wilkins; 1990.

VULNERABLE POPULATIONS

III

CHAPTER 19

ISSUES IN THE CARE OF ADOLESCENT CLIENTS

Wanda K. Mohr

*C*onfusion sur-
rounds the pathol-
ogy of adolescence, and
diagnostic errors of
commission and omis-
sion are often made by
the most experienced
and honest clinicians.
One reason for the con-
fusion is the difficulty
in distinguishing be-
tween normal adoles-
cent turmoil, turmoil
due to family dysfunc-
tion, and incipient men-
tal problems.

Chapter Overview

► INTRODUCTION

From the Christian confirmation and the Jewish bar mitzvah or bas mitzvah to the complicated marking or mutilating rituals of preliterate cultures, all cultures have historically acknowledged and celebrated the coming of puberty as a passage into adulthood. Despite the wonder that should be evoked by the process of adolescence, 20th century United States society has placed little value on this special group. People seldom seem to be dispassionate about adolescents, and many professionals would rather work with any other age group. Adolescents can be irritating and obnoxious, frequently doing everything possible to fly in the face of convention, and often seeming to go out of their way to insult their caregivers to the maximum degree possible. Perhaps it is these less endearing qualities that have led to the tragic neglect of adolescent health issues. In the 1990s adolescents are the single age group who have shown no improvement in overall morbidity and mortality rates. They are the first generation that is less healthy than their parents were at the same age. The leading causes of death in adolescents are homicide, suicide and accidents—all of which are directly related to behavior.

This chapter is an overview of adolescence, adolescent behavior and the problems that ensue from those behaviors. It deals with issues that are important for advanced psychiatric practice nurses to incorporate into their thinking and practice, focusing on some of the high-risk and deviant behaviors exhibited by this age group.

ADOLESCENCE

Adolescence is a process during which an individual changes from a child into an adult. During adolescence young people mature physically, begin to take responsibility for themselves, and start to confront the adult world on their own. From a purely physiological standpoint, the process is marked by the onset of puberty, which usually occurs between the ages of 11 and 14, and continues for approximately 6 to 10 years. In the past adolescence was defined solely by physiological changes, and for many years the child's entry into puberty was the most widely accepted indicator of the beginning of adolescence. Elliott and Feldman (1990), however, argue that, in addition to biological factors, social factors also define adolescence. Compulsory schooling, child labor laws prohibiting early entry into the job market, and the existence of a separate juvenile justice system define adolescence as a distinct stage of life. There are also other more confusing and ambiguous markers, such as paying full fare for transportation, restricting access to certain forms of entertainment, obtaining a driver's license, voter registration, and alcohol consumption.

In addition to cultural expectations, the divisions that mark junior high or middle school, high school, and college make adolescence more than simply a biologically defined time of life (Elliott and Feldman, 1990). Certain segments of society may also impose specific expectations that extend late adolescence, such as extended education. The construct of adolescence is thus a fluid and multifactorially determined, and that may change according to time and context.

Certain tasks must be completed during adolescence: becoming physically and sexually mature, acquiring skills needed to carry out adult roles, gaining varying degrees of autonomy from parents, and establishing and realigning other social interconnections with members of both the same and the opposite sex (Nicholi, 1988). In Western-based cultures, like the United States, there is a societal expectation that these tasks must be completed during the ages of 8 to 13. This is precisely the time when a decrease in self-ideal congruence and self-esteem begins to occur, a decrease that is often followed by a downward trend in the sense of self-worth.

Research on adolescence has been flawed in many respects, especially in terms of sampling. Inattention to girls has been noted as a significant shortcoming in the study of the adolescent experience (Gilligan, 1987). Minority youth also have been significantly underrepresented in studies (Elliott and Feldman, 1990). The growing awareness of serious flaws and gaps has resulted in a profusion of new findings about adolescent development, some of which have built on prior studies and others of which have raised critical doubts about previous beliefs. For example, until very recently adolescence was conceived of as a time of tremendous conflict, turmoil, ego instability, and upheaval. This view, introduced and elaborated upon by Hall in 1904 and refined by the psychodynamic schools (Freud, 1958), was asserted as dogma. It influenced understanding of the adolescent, and was reflected in psychiatric diagnoses for many years (Nicholi, 1988). In more recent years large-scale longitudinal studies have offered serious evidence that, in fact, adolescents are for the most part free of the turmoil that was described in the literature for more than half of the 20th century (Rutter et al., 1976).

The presupposition that self-sufficiency is the pinnacle of adolescent maturity has been challenged by research that questions traditional theories of children's cognitive and moral development. Baumrind (1987) and Gilligan (1987) posit that the Western emphasis on individualism at the expense of interdependence, coupled with flawed research models based on this emphasis, have shaped our presumptions about adolescent individuation. They argue that these premises have never been systematically validated. Current research reexamines previous assumptions and reflects a growing awareness of the complexity involved in human research and of the large role that multiple factors play in the course of human development (Elliott and Feldman, 1990).

Across cultures young people find the process of adolescence to be a time when pleasure and excitement are mixed with confusion and frustration. Because adolescence is also marked by ever-changing contexts, it is a period that can be fraught with confusion and frustration for parents as well. Changing contexts make it more and more difficult for intergenerational understanding to take place (Elliott and Feldman, 1990; Nicholi, 1988).

CONCEPTUAL FRAMEWORKS FOR ADVANCED PRACTICE WITH ADOLESCENTS

Conceptual models are useful as tools that guide systematic data gathering, intervention, and practice. They provide a framework that allows practicing professionals to focus in a certain way, rather than be overwhelmed by the sheer complexity of the natural world. They also provide a compass for decision making, facilitating a clinician's interpretations and evaluations as to what is appropriate or inappropriate given a patient's behavior, environment, and development.

Chapter 4 considered conceptual models and their role in providing the foundation of advanced practice. In implementing a comprehensive program of care for the adolescent patient and deciding on a conceptual model of care that is relevant to this population, the nurse must determine the specific constructs, principles, theories, terms, and concepts that are needed.

The construct of *development* is indispensable. It provides the key element in constructing a framework from which to view the adolescent client. Personality differentiation developmental tasks, and stressors differ in childhood, adolescence, and adulthood, and thus there are differences in maladaptive behavior patterns in these different periods. The characteristics that differentiate adolescent disorders are as follows.

- Differences in clinical picture that may be confounded by developmental processes. Adolescents may use a different conceptual schema than adults to explain what is happening to them.
- Vulnerability related to limited perspective and dependency on adults. Because adolescents have a finite amount of life experience, their world view is necessarily colored by a narrower range of informational tools that they might use in their evaluations and decision making. Moreover, most adolescents are financially and otherwise dependent on their parents. At the same time, they have a normal and healthy desire to break away, and to achieve autonomy and self direction. This predicament can result in serious conflict between family members that may precipitate or complicate any incipient disorders.
- Masking underlying problems. For example, depression in adolescents often is not expressed directly but may be masked by irritability, "acting out," or running away.

The concept of *learning* plays a central role in the development and resolution of human responses. However, humans do not respond to some disconnected "real" environment, but rather to a perceived environment. There is persuasive evidence that learning does not occur automatically but is cognitively mediated. These cognitions constitute private events (thoughts, feelings, images, and sensations); people may not be aware that some of these cognitions are connected to their ongoing behaviors. Cognitions as psychological constructs are another important addition to the conceptual framework.

Within the interpersonal realm family theorists supply the necessary concept of *systems* from which to view the dynamic environment within which the adolescent client is nested. Advanced practice nurses who have adolescents for clients will find a systems approach indispensable as they attempt to swing the focus of their attention back and forth between the child as an individual and the child within his or her social setting.

Because human beings are essentially biochemical/neurophysiological beings and because much new research data is constantly becoming available, advanced practice nurses must include *biophysiology* in their approach to care of clients.

Finally, the issue of personal knowledge is an important one in approaching the field of adolescent advanced practice. Lewis (1991) counsels therapists to be aware of the feelings that are aroused in the therapeutic encounter and asserts that the therapist's own feelings can serve as a vital instrument for understanding the teenage client.

Nurses in advanced practice are urged to be flexible about their conceptual models and theories. Adolescent psychology has been dominated by the personality theorists, and adolescent psychiatry has been dominated by the medical model. Nursing practice has been guided by both, with the result that some of the unique contributions that nurses can bring to the advanced practice arena has been lost. While there is no value in being parochial, it is important to remember that each practice discipline has a different emphasis that reflects a particular world view and discipline, and each has value. Bringing the contributions of many disciplines and approaches to the care of clients is most likely to best serve them and to allow them to choose from among a number of approaches that might work for them.

HIGH-RISK BEHAVIORS AND HEALTH ISSUES IN THE ADOLESCENT'S WORLD

Most textbooks and research reports indicate that there seems to be a peak in the incidence of mental disorders during the adolescent years. The entire range of psychopathology experienced by adults is seen in adolescents as well (Litt 1991). However, reports on adolescent mental illness rates, such as those represented by hospital admissions, are flawed and must be viewed with caution. A rash of overdiagnosing of mental illness and skyrocketing admission rates have resulted from the unregulated state of the mental health "industry" as well as from reimbursement practices that have led to diagnostic manipulation and the unnecessary hospitalization of adolescents (Mohr, 1994; Schwartz et al., 1984, 1989; Weithorn, 1988). Confusion surrounds the pathology of adolescence, and diagnostic errors of commission and omission are often made by the most experienced and honest clinicians. One reason for the confusion is the difficulty in distinguishing between normal adolescent turmoil, turmoil due to family dysfunction, and incipient mental problems (Cantwell and Baker, 1991).

Nurses, unlike physicians, are not obligated professionally to view patients through the "objectifying gaze" of the DSM (Kovel, 1988). Thus the advanced practitioner is free to focus efforts on problems and strengths rather than on diagnostic labeling, except that which is necessary for reimbursement. The difficulties and problems in living that result in the adolescent's referral to a mental health professional often are rooted in their engagement in high-risk behaviors. It makes sense to focus efforts at assessment and intervention in these areas. Overall, the health status of adolescents has declined over the past several decades (Wilson and Joffe, 1995). The causes for the decline are related primarily to social, environmental, and behavioral determinants rather than biomedical factors. From 1984 to 1995, factors related to violence posed the greatest health problems for young people. Major declines in health status can also be linked to substance abuse, accidental injuries, and the consequences of unprotected sexual activity resulting in teen pregnancies and sexually transmitted diseases, including AIDS.

ASSESSMENT OF THE ADOLESCENT CLIENT

In exceptional cases the adolescent client may be in so much psychic pain that he or she is agreeable to intervention and treatment. Most often, adolescents come to treatment manifesting overt distrust and hostility. They are likely to be crude, rude, and obnoxious. If they are accompanied by parents, they will invariably act in a way such as to maximally embarrass and provoke them. They may also attempt to antagonize and humiliate the nurse. Thus, major issues in working with adolescents are transference and countertransference. Working with adolescents requires a sense of humor and an awareness of the clinician's own adolescent experiences and comfort level with those past experiences. Advanced practice nurses must be aware of their feelings and reactions toward behavior that is often belligerent, impulsive, and obnoxious. It can be very exasperating to be on the receiving end of a barrage of verbal abuse. If nurses have unresolved issues within their own histories, they may overreact in ways that benefit no one and may potentially be harmful to all parties in the therapeutic relationship.

Working with adolescents is not difficult so long as the nurse keeps in mind that conveying a genuine and benign interest is essential. Experienced practitioners know that one way to cut off communication with teenagers is to transmit any hint of a judgmental or condescending attitude or to come off as an aloof expert. Assessment interviewing should be informed by an understanding of the developmental tasks and dynamics of adolescence. Adolescents are preoccupied with themselves and how they appear to others, and they will overreact to any perceived criticism. On the other hand, they will also react negatively to any form of "peering" by the clinician. Rather than using street jargon or referring knowingly to the latest fads or rock groups, it is better to let adolescents talk about their own special interests. Not only does this instill a sense of some control or parity in hypervigilant teens, but it also allows the nurse to elicit valuable information about adolescent interests.

Confidentiality is an issue that must be dealt with early and honestly. It is important for the clinician to make clear to both adolescents and parents that all interactions are confidential, except when the clinician believes that someone is in danger. Initially, parents and children should be seen separately, although at some point it may be valuable to bring the family together to get a better idea of the interpersonal dynamics.

Cohen (1991) suggests that an assessment should begin with the "least personal question" and follow a conversational style. The degree to which the clinician will perform a formal, rather than informal, mental status examination depends on such factors as the severity of the disorder, the reason for evaluation, the amount of time available, and the experience of the interviewer. A more formal approach is preferable when the presenting disorder is more severe.

Mishne (1986) suggests that the elements covered in the initial examination of the adolescent patient should include areas of difficulty, as well as other information about the teen as a person. Not only is this helpful in learning the contextual issues that are necessary for planning intervention, it is indispensable in getting a picture of the adolescent as a person, not only a patient. In order to begin the planning process for intervention, at the conclusion of the first interview, an advanced practitioner should be able to answer the following questions.

- Are there signs of a thought disorder (grossly bizarre or inappropriate behaviors, delusions, incongruity of affect)?
- What are the adolescent's present complaints and what precipitated them?
- Is there any evidence of self-harm, depression, or suicidal or homicidal tendencies?
- What was the adolescent's appearance: grooming, personal hygiene, physical health factors, manner of speaking, and attitude? Did the adolescent evidence any disturbed motor activity?

- What seemed to be significant antecedent factors in the adolescent's life?
- What seems to be maintaining the maladaptive behavior (secondary gain aspects, parental unwitting reinforcers, peer reinforcement)?
- Are the adolescent's expectations regarding the therapy clear?
- Are any indications apparent as to what therapeutic style the adolescent would prefer and thereby benefit from?
- Can a mutually satisfactory alliance be established, or should the client be referred elsewhere?
- What are some of the adolescent's positive attributes and strengths?
- Why is the adolescent seeking help now? Why not in the past? Is the therapy mandated or voluntarily entered into?
- Does the adolescent project with legitimate grounds for hope?

At the end of the initial assessment, it is desirable for the advanced practitioner to invite the teen to contribute anything else that he or she might think is important for the clinician to know. The nurse should then summarize the findings and ask for additional feedback, specifically obtaining the adolescent's perspective on how he or she believes that the therapeutic process should unfold. Once again, this will give the adolescent a sense of parity and will also lay out areas of potential disagreement and resistance for the clinician. There might be room for negotiation; if not, at least the clinician can deal with initial areas of divergence early and honestly. Research has shown that children as young as nine years of age are capable of participating meaningfully in personal health care decision making (Weithorn and Campbell, 1982).

Finally, in an increasingly multicultural society, it is crucial that the advanced psychiatric nurse be aware of the powerful role that culture plays in mental health. Mental behaviors vary with expressions and forms of illness and wellness in a culture. What is an aberration by the standards of Western psychiatric nomenclature is not necessarily abnormal within the context of a client's culture. The problems inherent in an adolescent's living with two or more conflicting value systems is also an important consideration. In such an instance, the nurse must be able to identify the unique demands of each culture.

ALCOHOL AND DRUG ABUSE IN ADOLESCENTS

The use of psychoactive drugs to alter perceptions, feeling states, or behaviors is common among young persons in Western societies. The use of these substances accounts for large numbers of emergency room visits, arrest rates, and drug-related deaths. The past two decades have seen an unprecedented increase in the abuse of alcohol and drugs by adolescents (Johnston et al., 1994). After a brief decrease of drug use during the 1980s, there has been an overall increase in drug use among all teenagers. Complicating the picture of adolescent drug use in the United States is the fact that patterns of drug use change so rapidly that surveys are often outdated by the time of publication.

Alcohol, which is a legal substance and well ingrained in Western cultural traditions, is the psychoactive substance most frequently used by adolescents. Other legal substances include tobacco products, nonprescription medications, anabolic steroids, and volatile inhalants. Marijuana is the most frequently used illicit substance; experimentation with marijuana has become almost a rite of passage in this country. Other illegal substances include cocaine (in the form of powder, freebase, and crack), heroin, hallucinogens, methamphetamine, and synthetic analogs (designer drugs).

The various forms of drug and alcohol abuse and addictions present very different clinical pictures. These profiles are extensively discussed and presented in the American Psychiatric Association's *Diagnostic and Statistical Manual of Mental Disorders* (DSM-IV, 1994). Because youthful substance abuse is the most commonly

missed pediatric diagnosis (Litt 1996), all advanced practice nurses who work with children and adolescents should become familiar with the clinical pictures. In addition to DSM-IV criteria, APNs should be aware in performing physical examinations that very often indicators of drug use include alterations in vital signs, weight loss, chronic fatigue, chronic cough, respiratory congestion, red eyes, deterioration in personal hygiene, constipation, general apathy, and malaise.

Substance use and abuse are frequently implicated in both violent behavior and accidents. More than half of all deaths among young people aged 10 to 19 are due to accidents. Most of these accidents involve motor vehicles (Pipkin et al., 1989). In over half of the motor vehicle fatalities involving an adolescent driver, the driver's blood alcohol level is above 0.10 percent (Centers for Disease Control, 1983a, 1983b; Insurance Institute for Highway Safety, 1984), twice the legal limit that is considered "under the influence" in some states. Nonfatal injuries resulting from vehicular accidents account for the largest number of hospital days among adolescents between the ages of 12 and 17. Most of these accidents involve the use of alcohol (Millstein and Irwin, 1988).

Violent behavior, including homicide, is also related to the abuse of alcohol (Busch et al., 1990). Alcohol and drug abuse has been implicated in other delinquent behaviors, such as destruction of property, violence against other people, and other behavior contrary to the rights of others and in violation of the society's rules. In addition, as many as 30 percent of adolescents who commit suicide are abusers of drugs and alcohol. Adolescents who use drugs and alcohol are three times more likely to attempt suicide than those who do not. Studies show that suicidal ideation increases dramatically after drug or alcohol use begins (Berman, 1991).

Of particular significance to the advanced practice nurse are studies that demonstrate that the drug experience is affected by, and in turn affects, the developmental phase of the adolescent user. Baumrind (1985) argues that recreational and chronic early adolescent drug use results in negative consequences that may either activate difficulties or intensify and exacerbate pre-existing problems. According to her research, negative consequences of adolescent drug use include impairment of attention and memory; developmental lag in cognitive, moral and psychosocial domains; and an amotivational syndrome (a pattern of apathetic withdrawal of energy and interest from effortful activity, uncertainty about long-range goals with resultant mental and physical lethargy, loss of creativity and withdrawal from demanding social stimuli). In addition, drug and alcohol use and the resulting negative reactions of family and other social groups can lead adolescent drug users to develop a negative identity, social alienation, and estrangement at a time when they need social support.

It is not known why some adolescents develop drug problems and others do not, despite recreational use or experimentation. Studies have identified variables that distinguish populations that use drugs from those who do not. These variables include family attitudes, personality, cognitive styles, and peer group orientation, but the available research is limited in its usefulness due to methodological flaws. Nevertheless, it is important for the advanced practice nurse to be aware of some of the determinants of drug use when the nurse is evaluating youngsters with suspected drug use and designing interventions and prevention programs. These determinants include maternal drug use, poor relationships with parents, and environmental substance use patterns (Harford and Grant, 1987; Newcomb et al., 1986; Semlitz and Gold, 1986).

Gangs, cults, and violence

Adolescent dependency on peer relationships and other nonfamily influences has increased over the past 25 years, while family influences have declined. Although most scholars are cautious when making attributional statements, many professionals in the field of adolescent psychology suggest that parental influence has declined because parents have chosen to withdraw from the lives of their youngsters (Baumrind, 1987; Nicholi, 1988; Uhlenberg and Eggebeen, 1986). Arguing that emotional withdrawal, irrespective of the makeup of the family unit, creates an emptiness in the life of the child, they contend that the groundwork is laid for feelings of abandonment and alienation. Gang and cult activity is the inevitable result of this alienation as adolescents seek comfort from those who welcome them and who reinforce their sense of belonging.

This has widespread implications for adolescents, for their caregivers, and for the larger community. Violence in all forms is a greater killer of children in the United States than diseases (Novello, 1991). Homicide accounts for 33 percent of deaths in those between the ages of 15 and 19 (Bureau of Justice Statistics, 1992). It is the leading cause of death among black males, particularly those living in impoverished, high-density urban areas—areas that are traditional breeding grounds for gang activity. National gang statistics show that once youths are pledged to gang membership, 63 percent end up imprisoned or dead (McNamara, 1994).

Other hate-related groups such as neo-Nazi skinheads have also grown in membership and have become increasingly more apt to engage in violent activity against racial and religious minorities (Williams, 1989). Gang activity has many mental health ramifications, from its impact on the adolescent who joins the gang to the community. Gang members are often found to have a high incidence of behaviors that are common to the DSM-IV diagnostic category of conduct disorder, whether or not they are formally diagnosed as having the condition. Retrospective studies note that conduct disorder occurs at a particularly high rate in adolescent boys who complete suicide (Berman, 1991). Gang violence is a problem for the community, which has to bear the expense of violent and nonviolent crime and bear the burden of caring for those who have been traumatized by gang activity. Exposure to violence related to gang and cult activities may result in a high incidence of severe post-traumatic stress disorder symptoms in both gang members and those on the periphery of the activities (Pynoos and Nader, 1989). Children and adolescents who witness injuries to others and who hear their cries for help are vulnerable to reexperiencing the violent events by way of traumatic dreams and other manifestations of PTSD. Gang and cult violence also poses a danger to caregivers who may get in the way of aggressive acting out during their caregiving efforts.

Adolescents who join cults generally are thrill seekers who have low self-esteem and poor social skills. Identification with, and loyalty to, a cause or leader gives their lives meaning. Unlike gangs, the cult often stands for noble values, with elements of idealism and elitism. As in gangs, once they become involved in the cult, adolescents become subject to powerful pressures from other group members, and may do whatever is necessary to prove their absolute commitment to the leader. This may include sleep deprivation, fasting and starvation, degrading sexual activity at the behest of the leader, begging and other ritualistic or personally demeaning behavior, and criminal activity (Galanter, 1989).

During assessment of adolescent clients, advanced practice nurses should be aware of the following indicators of pre-gang-cult and gang-cult activity: a sudden change of friends, using new words or nicknames, strange logos drawn on personal possessions or on the body, wearing the same color or pattern of clothing on a daily basis, solitary behavior, withdrawal from family, truancy or trouble with law enforcement, and bullying behavior (Short, 1990).

Efforts to prevent adolescent alienation can be undertaken by community-oriented practitioners who can initiate educational and intervention efforts within family groups, schools, and churches. Experiential programs are best geared to building self-esteem and teaching solid decision-making skills, as well as to engaging parents to provide structure and reinforcements

in the promotion of acceptable behaviors. With respect to other treatment or prevention modalities, incarceration fails to deter crime, and diversion programs have had disappointing results (Hawkins et al., 1987; McCord, 1988; Wolfgang et al., 1972). Job programs and counseling used as preventive techniques have also failed to live up to their promise (McCord, 1981).

Studies consistently point out the negative consequences of premature adolescent emancipation from parental control. It seems safe to say that postponing adolescent emancipation as long as possible may be one prescription in the prevention of deviant behavior. Steinberg (1987) presented data that supported this contention in one study which demonstrated that emotional distance from the family resulted in heightened susceptibility to negative peer influences and lessened parental influence correspondingly. Further support was demonstrated by Hawkins and associates (1987), who proposed that youth are more susceptible to negative peer influences when the social bonds of attachment and commitment to prosocial others (such as parents) are weakened. They concluded that parents who use authoritative management skills, including effective and open communication, consistent support, and firm enforcement of mutually agreed upon rules that respect the developmental needs of adolescents, are better able to prevent adolescent drug abuse than parents who are more lenient or more restrictive. The results of these studies can be helpful to the advanced practitioner in designing educational programs which emphasize family education and the importance of engaging the entire family in prevention and subsequent treatment efforts.

When the adolescent is already involved in a gang or cult, intervention and even clinical treatment may be necessary. The advanced practice nurse should be aware that it may take a considerable length of time to establish rapport with the adolescent; thus, patience is advised. Clark (1992) advises that it is crucial to assess the adolescent's level of fear and to determine when the gang or cult involvement began. Gang and cult activity is often preceded by a traumatic event, which can serve as a focal point for treatment interventions. If inpatient treatment is necessary, treatment staff should be made aware that the adolescent is engaged in a major coping strategy and that the strategy must be slowly replaced by healthier alternatives. Thus, the inpatient milieu should not be rigid, but should focus on accountability and responsibility, while discouraging destructive behaviors.

Adolescents with a history of violent, impulsive behavior pose a special challenge to nursing staff. Warning signs of potentially explosive episodes are a loud strident voice, tense posture, fist clenching, or inability to sit still. Nurses should be particularly careful when assessing adolescents who show no remorse or discomfort when discussing their violent acts. In the initial contact with the potentially violent adolescent, the nurse should never be alone. From the beginning, the nurse must calmly state (without issuing hostile directives or ultimatums) that violent acting out will not be tolerated. However, limit setting with no avenue that allows the adolescent to "save face" is counterproductive and could potentially be dangerous. Nurses should speak slowly and clearly and listen uncritically. An offer of a soft drink or snack can often help to reduce agitation when an adolescent is particularly belligerent (Howells and Hollin, 1989).

In addition to adolescents' impulsivity and acting out, the nurse must be cognizant that there may be many obstacles to treatment if it is involuntary. No one takes pleasure in being incarcerated, nor do they relish the perception that they are forced to obey the will of others. Part of the difficulty involved with involuntary treatment is that it heightens the disparity in power between the adolescent patient and staff member and exacerbates already existing conflicts over authority. Involuntarily committed adolescents who already have impulse control difficulties may be hostile, guarded, and suspicious or deceptively placating and submissive. Advanced practice nurses have multiple challenges to face when dealing with this group. They must also be acutely aware of their countertransference reactions, and they must be willing to exercise great patience and restraint when working with this difficult group of patients.

DEPRESSION AND SUICIDALITY

The incidence of depression in adolescents is difficult to determine because of variations in definition and measurement (Brage, 1995). Estimates range from 5 to 7 percent of high school students experiencing severe depression and 21 to 27 percent experiencing moderate depression (Teri, 1982; Worchel et al., 1987). Depression occurring as a psychiatric illness is a debilitating affective state that is characterized in the DSM-IV as consisting of dysphoric mood or loss of interest or pleasure in usual activities and marked by persistent symptoms such as hopelessness, irritability, or "feeling blue or sad" (APA, 1994). The clinical picture of depression in adolescents may express itself in ways that vary from the picture in adults, reflecting differences in stages of development. Signs of depression in the adolescent may include poor academic performance, restlessness, listlessness, and aggressive or sexual acting-out behavior. In addition, the adolescent may appear bored or engage in other high-risk behaviors, such as careless driving of vehicles or alcohol and drug use (Nicholi, 1988).

The immediate goals of intervention are to develop a working relationship with the depressed adolescent, to protect the individual from self-harm, and to decrease the amount of dysphoria. Treatment plans should focus on reducing the effects of psychopathology and maladaptive cognitions and behaviors, increasing self-esteem and self-worth, and enhancing instrumental skills. Cognitive therapy has been shown to be an effective treatment for adults with affective disorders, especially when depressive symptoms interfere with insight-oriented approaches (Beck et al., 1985).

Adolescent depression often goes unrecognized, and thus has been a neglected area of study. Differentiating pathology from mood fluctuations and transient depressive feelings that accompany hormonal and other neuroendocrine changes of puberty can present a challenge to practitioners. However, studies have shown that depression is the strongest discriminator of high suicide ideation. The statistics on adolescent suicide underscore the fact that depression can be a grave, life-threatening condition and one that merits serious study and consideration. Suicide accounts for 12 percent of deaths between ages 15 and 19. It is the second leading cause of death among white adolescents and the fifth leading cause of death among black teens (U.S. Dept of Health and Human Services, 1991). Adolescents who are at high risk for suicidal behavior and who experience high degrees of suicidal ideation are in considerable psychosocial distress (Thompson et al., 1994). Adolescents who complete suicide have usually made previous attempts. Those at risk for suicide include teens with a major psychiatric disorder (principally depression), antisocial behavior, affective instability, and a family history of suicide or psychiatric illness (Holinger et al., 1994; Shaffer, 1993). Other traits that are considered common risk factors indicating a need for suicide prevention are intense rage, impulsive behavior, and limited tolerance for frustration. Suicidal behavior is associated with a history of bipolar disorder, schizophrenia, character disorders, substance use, depression, and learning disorders. Perceived stressors, such as family conflicts and rejection by peers or by the subjects of romantic involvement, may be sufficient to trigger a suicidal gesture or attempt (Brent et al., 1988; Thompson et al., 1994).

Suicide prevention strategies require a knowledge of the factors that may lead to suicide. Primary prevention strategies, or those that are geared to prevent suicide, might include limitation of alcohol sales and restricting access to the means of suicide, such as by gun control. Secondary prevention strategies provide help for those who are already suicidal. Thus far, identifying an "at risk" group and direct case finding, with a follow-up assessment and intervention if necessary, holds the most promise. Preliminary data analysis of studies conducted by Shaffer and colleagues (1993) has shown promise of identifying at-risk high school students through computerized interviewing. Results show that adolescents with troubling suicidal preoccupation will identify themselves.

As far as other suicide prevention strategies, researchers conclude that many common approaches that have intuitive appeal are ineffective in preventing suicidal behavior (Shaffer, 1993; Shaffer et al., 1988). School programs are not cost effective and there is no evidence that they have any impact. Studies have shown that they are ineffective at changing unwanted attitudes toward suicide (Shaffer et al., 1993; Vieland et al., 1991). In addition, there is little knowledge as to their impact on students who are not considering suicide or those who constitute a disturbed subgroup of teens. The results of studies on hotlines and other crisis services are not encouraging. First, most teens are not aware of crisis hotlines; second, the advice given to callers to such hotlines is often inappropriate, stereotyped, and insensitive to specific needs of the caller.

Treatment of the suicidal adolescent can be conceptualized as having a twofold approach. The first aspect includes suicide crisis intervention, where interventions are designed to prevent death or injury by restoring a presuicidal equilibrium. In this approach, the advanced practice nurse helps to restore equilibrium as rapidly as possible by providing the resources and supports, both internal and external, necessary to allow a normal healing process to occur. Suicidal crisis in adolescents requires inpatient treatment in order to keep the child safe. The immediate task of the nurse will be to assess the adolescent's potential for self-destructive behavior, while concurrently acting to protect the individual from self-destructive impulses.

Following the resolution of the immediate crisis, the second approach will be to deal with the vulnerabilities that led to the suicidal crisis in the first place. This will include therapeutic interventions that are geared to reduce psychopathology and teach adaptive skills. Because most clinicians do not have any extensive training in clinical suicidology, the advanced practice nurse should engage professional assistance and use a team approach in longer-term treatment.

OTHER ADOLESCENT HIGH-RISK BEHAVIOR

BODY MARKING

Several recent fads among adolescents have the potential to cause injury or illness. One of these fads is the current form of expression known as body marking, which includes body piercing, scarring, and tattooing. No research is presently available on the meaning of body marking to adolescents, but since antiquity marking of bodies has served as a sign of group membership, pair bonding, and the achievement of a rite of passage (Litt, 1994). Tattooing proclaims affiliation with certain gang groups and members of gangs have multiple tattoo sites. They serve as signs of both power and acceptance. Some gang members may tattoo their girlfriends as a sign of ownership. Another use of tattooing can be an attempt to disguise the tracks of intravenous drug use.

Tattooing is done by introducing pigments through puncture marks in the skin to create patterns or pictures. Ornamental scarring, also known as cicatrization, is the induction of a scar, resulting in the formation and contraction of fibrous tissue. This is done through cutting or burning; often irritants are rubbed into the wounds in order to raise weals or keloids (Strathern and Strathern, 1971). Body piercing ranges from multiple ear piercing to the piercing of other body parts, including nipples, labia, eyelids, tongues, and noses. Because the needles and other instruments used by professional body artists are not disposable and sterilization is often inadequate, the potential health hazards of body marking include hepatitis B and HIV infection (Mercer, 1991). In addition, most adolescents do not get their bodies marked by professionals, but rather from amateurs or from each other, making the concerns of infection even more worrisome. However, by 1994 there had been no published cases of HIV contracted from these practices (Litt, 1994).

The psychological and social sequelae of adolescent body marking has not been examined in a scholarly manner from a mental health perspective. Nevertheless, it seems reasonable that after the impulse has passed, unwanted body marking can have an impact on a young person's job potential, as well as impacting on attempts to leave a gang or to overcome the stigma that the momentary lapse into wanting to "fit in" brings with it in the long term.

HIGH-RISK SEXUAL ACTIVITY

The United States leads the industrialized world in the rates of teenage pregnancy, abortion, and birth (Spitz et al., 1996). By the age of 19 over 77 percent of males and 62 percent of females have engaged in sexual intercourse (Hofferth and Hayes, 1987). Problems associated with teenage sexual behavior include infection with sexually transmitted diseases (STDs) and the social and economic consequences of pregnancy. High-risk sexual activity is particularly worrisome since AIDS joined the ranks of STDs. STD rates are higher among adolescent groups than any other groups, with 25 percent of sexually active adolescents becoming infected during their high school careers (Shaffer et al., 1984). Risk factors for STDs include low socioeconomic status, low educational attainment, minority status, history of poor family relationships, multiple partners, and failure to use condoms (Bell and Holmes, 1984).

It is challenging to provide preventative programming for adolescents because of their propensity to "live for the moment." Nevertheless much needs to be done, due to the vulnerability of this group and the enormous mental health and physical costs that are the consequences of unprotected sexual activity. Treatment efforts should be closely linked to drug treatment programs, family planning programs, programs for runaway and homeless youth, child protective services, perinatal and sexually transmitted disease clinics, and the juvenile justice system.

EATING DISORDERS

Eating disorders and the behaviors that accompany them pose great risk for the adolescent patient. Eating disorders typically refer to the syndromes of anorexia nervosa and bulimia nervosa. DSM-IV (1994) provides detailed descriptions and criteria for both of these conditions as well as the binge eating disorders. Populations most likely to be at risk for anorexia nervosa are those whose recreational and occupational areas of interest require highly focused attention on weight, appearance, and lean body mass. In addition, girls who have been sexually abused are at great risk of developing anorexia nervosa (Sloan and Leichner, 1986). Anorexia nervosa and bulimia may co-exist or one may manifest itself following the appearance or resolution of the other. In the two decades from 1965 to 1985, the incidence of anorexia nervosa doubled. It is estimated to occur in 0.5 percent of females between the ages of 12 and 18 (Kennedy and Garfinkel, 1985). Reports on the incidence of bulimia also indicate that it is widespread and increasing in prevalence, with at least 5 to 18 percent of young women in high school afflicted with the disorder (Herzog et al., 1985).

Drastically restricting caloric intake, purging through vomiting, fasting, laxatives, or diuretics, and excessive physical activity lead to rapid and extreme weight loss in the anorexic adolescent. As a result of complications related to starvation, anorexia nervosa has the highest reported morbidity and mortality rates among all psychiatric illness. Physical problems related to anorexia nervosa involve all body systems. Man-

ifestations include osteoporosis, cardiac arrhythmias, renal failure, endocrine imbalances such as hypothyroidism, skeletal complications due to loss of bone density, hematological changes, gastrointestinal complications, and amenorrhea. Anorexia is associated with a mortality rate of 10 to 15 percent (Herzog and Copeland, 1985). In assessing an adolescent who is suspected of having anorexia nervosa, the advanced practice nurse should be aware that three of the hallmarks of the disorder are secretiveness, massive denial that a problem exists, and a resistance to therapy or to any treatment that will lead to weight gain (Halmi, 1983). Clinical findings include complaints of cold intolerance, dizziness, constipation, abdominal discomfort, and bloating. Youngsters with anorexia nervosa often wear multiple layers of clothing and appear younger than their stated age. They present with cachexia, breast atrophy, dry skin, bradycardia, hypotension, alopecia, and facial hair, and they may have edema of their lower extremities. Psychological findings include a co-morbid depressive disorder, but the affective range of expression for anorexic patients is highly variable and they may present with a hypomanic rather than a hypoactive state (Herzog et al., 1985).

Bulimia occurs more typically in later adolescence, usually between the ages of 17 and 25, in young women who are concerned with weight control. Women have been under pressure to be thin for at least 40 years. The concept of psychosocial causation is well documented in eating disorders. Somehow, young girls discover that laxative abuse and vomiting can be a means of weight management and they begin to follow a pattern of binging on large amounts of usually high-calorie, starchy food followed by self-induced vomiting, diuretic or laxative use, vigorous exercise, or fasting (Herzog, 1982). Clinical findings in bulimia are largely dependent on the degree of purging, starvation, dehydration, and electrolyte imbalance (Drewnowski et al., 1988). Bulimics frequently develop salivary gland atrophy, gum recession, erosion of dental enamel, electrolyte imbalances, and esophagitis, but they do not experience amenor-rhea or severe weight loss (Halmi, 1983). Low-weight patients may manifest many of the same signs and symptoms as anorexics. The presence of frank blood in the patient's vomitus may her-ald the presence of a life-threatening gastric or esophageal tear and indicates that the advanced practice nurse must immediately seek profes-sional consultation.

A primary prevention measure would be the nurse becoming proactive in efforts to raise media consciousness and engaging in efforts to counteract the hegemony of thinness. They can also start support groups on high school and col-lege campuses to empower young women to ac-cept the bodies they have, instead of constantly striving to attain an unrealistic ideal.

On the treatment side, it should be noted that anorexia nervosa is an egosyntonic disor-der. Believing that nothing is wrong, young pa-tients do not present themselves for treatment. Most often they are referred for treatment by an adult, either a professional or their parents. The treatment of anorexia nervosa is guided by the severity of the disorder and can include in-patient as well as outpatient treatment. Irrespec-tive of the setting, the treatment program must have a rehabilitation protocol to which all of the treating clinicians agree. The goal of psy-chotherapy with anorexic patients is to help them achieve capacities for self-regulation that are more adaptive than the ones they are presently employing.

Treatment of bulimia nervosa remains controversial because of the complexity of the condition itself as well as the underlying psy-chopathology. All treatment modalities (group therapy, cognitive therapy, inpatient and outpa-tient treatment, and antidepressant medication) have been shown to be effective, but no regimen has been shown to be effective for all patients. Outpatient treatment of eating diseases is dis-cussed in more detail in Chapter 22. Irrespec-tive of the method chosen for treatment, the restoration of a normal eating pattern should al-ways be an initial goal of treatment.

RUNNING AWAY

Up to two million young people in the United States run away from home each year, and an-other 900,000 have no home. Studies indicate than less than 30 percent of children are true run-aways, meaning that they are absent from the family home without the approval of their parents (Shane, 1989). Sixty percent are thrown out ("throwaway kids"), agreed to leave their fami-lies, or were removed by authorities. Most chil-dren had been living with a biological mother before running away and about 40 percent had been living in two-parent families Almost 50 per-cent reported physical or emotional abuse at home and 10 percent reported sexual abuse. Other family problems included serious conflict, drug or alcohol abuse, violence, and poor physical or mental health. Shane (1989) argues that most run-away and homeless adolescents cannot go back to their families because of the high level of severe dysfunction. This group of runaway or throw-away youth is characterized by multiple and over-lapping problems, including substance abuse, drug dealing, prostitution, and a history of legal and mental health interventions (Wolf, 1990). This population is also at significant risk for the development of HIV infections and other sexu-ally transmitted diseases.

GUIDELINES FOR INTERVENTION

Planning and intervention should always involve a multidisciplinary team in order to reduce frag-mentation and offer a collaborative and more holistic approach to patient care. In addition to the professionals, the patient and family must be considered an integral part of the treatment team in order for interventions to be successful. The purpose of interventions can be remedial (to resolve a problem that has already developed), preventive (to develop skills and programs to prevent a specific problem from occurring), or de-velopmental (to educate or increase functioning or coping). Treatment modalities for adolescents include pharmacotherapy and medication management that targets individual symptoms. Pharmacotherapy should be integrated into the treatment plan as an adjunct to psychoeducational behavioral interventions rather than as an alternative to these interventions.

It is uncommon for any single form of therapy to be the only correct one for a particular disorder. Although opinions differ on therapy with adolescents, several generalities are agreed upon, including flexibility of approach, focusing on present functioning, and directiveness and directness, as opposed to interpretation and analysis (Shaffer et al., 1988).

Behavior modification represents a broad approach to treatment that encompasses over 160 different behavioral treatments and treatment variations, including operant conditioning, social skills training, problem-solving skills training, parent management training, and functional family therapy. All of these treatments share a common commitment to operationalization, assessment, and evaluation.

With recent pressures to limit psychotherapy and the time spent in therapy, there has been interest in outcome research regarding short-term psychotherapy. Favorable outcomes were dependent on rapid establishment of rapport, cooperative and warm feelings between family members, positive feelings of hope on the part of the therapist, recognition by the family and client of the time-limited nature of the treatment, and the ability to define a clear treatment focus.

As a result of the challenges of complex child and family pathology, together with the insights that are emerging from clinical and research efforts organized by a family systems perspective, family therapy is beginning to play an important part in the treatment of adolescent problems. Therapists have realized that adolescent turmoil and other symptoms may often be a direct reflection of disturbed family functioning. Although there have been conceptual differences between family therapy and psychiatry, with its focus on the individual and on confidentiality,

promising outcomes have emerged from family research that have significant implications for therapeutic practices with child and adolescent clients (Graham 1991).

Group therapy has also been found to be effective in treating adolescent patients. There is an enormous array of "helping" type groups designed for this age group. They are classified as group psychotherapy, therapeutic groups, human development and training groups, and self help/mutual help groups. Because of fragile adolescent self-images, the selection of teens for groups must be careful. Faced with peer pressures that are inherent in groups, the therapy may in fact confirm adolescents' worst fears about themselves. Groups seem to be most effective for adolescents whose problems manifest themselves primarily in interpersonal difficulties and who show a pattern of withdrawal and isolation or who become involved in gangs that are bound together by destructive behavior.

Summary

Adolescence is a period of development that is characterized by a number of tasks and shifts in learning. It is determined by chronological age as well as a variety of physical, sexual, and emotional factors, and by contextual factors such as historico-socio-cultural influences. A number of theories and models are available to the advanced practice nurse. The use of a conceptual model is useful as a heuristic device and as a guide for systematic assessment, planning, and intervention. Adolescent issues that can cause difficulties and disruptions include a number of high-risk behaviors, such as high-risk sexual activities, substance use and abuse, gang and cult activity, and running away.

Advanced practice nurses can utilize a number of primary, secondary, and tertiary interventions that are useful in working with adolescent populations. These should be underpinned by the nurses' strong sense of awareness of their own histories and responses as well as by data about adolescents' sense of identity, independence-dependence issues, strengths, self-images, impulsivity, sexuality, and support systems. Strategies for working with adolescents include pharmacotherapy; group, individual, and family therapies; psychopharmacology; and behavior modification.

REFERENCES

American Psychiatric Association. *Diagnostic and Statistical Manual of Mental Disorders–IV.* Washington, DC: APA, 1994.

Baumrind D. A developmental perspective on adolescent risk taking in contemporary America. In: Irwin C, ed. *Adolescent Social Behavior and Health.* San Francisco: Jossey Bass: New Directions for Child Development; 1987.

Baumrind D. Familial antecedents of adolescent drug use: A developmental perspective. In: Jones, CL, Battjes RJ, eds. *Etiology of Adolescent Drug Abuse: Implications for Prevention.* NIDA Research Monograph 56. Rockville, MD: National Institute on Drug Abuse; 1985.

Beck AT, Hollon SD, Young JE, et al. Treatment of depression with cognitive therapy and amitriptyline. *Arch Gen Psychiatry.* 1985;42:142–148.

Bell TA, Holmes KK. Age-specific risks of syphilis, gonorrhea and hospitalized pelvic inflammatory disease in sexually experienced U.S. women. *Sex Transmi Dis.* 1984;11:291–295.

Berman AL. *Adolescent Suicide: Assessment and Intervention.* Washington, DC: American Psychological Association; 1991.

Brage D. Adolescent depression: A review of the literature. *Arch Psychiatr Nurs.* 1995;9:45–55.

Brent D, Perper J, Goldstein C, et al. Risk factors for adolescent suicide: A comparison of adolescent suicide victims with suicidal patients. *Arch Gen Psychiatry.* 1988;45:581–588.

Busch KG, Zagar R, Hughes JR, et al. Adolescents who kill. *J Clin Psychol.* 1990;46:472–485.

Cantwell DP, Baker L. Manifestations of depressive affect in adolescents. *J Youth and Adoles.* 1991; 28:681–700.

Centers for Disease Control. Patterns of alcohol use among teenage drivers in fatal motor vehicle accidents: US, 1977–81. *MMWR.* 1983b;32:344–347.

Centers for Disease Control. Alchohol as a risk factor for injuries. *MMWR.* 1983a;32:61–62.

Clark CM. Deviant adolescent subcultures: Assessment strategies and clinical interventions. *Adolescence.* 1992;27:283–293.

Cohen E. HEADSS, a psychosocial risk assessment instrumen. Implications for designing effective intervention for runaway yourth. *J Adolesc Health.* 1991;12:539–544.

Drewnowski A, Yee KD, Krahn DD. Bulimia in college women: Incidence and recovery rates. *Am J Psychiatry.* 1988;145:753–755.

Elliott GR, Feldman SS. Capturing the adolescent experience. In: Elliott, GR, Feldman SS, (eds.) *At the Threshold.* Cambridge, MA: Harvard University Press; 1990.

Freud A. Adolescence. In: *Psychoanalytic Study of the Child.* Vol 13. NY: International Universities Press; 1958:255–278.

Galanter M. *Cults and New Religious Movements.* Washington, DC: American Psychiatric Press; 1989.

Gilligan C. Adolescent development reconsidered. In: Irwin C, ed. *Adolescent Social Behavior and Health.* San Francisco: Jossey-Bass; 1987.

Graham P. *Child psychiatry: a development approach* (2nd ed). New York: Oxford University Press; 1991.

Hall GS. *Adolescence: Its psychology and its relation to psychology, anthropology, sociology, sex, crime, religion and education.* Englewood Cliffs, N.J.: Prentice-Hall; 1904.

Halmi KA. The state of research in anorexia nervosa and bulimia. In: Guze J, Roth M, eds. *Psychiatric Development, Advances and Prospects in Research and Clinical Practice.* New York: Oxford University Press; 1983.

Harford TC, Grant BF. Psychosocial factors in adolescent drinking contexts. *J Stud Alcohol.* 1987; 48:551–557.

Hawkins JD, Lishner DM, Jenson JM, Catalano RF. Delinquents and drugs: What the evidence suggests about prevention and treatment programming. In: Brown BS, Mills AR, eds. *Youth at High Risk for Substance Abuse.* Rockville, MD: National Institute on Drug Abuse, 1987.

Herzog DB. Bulimia: The secretive syndrome. *Psychosomatics.* 1982;23:481–487.

Herzog DB, Copeland PM. Eating disorders. *N Engl J Med.* 1985;313:295–303.

Herzog DB, Pepose M, Norman DK, Rigotti NA. Eating disorders and social maladjustment in female medical students. *J Nerv Mental Dis.* 1985;173: 734–737.

Hofferth SL, Hayes CD. Risking the future: *Adolescent Sexuality, Pregnancy and Childbearing.* Washington, DC: National Academy Press, 1987.

Holinger PC, Offer D, Barter JT, Bell CC. *Suicide and Homicide Among Adolescents.* New York: Guilford Press; 1994.

Howells K, Hollin CR. *Clinical Approaches to Violence.* New York: Wiley; 1989.

Johnston LS, O'Malley PM, Bachman JG. *National Survey Results on Drug Use From the Monitoring the Future Study 1975–1993.* Rockville, MD: National Institute on Drug Abuse; 1994: Pub 94-3809.

Kennedy S, Garfinkel PE. Anorexia nervosa. In: Francis AJ, Hales RE, eds. *American Psychiatric Association Annual Review.* Washington DC: American Psychiatric Press; 1985.

Kovel J. A critique of DSM-III. *Res Law Deviance Social Control.* 1988;9:127–146.

Lewis M. Intensive individual psychodynamic psychotherapy: The therapeutic relationship and the technique of interpretation In: Lewis M, ed. *Child and Adolescent Psychiatry: A Comprehensive Textbook.* Philadelphia: Williams & Wilkins; 1991.

Litt IF. Adolescent Medicine. *JAMA,* 1991;265: 3100–3101.

Litt, IF. Self-graffiti? Self-image? Self destruction? *J Adolesc Health.* 1994;15:198.

Litt IF. Prevention of substance abuse, *J Adol Health,* 1996;18:58–65.

McCord J. Deterrence and the light touch of the law. In: Farrington DP, Gunn J, eds. *Reactions to Crime: The Public, the Police Courts and Prisons.* London: Wiley; 1988.

McCord J. Consideration of some effects of a counseling program. In: Martin WE, Sechrest LB, Redner R, eds. *New Directions in the Rehabilitation of Criminal Offenders.* Washington, DC: National Academy of Sciences; 1981.

McNamara D. Gang violence and the street smart nurse. *J Commun Health Nurs.* 1994;11:193–200.

Mercer NS. Tattoos. Marked for life. *Br Med J.* 1991; 303:389.

Millstein SG, Irwin CE. Accident-related behaviors in adolescents: A biopsychosocial view. *Alcohol Drugs Driving.* 1988;4:21–29.

Mishne JM. *Clinical Work With Adolescents.* New York: Free Press; 1986.

Mohr WK. The private psychiatric hospital scandal: A critical social approach. *Arch Psychiatr Nurs.* 1994; 8:3–8.

Newcomb MD, Maddahian E, Bentler PM. Risk factors for drug use among adolescents: Concurrent and longitudinal analysis. *Am J Public Health.* 1986; 76:525–531.

Nicholi AM. The adolescent. In: Nicholi AM, ed. *The New Harvard Guide to Psychiatry.* Cambridge, MA: Harvard University Press; 1988.

Novello AC. Violence is a greater killer of children than disease. *Public Health Rep.* 1991;106:231–232.

Pipkin NL, Walker LG, Thomason MH. Alcohol and vehicular injuries in adolescents. *J Adolesc Health Care.* 1989;10:119–121.

Pynoos RS, Nader K. Case study: Children's memory and proximity to violence. *Am Acad Child Adolesc Psychiatry.* 1989;28:236–241.

Rutter M, Graham P, Chadwick OFD, Yule W. Adolescent turmoil: Fact or fiction? *J Child Psychol Psychiatr.* 1976;17:35–56.

Schwartz IM. Hospitalization of adolescents for psychiatric and substance abuse treatment. *J Adolesc Health Care.* 1989;10:1–6.

Schwartz IM, Jackson-Beeck M, Anderson R. The hidden system of juvenile control. *Crime Delinquency.* 1984;30:371–385.

Semlitz L, Gold MS. Adolescent drug abuse: Diagnosis, treatment and prevention. *Psychiatr Clin North Am.* 1986;9:455–473.

Shaffer D. Preventing suicide in young people. *Innovations Res.* 1993;2:3–9.

Shaffer D, Blain B, Beck A, et al. Chlamydia trachomatis: Important relationships to race, contraceptive use, lower genital tract infection and Papanicolaou smears. *J Pediatr.* 1984;104:141–146.

Shaffer D, Garland A, Gould M, et al. Preventing teenage suicide: A critical review. *J Am Acad Child Adolesc Psychiatry.* 1988;27:675–687.

Shaffer D, Schwab-Stone M, Fisher PF, et al. The Diagnostic Interview Schedule for Children, revised version: Preparation, field testing, interrater reliability and acceptability. *J Am Acad Child Adolesc Psychiatry.* 1993;32:643–650.

Shane PG. Changing patterns among homeless and runaway youth. *Am J Orthopsychiatry.* 1989;59: 208–214.

Short JF. New wine in old bottles? Change and continuity in American gangs. In: Huff CR, ed. *Gangs in America*. Newbury Park, CA: Sage; 1990.

Sloan G, Leichner P. Is there a relationship between sexual abuse or incest and eating disorders? *Can J Psychiatry*. 1986;31:656–660.

Spitz AM, Velebil P, Koonin LM, Strauss LT, Goodman KA, Wingo P, Wilson JB, Morris L, Marks JS. Pregnancy, abortion, and birth rates among U.S. adolescents—1980, 1985, and 1990. *JAMA*. 1996; 275:989–94.

Steinberg J. Single parents, step parents and the susceptibility of adolescents to antisocial peer pressure. *Child Development*. 1987;58:269–275.

Strathern A, Strathern M. *Self-decoration in Mount Hagen*. London: Lippincott; 1971.

Teri L. Depression in adolescence: Its relationship to assertion and various aspects of self-image. *J Clin Child Psychol*. 1982;13:475–487.

Thompson EA, Moody KA, Eggert LL. Discriminating suicide ideation among high-risk youth. *J School Health*. 1994;64:361–367.

Uhlenberg P, Eggebeen D. The declining well-being of American adolescents. *Public Interest*. 1986; 82:25–38.

U.S. Department of Health and Human Services. *Healthy People 2000: National Health Promotion and Disease Prevention Objectives*. Washington, DC: Public Health Services; 1991.

Vieland V, Whittle B, Garland A, et al. The impact of curriculum-based suicide prevention programs for teenagers: An 18-month follow-up. *J Am Acad Child Adolesc Psychiatry*. 1991;30:811–815.

Weithorn LA. Mental hospitalization of troublesome youth: An analysis of skyrocketing admission rates. *Stanford Law Rev*. 1988;40:753, 773–838.

Weithorn LA, Campbell SB. The competency of children and adolescents to make informed treatment decisions. *Child Devel*. 1982;53:1589–1598.

Williams R (ed). *Klanwatch: A project of the Southern Povery Law Center*. Montgomery, AL; 1989.

Wilson MD, Joffe A. Adolescent medicine. *JAMA*. 1995;273:1657–1659.

Wolf S. The health care needs of homeless and runaway youths. *JAMA*. 1990;263:811.

Wolfgang ME, Figlio RM, Sellin T. *Delinquency in a Birth Cohort*. Chicago: University of Chicago Press; 1972.

Worchel F, Nolan B, Wilson V. New perspectives on child and adolescent depression. *J School Psychol*. 1987;25:411–414.

CHAPTER 20

PARAPHILIC DISORDERS

Shelly Lurie

*C*ognitive distortions are common in the paraphilic population. The two most frequently identified cognitive distortions are denial and rationalization. Others to be assessed for are intellectualization and minimalization.

Chapter Overview

► INTRODUCTION

Paraphiliacs experience recurrent, intense, unusual sexual thoughts and erotic fantasies about engaging in inappropriate sexual activity. Such activity may involve inappropriate sexual partners or unusual objects for sexual arousal. The frequent occurrence of these sexually arousing thoughts over a 6-month period will often lead the individual to engage in paraphilic activity. Paraphilic thoughts and activities frequently interfere with the individual's level of functioning at some time. The aforementioned are the diagnostic features that must be present to formulate a paraphilic diagnosis (APA, 1994).

By virtue of heightened media exposure, society has become more aware of the presence of paraphilic activities in the community. In the past, rarely did one hear or read about paraphilic activity in a school system or a house of worship.

The advanced practice nurse psychotherapist may become involved in diagnosing and treating individuals who are currently or have in the past engaged in various inappropriate (eroticized) sexual behaviors and activities. This chapter discusses the psychiatric syndrome of paraphilic disorders, previously referred to as sexual deviations.

EPIDEMIOLOGIC CONSIDERATIONS

The prevalence of sexual disorders (paraphilias) is difficult to determine because the frequency with which men and women engage in paraphilic activity may be unreported or undiagnosed. DSM-IV notes there may be more of these individuals in today's society than acknowledged by the general population (APA, 1994).

FORMULATION OF A DIFFERENTIAL DIAGNOSIS OF PARAPHILIA

Diagnostic assessment is frequently one of the most difficult aspects of working with an individual who is engaging in eroticized behaviors. The advanced practice nurse psychotherapist should assess the individual from a holistic perspective. Presenting behaviors need to be assessed with consideration of three elements: the inappropriate behaviors, their impact on others, and motivational factors that may precipitate the acts. These elements are further defined in Table 20–1.

The advanced practice nurse psychotherapist who is conducting an initial intake must also explore other areas relevant to the formulation of a paraphilic diagnosis. Information should be obtained regarding the patient's family history, social position, home atmosphere, personal history, medical history, previous psychiatric history, and history of present illness. A current mental status assessment should be performed as well. Assessments performed in these areas will provide pertinent data needed to establish a differential diagnosis and formulate a diagnosis of a paraphilic disorder. Table 20–2 indicates specific content to be obtained in each of the areas.

FAMILY HISTORY

When eliciting information regarding the patient's family history, it is important to consider not only the family health history (neurological,

TABLE 20–1. THREE ELEMENTS TO BE CONSIDERED WHEN ASSESSING FOR PARAPHILIC ACTIVITY

Presence of Sexually Arousing Behaviors
- Watching ("peeping") an unsuspecting stranger who is naked or engaged in sexual activity or disrobing (voyeurism).
- Exposing one's genitals to an unsuspecting person (exhibitionism).
- Sexual activity with a prepubescent (under the age of 13) child (pedophilia).
- Sexual activity with a postpubescent (ages 13 to 18) teenager who is developing secondary sex characteristics (ephebophilia).
- Sexual activity with animals (zoophilia).
- The infliction of pain, humiliation, or suffering onto another individual (sexual sadism).
- The infliction of or receipt of pain, humiliation, or suffering onto oneself (sexual masochism).
- Rubbing up against an unsuspecting stranger (frotteurism).
- The use of objects, such as black leather, silk lingerie, rubber sheeting (fetishism).
- Heterosexual males who cross-dress in female clothing for sexual arousal (transvestic fetishism).

Impact of Sexually Arousing Behaviors on Others
- Directly (victim).
- Indirectly (family).

Motivational Factors That May Have Precipitated Paraphilic Activity
- Psychotic symptomatology: hallucinations/delusions.
- Intoxication from ingestion of or withdrawal from drugs, alcohol, or other substances.
- Disregard for rights of others and a lack of appreciation of social boundaries.

Adapted from American Psychiatric Association (1994).

psychiatric, and medical) but also the quality of the relationships the patient has with family members. The patient's description of the quality of the relationship(s) he or she has with parents can be significant.

The nurse psychotherapist should consider how family relationships may have affected the patient in regard to paraphilic desires. It is important to note family relationships that allude to issues of power and control or expectations of perfection. Inquiry should also include an assessment of current or previous physical, emotional, sexual, or verbal abuse as well as early childhood neglect. Groth (1979) suggests that individuals who have been sexually abused during childhood may be at risk for developing a paraphilic disorder.

Information regarding parental role modeling may be significant to the diagnostic formulation. Parkin (1963) noted cases in which paraphilic behavior, including exhibitionism, voyeurism, and fetishism, was modeled directly after a parent's behavior. Biller (1971) studied the influence of the father on the male child's sense of identity

and found that the portion of the father's behavior the boy directly observes is the most significant in terms of his masculine development.

In discussing the neurological health history of the patient's family, one needs to be cognizant of disorders that present with symptomatology that may include sexually inappropriate behaviors. One such disorder is Tourette's syndrome, whereby the patient may present with sexually inappropriate behaviors and profane language with sexual content (APA, 1994).

Family psychiatric health history may be significant if there is a history of sexual abuse or a family member with a paraphilic diagnosis or an axis I diagnosis, such as schizophrenia, bipolar disorder, or substance use disorder, with the presence of psychotic symptoms.

Information regarding the patient's socioeconomic class may be helpful in gaining a better understanding of the patient. Inquiry about the patient's type of housing and the persons living in the home may assist in the identification of patient needs. Significant events occurring in the home will have an effect on the patient as well.

TABLE 20–2. INFORMATION TO BE OBTAINED FOR DIAGNOSTIC FORMULATION

Family Health History
- Relationship to the patient
- Health history: neurological, psychiatric, medical

Social Position and Home Atmosphere
- Socioeconomic class
- Type of housing
- Persons living in the home
- Significant events at home
- Emotional relationships of family members

Personal History
- Educational history
- Occupational history
- Living situation
- Sexual inclinations and practice
- History of victimization
- Marital history
- Children
- Nicotine/alcohol/substance use
- Legal history/current legal status
- Religious affiliation and interest
- Cultural variables

Medical History

Previous Psychiatric History

History of Present Illness
- Patient's level of insight
- Presence of cognitive distortions
- Victim empathy
- Changes in relationships

Mental Status Assessment

Penile Plethysmography

Significant events may be defined as changes in residence or lifestyle, employment status, terminal illness of a family member, and death of a family member.

It is important for the advanced nurse psychotherapist to ascertain the quality of familial relationships within the home. The nurse therapist should elicit the patient's description of relationships with parents and other family members living in the home, and should note the presence of conflictual relationships. If conflictual relationships are present, the nurse therapist needs to consider how these may have affected the patient in terms of paraphilic activity.

PERSONAL HISTORY

Information about the patient's personal history will provide most of the data that will determine the psychiatric diagnosis. The nurse therapist begins this inquiry with the gathering of details about the patient's academic performance. This should include information about the patient's grades, presence of learning disabilities, and the quality of relationships with teachers and classmates.

The patient's occupational history is also important data to obtain, particularly facts about the patient's current employment functioning and past history. The patient's present living situation should also be evaluated. Information regarding the family's sleeping arrangements and bathroom privacy may be significant. It is important to ask questions regarding any incestuous activities that may have occurred. The patient's level of instability regarding these areas should also be noted. Other areas to be explored are the patient's birth history, developmental milestones and the presence of unusual or abnormal childhood behaviors, such as enuresis. If the patient is a female, data must be obtained regarding her menstrual history.

When gathering information to be included in the formulation of an accurate diagnosis, the nurse psychotherapist will also want to assess the patient's habits concerning smoking, drinking, illicit substance use, and misuse of prescription medications. Ingestion of illicit substances or alcohol may decrease inhibitions and increase impulsivity, thereby increasing the potential for paraphilic activity.

While addressing the patient from a holistic perspective, it is necessary to also inquire about the patient's religious affiliations and interests. Religious beliefs may contribute to guilt, shame, and remorse, as well as to self-esteem issues.

A chronological account of the patient's medical history may affect the formulation of a paraphilic diagnosis. Of particular interest would be the presence of genitourinary difficulties or surgery, or testicular accidents. It is important to assess for brain injury targeting damage to the frontal lobe, which may cause the patient to become hypersexual. Knowledge of the patient's medication history may be significant, especially if medications present with side effects that affect areas related to sexuality. Thyroxine, for example, has been reported to enhance one's sexual desires. Medication side effects may also affect the patient's sexuality on a physiological level. For example, impotence may occur as a side effect of hypertensive treatment with alpha methyldopa.

A previous psychiatric history may contribute significantly to the diagnostic formulation of a paraphilic disorder. It is vital to obtain information as to whether the patient has received psychiatric inpatient or outpatient treatments, as well as to identify previous diagnoses and treatment regimes. The nurse psychotherapist should also inquire about the length of time the patient received treatment and about the patient's level of compliance and effectiveness of treatment regimes.

SEXUAL INTAKE EVALUATION

Before addressing the patient's sexual inclinations and practices, it is paramount for the advanced practice nurse psychotherapist to understand how to conduct a sexual intake evaluation. The nurse therapist must be cognizant of his or her own values, beliefs, attitudes, and conflicts, and must possess the ability to remain nonjudgmental of the patient being evaluated. Knowledge of state laws regarding mandatory reporting and confidentiality must be current, and the nurse therapist needs to inform the patient of these prior to the beginning of the assessment. Paraphilic patients generally will not voluntarily offer information necessary to assist the nurse therapist in formulating a paraphilic diagnosis; therefore, it becomes the responsibility of the advanced practice nurse psychotherapist to guide the intake in such a fashion as to obtain all necessary information.

During the sexual intake evaluation, the nurse therapist should use open-ended questions and follow up with direct questioning when further clarification is needed. The therapist should ask questions that specifically pertain to the patient's presenting behaviors. For example, in addressing the pedophilic patient, one might not want to ask questions regarding exhibitionistic or voyeuristic activities.

The data to be obtained during a sexual intake may include when and how the patient first learned about sex and who "taught" the patient; a description of the type of sexual play during childhood; the patient's age at the first sexual encounter and the type of encounter; information about the patient's partner and the patient's thoughts and feelings about the experience; age of first sexual intercourse experience and the type of intercourse (same sex or opposite sex partner, mutual consent or coercive); type and frequency of masturbatory activities; presence and content of sexual or erotic fantasies; and the history and type of inappropriate sexual activity.

Groth (1979) suggested that patients with a history of sexual victimization may be predisposed to develop a paraphilic disorder; therefore, it is imperative for the nurse psychotherapist to question the patient about victimization. It is important to assess for history of sexual, physical, and emotional abuse. This information may have already been obtained via earlier inquiry about family history.

Another component of the diagnostic assessment is the patient's marital history. If the patient has been married more than once or involved in other ongoing sexual relationships, the nurse therapist will need to elicit details about these relationships as well. Of importance is information regarding the duration of acquaintance(s) prior to marriage; parental attitudes regarding the patient's choice of partner; patient's statement of compatibility and sexual satisfaction with his or her partner(s); and the current status of the patient's marital relationship. If the patient has children, a chronological account of the children should be obtained, including ages, a description of the quality of relationships the patient has with them, and whether there is any history of abuse.

As previously stated, it is important to pay attention to possible etiologic factors that may precipitate paraphilic activity. Table 20–1 lists these factors and defines several paraphilic disorders.

LEGAL HISTORY

During the assessment, it is not uncommon to discover that the individual is seeking psychiatric services as a result of having been charged with a sexual offense. These individuals, referred to as sex offenders, may appear for an evaluation upon attorney referral. Due to the sensitive nature of the disorder and the presence of cognitive distortions, very few paraphiliacs voluntarily present themselves for evaluation and treatment of inappropriate sexual behaviors (APA, 1994). The existence and knowledge of mandatory reporting laws also affects the number of patients who will voluntarily seek treatment for recurrent inappropriate sexual thoughts or activity (Berlin et al., 1991).

A legal history of a paraphilic patient must include the number of prior arrests that involve the presenting behaviors, details of the current charges, and the status of these charges along with possible outcomes, if known. A possible outcome may be a suspended sentence or being placed on work release. The nurse psychotherapist also needs to assess whether all arrests were sexual crimes or if the patient was charged with other crimes, such as breaking and entering.

PATIENT'S PRESENT ILLNESS

The next part of the diagnostic assessment addresses the history of the patient's present illness and begins with the patient's acknowledgment of his or her paraphilic behavior(s). Often, the individual with a paraphilic disorder does not readily, if at all, acknowledge engaging in sexually inappropriate behaviors, or that these behaviors are indeed inappropriate.

Cognitive distortions are common in the paraphilic population. The two most frequently identified cognitive distortions are denial and rationalization. Others to be assessed for are intellectualization and minimalization (McCarthy, 1994).

The advanced practice nurse psychotherapist must also assess the patient for the presence of victim empathy. The paraphilic patient who is assessed as being ego-dystonic is disturbed by inappropriate sexual (eroticized) thoughts, desires, and activity and may be able to acknowledge the impact of the inappropriate sexual behavior on a victim. These patients are more likely to be remorseful and to experience feelings of guilt and shame. In contrast, a patient who is assessed as being ego-syntonic is not bothered by his or her paraphilic behaviors and, most often, does not express empathy towards the victim(s) (APA, 1980). Ego-syntonic patients are usually more difficult to treat and may be at a higher risk for treatment noncompliance.

When assessing the patient's present illness, it is also important to elicit information regarding the patient's ability to form or maintain age-appropriate relationships. The nurse therapist will also want to know how the patient perceives the effects of his or her paraphilic activities on current relationships with others.

As always, when performing a psychiatric intake for the purpose of diagnostic formulation, the advanced practice nurse psychotherapist must include a mental status assessment. The mental status assessment includes information in the following areas: general behavior and appearance; characteristics of talk; emotional state (mood and affect); nature of thought experiences; orientation; memory; intellectual functioning; and patient's level of insight and judgement (Trzepacz and Baker, 1993).

Occasionally the data collected from the diagnostic assessment are not sufficient or conclusive to form a paraphilic diagnosis. Penile plethysmography is a diagnostic aid that is used in determining a patient's sexual arousal pattern and level of sexual arousal (Simon and Schouten,

1991). This may be helpful in formulating a paraphilic diagnosis when the patient presents with cognitive distortions, and may reveal what arouses the patient and to what extent.

PARAPHILIC TREATMENT

Once a paraphilic diagnosis has been formulated, the advanced practice nurse psychotherapist needs to develop an individualized plan of treatment for the patient. Table 20–3 identifies various forms of treatment commonly used in the treatment of the paraphilic patient and target symptomatology.

The nurse therapist makes recommendations for treatment based upon all of the data collected during the diagnostic assessment. The treatment recommended by the nurse therapist must be patient specific.

When determining what form of treatment may produce the best results for the patient, the advanced practice nurse therapist needs to be cognizant of the presenting problems or symptoms, patient's level of motivation, and level of risk. The therapist also needs to assess the patient's expectations of treatment and determine if they are reasonable.

DESIRED PARAPHILIC TREATMENT OUTCOMES

The nurse psychotherapist must have knowledge of the paraphilic patient's care needs and be able to design a treatment plan that will meet those needs. The treatment provided should assist the patient in reaching identified outcomes. These outcomes must, at the very least, consist of acknowledgment of paraphilic behaviors; development of victim empathy, or confronting cognitive distortions; decreasing or stopping the frequency or intensity of paraphilic ideation or behaviors; identification of internal and external factors that lead to paraphilic activity (triggers); and the development of appropriate

relapse prevention strategies (safeguards) to avoid recidivism (Berlin et al., 1991a)

The literature contains many articles addressing efficacy of treating the paraphilic patient with anti-androgen medications in conjunction with group psychotherapy with a specific focus on the paraphilias (Berlin, 1991; Federoff et al., 1992, Kravitz et al., 1995) This is not to say that this treatment regimen will cure the patient or avoid, with certainty, sexual recidivism.

PHARMACOTHERAPIES

Federoff and associates (1992) reported that paraphilic patients who have attended and participated in group therapy dealing with issues common to the paraphilic population, and who have received antiandrogen medications, tend to improve more than those patients receiving a single form of treatment, such as specialized paraphilic group therapy. Adjunctive treatment of the paraphilic patient may be more beneficial than other forms of treatment.

Pharmacotherapies primarily used in the adjunctive treatment of paraphilic disorders consist of antiandrogen (testosterone-lowering) medications (Berlin et al., 1995, Maletzsky, 1991). These medications may provide the patient with a form of external control by lowering testosterone to a prepubescent level, which may result in a decrease in the frequency and intensity of paraphilic desires. Two commonly used anti-androgen medications are medroxyprogesterone acetate (Depo-Provera) and leuprolide acetate (Lupron Depot).

Paraphilic treatment with Depo-Provera usually starts at 500 mg intramuscularly every week. Dosing, titration, or discontinuation of this medication is based upon the patient's level of progress and/or the presence and type of side effects. Patients have reported a noticeable decrease in the frequency and intensity of inappropriate sexual desires when receiving Depo-Provera. Patients have also related they find themselves less focused on paraphilic thinking and are better able to control their behavior. In essence, Depo-Provera affords the

TABLE 20–3. THERAPEUTIC TREATMENT MODALITIES RELATED TO PARAPHILIC SYMPTOMATOLOGY

	Paraphilic Treatment Modalities								Desired Paraphilic Treatment Outcomes
			Behavioral Therapies						
Paraphilic Symptomatology	Antiandrogen Medications[a]	SSRIs/ Anti-obsessional Medications	Insight-oriented Therapy	Aversion Therapy	Cognitive Restructuring	Thought Blocking	SLAA (Sex & Love Addicts Anonymous)	Paraphilic Group Therapy/ Psychoeducation[a]	
Intense/frequent paraphilic thoughts/desires	x	x		x		x		x	Decreased intensity/ frequency of paraphilic ideation
Lack of control over paraphilic ideation/activity	x	x	x	x		x		x	Increased control; absence of paraphilic activity
Obsessive sexual preoccupation (noneroticized) and compulsive sexual behavior		x						x	Decreased obsessive-compulsive sexual behaviors
Lack of insight regarding paraphilic behavior			x	x	x	x	x	x	Cognizant of paraphilic disorder, symptomatology, and need to avoid engaging in paraphilic activity
Lack of victim empathy (ego-syntonic)					x			x	Ability to relate possible effect of paraphilic activity on the victim(s)
Presence of cognitive distortions					x			x	Development of appropriate, adaptive cognition; absence of cognitive distortions

Nursing Diagnosis					Outcome Criteria
Knowledge deficit regarding: • Identification of stimuli ("triggers") • Need for relapse prevention strategies ("safeguards")	X	X	X	X	Identification of triggers and development of appropriate relapse prevention strategies to avoid recidivism
Lack of assertiveness	X			X	Demonstrated utilization of assertiveness techniques
Inability to formulate/maintain "healthy" relationships	X			X	Increased awareness of altered relationship patterns and identification of appropriate methods to improve same
Ineffective coping skills	X			X	Development of appropriate coping strategies
Grieving (potential) loss of: • Family/friends support • Finances • Employment • Liberty • Self-esteem/self-respect • Paraphilic behaviors	X			X	Acceptance of current life situation

[a] Adjunctive treatment preferred.

► CASE EXAMPLE

Sam is a 43-year-old man who never married. He is the leader of a scout troop that consists of 10 young males ages 9 to 11. He lives alone and has been described by his neighbors as a loner who doesn't seem to socialize with adults, but is seen as a caring, nurturing guy with his scouts. He was recently charged with a fourth-degree sexual offense involving mutual masturbation, genital fondling, and nude photography of 6 of the 10 scouts in his troop. This was Sam's first arrest and he was released on his own recognizance. The patient appeared for an evaluation of a paraphilic disorder at the request of his attorney, preparatory to sentencing.

A comprehensive diagnostic assessment revealed Sam had been engaging in pedophilic activity "ever since I can remember." Sam further reported, "I didn't do anything wrong. I didn't force my scouts and they never seemed frightened and seemed to like it. The same was done to me by my father and my uncles when I was a kid. So, were they wrong, too?"

Sam's diagnosis is homosexual pedophilia: exclusive type. His evaluation also revealed a lack of victim empathy and the presence of cognitive distortions consisting of denial, rationalization, and minimalization. He had never been evaluated for a paraphilic disorder, and hence never received treatment.

After an intensive 3-week inpatient psychiatric admission on the sexual disorders unit, Sam will begin weekly outpatient group therapy. The sexual disorders group is based upon insight-oriented therapy to address the identification of triggers and development of safeguards. Outpatient treatment will also include behavioral therapy, specifically cognitive restructuring and thought blocking. Pharmacotherapy will involve the medication medroxyprogesterone acetate (Depo-Provera) 500 mg, to be given intramuscularly every week.

---

patient the opportunity to develop his or her own internal controls to avoid engaging in paraphilic activity by lowering the sex drive, thereby possibly lowering the risk.

The nurse therapist needs to be cognizant of the nontherapeutic side effects that do exist and may precipitate other difficulties for the patient. Patients have reported an inability to obtain and/or maintain an erection. This sometimes has created difficulties with the quality of appropriate sexual relations with an appropriate partner. If difficulties occur, reassessment of the risks versus the benefits of continued treatment with antiandrogen medications would be required. Depo-Provera, because of its testosterone-lowering properties, also reduces sperm production, and thus may create the possibility that the paraphilic patient may not be able to reproduce. This, too, may become problematic for the patient. However, clinical experience has shown a few cases where men receiving Depo-Provera as part of paraphilic treatment have been able to father "normal," healthy offspring (Meyer et al., 1985).

Common side effects noted in paraphilic patients receiving Depo-Provera are weight gain and hypertension (Bradford, 1993). Some patients have reported experiencing intermittent night sweats and nightmares. There have been a few reported cases of the development of gynecomastia as a result of treatment with Depo-Provera; however, these side effects are not well documented.

The nurse therapist, knowing that a possible side effect of paraphilic treatment with Depo-Provera may be hypertension, will want to monitor the patient's blood pressure prior to medication administration, and may find it prudent to hold the medication if the diastolic reading is greater than 100 mm Hg. In this case, the nurse therapist will want to evaluate or initiate the appropriate referral for evaluation of the patient regarding elevated blood pressure readings.

The therapist needs to assess the benefits versus the risks to the hypertensive patient for continuing treatment with Depo-Provera. This needs to be done on a case-by-case basis and is based upon the expert clinical judgment of the nurse therapist.

Leuprolide acetate (Lupron Depot) is a relatively new antiandrogen medication being used in the treatment of paraphilic disorders. A review of the literature shows a lack of double-blind controlled studies regarding the use of this medication in the treatment of paraphilic disorders; studies in this area would be warranted. The recommended starting dose of Lupron Depot as a form of paraphilic treatment is 7.5 mg intramuscularly once a month (Riley et al., 1993). Initially, treatment with Lupron Depot causes an increase in testosterone production, which could cause a temporary increase in the patient's sex drive. Therefore, it is recommended that the nurse therapist also prescribe concurrent treatment with Flutamide 250 mg orally, three times a day (Riley et al., 1993). Flutamide acts to block testosterone receptors, thereby preventing the potential for a temporary increase in the patient's sex drive. This medication should be given during the first 2 weeks of starting treatment with Lupron Depot.

Lupron Depot decreases testosterone levels and can precipitate similar side effects as identified with Depo-Provera. The desired effect of treatment with Lupron Depot is a decrease in the patient's sex drive. A review of the literature revealed documentation addressing a correlation between testosterone levels at prepubescent or very low levels and a decrease in libido (Hucker and Bain, 1990). An individual who has an elevated testosterone level may not necessarily be suffering from a paraphilic disorder.

Antiandrogen medications can be costly for the paraphilic patient. The nurse psychotherapist may want to prescribe a monthly injection of Lupron Depot as opposed to a weekly injection of Depo-Provera due to the invasive properties inherent in the administration of intramuscular injections. The nurse psychotherapist must be sensitive to the patient's financial status as it relates to ability to pay for this medication. In today's market, the cost of Depo-Provera is significantly lower than that of a monthly injection of Lupron Depot. This tends to be the primary, if not the only, reason that Lupron Depot is not prescribed with as much frequency as Depo-Provera as part of an adjunctive treatment plan for the paraphilic patient.

A few single case reports have recently been documented that explore the use of selective serotonin reuptake inhibitors (SSRIs) in the treatment of paraphilic disorders (Bradford and Gratzner, 1995; Kafka, 1995). This may be based upon the idea that there are similarities between the paraphilias and obsessive-compulsive disorders. For example, a patient diagnosed with telephone scatalogia (obscene phone calling) may find their recurrent, intense, erotic sexual thoughts and fantasies to be unwanted and interfering with his or her level of functioning, similar to that of a typist's obsessive-compulsive handwashing. This patient may relate that he or she cannot stop these thoughts and may report intense urges that lead to engaging in paraphilic activity.

If the therapist has assessed the patient's sexual behavior as obsessive in nature and the patient has reported feeling driven (compelled) to engage in inappropriate sexual activity, one could easily understand the idea of treating this patient with SSRIs or antiobsessional medications such as clomipramine.

A review of the literature revealed a few single case reports addressing the treatment of exhibitionism, voyeurism, sexual masochism, transvestic fetishism, paraphilic coercive disorder, pedophilia, and frotteurism with fluoxetine (Prozac) or sertraline (Zoloft). Currently, there are no documented outcome or double-blind placebo-controlled studies that address the efficacy of paraphilic treatment with SSRIs.

It would be wise for the nurse psychotherapist to remember that the frequent, intense sexual thoughts experienced by a paraphilic patient are eroticized in nature. Therefore, consideration should be given to adjunctive treatment of the paraphilic patient with antiandrogen medications versus SSRIs by virtue of the testosterone-lowering effects of antiandrogen medications. Further clinical trials will help determine the efficacy of these medications effective for patients.

VOLUNTARY CASTRATION

Voluntary castration, another treatment option, remains a controversial issue. Incarcerated sexual offenders such as rapists or fixated pedophiles have requested castration secondary to their fear of recidivism upon release. These inmates must undergo a comprehensive evaluation and seek legal counsel to assist them in making an informed decision.

COLLABORATIVE RELATIONSHIPS

Adjunctive treatment of a paraphiliac may also involve collateral therapists, such as a spouse's therapist or the family internist, who may be prescribing medications for medical reasons. Therefore, it is of importance for the advanced practice nurse psychotherapist to be aware of other therapies and treatment in which the patient is engaged.

The nurse therapist must obtain the patient's permission to exchange information with collateral practitioners. This may be done by requesting that the patient sign a release of information document that will permit collaborative relationships. This will allow for communications with others involved in the care of the patient and will promote a holistic approach to the patient's treatment.

As stated previously, individuals may seek psychiatric services as a result of being arrested and charged with a sexual offense. Depending upon the sentence received, the nurse therapist may become involved in a collaborative relationship with the department of parole and probation. Probation officers will want to know if the patient attends and participates in assigned treatment(s) and how he or she is doing in terms of progress, risk of relapse, or actual recidivism.

ETHICAL AND LEGAL ISSUES

The need for the nurse psychotherapist to be acutely aware of the individual state laws that affect the sexual offender cannot be emphasized enough. These laws may address confidentiality, mandatory reporting, and sexual offender registration and neighborhood notification of a sexual offender's return to the community ("Megan's law"). It is critical to have this fund of knowledge when working with the paraphilic population. As of April 1996, 47 states had sexual offender registration laws and 30 had sexual offender public notification laws (Freeman-Longo, 1996).

It is also wise to familiarize oneself to the laws governing forensic psychiatry regarding issues related to criminal responsibility and level of dangerousness. When performing a psychiatric evaluation for the presence of a paraphilic disorder, the nurse psychotherapist must inform the patient of the nonconfidential nature of the evaluation and its potential uses. The patient also needs to know that copies of the evaluation may be sent to the patient's attorney, state's attorney, and perhaps the judge. The therapist should be certain to elicit evidence of comprehension that the patient understood this confidentiality warning and to document this in the evaluation.

Mandatory reporting laws have taken their toll on the diagnosing and treatment of individuals with a potential paraphilic disorder. During outpatient group therapy, the nurse psychotherapist will want to emphasize the importance of patients' candidness in an effort to provide the best possible treatment. Prior to the onset of mandatory reporting laws, patients were encouraged to report any difficulties they might be experiencing in their ability to control paraphilic thoughts and desires, as well as any sexual recidivistic activity.

The existence of mandatory reporting laws has made it more difficult for the nurse therapist to effectively treat the paraphilic patient from a preventive perspective. For example, take a heterosexual pedophile who informs the therapist of touching the bottom of a 5-year-old girl while swimming in the community pool, but who was not "caught." There has been no report filed and no charges pending. Surely the nurse therapist would want to know this information. The therapist may then recommend hospitalization for the patient so that he can receive more intensive psychiatric treatment, thereby promoting societal safety by removing the patient from the community. This action would potentially decrease the possibility of further sexual recidivism.

Knowledge of the obligation to report such occurrences has greatly affected honest, open communications between the therapist and the pedophilic patient (Berlin et al., 1991). Think of it this way—what pedophilic patient would voluntarily admit to committing a sexual crime, knowing that the consequences of this disclosure may be further involvement in the criminal justice system? Furthermore, if pedophiles are hindered from disclosing critical information, how does the nurse psychotherapist provide effective treatment to that patient?

The neighborhood notification law, known as Megan's Law, has received much recent media exposure. It became part of the federal crime bill passed in 1994 and mandates that convicted sexual offenders, upon release or when moving into a neighborhood, must register themselves with the local authorities for the purposes of notifying the community of the patient's release. The management of this registration and notification remain unsettled and many states continue to work out the logistics. Currently, there are no federally mandated criteria regarding notification, which is presently based upon the judgment of the local authorities as to who will be notified and how. This requirement may present problems for the paraphilic patient who is returning to the community.

To date, there have been a few documented reports of vigilante actions toward sexual offenders who have returned to the community. In one state where there is community notification, a house in which a heterosexual pedophile was to live was burnt down (AP Wire, 1993). In another report, an innocent victim, staying in the same home as a heterosexual pedophile, was beaten in his sleep by two intruders who mistook this person as the offender (Nordheimer, 1995). The possibility of such incidents should not go unnoticed and the nurse therapist needs to be prepared to address this issue, should it arise.

NURSE PSYCHOTHERAPIST AS EXPERT WITNESS

The advanced practice nurse psychotherapist may be called upon by the patient's attorney to offer expert testimony on behalf of the patient. The judge, in an effort to recognize the nurse therapist as an expert witness, may ask the therapist to explain the types of degrees or credentials held, title, and the extent of clinical practice in the specialty of paraphilic disorders. The judge will use this information to determine the therapist's level of competency to serve as an expert witness.

There are several "rules" that the advanced nurse psychotherapist must pay attention to when testifying in a court of law (Table 20–4).

TABLE 20–4. RULES FOR THE ADVANCED NURSE PSYCHOTHERAPIST WHEN TESTIFYING AS AN EXPERT WITNESS

- You are the expert and will always know more about the paraphilias than others in the courtroom. If you become nervous, stop and remind yourself that you are the expert!
- You MUST be prepared! Preparation may include a review of the patient's medical records and the case itself, a practice session giving your answers out loud, and making notations on what you are going to say in your testimony.
- Dress in conservative clothing (a suit) and do not wear flashy jewelry. You will want the content of your testimony to be the most lasting impression on the person(s) listening to you.
- Avoid using slang, medical terminology, or "psychobabble."
- Be fearless! Exude confidence! Speak up with authority. Use, "I don't know" or pause when you have to. Don't be afraid to say, "I need to look at my notes" or "I need to review the record." You must bear in mind that your notes are subject to be looked upon by the attorneys and may be entered into evidence. Don't doodle or make derogatory remarks on your notes.
- Address your audience, whether it be judge or jury, and be certain to maintain eye contact with that audience.
- Obtain a written transcript of your testimony and review your courtroom experience. If the court videotaped the courtroom experience, you might request a copy of the tape for your review.
- Keep your cool!

It is important for the therapist to remember that he or she is being called on as an expert in diagnosing and treating paraphilias and to maintain confidence in his or her knowledge and ability to testify. Regardless of the sentence the patient receives, the nurse therapist must not assume responsibility. It would be helpful for the nurse psychotherapist to participate in clinical supervision with a peer or another professional who is proficient in working with the paraphilic population.

► CASE EXAMPLE

Mr. Ruby Jewels, a 68-year-old pet shop owner, lives in a suburban community and is well respected and well liked. He has been recognized on numerous occasions for his philanthrophic efforts and has received several awards for his community activism. His wife of 40 years and their two children are very proud of Ruby.

The members of the community and his family were shocked when they learned of Mr. Jewels' recent arrest for molesting two young girls, ages 7 and 11, approximately 3 years ago. These two girls, now ages 10 and 14, have filed criminal charges against Mr. Jewels for fondling them and attempting to insert his finger inside their vaginas. They also reported Mr. Jewels made them touch his genitals during that time. A search of his home revealed numerous child pornographic materials, which were confiscated by the authorities. He has no prior arrests as confirmed by "rap sheets."

Mr. Jewels was charged and found guilty on four counts of child sexual assault. He is currently awaiting sentencing for a crime that was allegedly committed approximately 3 years ago (criminal charge) and for possession of child pornography (federal offense).

▶ DIAGNOSTIC FORMULATION

A comprehensive psychiatric evaluation was performed by the nurse psychotherapist to assess for the presence of a paraphilic disorder. Mr. Jewels reported he had engaged in similar behaviors with one other young girl around the same time. He denied any other similar occurrences.

He reported he felt driven to engage in such behaviors and was too embarrassed, back then, to talk about it with anyone, but did disclose this to his minister when seeking absolution. He stated he felt terrible for what he had done and could never understand what caused him to behave in such a way. He expressed concern regarding the young girls' well-being and added he wished he could "make it up to them and let them know how truly sorry I am and explain to them I just could not control myself." Ruby also stated he knew that being sorry for his actions would not excuse his behavior.

In an effort to cope with this problem, Mr. Jewels began sending away through the mail for child pornography depicting naked young girls engaging in sexual activities with various sexual partners. He thought this would be a better way to avoid touching children and believed he could secretly masturbate to these materials when his sexual desires became too intense to do anything else. Ruby also told the nurse therapist that after each occurrence, he would stick a pin into his penis to punish himself, hoping the pain would help him stop these unwanted, erotic thoughts of engaging in sexual activity with young girls. Mr. Jewels tearfully pleaded for "help to make these thoughts go away."

Based upon data obtained from Mr. Jewels during the psychiatric evaluation, the nurse psychotherapist formulated a diagnosis of heterosexual pedophilia: nonexclusive type.

▶ COURSE OF TREATMENT

Mr. Jewels spent 3 weeks on an inpatient psychiatric unit that specialized in the treatment of paraphilic disorders. Through the group therapy process, he had learned that it was all right to talk about his problem without being rejected or judged. He was able to recognize what stimulated him to engage in such behaviors and was able to identify appropriate, realistic relapse prevention strategies. He was receiving Depo-Provera 500 mg intramuscularly every Monday.

Ruby reported he'd "never felt so good" and related this to a decrease in the frequency and intensity of unwanted erotic pedophilic thoughts and desires. He further added, "I can actually concentrate on what's before me without needing to go masturbate or look at pornographic materials." He was very involved in his treatment, and his family remained by his side in support.

Mr. Jewels was discharged from the hospital, and his outpatient treatment consisted of weekly outpatient group therapy and weekly injections of Depo-Provera. He has been compliant with group attendance and is an active participant. Mr. Jewels has gained much insight into his illness and ways to avoid recidivism.

▶ SENTENCING AND NURSE PSYCHOTHERAPIST'S TESTIMONY

The nurse psychotherapist was subpoenaed by Mr. Jewels' attorney to testify at sentencing. Nurse psychotherapists are usually hired to give their opinion during sentencing. The therapist is not called upon to testify during the trial regarding the determination of guilt versus innocence, but may be asked to testify regarding forensic issues such as the patient's criminal responsibility or competency to stand trial.

The advanced practice nurse psychotherapist should prepare for testimony prior to the sentencing. This preparation should include a review of the patient's medical record and making notations to refer to when rendering testimony. These notations may consist of the diagnostic criteria, per DSM-IV, which the therapist used to help formulate the diagnosis of heterosexual pedophilia: nonexclusive type for Mr. Jewels. It would also be helpful for the nurse therapist to make notations of references indicating statistical data that may support various aspects of testimony, such as treatment methodologies and effects of treatment on rates of sexual recidivism. Information regarding collaboration with other disciplines may also be noted, such as psychological testing performed by a psychologist.

Once the court has recognized the advanced practice nurse psychotherapist as an expert witness, the testimony begins. The nurse psychotherapist will testify to the psychiatric evaluation that was performed and to the diagnostic formulation that was made. The nurse therapist needs to be very clear as to the diagnostic criteria as stated in DSM-IV for paraphilic disorders. The diagnosis needs to be explained in terms that would be understood by all those present in the courtroom and the therapist should avoid psychiatric jargon to the extent possible.

At this time, the nurse psychotherapist would attempt, in testimony, to educate those present about why a paraphilia is a disorder, factors that may have contributed to Mr. Jewels' paraphilic disorder, the therapist's rationale for the course of treatment identified and the types of treatment recommended, the potential effects of this form of treatment on sexual recidivism, and identification of potential risks to others if treatment were no longer available to Mr. Jewels or was ineffective.

The nurse psychotherapist needs to be prepared to respond to questions posed by the prosecution during cross-examination. These questions may pertain to the level of risk, in general, from the paraphilic population; how the therapist knows the patient is a reliable source of information versus being dishonest; whether the evaluation reflects an accurate account of the patient's paraphilic history; and what means were used with Mr. Jewels to validate the effects of treatment and support the therapist's statement regarding level of risk.

The court may also want to know the therapist's opinion of Mr. Jewels' level of compliance and understanding of his disorder. One should be cautious if and when asked for a prognosis. As with anything, there are no guarantees. The best that could be said might be that Mr. Jewels' risk to society may be lessened by his compliance with continued treatment, to be continuously monitored by the therapist during weekly group therapy sessions. At this time, the nurse psychotherapist may want to refer to the notations made preparatory to testimony that may support the therapist's position.

▶ SENTENCING OUTCOME

Despite the therapist's testimony regarding Mr. Jewels' paraphilic disorder, compliance with treatment, and the reported positive effects of treatment, Mr. Jewels was sentenced to a 30-year prison sentence. The judge suspended 25 years of this sentence and ordered Mr. Jewels to serve 5 years in the state penitentiary. The judge stated that Mr. Jewels was charged with a federal offense as well, which "deserved" a heavier sentence.

SEXUAL RECIDIVISM

Berlin and associates (1991) performed a 5-year follow-up survey of recidivism among 600 paraphiliacs who were treated with antiandrogen medications and who participated in group therapy with others who had a sexual disorder. The sexual recidivism rate (repeated sexual offense involving paraphilic behaviors) of these patients was less than 8 percent. The nurse psychotherapist should be cognizant that not all paraphilic patients will benefit from the form of adjunctive treatment previously described.

Kravitz and co-workers (1995) noted that treatment of paraphilic patients with testosterone-lowering medication (Depo-Provera), in addition to participation in a specialized sexual disorders group, decreased the patient's paraphilic desires. They acknowledged the need for further long-term clinical studies involving controlled trials regarding efficacy of paraphilic treatment and its effects on sexual recidivism rates.

SUMMARY

The ability to appropriately diagnose the presence of a paraphilia is critical to the planning of treatment. Evaluation of an individual exhibiting paraphilic behaviors may also include concepts pertinent to a forensic evaluation. In working with this population, the advanced practice nurse psychotherapist may also have the opportunity to work with issues regarding psychiatry and the law.

More controlled studies are warranted to determine the efficacy of paraphilic treatment, over time, with antiandrogen medications and group psychotherapy as well as the use of SSRIs. No one can determine which paraphilic patient may be "rehabilitated," who to hospitalize, who to incarcerate, or what method to use to assure a societal safety from the risks posed by the paraphilic patient. The nurse therapist should not formulate a prognosis for a paraphilic patient and must be ever aware that no cure is known for paraphilic disorders.

Diagnosing and treating paraphilic patients can be a challenging clinical specialty for the advanced practice nurse psychotherapist. This area of clinical specialization has many issues yet to be explored and researched, creating an opportunity for nurse therapists to conduct paraphilic research. The advanced practice nurse psychotherapist, by engaging in paraphilic research, would contribute significantly to the field of advanced psychiatric nursing practice and to society as well.

REFERENCES

American Psychiatric Association. *Diagnostic and Statistical Manual of Mental Disorders*, 4th ed. Washington, DC: American Psychiatric Association; 1994.

American Psychiatric Association. *Diagnostic and Statistical Manual of Mental Disorders*, 3rd ed, rev. Washington, DC: American Psychiatric Association; 1980.

AP Wire. Driven out, sex offender returns to town. *New York Times*. Aug. 15, 1993; section 1:23.

Berlin FS. The paraphilias and depo-provera: Some medical, ethical and legal considerations. *Bull Am Acad Psychiatry Law*. 1989;17:233–239.

Berlin FS. Laws on mandatory reporting of suspected child sexual abuse. *Am J Psychiatry*. 1988;145:1039.

Berlin FS, Hunt WP, Malin HM, et al. A five year plus follow-up survey of clinical recidivism within a treated cohort of 406 pedophiles, 111 exhibitionists and 109 sexual aggressives: Issues and outcome. *Am J Forensic Psychiatry*. 1991;12:5–28.

Berlin FS, Malin HM. Media distortion of the public's perception of recidivism and psychiatric rehabilitation. *Am J Psychiatry*. 1991;148:1572–1576.

Berlin FS, Malin HM, Dean S. Affects of statutes requiring psychiatrists to report suspected sexual abuse of children. *Am J. Psychiatry*. 1991;148:449–453.

Berlin FS, Malin HM, Thomas K. Treatment of the non-pedophilic and non-transvestic paraphilias. In: Gabbard GO, ed. *Treatments of Psychiatric Disorders*. 2nd ed. Washington, DC: American Psychiatric Press; 1996.

Biller HB. Sex role patterns, paternal similarity and personality adjustment in college males. *Develop Psychol*. 1971;4:107.

Bradford JM, Gratzner TG. A treatment for impulse control disorders and paraphilia. *Can J Psychiatry*. 1995;40:4–5.

Federoff JP, Berlin FS, Wisner-Carlson R, Dean S. An open five-year follow-up of paraphilic men treated with psychotherapy and medroxyprogesterone acetate (poster presentation). International Academy of Sex Research, 1992.

Freeman-Longo RE. Prevention or problem. *Sex Abuse*. 1996;8:91–104.

Groth AN. *Men Who Rape*. New York: Plenum; 1979.

Hall GC Nagayama. Sexual offender recidivism revisited: A meta-analysis of recent treatment studies. *J Consult Clin Psychol*. 1995;63:802–809.

Hucker J, Bain J. Androgenic hormones and sexual assault. In: Marshall WL, Laws DR, Burburee HE, eds. *Handbook of Sexual Assault: Issues, Theories and Treatment of the Offender*. New York: Plenum; 1990.

Kafka MP. Sertraline pharmacotherapy for paraphilias and paraphilia-related disorders: An open trial. *Ann Clin Psychiatry*. 1995;6:189–195.

Kravitz HM, Haywood TW, Kelly J, et al. Medroxyprogesterone treatment for paraphiliacs. *Bull Am Acad Psychiatry Law*. 1995;23:19–33.

McCarthy BW. Sexually compulsive men and inhibited sexual desire. *J Sex Marital Ther*. 1994;20:200–209.

Maletzky B. The use of medroxyprogesterone acetate to assist in the treatment of sexual offenders. *Ann Sex Res.* 1991;4:117–129.

Meyer WJ, Walker PA, Emory LE, et al. Physical, metabolic, and hormonal effects on men of long-term therapy with medroxyprogesterone acetate. *Fertil Steril.* 1985;43:102–109.

Nordheimer J. Vigilante attack in New Jersey is linked to sex-offenders law. *New York Times.* Jan. 11, 1995; section A:1.

Parkin A. On fetishism. *Int J Psychoanal.* 1963;44:352–361.

Riley A, Peet M, Wilson C. *Sexual Pharmacology.* Oxford, England: Clarendon Press; 1993

Simon WT, Schouten PG. Plethysmography in the assessment of sexual deviance: An overview. *Arch Sexual Behav.* 1991;20:75–91.

Trzepacz PT, Baker RW. *Psychiatric Mental Status Examination.* Oxford, England: Oxford University Press; 1993.

CHAPTER 21

GENDER IDENTITY DISORDER

Pamela E. Marcus

*I*ndividuals with gender identity disorder are often incorrectly identified as being homosexual. In reality, people who have gender identity disorder may be heterosexual or homosexual.

Chapter Overview

- Symptoms of Gender Identity Disorder
- Etiology
- Terminology
- Case Examples
- Life Course of Symptom Development
- Treatment
    Supporting Transition
    Hormone Replacement Therapy
    Surgery
    Psychotherapy
- Organizations for the Transgendered Community
- Publications for the Transgendered Community
- References

MY NAME IS ZYTHYRA

My name is Zythyra, I'm here to speak
You've nothing to fear, I'm not a freak
Of nature or God, it's just that my body
Needs modification to match the creation
Of my spirit inside. I can no longer hide
From my true nature, I must nurture to grow
From a scared little girl, who's afraid of the
     world
And how they'd hurt her if they discovered
     this pearl
This beautiful stone that she carried alone
In her heart, in her soul. It's always been a
     part of the whole
Person I am.

Who is this woman, this powerful woman
With a voice so strong, resonating in songs
That shatter the silence of lies. She cries
In the middle of the night. Chase away the
     tears
Built up over the years, constructed of fear.
Now I allow myself permission to unfold.
Behold!
The birth of Zythyra, an ethereal being
No longer fleeing, I'm finally seeing
With child-like eyes, filled with awe and
     surprise
And wonder at the world hidden under
The crevices of her dreams. It seems

There's a magical forest, enchanted, of
     course
Inhabited by a mystical creature with deli-
     cate features
A girl-child, hair flying wild
Eyes afire with wisdom acquired
From the ages of old. Now I am so bold
As to declare her name out loud. I am proud
To be this woman Zythyra. Now it's all so
     clear.
I've experienced rebirth, I'm a child of the
     earth
I accept my worth as a beautiful woman
Who tried to be the boy that others see
Well, I tell you they're wrong, 'cause I
     belong
To a different gender, No one can bend her.
There's no need to defend, we've just come
     to the end
Of a life known as Seth. He's exhaled his
     last breath.
Please don't mourn his death.

Now created from his ashes, from his love
     and his passions
Meet the woman Zythyra. My name . . . is
     Zythyra.

I AM ZYTHYRA!

(Copyright 1993, Seth Austen,
Sethstrings Music BMI.)

SYMPTOMS OF GENDER IDENTITY DISORDER

Gender identity disorder is a disorder described in DSM-IV (APA, 1994) as a "strong and persistent cross-gender identification accompanied by persistent discomfort with one's assigned sex."

The symptoms are often seen in childhood; the following are most common:

- The child states that he or she would rather be the opposite sex, or views self as the opposite sex. As an adult, the individual feels inappropriate and uncomfortable about his or her biological sex and views self as the opposite sex.

- The child plays with toys that are preferred by the opposite sex or are gender neutral. As an adult, the male individual has fantasies about being a female, including pregnancy. This individual is often interested in work areas or hobbies that are often associated with the opposite sex.
- The child's taste in clothing reflects a desire to wear clothing generally worn by the opposite sex. As an adult the individual may wear clothing that is appropriate for the opposite sex, and may feel very uncomfortable wearing traditional clothing of his or her biological sex.
- The child identifies as a role model someone who is the opposite sex. As an adult, the individual identifies with people of the opposite sex or peers with gender identity disorder.
- The child demonstrates mannerisms that are gender opposite, and may demonstrate anatomic dysphoria. Male to female individuals with gender identity disorder often tuck the penis. Female to male individuals with gender identity disorder may bind the breasts, and despise menstruation. Individuals with gender identity disorder are often desirous of wanting to live full-time as the preferred sex. These individuals seek electrolysis, hormonal reassignment, and surgical intervention (APA, 1994; Zucker, 1990).

ETIOLOGY

The etiology of gender identity disorder is not known. Some speculate that biological factors cause this disorder. For example, a hormonal change may occur during embryonic development; however, adult endocrine levels are usually normal in individuals with gender identity disorder (Beemer, 1996). Zhou and associates (1995) studied the bed nucleus of the stria terminalis (BST) due to the size difference in those of men and women (the measurement of the caudal part of the BST is 2.5 times larger in men than women); this is an area of sexual hormonal receptor sites in rats. In autopsies of six male to fe-

male transsexuals, Zhou and associates found the caudal part of the BST was within the range of a normal female sized BST, and therefore smaller than what would be normal for a male BST. These authors conclude that gender identity alterations in the brain may occur due to a change in the interaction between the development of the brain and sex hormones. The small caudal part of the BST in the transsexual's brain was the only difference noted on autopsy from the rest of the brain structure. The authors are continuing to study the distribution of sex hormone receptors and the aromatase activity in hypothalamic nuclei as it relates to sexual orientation and gender identity issues.

TERMINOLOGY

Having an understanding of the following terms will help in providing care for this population of patients.

Gender identity disorder: A term used to describe individuals who have conflicting feelings and feel inappropriate living as the gender assigned at birth. Described in DSM-IV as a "strong and persistent cross-gender identification accompanied by persistent discomfort with one's assigned sex."

Transsexual: An individual who has the symptoms of gender identity disorder.

Gender dysphoria: A feeling of conflict or a sense of feeling inappropriate living as the individual with the gender assigned at birth. This person experiences an internal view of self as gender opposite from the biological gender.

Transgender: A term that encompasses all individuals dealing with issues related to gender identity conflict; for example, people who cross-dress, transvestites, drag queens, or those individuals who practice gender bending.

Androgyny: Dress and appearance that is specific to neither males or females.

Transvestite: An individual who becomes sexually aroused or comforted by wearing clothing, makeup, and/or jewelry of the opposite gender. Most transvestites are heterosexual males who use this activity as a sexual or emotional release, and the behavior may increase during times of stress; a transvestite does not generally have gender dysphoria and is not interested in reassignment surgery.

Gender bending: Dressing and living in both male and female gender roles; for example, a male individual may have a full beard, but wear makeup and female clothing.

Drag queen: Gay men who cross dress. The public may have seen a drag queen in a stage performance.

Transition: When an individual with gender identity disorder begins to live full-time as the gender of choice.

Sexual preference: Whether an individual is sexually attracted to someone who is heterosexual, bisexual, or homosexual. Individuals with gender identity disorder are often incorrectly identified as being homosexual. It is important to distinguish gender identity disorder from sexual preference; individuals who have gender identity disorder may be heterosexual or homosexual (APA, 1994; Beemer, 1996; Blanchard, 1990a,b; Stuart, 1983).

► CASE EXAMPLE: MALE TO FEMALE TRANSSEXUAL

Andrea is a 37-year-old male to female individual with gender identity disorder. She has been living full-time as a female for 8 months and has remained at her job as a computer programmer for a local company. Andrea states that she first began to view herself as female around age 5, when she began to dream that she was a girl. She played with dolls during her childhood and had fantasies of being a beautiful bride on the day of her marriage. She would sneak into her sister's room and take some of her underwear or stockings and wear these items under her clothes at age 6. She reports no sexual feelings attached to wearing women's clothing, but states she feels more comfortable.

As a teenager, she tried to block out any thoughts of wanting to be a girl. She felt particularly uncomfortable when she experienced erections and ejaculations. She tried to become more masculine and joined the marines at age 19, where she was placed in computer training to write programs for procurement of supplies. It was during her tour of duty at Camp LaJune that she met her wife, Jean. They were married 6 months after meeting. Andrea loved Jean's femininity and would wear some of her clothing when Jean was out of the house. One year ago, Andrea told Jean about the gender identity problem. Jean became enraged and separated from Andrea, stating, "I am not a lesbian, I can't live with you! You will never see our children! You are a liar, a pervert, I consider you dead!" After Jean left, Andrea decided she would try to live as a woman full-time. She used the gender chat room on the Internet to get advice. She learned that she would need psychotherapy in order to obtain reassignment hormones and surgery. Andrea felt that she could no longer fight her true identity, and would rather die than live as a man.

▶   CASE EXAMPLE: FEMALE TO MALE TRANSSEXUAL

Max is a 27-year-old female to male transsexual who has sought treatment to begin transition to live full-time as a male. He began to "feel like a boy" when he was 4, and used to refer to himself as "that boy, Max." His mother would become angry at him, and correct him, using the birth name, Maxine. Max had several male friends during his youth who saw him as a tomboy, and he would do adventurous activities, such as climb trees, go hiking in the cavern in their hometown, and dare each other to dive into the cold water they found outside the cave. During high school, Max did not date, and some of the girls would tease Max for being so "butch." Max would insist on wearing pants bought in the male section of the store and would not wear blouses, skirts, or dresses. If challenged by an authority—for example, at school—Max would recite the constitutional right to free speech, and thereby free expression. Max attended the fire academy after graduation from high school, and became a firefighter. He sees his role in life as "helping others." It was at a fund-raising dance at the fire station that Max met Julie. Max told Julie that he sees himself as male, that he would like to date her, but that she must understand that he will eventually be able to take testosterone and become more masculine. Julie agreed to this part of the relationship, feeling relieved that she is not lesbian.

Max began therapy to begin the transition from female to male. He told his mother about his gender identity disorder, and his mother refused to talk to him unless he agreed never to discuss this subject again, and to refer to himself only as Maxine. Max stated he could not do that. He decided to continue the transition even if the consequences are that he is cut off from his mother. His sister and brother were rather distant and have become more unavailable. His father has been absent from the family since Max was 2 years old. Julie became more supportive and has moved in with Max.

People at work have been rather sympathetic, as most of the fire crew saw Max as a "butch." They have decided that if Max wants to present himself as male, they do not have a problem with that.

LIFE COURSE OF SYMPTOM DEVELOPMENT

Individuals with gender identity disorder usually begin to experience self as gender opposite in early childhood. An individual who is male to female may wear some of their mother's or sister's clothing and feel comforted and elated by the act. During adolescence, the individual often attempts to cope with the gender dysphoria by hiding the problem from others. Many male to female transsexuals exhibit hypermasculine behavior to try to reduce the desire to be female. Brown (1988) states that the prevalence of individuals with gender identity disorder may be higher in the armed services than in the general population due to the hypermasculine environment. This environment gives the male to female transsexual individual a place to purge the identification with femininity. Periods of buying female clothing and then purging them often occur with people who are male to female transsexuals.

As young adults, many transsexuals marry. Many marriages involve a deep friendship between the husband and wife, but often the transsexual spouse does not disclose to his or her spouse prior to marriage the gender identity conflict. During the marriage, an individual with male to female gender identity disorder may secretly cross-dress. As the internal pressure mounts inside the person to feel less conflicted, the spouse may increase wearing gender-opposite clothing and talk to other individuals with gender identity disorder. The individual may attend support groups in the community or use the Internet chat rooms. Generally, an individual with gender identity disorder reads as much information about the disorder as he or she can find. After determining that the disorder is the source of internal conflict, the individual seeks psychotherapy.

TREATMENT

Usually the first goal of therapy is to determine the diagnosis, which is accomplished by conducting a thorough assessment interview. In addition to the usual assessment questions, information must be directly elicited about the individual's view of self, fantasies of self, and sexual history, including information regarding the actual sexual activity in which the patient engages. Individuals with gender dysphoria generally avoid direct genital contact. Often, the individual may fantasize while having sexual relations that he or she is of the opposite sex. It is important to ask the patient when the first time was that he or she dressed in clothing usu-

ally considered appropriate for a member of the opposite sex and whether the individual was sexually aroused by the experience. Also ask what toys and games the individual preferred as a child and what the current areas of interest are (Steiner, 1990). Assess the individual for complications, such as alcohol and substance abuse, depression, and childhood abuse that was verbal, physical, sexual, and/or neglect. It is important to assess the individual for a personality disorder. Determine the thought pattern; are there symptoms of loosening of associations, delusions, and/or hallucinations? Are symptoms of dissociative identity disorder evident? Has the patient ever had suicidal ideation? Is the patient currently experiencing suicidal thoughts? Has the patient ever attempted suicide? What were the issues involved that caused that level of psychological pain?

SUPPORTING TRANSITION

Once the patient, along with the psychotherapist, has determined that he or she has gender dysphoria, the course of treatment is to support the patient while he or she begins the transition to the gender of choice. The individual begins the transition by disclosing the gender conflict to spouse, parents, siblings, and/or children. It is a very emotional period, as some family members and friends reject the patient based on the new information. Marriage often ends, as the spouse who has the gender identity disorder begins to dress and behave as the gender of choice. The other spouse frequently expresses feelings of anger and loss of the marital friendship, and denies being homosexual because the problem is often misinterpreted as one of sexual preference. In many instances, there are custody battles where the spouse tries to block the spouse with gender identity disorder from seeing the children once transition has begun.

The transition involves living full-time as the gender of choice. Patients often begin by cross-dressing on weekends or when not at work. The early goal of transition is to become accustomed to how the individual moves, talks, phrases sentences, and perceives the world in the gender of choice. While the patient who is male to female transsexual is beginning to cross dress, electrolysis reduces body hair and the need to shave often. Patients often describe this time as reliving an adolescence. Having the support of the psychotherapist, friends, and peers is important during the early transitional period. Support groups in the community are also helpful during the transition.

Testing Real Life

As the individual becomes more sure of self in the gender role, a trip to the grocery store or a shopping mall may build confidence. It is important for an individual who is beginning the real life test to obtain a letter from the psychotherapist explaining the gender dysphoria and cross-dressing in case of an accident or arrest. This letter points out that the patient has gender identity disorder and is wearing clothing and living full-time as the opposite gender as part of the therapeutic treatment for this disorder, rather than due to any illegal act. The letter further states that if there are any questions about this behavior, the therapist can be reached to assist in this matter (Denny, 1994).

Transition to Work

As the transition progresses, and the individual begins to strengthen in the preferred sexual role,

plans may be made for transition to occur at work. Some patients elect to change jobs to a more gender-appropriate role, while others decide to transition in the current job. It is most helpful to inform the supervisory staff, personnel department, and employee assistance program staff to discuss when the transition can occur, how the staff will be informed, and what restroom accommodations will be made. It is helpful if the psychotherapist teaches the supervisory staff of the organization about gender identity disorder. Although some co-workers will have strong feelings about the transition, providing education to the organization decreases some of the conflict (Cole, 1992).

HORMONE REPLACEMENT THERAPY

After the individual has successfully lived full-time as the gender of choice, hormone replacement therapy can begin. If the individual is still in a marriage, written permission must be obtained from the spouse (Fig. 21–1).

The therapist must become familiar with the Harry Benjamin standards for care of the individual with gender identity disorder (Walker et al., 1985) These standards were developed as a comprehensive set of principles for professionals who treat individuals with gender identity disorder by the Harry Benjamin International Gender Dysphoria Association (1990). The standards

---

We realize the potential for disruptions in our marital relationship resulting from _____ undergoing estrogen treatments. We agree, jointly and severally, to waive any and all claims against _____ for alienation of affection and/or loss of consortium. This waiver is limited in its effect to tort claims involving disruptions in the quality and duration of our marital relationship and does not release _____ from liability for negligence, malpractice, or any other tort claims other than alienation of affection and/or loss of consortium.

Signature _____

Signature _____

Witnessed by _____

Date _____

Figure 21–1. Limited waiver of tort liability.

specifically address the minimum time in therapy and real life test that the individual must meet prior to obtaining reassignment hormones and reassignment surgery. It is important that reassignment hormonal therapy not begin based only on the patient's request.

The therapy is a conflictual subject for this patient population. A segment of this population would like DSM-IV to delete this category from the diagnostic labeling and not view gender identity disorder as an illness. Other members of this group feel the therapist should not be the gatekeeper of whether the individual should have reassignment hormones and/or reassignment surgery. It is important to consider the patient's level of functioning within the new role prior to beginning reassignment hormones. The hormones have effects that are irreversible should the individual decide not to continue to live his or her life as the gender of choice. The Benjamin standards recommend that the reassignment hormonal therapy be instituted prior to reassignment surgery as an important factor determining whether the individual wants to continue to live full-time in the gender of choice. The standards specify that the patient must demonstrate the desire to be gender opposite for at least 2 years prior to obtaining therapeutic intervention. This must be verified by a family member, significant other, or close friend. The therapist must have treated the patient for 3 months prior to referring the individual for reassignment hormonal therapy (Harry Benjamin International Gender Dysphoria Association, 1990). Clemmensen (1990) suggests that the patient delay reassignment hormonal replacement for 1 year after beginning therapy while initiating the real-life test. This time is spent working or going to school in the opposite gender role and learning how to problem solve issues related to seeking employment or attending school in this role. Some therapists require a 3 month real-life test prior to assisting the patient to obtain hormonal therapy. The important thread of the treatment is assisting the patient to function productively in the new gender role

prior to making actual physical changes that may be irreversible.

Hormone Preparations

Currently, the male to female transsexual patient can obtain hormonal replacement therapy with oral preparations, injections, or by patch. The oral preparations that are used most often for the male to female transsexual are estinyl estradiol 0.5 mg qd, estrace 2.0 mg qd, or premarin 1.25 to 5.0 mg qd (Dickey and Steiner, 1990; Kirk, 1994). An additional medication may include an androgen blocker; spironolactone 200 mg to 400 mg qd, which helps to enhance femininization; it reduces facial and body hair, redistributes body fat, and enlarges some breasts somewhat (Beemer, 1996; Kirk, 1994).

Progesterone may be injected or given orally. Although its use is controversial, Provera (medroxyprogesterone) 10 mg may be used the last 10 days of each month (Kirk, 1994). Some physicians may dose the patient daily with Provera. Deproprovera (aqueous suspension of progesterone) may be given 100 to 200 mg IM once a month (Kirk, 1994). Injectable estrogens are sometimes given; Estradurin 40 mg may be given IM every 2 to 4 weeks or Delestrogen (oil preparation) 20 to 40 mg every 2 to 4 weeks. The Estroderm patch is useful for patients older than 40 years, as it does not have the blood clotting potential of oral or injectable estrogen (Kirk, 1994). The female to male transsexual receives testosterone enanthate or testosterone cypionate, 200 mg every 2 weeks or 400 mg every 4 weeks (Dickey and Steiner, 1990). Prior to receiving hormonal reassignment therapy, a patient must have a thorough physical assessment. Follow-up tests are important, particularly liver and kidney function studies, as well as cardiovascular functioning.

Follow-up by an endocrinologist is essential for patients receiving any hormonal reassignment treatment.

SURGERY

Reassignment surgery is recommended after the patient has been able to live full-time functioning as the gender of choice; for example, the patient has worked or gone to school for a minimum of 1 year. The psychotherapist must have treated the patient for a minimum of 6 months prior to recommending reassignment surgery. Before reassignment surgery is done, a peer review in the form of a second opinion must take place, with one of the psychotherapists having a PhD or MD credential (Harry Benjamin International Gender Dysphoria Association, 1990). Some practitioners require a minimum of 2 years living and functioning in the gender of choice prior to surgery (Dickey and Steiner, 1990). Patients who do not live full-time in the gender of choice have more psychological complications in their postoperative course.

The surgical intervention for a male to female transsexual involves a procedure known as penile inversion; the resected penis is used to create a neovagina and the scrotal skin to create labia (Beemer, 1996; Dickey and Steiner, 1990). Another surgical intervention for the male to female transsexual is to use a part of the rectosigmoid colon to form a neovagina (Beemer, 1996). The procedures for the female to male transsexual involve a bilateral mastectomy, with construction of a male chest contour, bilateral oophorectomy, and hysterectomy. A neophallus is constructed by using a full-thickness skin graft from the upper or lower forearm, abdomen, or thigh and a tissue expander. The urethra is made longer using endothelial tissue from other parts of the body. The scrotum is made from labial tissue and synthetic implants are used for the testicles (Beemer, 1996). The construction of a neophallus is often complicated by many postoperative problems, and many gender clinics counsel against attempting the procedure (Dickey and Steiner, 1990). An alternative to phalloplasty surgery would be to release the clitoral hood after testosterone has been administered. This surgery is less risky and can be done as an outpatient procedure (Dickey and Steiner, 1990).

Patients with gender identity disorder do not have to have surgical intervention in order to be "true transsexuals." A patient with this disorder needs to think through each step of the treatment and make decisions based on what is best for the individual rather than what other transgendered individuals or society see as the best intervention. Many individuals with gender identity disorder elect not to have surgical intervention.

PSYCHOTHERAPY

Psychotherapy continues for 6 months to a year following surgery or after the patient has made the decision to live full-time in the gender of choice without surgical intervention. The purpose of the therapy is to provide support in the new role, monitor any psychological side effects of the patient's surgery, and to assist with any new adjustments in new intimate relationships. The frequency of therapy is dependent on the patient's adjustment. Stabilized patients are seen once a month for support in the new role.

During the course of his or her life, many transgendered individuals may need psychiatric care or hospitalization. It is important that the nursing staff attend to the primary reason for hospitalization, such as a suicide attempt after the loss of a marriage. The emphasis on the transition to the opposite gender as one causal factor in the crisis may be part of the therapy. However, limit setting by using the pronoun of the biological gender after the individual has started the real-life test is countertherapeutic. The individual who is transgendered should be placed in a private room. A good rule of thumb is to call the patient by the name he or she requests and the gender that is appropriate to the patient's presentation or request. It offends the patient to be called by his or her biological name and gender once the real-life test has begun. It could damage the trust that is an inherent part of the therapeutic relationship. If a patient who is transgendered is admitted to the hospital or a program such as a partial-hospitalization program, staff should seek assistance from a clinician who is familiar with the population.

ORGANIZATIONS FOR THE TRANSGENDERED COMMUNITY

AEGIS (American Educational Gender
   Information Service)
P.O. Box 33724
Decatur, GA 33033-0724
(770) 939–0212

Gender Identity Clinic
Clarke Institute of Psychiatry
250 College Street
Toronto, Ontario M5T 1RB

IFGE (International Foundation for
   Gender Education)
P.O. Box 367
Wayland, MA 01778-0367
(617) 899–2212

Ingersoll Gender Center
1812 East Madison
Seattle, WA 98122

Renaissance Education Association
P.O. Box 60552
King of Prussia, PA 19406

PUBLICATIONS FOR THE TRANSGENDERED COMMUNITY

Chrysalis Quarterly
AEGIS
P.O. Box 33724
Decatur, GA 33033-0724

*Tapestry Journal: For All Persons Interested in
   Crossdressing and Transsexualism*
The International Foundation for Gender
   Education
P.O. Box 367
Wayland, MA 01778-0369

*Transsexual * News * Telegraph: The Magazine
   of Transexual Culture*
TNT
41 Sutter Street, no. 1124
San Francisco, CA 94104-4903

Trans Sisters: A Journal of Transsexual Feminism
4004 Troost Ave
Kansas City, MO 64110
(816) 753–7816

REFERENCES

American Psychiatric Association. *Diagnostic and Statistical Manual of Mental Disorders. 4th ed.* Washington, DC: APA; 1994.

Beemer BR. Gender dysphoria update. *J Psychosoc Nurs Ment Health Serv.* 1996;34:12–19.

Blanchard R. Gender identity disorders in adult men. In: Blanchard R, Steiner BW, eds. *Clinical Management of Gender Identity Disorders in Children and Adults.* Washington, DC: American Psychiatric Press; 1990a:47–77.

Blanchard R. Gender identity disorders in adult women. In: Blanchard R, Steiner BW. *Clinical Management of Gender Identity Disorders in Children and Adults.* Washington, DC: American Psychiatric Press; 1990b:78–92.

Brown GR. Transsexuals in the military: Flight into hypermasculinity. *Arch Sexual Behav.* 1988;17:527–537.

Clemmensen LH. The "real-life test" for surgical candidates. In: Blanchard R, Steiner BW, eds. *Clinical Management of Gender Identity Disorders in Children and Adults.* Washington, DC: American Psychiatric Press; 1990:119–136.

Cole D. *The Employer's Guide to Gender Transition.* Wayland, MA: International Foundation for Gender Education; 1992.

Denny D. *Identity Management in Transsexualism: A Practical Guide to Managing Identity on Paper.* King of Prussia, PA: Creative Design Services; 1994.

Dickey R, Steiner BW. Hormone treatment and surgery. In: Blanchard R, Steiner BW, eds. *Clinical Management of Gender Identity Disorders in Children and Adults.* Washington, DC: American Psychiatric Press; 1990:139–154.

Harry Benjamin International Gender Dysphoria Association. *Standards of Care: The Hormonal and Surgical Sex Reassignment of Gender Dysphoria Persons*, revised. Palo Alto: Harry Bender International Gender Dysphoria Association; 1990.

Kirk S. *Hormones for the Male to Female Transgendered Individual*. Wayland, MA: International Foundation for Gender Education; 1994.

Steiner BW. Intake assessment of gender-dysphoric patients. In: Blanchard R, Steiner BW, eds. *Clinical Management of Gender Identity Disorders in Children and Adults*. Washington, DC: American Psychiatric Press; 1990:93–106.

Stuart KE. *The Uninvited Dilemma: A Question of Gender*. Portland. OR: Metamorphous Press; 1983.

Walker PA, Berger JC, Green R, et al. Standards of care: The hormonal and surgical sex reassignment of gender dysphoria persons. *Arch Sexual Behav.* 1985;14:79–90.

Zhou JN, Hofman MA, Gooren LJG, Swaab DF. A sex difference in the human brain and its relation to transsexuality. *Nature*. 1995;378:68–70.

Zucker KJ. Gender identity disorders in children: Clinical descriptions and natural history. In: Blanchard R, Steiner BW, eds. *Clinical Management of Gender Identity Disorders in Children and Adults*. Washington, DC: American Psychiatric Press; 1990:3–23.

CHAPTER 22

OUTPATIENT TREATMENT OF CLIENTS WITH ANOREXIA AND BULIMIA NERVOSA

Barbara E. Wolfe

*T*he focus of cognitive-behavioral therapy is to change targeted behaviors by challenging and restructuring sustaining beliefs, a useful approach in the treatment of bulimia. Behavioral therapy takes a more traditional stimulus-response approach, primarily focusing on extinguishing targeted behavior. It does not actively address the underlying cognitive functions that sustain the behavior. Interpersonal therapy focuses on particular interpersonal difficulties and relationships, drawing upon techniques developed to treat depression.

Chapter Overview

- Epidemiology
- Case Example
- Plan of Care: Outpatient Treatment Approaches
    Psychological Therapies
    Nutritional Counseling and Management
    Family Therapy
    Group Therapy
    Psychopharmacotherapy
    Client Education
    Resources
- Collaboration with Other Disciplines
- Ethical and Legal Implications
- Outcome Measures and Evaluation
- Follow-up and Referral
- Summary
- References

Supported in part by USPHS grant K07 MH00965 from the National Institute of Mental Health.

► INTRODUCTION

Treatment of eating disorders is commonly done on an outpatient basis, with hospitalization generally reserved for cases involving significant co-morbidity, suicidality, detoxification from substance abuse, or refractory illness. Cognitive-behavioral, interpersonal, and psychodynamic perspectives are typically used as grounding frameworks for outpatient therapy. Therapy often incorporates aspects of several of these modalities, and thus the treatment approach is not an "either/or" phenomenon. This chapter provides a brief overview of the epidemiology and diagnostic characteristics of anorexia nervosa and bulimia nervosa, followed by a description of outpatient therapies. Therapeutic approaches covered in this chapter include individual psychological therapies, nutritional counseling, family therapy, group therapy, pharmacotherapy, and patient education.

EPIDEMIOLOGY

Up to 1 percent of the young adult female population has anorexia nervosa. This disorder occurs more frequently in women; the average age of onset is late adolescence. Childhood anorexia nervosa is also more common in girls than boys. Characteristic of anorexia nervosa is a low body weight, less than 85 percent of that normally expected for the individual's age and height (American Psychiatric Association, 1994). Accompanying features include preoccupation with food, intense fear of gaining weight and the loss of at least three consecutive menstrual cycles (for females beyond menarche) (American Psychiatric Association, 1994).

Bulimia nervosa affects up to 3 percent of the young adult female population and occurs approximately ten times more frequently in women than in men. The average age of onset is during late adolescence. Binge eating episodes, the hallmark feature, typically consist of sweet-tasting, high-carbohydrate, high-fat foods. Episodes typically occur in less than 2 hours and the amount of food consumed is excessive relative to that of an average person in a similar situation. Although binge eating is characteristic of bulimia, approximately half of all persons with anorexia nervosa will also experience binge eating. Unlike anorexia, individuals with bulimia are usually in a normal weight range.

Compensatory behaviors to prevent weight gain are common in patients with anorexia or bulimia nervosa, reflecting the prominent fears of weight gain. Excessive exercising, fasting, self-induced vomiting, and the inappropriate use of laxatives and diet pills are common. Misuse of diuretics and syrup of ipecac, as well as frequent diets, are characteristic of this patient population.

PLAN OF CARE: OUTPATIENT TREATMENT APPROACHES

Several different therapeutic approaches may be appropriate in the outpatient treatment of individuals with an eating disorder. An initial evaluation often involves a thorough medical and psychosocial assessment. Unless warranted by the presence of significant comorbidity or debilitating symptoms, less invasive modalities are the initial treatment of choice (American Psychiatric Association, 1993).

► CASE EXAMPLE

Cindy is a 21-year-old college student seeking outpatient therapy. She is bright, articulate, and insightful. Her chief complaint is "my eating is too out of control." When talking about her eating patterns, she frequently looks down at the floor, displaying poor eye contact. She is ashamed of her symptoms and at times is slow to reveal information. The frequency of binge eating and self-induced vomiting averages 12 times per week. She is bothered by being distracted from her studies and fearful that her scholastic achievements will soon suffer. She is increasingly isolated, in part due to the secrecy of her symptoms and her feeling of disgust with her body shape and weight. Her most recent binge episode included one-half gallon of chocolate ice cream, one large bag of potato chips, three bowls of corn flakes cereal, one slice of chocolate cake, two slices of pizza, four bran muffins, a large box of pasta, and two liters of diet soda. Binge eating episodes have become a financial burden on her student allowance.

Cindy is currently 172.7 cm (5'8") tall and weighs 64.9 kg (143 lb), a BMI of 21.8. To prevent further weight gain, she runs 20 to 30 miles per week and spends an additional 2 hours a day exercising at the gym. In addition to vomiting, she fasts at least one day a week and is taking five laxative tablets three times a week. On a few occasions in the past, she has used syrup of ipecac to induce vomiting. She currently reports experiencing periodic dizziness when changing from a sitting to a standing position.

The onset of bulimia nervosa dates back to age 17, followed by an episode of anorexia at ages 18 to 19. Cindy has been in several outpatient therapies over the past few years. She has been hospitalized once for depression, coinciding with the anorexic episode.

The clinician conducts a complete psychosocial assessment and refers the client for a physical examination. In addition to a thorough assessment, the above description of the client points to the need for specific inquiry regarding the following: presence of depression, medical stability, social isolation, weight changes over the past six months, recent tendencies toward anorexic behavior, the nature of previous outpatient therapies including strategies used, interventions perceived as helpful or not helpful by the patient and treating clinician, and the circumstances surrounding the client's disengagement from previous therapies. Based on the clinician's assessment and physical exam results (including laboratory studies), it is determined that outpatient therapy is indicated.

Cognitive-behavioral therapy (CBT), interpersonal psychotherapy (IPT), behavioral therapy (BT), or psychodynamic therapy are possible interventions with this client. In deciding with which treatment approach to proceed, the clinician considers several factors including the client's motivation, capacity for insight, current situational influences (for example, school semesters, moving home for summer break), resources, and experiences with previous related treatments. Given the client's desire and motivation for symptom management, and current level of social isolation, short-term CBT or IPT group therapy is a likely treatment intervention at this time.

PSYCHOLOGICAL THERAPIES

Cognitive-Behavioral Therapy

Studies examining the efficacy of psychological treatments with eating disorders have focused on the use of cognitive-behavioral therapy (CBT), particularly with bulimia nervosa. The focus of CBT is to change targeted behaviors by challenging and restructuring sustaining beliefs. Results to date show that CBT is a useful approach in the treatment of bulimia (Agras et al., 1992; Fairburn et al., 1995; Garner et al., 1993), with positive results maintained at 1 year follow-up (Agras et al., 1994; Fairburn et al., 1993a; Wilfley, et al., 1993). Initial studies suggest that group CBT is more effective than medication treatment alone (Agras et al., 1992; Leitenberg et al., 1994; Mitchell et al., 1990). Other investigators have found that a program in which the client uses a self-directed treatment manual for 8 weeks followed by up to 8 sessions of CBT results in a comparable remission rate at 18 months follow-up when compared with the effects of 16 CBT sessions (Treasure et al., 1996). Thus, a combination of CBT and an educational component has the potential for reducing the number of therapy sessions while being equally helpful. In general, studies suggest that 50 percent or more of patients with bulimia nervosa may respond to CBT. The usefulness of CBT in the treatment of anorexia nervosa remains unknown. Some components of CBT may be beneficial for anorexia; however, this area is in need of further study.

Several CBT strategies for eating disorders have been described in the literature (Fairburn et al., 1993b; Garner and Bemis, 1985). The crux of CBT is the use of cognitive exercises—for example, homework assignments—requiring the patient's active participation. Assignments completed by the patient provide the therapist with information about behavioral response patterns. This data shapes successive homework assignments. Listing the advantages and disadvantages of the maladaptive behavior assists in assessing the client's experience of the illness, motivational factors, capacity for insight, underlying belief system, and understanding of the consequences of symptomatology. Teaching patients to test the validity of each described advantage and disadvantage helps challenge their underlying beliefs.

Subsequent assignments include addressing the patient's identification of "taboo" foods. The therapist asks the patient to list "good" and "bad" foods and the list is then used to show the rigidity of cognitive patterns. The therapist encourages and supports the person's ability to challenge such dichotomous thinking. Exploring fears of eating forbidden foods provides a basis for tasks directed at testing the validity of these beliefs. Asking about these fears can be empathic in acknowledging the presence of such concerns. Reintroduction of forbidden foods into the daily diet occurs gradually, starting with tasting avoided foods. As therapy progresses, forbidden foods are steadily added to the daily dietary intake.

Education is another important aspect of cognitive restructuring. The patient needs to relearn normal psychosocial and physiological cues related to eating behavior. Identifying where and when meals will take place and how much to eat offers structure and sensitizes the individual toward more normalized meal patterns. Patients need help in learning to recognize normal physiological signals associated with hunger and satiety, including cues such as stomach rumbling and a feeling of fullness. Patients with bulimia keep a self-monitoring diary to identify circumstances surrounding eating behavior, including the environment and the time of day. Diaries identify precipitants of binge episodes and the patient's associated feelings. The diaries also provide a source of data for challenging illogical assumptions and thoughts about eating behavior. Food diaries are commonly accepted to be helpful in the treatment of bulimia nervosa. Their use appears to be less common in therapeutic work with anorexic patients.

Although CBT initially focuses on decreasing symptoms and normalizing eating behavior, the maintenance of recovery and prevention of relapse becomes the focus as therapy progresses. In this latter phase, strategies include addressing underlying themes of low self-esteem, interpersonal issues, and individuation. Patients are encouraged to explore ways of defining self-worth other than through measurement of body weight and shape or display of rigid dietary control.

Generally, CBT occurs in weekly, individual, 50-minute therapy sessions, although groups are an alternate format. Frequency of therapy is often greater in the beginning of treatment for individuals presenting with increased symptom severity. Frequency of therapy declines as the end of treatment approaches, in an attempt to promote autonomous functioning. CBT, in the treatment of bulimia nervosa, tends to be brief (12 to 24 sessions). Factors such as degree of comorbidity, motivation for change, compliance, and degree of active participation will influence length of treatment.

Behavioral Therapy

Unlike CBT, behavioral therapy (BT) takes a more traditional stimulus-response approach, primarily focusing on extinguishing targeted

behavior. BT does not actively address the underlying cognitive functions that sustain the behavior. Although BT is helpful in short-term management of the symptoms of bulimia, it is less effective in modifying dieting behavior and attitudes toward body shape and weight than is CBT (Fairburn et al., 1991). BT alone is associated with a greater rate of attrition (Fairburn et al., 1993a) and relapse (Fairburn et al., 1995) when compared to CBT.

Interventions characteristic of BT include the use of food diaries and self-monitoring to identify antecedents or stimuli provoking the targeted behavior. Self-monitoring activities may also include the use of graphing techniques to track binge and purge activity over time. Diaries may be targeted at monitoring thoughts of self-worth and body image. BT also addresses the use of alternate responses to anxiety-provoking stimuli. Devising a list of substitute behaviors to carry out in the presence of the stimuli helps the patient to interrupt the targeted behavior.

Other more traditional BT interventions include the use of positive and negative reinforcements. Positive reinforcements provide motivation or incentive. Attached to the goal of successful attainment of the desired behavior, or extinguished behavior, is an identified reward. The reward reflects something valued by the patient. Thus, it will differ from person to person. As an example, a patient who has a week without binge/purge episodes might reward herself by going to the movies. While rewards reinforce desired behaviors, negative reinforcements deter targeted behaviors. Use of negative reinforcement is complicated and requires extreme care, as reinforcements should not be self-destructive or jeopardize the patient's personal integrity.

"Exposure plus response prevention" (EPRP) is another form of behavioral therapy. EPRP involves exposing the patient to problematic circumstances and challenging the patient to develop alternate strategies for responding to these circumstances. With people who binge and self-induce vomiting, exposure to an excessive food intake is instituted to teach the client alternate methods for dealing with the desire to purge. Although studies show EPRP to be effective in the treatment of bulimia nervosa (Gray and Hoage, 1990; Leitenberg et al., 1988), patients do not particularly like this form of therapy given the anxiety associated with "exposure" exercises.

Interpersonal Therapy

Interpersonal therapy (IPT) focuses on particular interpersonal difficulties and relationships, drawing upon IPT techniques developed to treat depression (Klerman et al., 1984). Initial studies suggest that patients with bulimia nervosa benefit from IPT (Fairburn et al., 1995; Wilfley et al., 1993). Although comparative studies are few, after 18 weeks of treatment IPT may lag behind CBT in terms of immediate impact on bulimic symptoms (Fairburn et al., 1991). However, at 1 year follow-up, IPT seems to catch up, having an equivalent effect on symptoms when compared to CBT (Fairburn et al., 1993a). In an initial comparison of three treatment modalities, IPT and CBT were associated with a better outcome at 12-month or longer follow-up compared with behavioral therapy (Fairburn et al., 1995). These initial results suggest that successful treatment of bulimia nervosa does not need to focus directly on the eating behavior and related attitudes. To date, data are scarce on the effect of IPT with anorexia nervosa.

Psychodynamic Psychotherapy

Psychodynamic psychotherapy focuses largely on interpersonal dynamics and relationships. Anecdotal literature and clinical experience provide the primary basis for its use in patients with an eating disorder. Psychodynamic psychotherapy helps patients understand the meaning and origin of symptoms. Therapy is typically long term and expensive. Psychodynamic psychotherapy requires that the client have the capacity for insight—a critical factor in deciding the appropriateness of this form of therapy for a particular client.

Over the years, several psychodynamic explanations for symptoms of binge eating and

self-induced vomiting have emerged (Johnson, 1991). Considerations of early childhood development have led to theories of stagnation at the sensory-oral phase of infancy, resulting in disturbed object-relations. Theories of psychosexual arrest, including the fear of sexual development, emerge from the refusal to maintain a body weight adequate for normal maturation, as in anorexia. Given that adolescence is the typical age of onset of eating disorders, issues concerning identity are a consideration. Reflecting many of these theories, common topics of focus during therapy include sexuality and development, individuation and separation, intimacy and isolation, control, and role confusion.

Initial efforts are directed at establishing a therapeutic relationship. Given the secrecy and shame frequently associated with eating disorders, guardedness and reluctance to share experiences are common. A neutral stance by the therapist is important in engaging the patient, although some individuals may interpret this as aloofness. Avoiding a controlling or dogmatic demeanor is critical, as self-control is a central issue for many individuals.

Attention to transference and countertransference is integral to the therapeutic work. The patient–therapist interactions are a way to observe the reenactment of early childhood interactions with the parent. Transference issues include the patient viewing the therapist as an austere figure of authority, as an idealized role model, or as a parent who is either controlling or submissive. Provocative or seductive feelings for the therapist may emerge. Countertransference issues include the therapist feeling as though the patient is not making progress as quickly as the clinician desires, fostering dependency, and experiencing diffused professional–client boundaries. The role of the therapist is to listen and offer interpretations of the transference to increase the client's awareness of conscious and unconscious interpersonal and behavioral patterns.

The focus of psychodynamic psychotherapy often extends beyond the eating disorder symptoms. Duration of treatment with weekly psychodynamic psychotherapy is of a wide range (1 to 10 years), and as with other therapies, is influenced by the degree of comorbidity and severity of illness. Psychodynamic psychotherapy continues to be the most common treatment for anorexia nervosa and is often used as an adjunct to other treatment modalities (Herzog, 1995). Psychodynamic therapy is particularly useful for persons who do not respond to short-term interventions or medication intervention, or who have significant character pathology.

NUTRITIONAL COUNSELING AND MANAGEMENT

Historically, many clinicians avoided discussing nutritional needs with the patient with an eating disorder for fear of emphasizing symptomatic behavior. However, more contemporary views stress the importance of nutritional counseling concerning normalized eating patterns and nutritional requirements. Nutritional counseling often involves a nutritionist, either as a consultant or counselor. Nutritional management can be particularly helpful as an adjunct to psychotherapy. It often provides an avenue for addressing nutritional needs while allowing psychotherapy to simultaneously focus on other issues.

Nutritional counseling directed at normalizing eating patterns uses strategies similar to those used in CBT. Education regarding macronutrient selection and amount of food required to provide energy for bodily functions is important. Sessions include discussions of reading assignments, including articles on food choices and shopping strategies (Hsu et al., 1992). Use of normal foods is encouraged as is avoiding diet supplements/products and prescribed diets, because these only reinforce abnormal eating. Meeting with family members provides information on family attitudes and beliefs influencing the patient's ability to normalize eating patterns.

For weight restoration and monitoring, normal adult body weight estimates are determined using the body mass index (BMI), cal-

culated by dividing body weight in kilograms by height in meters squared (kg/m^2). A BMI range of approximately 19 to 25 is considered normal. A greater risk for protein-energy malnutrition exists as BMI values fall below 18. For children and adolescents, reference to a pediatric/adolescent weight chart provides normal body weight estimates.

For low-weight patients, it is often advantageous to monitor body weight at least weekly. During the weight restoration phase of therapy, the target rate of weight gain is approximately 1 to 1.5 kg per week for the anorexic patient at a very low weight. Consideration of energy expenditure is important in determining caloric intake requirements. In general, during the weight restoration phase, daily caloric intake begins at 1500 kilocalories/day and gradually increased up to 3500 kilocalories/day (Beumont and Touyz, 1995). Patients need to be prepared for this change in calories and the anxiety related to weight gain during this phase.

FAMILY THERAPY

Observations of family interactions prompted the use of family therapy in eating-disordered patients (Bruch, 1973). In a controlled study, Russell and colleagues (1987) found family therapy to be helpful for eating-disordered patients, particularly for individuals with disorders of early onset and limited chronicity.

Family therapy typically employs joint sessions with the patient, family, and therapist. Separate sessions may be more appropriate with younger patients. Therapy initially focuses on the management of targeted eating-related behaviors, shifting to family issues as therapy progresses. Children whose parents remain critical of them throughout the treatment are likely to have a poorer outcome (LeGrange et al., 1992). Thus for families displaying overt criticism at the onset of treatment, initial separate sessions focusing on parent-child communication may be helpful.

As with any illness, family members often feel helpless, self-blaming, or blaming of the symptomatic child for his or her behavior. Because of the complexity of these emotions, family members often feel defensive about entering into family therapy. Thus, family members need to be engaged in a nonjudgmental and supportive manner. Reassurance that the goal of family therapy is to help members deal with and grow from the current situation, rather than to provide a forum to determine blame, is helpful. Family members often have educational needs about the eating disorder. Inviting questions and discussion of concerns helps the members and assists in consolidating support for the patient.

GROUP THERAPY

Group therapy provides an alternate format to individual therapy, or may serve as an adjunct intervention. Group therapies have varying focuses and purposes. For example, some groups focus on eating-related experiences, including meal planning, shopping, and eating in a group setting (Franko, 1993). Other groups, including those for parents, significant others, and siblings, focus on providing support and education.

When group therapy is used as a primary treatment modality, the framework is typically cognitive-behavioral, behavioral, or interpersonal. Studies of group therapy in bulimia have noted a beneficial effect, with better outcomes observed when used in combination with other treatment modalities (Fettes and Peters, 1992).

The purpose of adjunctive group therapy is often psychoeducational and may include a participant manual (Davis et al., 1992). Olmsted and colleagues (1991) found that psychoeducational group therapy, involving five lecture/slide presentations, had a beneficial effect, especially in the less symptomatic patients with bulimia. Although response rates were slightly lower, results were comparable to abstinence rates observed in persons receiving 18 weeks of individual CBT (21 versus 36 percent). The long-term effects of a psychoeducational approach are unknown.

PSYCHOPHARMACOTHERAPY

Although it is beyond the scope of this chapter to review in detail the controlled medication trials in anorexia and bulimia nervosa and related neurobiological mechanisms, the role of psychopharmacologic agents is summarized in the following section. For a more comprehensive review of the psychopharmacology and neurobiology of eating disorders, the reader is referred to references listed at the end of this chapter (Halmi, 1992; Hoffman and Halmi, 1993; Jimerson et al., 1996).

Anorexia Nervosa

Psychopharmacology is often of limited use in the treatment of anorexia nervosa unless, however, it is indicated by co-morbid characteristics such as psychosis or depression (American Psychiatric Press, 1993). Prompted in part by distorted patient perceptions of body weight and shape, initial controlled trials explored the potential role of antipsychotics, with little clinical improvement noted. Because of the lack of supporting scientific data, and concerns regarding side effects, antipsychotic agents are generally not used in the treatment of anorexia nervosa. However, the presence of psychotic co-morbidity and/or severe refractory illness may warrant their use in this patient population.

The presence of depressive symptoms in anorexia nervosa stimulated an exploration of the role of antidepressant medications. However, depression can be a consequence of starvation, and frequently remits with weight restoration. Controlled trials with tricyclic antidepressants show no or small improvement of symptoms, although open trials of the selective serotonin reuptake inhibitor (SSRI) fluoxetine (Prozac) show potential benefit (Gwirtsman et al., 1990; Kaye et al., 1991).

Other agents studied in controlled trials with anorexia nervosa include lithium and cyproheptadine. Lithium has not been shown to be effective in treating anorexia (Gross et al., 1981). Lithium is also avoided due to the extreme caution required in patients already prone to alterations in electrolyte functioning. Controlled studies using cyproheptadine, an antihistaminic and antiserotonergic drug, suggest potential increase in weight gain at high doses (32 mg/day) for persons with nonpurging anorexia nervosa, although accompanied by considerable sedation (Halmi et al., 1986).

Bulimia Nervosa

Controlled medication trials in bulimia nervosa have focused on antidepressant agents. These trials have been primarily prompted by depressive co-morbidity. Antidepressant medications may interact with serotonergic systems, which are thought to be dysregulated in this patient population (Jimerson et al., 1992). Although several antidepressant agents decrease binge eating and purging as well as depressive symptoms, improvement in depression is not necessarily correlated with improvement in binge eating frequency.

Of the antidepressant agents, the SSRIs are promising in that they often have fewer side effects. The largest of the controlled trials has been with fluoxetine (Prozac, 60 mg/day), and has shown a significant decrease in binge eating and purging over the course of 8 weeks (Fluoxetine Bulimia Nervosa Collaborative Study Group, 1992). Tricyclics may be an alternative for persons unresponsive to SSRIs. Although monoamine oxidase inhibitors are an alternative for those who are unresponsive to other agents, their use in bulimia is complicated by the difficulties that patients may have in adhering to the low-tyramine dietary regimen. Because of inconsistent results in controlled studies, lithium and fenfluramine are not generally used in the treatment of bulimia nervosa.

In reviewing the controlled trials, it is important to note that while symptoms decreased, few patients achieved full remission. In addition, studies comparing medication intervention to less invasive interventions have often shown a more favorable response to nonpharmacologic interventions such as CBT (Agras et al., 1994; 1992; Mitchell et al., 1990). Further research is needed about the long-term efficacy of medication treatments.

CLIENT EDUCATION

Some important topics for client education include the following.

- Etiology/contributing factors
- Normal body weight range/regulation theories
- Nutritional requirements
- Medical and psychosocial consequences
- Medications
- Resources for additional assistance
- Relapse prevention

Explanation of the multifaceted etiologic factors of eating disorders is important, as is discussion of a realistic and appropriate weight range, rather than a specific weight. The clinician often reviews the consequences of dieting behavior, including constipation and dehydration, in addition to providing nutritional counseling. Psychosocial consequences include increased risk for social isolation and depression. Medical consequences more commonly include fluid and electrolyte abnormalities. Medical complications are many, ranging from dental enamel erosion to uncommon medical emergencies such as esophageal tear (for comprehensive reviews see Fisher et al., 1995; Kaplan and Garfinkel, 1993). Relapse prevention includes identification of vulnerable circumstances, anticipation of symptom exacerbation, and strategic planning for reapproaching, achieving, and maintaining remission.

RESOURCES

Several national organizations can be helpful in identifying local community resources (Table 22–1). Local organizations often provide support groups for both the patient and family members, and are also involved in sponsoring educational activities. Some of these organizations may also be helpful in identifying local therapists specializing in the treatment of eating disorders.

TABLE 22–1. SELECTED ORGANIZATIONAL RESOURCES

American Anorexia/Bulimia Association, Inc. 293 Central Park West, Suite 1R New York, NY 10024 (212) 501–8351	National Association of Anorexia Nervosa & Associated Disorders Box 7 Highland Park, IL 60035 (847) 831–3438
Anorexia Nervosa & Related Eating Disorders, Inc. P.O. Box 5102 Eugene, OR 97405 (503) 344–1144	National Eating Disorder Organization 6655 South Yale Avenue Tulsa, OK 74136 (918) 481–4044

COLLABORATION WITH OTHER DISCIPLINES

Treatment often involves and necessitates collaboration with other nursing specialties and other disciplines. Medical evaluation and follow-up frequently include the patient's primary careperson, who is either a nurse practitioner or physician. Graduate level social workers, psychologists, and advanced practice psychiatric nurses often lead adjunctive group or family therapies. Nutritionists often provide dietary counseling or consultation. Nonprescribing therapists considering a medication intervention for a client need to collaborate with another advanced practice psychiatric nurse with prescriptive authority or with a psychiatrist. Although the role of the advanced practice psychiatric nurses includes that of therapist, some nurses may be primarily in a psychopharmacology role requiring collaboration with the patient's primary therapist, who may be of another discipline.

ETHICAL AND LEGAL IMPLICATIONS

Ethical standards and legal implications in the treatment of eating-disordered patients are the same as with other psychiatric populations. The therapist needs to discuss the standard treatment approaches for the condition with the patient. Obtaining informed consent needs to occur be-

fore the initiation and delivery of any such treatments. Parental involvement/consent should be solicited according to standard practice in the psychiatric treatment of minors. In the presence of compromised safety or medical instability, legal intercession may be necessary.

OUTCOME MEASURES AND EVALUATION

In the initial phase of treatment, the therapist and patient identify targeted outcomes. Outcome measures related to symptomatology include self-report of the frequency of binge eating and purging episodes, frequency of compensatory behaviors used to prevent weight gain, and body weight (with anorexic clients). Although these outcomes may be relatively easily identified, other dimensions of response also need to be considered (Wolfe, 1995). Use of standardized rating scales can be helpful in establishing baseline ratings and ratings at subsequent timepoints. Self-report pencil/paper measures of eating-related attitudes and preoccupations include the Eating Attitudes Test (Garner et al., 1982) and Eating Disorder Inventory (Garner, 1991). Use of standardized measures of depression and anxiety assist in monitoring associated clinical characteristics. In addition, consideration needs to be given to potential changes in functional activity (e.g., activities of daily living, socialization, school performance).

Evaluation of treatment needs to occur in the context of the known efficacy of the particular treatment modality. For example, although controlled medication trials report a decrease in binge/purge episodes, few patients achieve full remission of symptoms following drug intervention. Thus, it may not be realistic to expect complete abstinence in the clinical setting. Other factors influencing outcome include the complexity and severity of presenting problems.

FOLLOW-UP AND REFERRAL

Referrals from outpatient therapy may include hospitalization or a day-hospital setting. Comorbid psychopathology often influences the need for hospitalization. Medical instability, suicidality, or drug detoxification are the more common indicators for hospitalization in this patient population.

SUMMARY

A trial of outpatient psychotherapy is generally used with individuals for whom safety and medical stability do not warrant hospitalization and when the additional structure provided by a day-hospital program is not needed. Therapeutic approaches are based on an initial comprehensive assessment and typically involve CBT, BT, or psychodynamic psychotherapy. Nutritional counseling, family therapies, psychoeducational group therapies, and pharmacology may be helpful adjunctive treatments. Consideration of the patient's motivation, ability to participate in the treatment of choice, and perception of the treatment plan are important in addition to the complexity and severity of the illness.

REFERENCES

Agras WS, Rossiter EM, Arnow B, et al. Pharmacologic and cognitive-behavioral treatment for bulimia nervosa: A controlled comparison. *Am J Psychiatry.* 1992;149:82–87.

Agras WS, Rossiter EM, Arnow B, et al. One-year follow-up of psychosocial and pharmacologic treatments for bulimia nervosa. *J Clin Psychiatry.* 1994;55:179–183.

American Psychiatric Association. *Diagnostic and Statistical Manual of Mental Disorders. 4th ed.* Washington, DC: APA; 1994.

American Psychiatric Association. Practice guidelines for eating disorders. *Am J Psychiatry.* 1993;150: 207–228.

Beumont JV, Touyz SW. The nutritional management of anorexia and bulimia nervosa. In: Brownell KD, Fairburn CG, eds. *Eating Disorders and Obesity: A Comprehensive Handbook.* New York: Guilford Press; 1995.

Bruch H. *Eating disorders: Obesity, Anorexia and the Person Within.* New York: Basic Books; 1973.

Davis R, Dearing S, Faulkner J, et al. The road to recovery: A manual for participants in the psychoeducational group for bulimia nervosa. In: Harper-Guiffre H, MacKenzie KR, eds. *Group Psychotherapy for Eating Disorders.* Washington, DC: American Psychiatric Press; 1992.

Fairburn CG, Jones R, Peveler RC, et al. Three psychological treatments for bulimia nervosa. *Arch Gen Psychiatry.* 1991;48:463–469.

Fairburn CG, Jones R, Peveler RC, et al. Psychotherapy and bulimia nervosa. Longer-term effects of interpersonal psychotherapy, behavior therapy, and cognitive behavior therapy. *Arch Gen Psychiatry.* 1993a;50:419–428.

Fairburn CG, Marcus MD, Wilson GT. Cognitive-behavioral therapy for binge eating and bulimia nervosa: A comprehensive treatment manual. In: Fairburn CG, Wilson GT, eds. *Binge Eating: Nature, Assessment, and Treatment.* New York: Guilford Press; 1993b.

Fairburn CG, Norman PA, Welch SL, et al. A prospective study of outcome in bulimia nervosa and the long-term effects of three psychological treatments. *Arch Gen Psychiatry.* 1995;52:304–312.

Fettes PA, Peters JM. A meta-analysis of group treatments for bulimia nervosa. *Int J Eat Disord.* 1992; 11:97–110.

Fisher M, Golden NH, Katzman DK, et al. Eating disorders in adolescents: A background paper. *J Adolesc Health.* 1995;16:420–437.

Fluoxetine Bulimia Nervosa Collaborative Study Group. Fluoxetine in the treatment of bulimia nervosa: A multicenter, placebo-controlled, double-blind trial. *Arch Gen Psychiatry.* 1992;49: 139–147.

Franko DL. The use of a group meal in the brief group therapy of bulimia nervosa. *Int J Group Psychother.* 1993;43:237–242.

Garner, DM. *Eating Disorder Inventory-2P. Professional manual.* Odessa, FL: Psychological Assessment Resources; 1991.

Garner DM, Bemis KM. Cognitive therapy for anorexia nervosa. In: Garner DM, Garfinkel PE, eds. *Handbook of Psychotherapy for Anorexia Nervosa and Bulimia.* New York: Guilford Press; 1985.

Garner DM, Olmsted MP, Bohr, Garfinkel PE. The eating attitudes test: Psychometric features and clinical correlates. *Psychol Med.* 1982;12:871–878.

Garner DM, Rockert W, Davis R, et al. Comparison of cognitive-behavioral and supportive-expressive therapy for bulimia nervosa. *Am J Psychiatry.* 1993; 150:37–46.

Gray JJ, Hoage CM. Bulimia nervosa: A group behavior therapy with exposure plus response prevention. *Psychol Rep.* 1990;66:667–674.

Gross H, Ebert MH, Fadem VB, et al. A double-blind controlled trial of lithium carbonate in primary anorexia nervosa. *J Clin Psychopharmacol.* 1981; 1:376–381.

Gwirtsman HE, Guze BH, Yager J, Gainsley B. Fluoxetine treatment of anorexia nervosa: An open clinical trial. *J Clin Psychiatry.* 1990;51:378–382.

Halmi KA, ed. *The Psychobiology and Treatment of Anorexia Nervosa and Bulimia Nervosa.* Washington, DC: American Psychiatric Press; 1992.

Halmi KA, Eckert E, LaDu TJ, Cohen J. Anorexia nervosa: Treatment efficacy of cyproheptadine and amitriptyline. *Arch Gen Psychiatry.* 1986;43: 177–181.

Herzog DB. Psychodynamic psychotherapy for anorexia nervosa. In: Brownell KD, Fairburn CG, eds. *Eating Disorders and Obesity: A Comprehensive Handbook.* New York: Guilford Press; 1995.

Hoffman L, Halmi K. Psychopharmacology in the treatment of anorexia nervosa and bulimia nervosa. *Psychiatr Clin North Am.* 1993;16:767–778.

Hsu LK, Holben B, West S. Nutritional counseling in bulimia nervosa. *Int J Eat Disord.* 1992;11:55–62.

Jimerson DC, Lesem MD, Kaye WH, Brewerton TD. Low serotonin and dopamine metabolite concentrations in cerebrospinal fluid from bulimic patients with frequent binge episodes. *Arch Gen Psychiatry.* 1992;49:132–138.

Jimerson DC, Wolfe BE, Brotman AW, Metzger ED. Medications in the treatment of eating disorders. *Psychiatr Clin North Am.* 1996;19:739–754.

Johnson C, ed. Psychodynamic treatment of anorexia nervosa and bulimia. New York: Guilford Press; 1991.

Kaplan AS, Garfinkel PE, eds. *Medical Issues and the Eating Disorders: The Interface.* New York: Brunner/Mazel; 1993.

Kaye WH, Weltzin TE, Hsu LK, Bulik CM. An open trial of fluoxetine in patients with anorexia nervosa. *J Clin Psychiatry.* 1991;52:464–471.

Klerman GL, Weissman MM, Rounsaville BJ, Chevron ES. *Interpersonal Psychotherapy of Depression.* New York: Basic Books; 1984.

LeGrange D, Eisler I, Dare C, Hodes M. Family criticism and self-starvation: A study of expressed emotion. *J Fam Therapy.* 1992;14:177–192.

Leitenberg H, Rosen JC, Gross J, et al. Exposure plus response-prevention treatment of bulimia nervosa. *J Consult Clin Psychol.* 1988;56:535–541.

Leitenberg H, Rosen JC, Wolf J, et al. Comparison of cognitive-behavior therapy and desipramine in the treatment of bulimia nervosa. *Behav Res Ther.* 1994;32:37–45.

Mitchell JE, Pyle RL, Eckert ED, et al. A comparison study of antidepressants and structured intensive group psychotherapy in the treatment of bulimia nervosa. *Arch Gen Psychiatry.* 1990;47:149–157.

Olmsted MP, Davis R, Rockert W, et al. Efficacy of a brief group psychoeducational intervention for bulimia nervosa. *Behav Res Ther.* 1991;29:71–83.

Russell GF, Szmukler GI, Dare C, Eisler I. An evaluation of family therapy in anorexia nervosa and bulimia nervosa. *Arch Gen Psychiatry.* 1987;44: 1047–1056.

Treasure J, Schmidt U, Troop N, et al. Sequential treatment for bulimia nervosa incorporating a self-care manual. *Br J Psychiatry.* 1996;168:94–98.

Wilfley DE, Agras WS, Telch CF, et al. Group cognitive-behavioral therapy and group interpersonal psychotherapy for the nonpurging bulimic individual. A controlled comparison. *J Consult Clin Psychol.* 1993;61:296–305.

Wolfe BE. Dimensions of response to antidepressant agents in bulimia nervosa: A review. *Arch Psych Nsg.* 1995;9:111–121.

CHAPTER 23

PERSONALITY DISORDERS

Pamela E. Marcus

*A*n individual with a personality disorder has difficulty identifying self; interpersonal relationships are often affected by the disorder; and the person's behavioral patterns, views, and expressions of emotions are different from those of others in the individual's cultural milieu.

Chapter Overview

► INTRODUCTION

Individuals with severe forms of personality disorders present a complex picture of symptoms that are often difficult for the nurse to understand and to work with. Once the advanced practice nurse understands the etiology, which includes the individual's relationship with self and others as well as the biological changes suspected in individuals with personality disorders, care can be delivered efficiently and effectively. The advanced practice nurse provides care in a primary care setting and educates the patient and family members to assist the patient to learn new coping mechanisms. This chapter discusses the etiology, theoretical principles, and treatment strategies for patients with a personality disorder.

DSM-IV (APA, 1994) outlines several symptoms that indicate the existence of a personality disorder. The individual is inflexible and maladaptive in traits that cause the individual to have significant difficulties functioning. The person also feels subjective distress. DSM-IV states that an important characteristic of an individual with a personality disorder is that his or her subjective thoughts, feelings, and behavior differ markedly from the expectations of others of the same culture and background. Personality disorder is manifested by the following criteria.

- The individual's thought process, emotional reactivity, interpersonal relationships, and impulse control are markedly different from others of his or her culture and peer group.
- The different patterns of thoughts, emotionality, and behavior are enduring and inflexible and are demonstrated consistently in most personal and social situations.
- Personal distress and/or impairment is significant during interactions within the family and with others in a social or occupational setting.
- The patterns of persistent thoughts, emotions, and behavior are long standing and are evident during adolescence and early adulthood.
- The cognitive, emotional, and behavioral patterns are not due to any other psychiatric disorders or physiological effects of a substance, as in substance abuse, or the side effects of medications, or exposure to toxic chemicals.

THEORETICAL PERSPECTIVES

Theorists such as Freud, Erickson, Kernberg, Mahler, and Masterson have theorized about why individuals with personality disorders have cognitive, emotional, and behavioral reactions that vary from other individuals in the same population. Freud (1905, 1917, 1923, 1924) began to postulate how the personality develops and what causes problems by conceptualizing developmental stages and the internal psychic structures that are made up of the id, ego, and superego. Erickson studied Freud and expanded his theory by labeling stages with explicit conflicts that must be resolved in order to relate to others in a healthful manner. Erickson's (1950) personality development theory includes stages of adult development. Recently, several theorists have studied object relations, which is the study of how the individual views himself or herself in relationship to other significant people.

OBJECT RELATIONS

Object Relations is a theoretical framework that explores how an individual views the self and relationships with others. This conceptual framework is particularly useful when working with patients who have a severe personality disorder. These individuals have grave disturbances in their view of self and problems relating to others. These relationship problems are exhibited in the therapeutic relationship and sometimes can block the patient's progress in problem solving. It is helpful to use the theory of object relations to understand the patient's view of self and interaction with others to provide interventions that will be useful and understandable to the patient.

Kernberg defines object relations as the "stability and depth of the patient's relations with significant others as manifested by warmth, dedication, concern and tactfulness. Other qualitative aspects are empathy, understanding and the ability to maintain a relationship when it is invaded by conflict or frustration" (Kernberg, 1984). Kernberg used his study of object relations to develop an understanding of borderline personality disorder and define this personality disorder in depth. He also utilized this theory to understand the narcissistic personality disorder. He developed a list of symptoms and behaviors that underline the interactive and inner thought and feeling process of both of these diagnoses. One symptom that is particularly useful to understand when providing patient care is *splitting*. Splitting is when the individual is unable to integrate "good" and "bad" images of self and others. This symptom is exhibited by an individual with borderline personality disorder who views self and others as either all good or all bad. An example of this would occur when a patient describes his mother as the most positive influence in his life, but when discussing his wife, he is unable to discuss any positive characteristics about her.

Another symptom that is important to understand when caring for individuals with severe personality disorders is the ability of the person to obtain *object constancy*. Mahler and associates (1963) observed mothers and their infants in a laboratory setting. During this time, she began to identify patterns of interaction between the mothers and their babies. Mahler developed a theory of separation and individuation that helps to define the child's intrapsychic self-representation and the separate representation of the mother. The child's task during the first 3 years of life is to develop a separate identity that is unique to that individual. Inherent in this process is the development of object constancy that occurs around 25 months of age. Object constancy is the ability to maintain a relationship, even during times of frustration and changes in the relationship. The child learns that when his or her needs are not met directly by the mother, comfort can occur by using something to self-soothe that represents the mother, such as a stuffed animal. Individuals with severe personality disorders did not fully develop object constancy. For example, when someone significant in his or her life leaves for work, the individual with a severe borderline personality disorder cannot picture their return at the end of the work day. The person with the severe borderline personality disorder may call the significant other multiple times during the day, become very emotional, and think that the person will never return home. This individual cannot use any self-soothing mechanism to calm his or her fears, and emotions take over the behavior.

Masterson (1976) identified four defenses that block the patient's developmental growth from Mahler's stages of separation-individuation to autonomy: projection, clinging, denial, and avoidance. Masterson points out that the individual with problems with object constancy does not relate to people as wholes, but as parts. This person is unable to sustain a relationship through the frustration of everyday living, and tends to experience feelings of anger and rage when feeling rejected or ignored. The individual who has not fully developed object constancy is unable to evoke the image of the other when they are not present, as described above. This individual is unable to use transitional objects, which are things that represent the other person. If the person in the above example could use a picture of the significant other to calm his or her fears of abandonment while the individual is at work, the picture would be the transitional object. If a significant person in his or her life dies, the patient with a severe personality disorder, such as borderline personality disorder, cannot mourn, but may exhibit one or more of what Masterson calls the six constituent states: depression, anger and rage, fear, guilt, passivity and helplessness, and emptiness and void. It is often these states and the consequences from the patient's behavior that lead to the symptoms that cause the patient to seek psychiatric help.

Linehan (1993) characterizes the main symptom to assess and treat when working with a patient with borderline personality disorder as *emotional dysregulation*. She attributes this symptom as caused by biological constitution, environmental factors, and the transition between these two factors during early development. She assesses the patient's family system to determine whether the communication patterns demonstrate an invalidating environment. Emotional dysregulation is present in one who responds in an emotional reactive and unpredictable manner to private experiences, such as beliefs, thoughts, or feelings.

Biological considerations for personality disorder development

Several types of ongoing biological studies are aimed at understanding the role that the brain and genetics play in psychiatric disorders. One research finding in the area of family studies demonstrates a strong genetic influence in several of the personality disorders, suggesting there are some ties between biological factors and personality organization (Coryell and Zimmerman,

1989; Kavoussi and Siever, 1991; Marin et al., 1989; Siever, 1992; Siever and Davis, 1991).

Two biological tests that were used to study individuals with schizotypal personality disorder demonstrate the role of the brain in abnormal interpersonal relations. One of these tests is called smooth-pursuit eye tracking. This examination tests the ability of the eyes to track a smoothly moving target (Siever, 1992). The smooth-pursuit eye tracking is important for cognitive interpretation of information in the environment. Individuals with schizophrenia demonstrate difficulty with smooth-pursuit eye movements, which is thought to reflect disrupted neurointegrative functioning of the frontal lobes (Siever, 1992). The impaired eye-tracking studies are associated with the "deficit" traits of schizophrenia: social isolation, detachment, and inability to relate to others. Lencz and associates (1993) studied impaired eye tracking in undergraduate students with schizotypal personality disorder. This study found that the 32 subjects with schizotypal personality disorder demonstrated an impairment in eye tracking movements.

Backward masking is another biological test that is indicative of cognitive-perceptual difficulties often seen with patients who have schizotypal personality disorder. This test of neurointegrative functioning involves showing the individual a visual stimulus, which is immediately followed by a different visual stimulus. The person is then asked to identify the first object that was the visual stimulus (Kavoussi and Siever, 1991). Siever (1985) noted that individuals with schizotypical personality disorder have results that are similar to those noted in individuals with schizophrenia, but not as severe.

A group of studies were done with cerebrospinal fluid homovanillic acid by Siever (1992) and Kavoussi and Siever (1991). Both of these studies reported an increase of cerebrospinal fluid homovanillic acid in studies of schizotypal patients and correlates with positive psychotic-like criteria for schizotypal personality.

Several studies demonstrate disturbances in central serotonergic neurotransmission. Brown and colleagues (1982) did research that demonstrated aggressive and suicidal behaviors in individuals with a personality disorder correlate with reduced levels of the cerebrospinal fluid 5-hydroxyindoleacetic acid, a major metabolite of serotonin, which indicates a reduction in serotonin activity. Mann and associates (1986) found increased postsynaptic serotonergic receptors in suicide victims, while Stanley and Stanley (1990) found a reduction in serotonin neurotransmission, which is interpreted as an underlying biochemical "risk factor" for suicide. Marin and associates (1989) and Kavoussi and Siever (1991) hypothesize that there seems to be serotonergic reduction in behaviors such as impulsiveness, motor aggression, and suicidal tendencies. Brown and Linnoila (1990) demonstrated that there is a relationship between reduced serotonergic activity and aggressive and impulsive behavior.

Siever and Davis (1991) suggest that there may be a dysfunction of the brain system's ability to modulate and inhibit aggressive responses to environmental stimuli. They found EEG slow-wave activity and a low threshold for sedation discrimination among individuals with antisocial personality disorder as opposed to individuals with a long-term depression (Siever and Davis, 1991).

PERSONALITY ASSESSMENT AND CLINICAL EXAMPLES

Assessment is an essential part of providing nursing care, as a thorough assessment lays the foundation for the nursing diagnosis, DSM-IV diagnosis, expected patient outcomes interventions, and evaluation of the nursing care provided to the patient. Patients with personality disorders, particularly those with Cluster B disorders, are often seen several times in a mental health setting over the course of their lives.

When determining the methodology for assessing personality disorder, two major forms are suggested: (1) open-ended questions for the clinical interview, and (2) self-report survey instruments. Responses to both the clinical interview and survey instruments are reviewed in making a DSM-IV diagnosis.

CLINICAL INTERVIEW

When determining what questions will yield significant data, it is important to consider some characteristics of an individual with a personality disorder. That person has difficulty identifying self, his or her interpersonal relationships are often affected by the disorder, and the person's behavioral patterns, views, and expressions of emotions are different from those of others in the individual's cultural milieu. These patterns of thought and behavior lay the foundation for the assessment and interventions for this patient population.

The following questions will assess the areas that are disturbed in an individual with a personality disorder. These questions are asked after the person has identified the problem areas that brought him or her to the treatment setting.

The Patient's Identification of Self

1. How does the patient take care of his or her physical needs? Does the patient appear clean and appropriately dressed? Is the person getting sufficient sleep, nourishment, and exercise?
2. Does the patient exhibit an inappropriate or flat, constricted affect?
3. Ask the patient to describe himself or herself, elaborating on the person's strengths and weaknesses. Does the patient often focus on the weakness in a critical manner without acknowledging the strengths? Does the patient inflate his or her importance? What are the patient's likes and dislikes?
4. How anxious is the patient? Are his or her vital signs elevated? Is the person pacing, glancing about, or fidgeting? What is the

patient worrying about, and how often does the person think about these worries?

5. Ask the patient to describe what he or she does to calm down when feeling anxious, upset, or sad. Does the patient ever use alcohol or other drugs, engage in sex with multiple partners, eat an excessive amount of food, or harm himself or herself in any way?

6. Ask the patient if he or she ever felt like killing himself or herself or anyone else. Does the patient feel that way now? Does the patient have a plan? How often does he or she think about this plan? Is there a weapon available? How does the patient prevent himself or herself from acting on these thoughts?

7. Ask the patient if there has ever been a time when he or she hurt himself or herself by self-mutilating, such as cutting the skin until it bleeds, burning the skin with cigarettes, or pulling out a significant amount of hair. When did these incidents occur? Are these behaviors ongoing?

8. Does the patient deny strong emotions, such as anger and joy?

The Patient's Interpersonal Relationships

1. How does the patient interact with family members? Does the patient have friends? How does the patient interact with friends? Can the patient tolerate frustrations and disappointments in the relationship without resorting to vindictive behavior, or to hurting others either verbally or by exhibiting aggressive behavior?

2. How does the patient function in the workplace? Does the patient need constant supervision to complete a task? Does the patient complain about his or her boss or supervisor? Are the themes of the complaints centered around resenting assignments and having to provide accountability for the patient's work performance?

3. Can the patient identify with other people? Does the patient lack empathy? Does the patient constantly behave in a manner that

places him or her in the center of attention? Does the patient demonstrate critical behavior towards others? Is the patient concerned about how others will evaluate him or her?

4. Does the patient demonstrate a low frustration tolerance? What does the patient do when he or she feels frustrated with others? (Ask the patient how he or she reacts when driving and suddenly is struck in a traffic jam as an example of a commonly experienced frustration.)

5. Does the patient identify himself or herself in the context of a relationship? Does the patient indicate a dependence on family members or a significant other to meet most of his or her needs?

6. Does the patient have any friends? What is the nature of the friendship? Does the patient have an intimate relationship? Describe that relationship. Does the patient have multiple sexual relationships? (This question will assist the nurse to assess the ability of the patient to form friendships and whether these relationships are intense and stormy or supportive and reciprocal.)

The Patient's Behavioral Patterns

1. How does the patient describe the problem areas that caused the patient to seek help? Does the patient demonstrate the ability to identify the problems and discuss some possible options to problem solve? Does the patient blame others and/or indicate a plan of retaliation? Does the patient indicate a sense of entitlement when discussing the problem areas?

2. Does the patient engage in illegal activities? How does the patient view these activities? Has the patient ever been arrested? If so, has the patient ever been convicted? What was the punishment? How did the patient handle the sentence?

3. Has the patient experienced a lack of consensual validation? Has the patient ever experienced any ideas of reference? During the assessment interview, does the patient dis-

cuss any odd beliefs or magical thinking that influences his or her behavior?

4. Does the patient read hidden meanings into benign remarks of others? Is the patient suspicious of others? Does the patient question the fidelity of his or her significant other?

5. Is the patient impulsive? Does the patient have difficulty learning from mistakes? (This would be reflected by a patient experiencing the same problem repeatedly, without a change in the understanding of the problem and how he or she reacted to the issues.)

6. Does the patient have a history of failing to honor financial obligations? Does the patient plan ahead, such as securing a new job prior to quitting the current position?

7. How does the patient view his or her parenting responsibilities? Is there a history of child neglect or abuse (physical, verbal, sexual)? Does the parent provide adequate care for the children?

8. Does the patient use drugs or alcohol? Has the patient ever gotten into trouble with the law due to drugs or alcohol (including driving when intoxicated violations)?

PERSONALITY ASSESSMENT SURVEY

The Personality Assessment Survey (see Figure 23-1 on pages 367–369) is a ninety item self-report instrument, structured to assist in making a DSM-IV Personality Disorder diagnosis. This survey is completed by the patient and provides enough information to suggest the presence of a personality disturbance, if one exists. This survey allows the advanced practice nurse to skip all of the items that the patient has not affirmed as characteristic of his or her behavior or feelings over the past several years. The nurse should also ask about the negative items within a diagnostic category if there is either a clinical basis to suspect that the item is true, or to clarify, within a diagnostic category, if other items are true. To clarify the positive responses to the survey, use questions such as:

What is that like?
Give me the most extreme example.
Does that happen in a lot of different situations?
Have you always been that way?
Do you think you are more this way than most people?
Do you regard this as a problem for you?

Be sure that there is clear evidence from behavior during the interview or from other sources that the item is true.

SCORING THE PERSONALITY ASSESSMENT SURVEY

This section describes the number of items needed to make a DSM-IV diagnosis, behavior to observe during the interview, and a brief example.

Paranoid Personality Disorder

The person indicates a pervasive distrust and suspiciousness of others such that their motives are interpreted as malevolent. It begins by early adulthood and may present in a variety of contexts. These personality traits are indicated by four or more yes answers to items 1–8.

1. Are you sometimes not sure whether you can trust your friends or the people you work with?

2. Do you often have to keep an eye out to stop people from using you or hurting you?

3. Do you often pick up hidden meanings in what people say or do?

4. Are you the kind of person who holds grudges or takes a long time to forgive people who have insulted or slighted you?

5. Do you find it is best not to let other people know too much about you?

6. Do you often get angry because someone has slighted you or insulted you in some way?

7. Have you suspected that your spouse or partner has been unfaithful?

8. When you see people talking, do you often wonder if they are talking about you?

For example, Aaron has always been suspicious. He does not trust anyone, even his family members. Everyone was surprised when he got married, but he had decided to marry Dee so that she would not date anyone else. Within a month after their marriage, he began to suspect that she was being unfaithful. He began to go through her mail, check the numbers of her telephone calls with "Caller ID," and look through her purse for clues pointing to an affair. He became angry and vindictive when interacting with Dee. The more she tried to prove her innocence, the more suspicious and angry he became. Dee begged him to come to couples sessions with her to save the marriage.

Schizoid Personality Disorder

The person indicates a pattern of detachment from social relationships and a restricted range of expression of emotions in interpersonal settings. Behavior observed through the interview includes constricted affect; he or she may be aloof, cold, and rarely make reciprocal gestures or facial expressions, such as smiling or nodding. These personality traits are indicated by four or more yes answers to items 9–14.

9. Do you not need close relationships with other people, like family or friends?

10. When you are not doing anything in particular, do you think about things and ideas rather than people?

11. Would you rather do things alone than with other people?

12. Do you never seem to have really strong feelings, like being very angry or very happy?

13. Could you be content without being sexually involved with another person?

14. Do you not care much about what people think of you?

For example, Steve is 40 years old, single, lives alone, and has no close friends. He is quiet and rarely speaks to his co-workers or neighbors. He visits his parents' home when his mother invites him, but he rarely participates in the family conversations. He looks down at the ground when there are other people present. His face shows no emotion. Steve works hard and produces a good product; however, he rarely responds to compliments. His hobbies are solitary. After work, he goes home and watches TV or plays computer games. He does not date. If asked how he views his life, he indicates, in as few words as possible, that he is satisfied.

Schizotypal Personality Disorder

This person indicates a pattern of social and interpersonal deficits marked by acute discomfort with, and reduced capacity for, close relationships as well as by cognitive or perceptual distortions and eccentricities of behavior. Behavior observed during the interview includes:

odd speech—speech that is impoverished, digressive, vague, inappropriately abstract inappropriate or constricted affect—silly, aloof, rarely makes reciprocal gestures or facial expressions, such as smiling or nodding

odd, eccentric, or peculiar behavior or appearance—is unkempt, has unusual mannerisms, talks to self

These personality traits are indicated by five or more yes answers to items 15–21.

15. Have you often felt that the way things were arranged had a special significance for you?
16. Do you often feel nervous in a group of more than two or three people you don't know?
17. Have you ever felt that you could make things happen just by making a wish or thinking about them?
18. Have you had experiences with the supernatural, astrology, seeing the future, UFOs, ESP, or a personal experience with a "sixth sense"?
19. Do you often mistake objects or shadows for people, or noises for voices?
20. Have you had the sense that some person or force is around you, even though you cannot see anyone?
21. Have you had the experience of looking at a person or yourself in the mirror and seeing the face change right before your eyes?

For example, Alice is a 27-year-old single woman who works as a computer information analyst. She has a reputation of "being hard to approach because she is weird." She has a different interpretation of events that are occurring around her than other people experience. She often states that she has a sixth sense and can tell what is going to happen prior to its occurrence. She is vague in her speech pattern and thinks that when people are talking around her, they are discussing her. Her face is usually devoid of emotion. When Alice attends a meeting of her workgroup involving a special aspect, such as a luncheon or a meeting with another workgroup to brainstorm, Alice becomes very anxious. This anxiety builds as the meeting continues and Alice feels overwhelmed. Her associations become loose and her thought process concrete. She recently experienced a major depression after her cat died. She interpreted her cat's death as a warning from the spirit world.

Antisocial Personality Disorder

This person indicates a pattern of disregard for and violation of the rights of others occurring since age 15 years, as indicated by yes answers to three or more of the following items 22–33.

22. Did you often skip school?
23. Did you ever run away from home and stay out overnight?
24. Did you ever start fights?
25. Did you ever use a weapon in a fight?
26. Did you ever force someone to have sex with you?
27. Did you ever hurt an animal on purpose?
28. Did you ever hurt another person on purpose (other than in a fight)?
29. Did you deliberately damage things that weren't yours?
30. Did you set fires?
31. Did you lie a lot?
32. Did you ever steal things?
33. Did you ever rob or mug someone?

For example, Larry, age 34, is a patient in a forensic psychiatric unit. He was committed to the unit after beating two men and resisting arrest. Larry has a prior record of breaking and entering from age 14. At the time of his first arrest, he was living in a foster home, as his mother felt she could not control his truancy from school and his propensity to start small fires. Larry is angry, threatening, intimidating to staff and patients, and believes he was unjustly arrested. "Those men approached me first. They started the fight. The cop wouldn't listen, so I thought I'd teach him a lesson, but he arrested me and made me come here. I don't think you can help, you don't know anything about me, and you don't care. I'm just a prisoner to you."

Borderline Personality Disorder

This person indicates a pattern of instability of interpersonal relationships, self-image and affects, and marked impulsivity. These traits are indicated by five or more yes answers to the following items 34–46.

34. Do your relationships with people you really care about have lots of ups and downs?
35. Have you often done things impulsively?
36. Are you a "moody" person?
37. Do you often have temper outbursts or get so angry that you lose control?
38. Do you hit people or throw things when you get angry?
39. Do even little things get you very angry?
40. Have you tried to hurt or kill yourself or threatened to do so?
41. Are you different with different people or in different situations so that you sometimes don't know who you really are?
42. Are you often confused about your long-term goals or career plans?
43. Do you often change your mind about the types of friends or lovers you want?
44. Are you often not sure about what your real values are?
45. Do you often feel bored or empty inside?
46. Have you often become frantic when you thought that someone you really cared about was going to leave you?

For example, Cheryl was admitted to the psychiatric unit after taking an overdose of Valium after her husband left her following an intense verbal and physical fight. "Don and I have been fighting since shortly after we got married. Today, he wouldn't listen, so I grabbed his collar around his neck, and he threw me up against the wall. He yelled he had enough of this marriage, got his coat, and left the house. I was so empty, all I could do was cry. He may never come back to me. I can't go on without him. I decided to take my nerve pills and kill myself, because with Don gone, there is nothing left of me." Cheryl has a history of relationship problems. When exploring whether she has any family or friends that would help her during this crisis, she gave a history of relationships that were ended due to the other person not satisfying her needs. Her mother has a history of suicidal ideation and depression, and her father is an alcoholic who was abusive when Cheryl was a child.

Histrionic Personality Disorder

This person has a pattern of excessive emotionality and attention seeking. Behavior observed during interview includes a style of speech that is excessively impressionistic and lacking in detail; for example, when asked to describe his or her mother, the answer is no more specific than, "She was a beautiful person." These traits are indicated by yes answers to five or more of the following items 47–52.

47. Do you often go out of your way to get people to praise you?
48. Do you flirt a lot?
49. Do you often dress in a sexy way even when you are going to work or doing errands?
50. Does it bother you more than most people if you don't look attractive?
51. Are you very open with your emotions, for example, hugging people when you greet them or crying easily?
52. Do you like to be the center of attention?

For example, Robert is an actor with a local Shakespeare company. He is 27 years old and is reviewed as an excellent Hamlet, his current role. He has had difficulty recently in his relationship with Karen. He needs to be the center of attention, on- and off-stage. He tells Karen that he is an "entertainer" and will always want attention. He recently had an intense argument with Karen due to his criticism of another actor's work. Karen told him she would no longer go to any other types of live entertainment with him. He became enraged, and yelled to the whole theater that he was an actor and that he and his girlfriend were having an argument. Karen walked out, and Robert turned to the people in the foyer of the theater, telling them the story of his relationship problems, as though they were an audience.

Narcissistic Personality Disorder

This person has a pattern of grandiosity (in fantasy or behavior), need for admiration, and lack of empathy. These traits are indicated by five or more yes answers to the following items 53–62.

53. When you're criticized, do you often feel very angry, ashamed, or put down, even hours or days later?
54. Have you sometimes had to use other people to get what you wanted?
55. Do you sometimes "sweet talk" people just to get what you want out of them?
56. Do you feel you are a person with special talents or abilities?
57. Have people told you that you have too high an opinion of yourself?
58. When you have a problem, do you almost always insist on seeing the top person?
59. Do you often daydream about achieving great things or being famous?
60. Do you often daydream about having a "perfect" romance?
61. Have people said that you are not sympathetic or understanding about their problems?
62. Are you often envious of other people?

For example, Martha is an accountant in a big firm. She is known for asking people to help her in such a way that they end up completing the project for her, while Martha gets the credit, and sometimes a raise. Martha is very verbal at most office staff meetings, usually bragging about what she has accomplished. She never acknowledges the individuals who have assisted her in the projects. She views herself as one of the top accountants in the region and expects to be treated as such. When other staff members assist in project completion, Martha views it as if they are interning under her direction. Martha sees herself as entitled to an expensive car, a big house, jewelry, a housekeeper, and someone who will tend her garden. She is married, but the relationship seems to have lost its spark. When she mentions her husband, it usually is followed by a criticism, and an explanation of how she can do better.

Avoidant Personality Disorder

This person has a pattern of social inhibition, feelings of inadequacy, and hypersensitivity to negative evaluation. These traits are indicated by five or more yes answers to the following items 63–79.

63. Are your feelings more easily hurt than most people's if someone criticizes you or disapproves of something you say or do?
64. Are there very few people that you are really close to outside of your immediate family?
65. Do you avoid getting involved with people unless you are certain they will like you?
66. Do you avoid social situations in which you might have to talk with other people?
67. Have you avoided jobs or assignments that involved having to deal with a lot of people?
68. Are you often quiet in social situations because you're afraid of saying the wrong thing?
69. Have you often been afraid that you might look nervous or tense, might cry, or blush in front of other people?

70. Do a lot of things seem dangerous or difficult to you that do not seem that way to most people?
71. Do you need a lot of advice or reassurance from others before you can make everyday decisions?
72. Have you allowed other people to make very important decisions for you?
73. Do you often agree with people even when you think they are wrong?
74. Do you find it hard to start or work on tasks when there is no one to help you?
75. Have you often done unpleasant or demeaning things to get other people to like you?
76. Do you generally prefer not to be by yourself?
77. Do you often do things to avoid being alone?
78. Have you ever felt helpless or devastated when a close relationship ended?
79. Do you worry a lot about people that you care about leaving you?

For example, Beth is a 39-year-old woman who works as a bookkeeper in a small printing company. She has worked in this same company since she graduated from high school. Prior to this year, all of the books were done by hand, using a calculator. Due to the ease and accuracy of computer programs, Beth's boss bought a computer and a software package that keeps track of the expenditures and profits the company is generating. Beth views the computer as the end of her job with this company. Even though the boss has given her encouragement that he is not planning to terminate her or her position, Beth remains emotionally paralyzed, unable to learn the new computer system. Beth is certain she will make mistakes that will "make her look dumb"; she is certain she will be fired. She further worries that if she were to be fired, she would lose her condominium, as she lives alone. She sees herself as worthless, unable to try anything new, and she is often anxious, particularly around people. Beth has only two friends she speaks to, and has not shared this problem with them, for fear that the friends will label her as stupid.

Obsessive–Compulsive Personality Disorder
This person has an excessive need to be taken care of that leads to submitting and clinging behavior and fears of separation. These traits are indicated by five or more yes answers to the following items 80–90.

80. Do you have trouble finishing jobs because you spend so much time trying to get things exactly right?
81. Are you the kind of person who focuses on details, order, and organization, or who likes to make lists and schedules?
82. Do you sometimes insist that other people do things exactly the way you want?
83. Do you sometimes do things yourself because you know that no one else will do them exactly right?
84. Are you, or does your family feel that you are, so devoted to work (or school) that you have no time left for other people or for just having fun?
85. Do you sometimes have trouble making decisions because you can't make up your mind what to do or how to do it?
86. Do you have higher standards than most people about what is right and what is wrong?
87. Do you often get angry at other people for breaking rules?
88. Have people complained that you are not affectionate enough?
89. Do you rarely give presents, volunteer time, or do favors for other people?
90. Do you have trouble throwing things out because they might come in handy some day?

For example, Vince is a dentist who has a large private practice. He is known as a good, careful dentist. His personal life presents some areas of conflict. He is married and has three children. He and his wife decided early in their marriage that she would stay home after the children were born and take care of the childrearing. Vince is now frustrated and angry with his wife, as he feels she is not setting a good example for the children. He feels they spend too much time in play activities when they should be studying or practicing piano or ballet. He thinks their world should be more disciplined and structured. Vince is particularly upset with how his wife spends money. He gives her a $20 weekly allowance, and he expects her not to ask for any more money. She has been using her ATM card to purchase gas for the car, groceries at the end of the week, and occasionally to do something fun with the kids. He handles his anger with his wife by refusing to speak to her. She becomes upset and tearful. He then tells her to control her emotions, particularly in front of the children.

Personality Disorder Not Otherwise Specified

This category is for disorders of personality functioning that do not meet the criteria for any specific personality disorder. An example is a person who has features of more than one personality disorder or the category may be used to include depressive personality disorder and passive–aggressive personality disorder which are still under consideration for the next DSM. A case example of Personality Disorder NOS is in Chapter 29.

NURSING INTERVENTIONS AND TREATMENT

The patients who are most likely to be seeking treatment from nurses in advanced practice are individuals with antisocial or borderline personality disorders. With this in mind, this section will concentrate on interventions for those two types of individuals.

Antisocial Personality Disorder

After determining that an individual has an antisocial personality disorder, the primary symptom complex that requires intervention is rageful, aggressive, and intimidating behavior. This behavior is often rationalized by the patient and can be used in a manipulative manner. The individual with antisocial behavior demonstrates symptoms such as lying, superficial charm, unreliability, lack of guilt, inability to learn from experiences, an incapacity to have intimate relationships, and a chaotic sexual life with multiple partners (Akhtar, 1992; APA, 1994; Widiger et al., 1992). Understanding the multiple symptoms that are part of this personality disorder can assist the therapist in planning intervention strategies to decrease the symptoms of aggressive and intimidating behavior.

► CASE EXAMPLE

Tom is a 25-year-old unmarried male, father of one, who was referred by the court for psychotherapy due to a recent incident of physically abusing his girlfriend, who is the mother of his child. He is angry and resentful towards the court for his sentence of 1 year probation and weekly psychotherapy. He does not understand why psychotherapy is warranted or would be helpful. "I get to stare at you for 45 minutes each week, for what!" He does not view the incident of abuse as something he should have gotten arrested for. "I was trying to get away from a nagging woman. She kept on bugging me to take care of Tommy. I just started my car, I was ready to leave, she hung on and got herself dragged. It wasn't my fault!"

Tom has a history of brushes with the law. When he was 10 he was caught setting a fire at a local elementary school. He lied about the incident and was released. At age 12 he was caught shoplifting with a friend. The store was willing to let him go, but banned him from ever coming into the store again. When he was 15, he was caught by the police driving without a license in his brother's car, which he had taken without his brother's knowledge. He had been speeding and ran a red light. He had purchased some beer which was found in the car. He was placed on supervisory court probation for a year. He dropped out of school at age 16, after failing to pass several courses. He has difficulty establishing relationships and becomes angry and threatening if the woman he is with does not do what he wants her to do. He has a history of physically abusing women who he considers his girlfriends.

Tom's parents separated when he was 3. His father was physically abusive to his mother as well as to Tom and his brother. His father abused alcohol and cocaine. His mother is a chronically depressed woman who views the world in negative terms. She drinks alcohol nightly to help her fall asleep. Tom sees his mother as "always needing something."

During the assessment it is evident that Tom's participation in therapy is court mandated. This is one of the first obstacles to explore when working with a person who is directed to attend therapy by the court or the workplace. Frequently, individuals with antisocial personality disorder are mandated to attend psychotherapy. The second area of concern is Tom's history of violence. It is important to attend to this issue early in the therapy work and explore alternative ways of expressing anger. The third area of concern that would be important to attend to while working with Tom is assisting him to use alternative communication patterns rather than intimidation when asking another individual for something.

Expectations for Intervention. It is critical for the advanced practice nurse to have realistic expectations for individuals with an antisocial personality disorder. Widiger and associates (1992) note that often the intensity of the symptoms of antisocial behavior decrease with age. These authors state that specialized residential therapeutic communities, such as wilderness programs, are the most effective programs due to the consistent milieu, close supervision, and confrontations of behaviors that are symptomatic of the antisocial personality-disordered individual. They believe that traditional psychiatric inpatient units are not as successful in reducing the behavioral symptoms, due to the ease with which the patient can manipulate the staff and patient peers. Outpatient treatment does not usually result in facilitating behavioral change, due to the patient's inability to commit himself or herself to the process of self-examination and limit setting. This information is important to keep in mind when assessing appropriate outcome expectations to measure the patient's progress.

If a patient, like Tom, demonstrates aggressive or violent behavior, use interventions that encompass the least restrictive modality possible to assist the patient and maintain safety. When the patient is in an inpatient setting, preplan with the health care team an organized plan of action that can be put into place immediately if a patient becomes aggressive and potentially violent. Set limits in a firm, nonpunitive, clear manner that provides structure and assists the patient to control his or her impulses. Patients must be held responsible for their aggressive or violent behavior. This can be communicated by stating a clear expectation that violence in this setting is unacceptable. Morrison (1993) suggests that a contract for safety is a helpful tool to reinforce the patient's responsibility for his or her impulse control. The contract must have information about the unacceptable patient behaviors, appropriate behaviors, consequences for breaking the contract, and the health care provider's contribution to the care of the patient. The focus should be on the safety of the patient and others in the environment (Morrison, 1993, 1994).

Pharmacotherapy. If the patient is beginning to lose control, the use of psychopharmacological agents may be helpful to prevent a violent outburst. The follow medications and dosages are most often recommended and are based on the patient's level of agitation and the degree of aggressive and violent behavior exhibited.

- A benzodiazepine can be administered orally and works rapidly. The recommended dosage is to use low-potency agents, such as oxazepam (Serax) 15 to 30 mg or diazepam (Valium) 5 to 10 mg (Keltner and Folks, 1993).
- Antipsychotic agents, such as a high-potency neuroleptic, can be used when a patient is agitated as well as when the patient is demonstrating aggressive behavior. Give the patient a choice of an oral elixir or an IM medication. Haloperidol (Haldol) 10 mg PO with a usual daily range of 15 to 100 mg/day would be an appropriate dosage for prevention of an aggressive outburst. Use rapid neuroleptization if the patient is unable to regain control after

the initial dosage. Haloperidol (Haldol) 5 mg IM every 4 hours is used for low-dose rapid neuroleptization. For a high-dose rapid neuroleptization, haloperidol (Haldol) 5 mg IM at 30- to 60-minute intervals is used. Monitor the patient for response to the medication 20 minutes after giving the dose, and observe for any side effects. Document levels of consciousness and vital signs before administering the next dose. Observe the patient closely for changes in behavior and mental status (Keltner and Folks, 1993).
- Short-term anesthetizing agents may be used to assist the patient to sleep, rather than act on the aggressive impulse. Sodium amytal 200 to 500 mg may be given by slow IV push as a 2.5 or 5-percent solution at the rate of 1 ml/min until sleep occurs. Diazepam (Valium) 5 to 10 mg IV may also facilitate sleep in an aggressive patient (Keltner and Folks, 1993).

Borderline Personality Disorder
The patient with a borderline personality disorder is a challenge for the advanced practice nurse. Often, the patient is referred for outpatient psychotherapy after a loss of a significant relationship or when the relationship is very rocky and conflictual. The patient may become suicidal or self-mutilate during this time of intense emotional pain, as an individual with borderline personality disorder is unable to mourn the end of a relationship due to difficulties achieving object constancy. Another common reason a person with borderline personality disorder seeks a referral for psychotherapy is that the individual has conflict within himself or herself regarding role, life purpose, love preference, and/or gender confusion. Often the individual with borderline personality disorder has a depression and may abuse alcohol or another drug when feeling anxious or empty.

Suicide Potential. Suicidal ideation and gestures are common among individuals with borderline personality disorder. Isometsa and coworkers (1996) found that 95 percent of the individuals in their study who completed suicide and had a personality disorder also had symptoms of a depressive disorder or a psychoactive substance use disorder. Soloff and associates (1994) state that one important risk factor to consider when treating patients who have suicidal thoughts is whether the patient has borderline personality disorder. In their research, they concluded that suicidal impulses are most common when the patient with borderline personality disorder is experiencing anger and impulsivity. The patient is most at risk for suicidal completion if the patient is older, has a history of impulsivity, has a borderline or antisocial personality disorder, experiences depressed moods, and has made prior suicide attempts (Soloff et al., 1994). It is important to assess the patient's potential for suicidal completion, and link the suicidal ideation with other emotional responses in the patient's life rather than to label the patient as "acting out" or "attention seeking."

Self-mutilation.

Self-mutilation is common with individuals who have a borderline personality disorder, particularly if there was a history of early psychological trauma. Dulit and colleagues (1994) culled the literature and highlight that individuals who self-mutilate have impulsivity, aggression, suicidal behavior, eating disorders, child abuse, depression, and anxiety. Their research showed that individuals who self-mutilate tend to have been in outpatient treatment with prior usage of psychotropic medications. Often this population of patients has a major depression or bulimia nervosa or anorexia nervosa. The individuals who frequently self-mutilate have acute and chronic suicidal ideation and have made several suicidal attempts. People who self-mutilate frequently have reported less sexual activity and less interest in having a sexual relationship (Dulit et al., 1994)

A concept that is helpful in understanding the individual who self-mutilates is alexithymia. Alexithymia is a term derived from the Greek "a" for "lack," "lexis" for "word," and "thymos" for "feeling" (Sifneos, 1996). Alexithymia means that the person is unable to find words for what

they are feeling. The patient acts out the feelings, due to the inability to express or process those feeling states. The individual has no fantasies that accompany an emotional arousal. In this disturbance there is difficulty in affective and cognitive functioning when the individual is interpreting feelings. With alexithymia, the emotions are experienced in an undifferentiated somatic form (APA, 1984; Sifneos, 1996). For example, Joan has had problems with her perception of self, particularly when it comes to eating. She often binge eats when feeling "empty." She is unable to identify her other feelings, and cannot identify a time when she felt good or happy. She has disclosed that she feels feelings in her stomach, especially when upset or fearful. Joan cannot identify why she binge eats, and does not cognitively tie the eating to the feeling of emptiness.

Defenses Against Anxiety.

When working with individuals who have borderline personality disorder, it is important to understand some of the defenses that are unconsciously used to deal with overwhelming feelings associated with abandonment, anxiety, and fear. The two primary defenses that disturb interactions with others are splitting and projective identification. Splitting is defined by Kernberg (1985) as the inability of the individual to deal with both positive and negative parts of self and others. The person can only recognize one part of self and others at a time. Therefore, when the individual with borderline personality disorder recognizes the "good" part of self or others, there is no other aspect to that person, and the person is idealized. When the individual who is splitting focuses on the negative aspect to self or others, that is the sole focus, and no positive attributes are recognized. This defense greatly disturbs relations with others and is particularly important to recognize in the therapeutic relationship, where the material disclosed is emotionally charged.

Projective identification is another defense against the patient's anxiety that is important to understand when providing psychotherapeutic care to the individual who has borderline personality disorder. This defense is a form of projection and was defined by Kernberg (1984). The person who is using the defense of projective identification:

- Has an intense feeling and simultaneously projects it to another person.
- Then begins to fear the other person involved in the projective identification.
- Attempts to decrease the anxiety and fear by striving to control the other person involved in the projection by his or her behavior and verbal output.

Psychopharmacotherapy. Patients with borderline personality disorder can benefit from the use of psychopharmacological agents. Davis and associates (1995) surveyed the literature to determine the best psychopharmacotherapy for patients with personality disorders. They suggest that small doses of antipsychotics are helpful for patients who have transient psychosis or paranoia; antidepressants, such as the SSRIs (selective serotonin reuptake inhibitors) for concurrent panic attacks, phobias, compulsive symptoms with depressive syndromes; and mood stabilizers (carbamazepine, or Tegretol) for cyclothymic presentations.

Soloff and associates (1991) reported that haloperidol assisted the patient with borderline personality disorder to decrease hostility and increase impulse control. This study also demonstrated that amitriptyline was found to decrease hostility and increase impulse control for patients with borderline personality disorder who were evaluated as being "unstable."

Staff Conflict. Often, when a patient with a borderline personality disorder is admitted to an inpatient unit there is staff conflict. An advanced practice psychiatric nurse may act in a consultative role for the unit to decrease the staff conflict or may be the attending psychotherapist for the patient. It is therefore important to understand the dynamics of this dispute. Part of the staff dissension can be traced to the patient's use of the primitive defense of splitting; the other contributing factor is differing philosophies of treatment. Staff members react to individuals with borderline personality disorder according to their understanding of the basis for the patient's behavior, comprehension of their own reactions to the patient's actions, and the integration of a theoretical model to clinical practice. Some staff members experience the patient as having a great deal of psychological pain and therefore unable to identify his or her own needs and feeling states, while other staff members view the patient as demanding, manipulative, and sabotaging of the nursing care.

THEORETICAL POSTURES THAT SHAPE TREATMENT GOALS

There are several theoretical schools of thought that shape the goals for treatment of the patient with a severe personality disorder. The theorists who utilize object relations, such as Kernberg (1984, 1985) and Masterson (1976) suggest long-term hospitalization or treatment when providing care. This treatment is designed to promote structural change within the patient's psychological makeup. The therapist with this belief explores issues, such as abandonment anxiety, the patient's view of self and others, and how the patient deals with losses. Patients are hospitalized when they become suicidal and need a supportive environment to prevent acting on this self-destructive impulse. Hospitalization is seen as providing a supportive environment, where the patient is protected from acting on self-destructive impulses, and the staff provides empathy, nuturance, and firm, consistent limit-setting. The patient's defenses, such as regression, alexithymia, and projective identification, are symptoms of the patient's attempt to deal with overwhelming stress. The therapeutic milieu is utilized by the staff members to help the patient learn how to deal with issues by exploring the presenting problems, assisting the patient to improve the ability to recognize his or her feelings, and to be better able to tolerate delayed gratification without anger and fears of abandonment.

► CASE EXAMPLE

The following is an example of an individual with a borderline personality disorder who sought treatment due to feeling overwhelmed with anger, depressed and suicidal.

Jayne is a 26-year-old single woman who lives with her brother. She has been having an affair with Ed, a married professional man, for the last 2 years. Jayne is also dating a woman, Andrea, who she had met at a women's basketball game. One evening, Jayne was feeling lonely and scared, so she beeped Ed. When he responded, he said he could not talk to her at that time, as he was having dinner with his wife. Jayne became enraged, yelled at him on the phone, called him names, and told him she did not want to see him again. After she hung up, she began to drink the alcohol that her brother had bought for a party he was planning. She was sobbing, became suicidal, and cut her wrist with a knife in the kitchen. Jayne called Andrea to say good-bye. Andrea rushed over to Jayne's house and took her to the emergency room. Jayne was treated for the wrist wound and was released, with a signed contract for safety and a referral for an appointment with an advanced practice nurse the next day.

One of the key issues to highlight when working with Jayne is the expectations of availability she has regarding the individuals with whom she has a significant relationship. She expected Ed to be able to talk to her when she beeped him, when by nature of his marital relationship, he was unavailable. It would be important to explore her expectations of Andrea when she made the call to say good-bye. Gunderson (1996) points out the difficulty individuals with borderline personality disorder have with feeling and being alone. He states that due to difficulties with object constancy, the individual with borderline personality disorder needs reassurance that he or she is cared for. When this reassurance does not occur, Masterson's (1976) work identifies the behaviors an individual exhibits in response to the feelings of abandonment: depression, rage, panic, guilt, passivity and helplessness, and emptiness and void. Jayne exhibited these behaviors as well as the impulsive behavior of drinking alcohol and the suicidal gesture. Understanding her behavior in this context can lead to patient teaching about how to deal with overwhelming feelings of loneliness, emptiness, rage, and suicidal ideation without acting on these impulses. Linehan (1993) has devised a course for individuals with borderline personality disorder that teaches the patient skills that can assist the patient to better cope with the overwhelming feelings described above.

By the nature of Jayne's relationships, she demonstrates having difficulty determining healthy boundaries. This is an important concept that can be discussed with the patient as it relates to her relationship with Ed, as well as by demonstrating healthy boundary setting by example in the psychotherapy. Boundaries provide a container, a definition of roles for each of the participants in the therapeutic relationship. For example, when discussing the patient's expectations of the therapeutic encounter, establishment of boundaries assists the discussion of nursing goals for the therapy. Establishment of boundaries refers to the definition of the context of the therapeutic encounter; how the patient and nurse refer to one another (by name); when they will meet (milieu groups, individual time approximately 10 to 15 minutes per shift when the nurse is on duty on an inpatient unit); what will be accomplished (the patient will discuss some of the issues that caused the hospitalization or the reason the patient entered therapy). If the patient is seen by an advanced practice psychiatric nurse in an outpatient setting, the therapeutic boundaries include where the therapy meetings will be held, length of the session, permission for the advanced practice nurse to discuss the case (without identification of the patient) in clinical supervision, when medication evaluation may be indicated, and arrangements to pay the fee established by the nurse psychotherapist. All therapeutic boundaries include a protection for both the therapist and the patient against socializing out of the therapeutic setting, and a prohibition against dating or any physical or sexual encounters. The therapeutic relationship is a relationship where the nurse assists the patient to explore problems, identify options for change, and evaluate how these new behaviors helped the patient accomplish some relief from symptoms. In light of this principle, it is important to decline treating someone one knows, no matter how informally, such as a neighbor, former boyfriend's sister, or a fellow professional colleague (Gutheil and Gabbard, 1993).

Recently, with the advent of managed care, short-term hospitalization is viewed as the most cost-effective use of the patient's insurance dollar. A short-term hospital stay emphasizes the patient's behavior and consequences of that action rather than the interpsychological dynamics and defenses. Limit setting, problem solving, patient teaching, and clear expectations of patient functioning are interventions that are used to promote control of impulsive behavior. The aim of the adaptational approach is to prevent the patient from regressing and encourage the patient to take more responsibility for his or her behavior (Gallop, 1992).

When there are staff members who represent these two schools of thought working with the same patient, a natural theoretical split occurs. The patient may view the staff who are working for structural change as being supportive, as opposed to the staff who view adaptation as the goal for treatment and who may be seen as angry and/or punitive when they set limits. This split is countertherapeutic for the patient and the staff milieu. It is important that the staff and attending practitioner agree on the purpose for the hospitalization, how to treat the precipitating event, and which therapeutic philosophy will be operational in the care of the patient. Staff disagreements should be aired and discussed at regular staff meetings. A peer supervision group should be a regular feature on an inpatient psychiatric unit. This group provides an avenue to review the nurse's countertransference towards difficult patients, assist the staff member to have a safe place to discuss these feelings and discuss plans to provide consistent therapeutic nursing interventions (Bonnivier, 1992).

Summary

One role of the advanced practice psychiatric nurse is to provide efficient and effective primary care to psychiatric patients. It is important for the advanced practice psychiatric nurse to be able to recognize individuals who have a personality disorder in order to be able to plan and execute a comprehensive plan of care. The nurse must keep in mind that these individuals have difficulty relating to others; therefore the therapeutic relationship will require patience and a desire to teach the patient a more effective way of communicating and coping. People who have personality disorders have different interpretations of the events around them, and therefore it is important for the advanced practice nurse to ascertain these ideas without judging the patient. Often the individual with a personality disorder has difficulty with impulse control, and therefore part of the treatment plan involves consistency in assisting the patient to devise new strategies to problem solve rather than the impulsive behavior pattern. Growth in these areas occurs slowly, and the patient teaching will need to include practical repetition of new ways to cope and relate. If the nurse in advanced practice can keep these principles in mind, the therapeutic work with an individual with a personality disorder is very satisfying for both the patient and the nurse psychotherapist.

INSTRUCTIONS

These questions are about the kind of person you generally are, that is, how you usually have felt or behaved over the past several years. Circle "Yes" or "No." If you do not understand a question, leave it blank.

1. Are you sometimes not sure whether you can trust your friends or the people you work with?	NO YES
2. Do you often have to keep an eye out to stop people from using you or hurting you?	NO YES
3. Do you often pick up hidden meanings in what people say or do?	NO YES
4. Are you the kind of person who holds grudges or takes a long time to forgive people who have insulted or slighted you?	NO YES
5. Do you find it is best not to let other people know too much about you?	NO YES
6. Do you often get angry because someone has slighted you or insulted you in some way?	NO YES
7. Have you suspected that your spouse or partner has been unfaithful?	NO YES
8. When you see people talking, do you often wonder if they are talking about you?	NO YES
9. Do you not need close relationships with other people, like family or friends?	NO YES
10. When you are not doing anything in particular, do you think about things and ideas rather than people?	NO YES
11. Would you rather do things alone than with other people?	NO YES
12. Do you never seem to have strong feelings, like being very angry or very happy?	NO YES
13. Could you be content without being sexually involved with another person?	NO YES
14. Do you not care much about what other people think of you?	NO YES
15. Have you often felt that the way things were arranged had a special significance for you?	NO YES
16. Do you often feel nervous in a group of more than two or three people you don't know?	NO YES
17. Have you ever felt that you could make things happen just by making a wish or thinking about them?	NO YES
18. Have you had experiences with the supernatural, astrology, seeing the future, UFO's, ESP, or a personal experience with a "sixth sense"?	NO YES
19. Do you often mistake objects or shadows for people, or noises for voices?	NO YES
20. Have you had the sense that some person or force is around you, even though you cannot see anyone?	NO YES
21. Have you had the experience of looking at a person or yourself in the mirror and seeing the face change right before your eyes?	NO YES

Questions 22–33 are about things you may have done before you were fifteen.

22. Did you often skip school?	NO YES
23. Did you ever run away from home and stay out overnight?	NO YES

(continued)

Figure 23–1. Personality Assessment Survey

24. Did you ever start fights?	NO	YES
25. Did you ever use a weapon in a fight?	NO	YES
26. Did you ever force someone to have sex with you?	NO	YES
27. Did you ever hurt an animal on purpose?	NO	YES
28. Did you ever hurt another person on purpose (other than in a fight)?	NO	YES
29. Did you deliberately damage things that weren't yours?	NO	YES
30. Did you set fires?	NO	YES
31. Did you lie a lot?	NO	YES
32. Did you ever steal things?	NO	YES
33. Did you ever rob or mug someone?	NO	YES
34. Do your relationships with people you care about have lots of ups and downs?	NO	YES
35. Have you often done things impulsively?	NO	YES
36. Are you a "moody" person?	NO	YES
37. Do you often have temper outbursts or get so angry that you lose control?	NO	YES
38. Do you hit people or throw things when you get angry?	NO	YES
39. Do even little things get you very angry?	NO	YES
40. Have you tried to hurt or kill yourself or threatened to do so?	NO	YES
41. Are you different with different people or in different situations so that you sometimes don't know who you really are?	NO	YES
42. Are you often confused about your long-term goals or career plans?	NO	YES
43. Do you often change your mind about the types of friends or lovers you want?	NO	YES
44. Are you often not sure about what your real values are?	NO	YES
45. Do you often feel bored or empty inside?	NO	YES
46. Have you often become frantic when you thought that someone you really cared about was going to leave you?	NO	YES
47. Do you often go out of your way to get people to praise you?	NO	YES
48. Do you flirt a lot?	NO	YES
49. Do you often dress in a sexy way even when you are going to work or doing errands?	NO	YES
50. Does it bother you more than most people if you don't look attractive?	NO	YES
51. Are you very open with your emotions, for example, hugging people when you greet them or crying easily?	NO	YES
52. Do you like to be the center of attention?	NO	YES
53. When you're criticized, do you often feel very angry, ashamed, or put down, even hours or days later?	NO	YES
54. Have you sometimes had to use other people to get what you wanted?	NO	YES
55. Do you sometimes "sweet talk" people just to get what you want out of them?	NO	YES
56. Do you feel you are a person with special talents or abilities?	NO	YES
57. Have people told you that you have too high an opinion of yourself?	NO	YES
58. When you have a problem, do you almost always insist on seeing the top person?	NO	YES
59. Do you often daydream about achieving great things or being famous?	NO	YES
60. Do you often daydream about having a "perfect" romance?	NO	YES
61. Have people said that you are not sympathetic or understanding about their problems?	NO	YES
62. Are you often envious of other people?	NO	YES
63. Are your feelings more easily hurt than most people's if someone criticizes you or disapproves of something you say or do?	NO	YES
64. Are there very few people that you are really close to outside of your immediate family?	NO	YES
65. Do you avoid getting involved with people unless you are certain they will like you?	NO	YES
66. Do you avoid social situations in which you might have to talk with other people?	NO	YES
67. Have you avoided jobs or assignments that involved having to deal with a lot of people?	NO	YES
68. Are you often quiet in social situations because you're afraid of saying the wrong thing?	NO	YES
69. Have you often been afraid that you might look nervous or tense, might cry, or blush in front of other people?	NO	YES
70. Do a lot of things seem dangerous or difficult to you that do not seem that way to most people?	NO	YES

(continued)

Figure 23–1. Personality Assessment Survey (continued)

71. Do you need a lot of advice or reassurance from others before you can make everyday decisions?   NO YES
72. Have you allowed other people to make very important decisions for you?   NO YES
73. Do you often agree with other people even when you think they are wrong?   NO YES
74. Do you find it hard to start work on tasks when there is no one to help you?   NO YES
75. Have you often done unpleasant or demeaning things to get other people to like you? NO YES
76. Do you generally prefer not to be by yourself?   NO YES
77. Do you often do things to avoid being alone?   NO YES
78. Have you ever felt helpless or devastated when a close relationship ended?   NO YES
79. Do you worry a lot about people that you care about leaving you?   NO YES
80. Do you have trouble finishing jobs because you spend so much time trying to get things exactly right?   NO YES
81. Are you the kind of person who focuses on details, order, and organization, or who likes to make lists and schedules?   NO YES
82. Do you sometimes insist that other people do things exactly the way you want?   NO YES
83. Do you sometimes do things yourself because you know that no one else will do them exactly right?   NO YES
84. Are you, or does your family feel that you are, so devoted to work (or school) that you have no time left for other people or for just having fun?   NO YES
85. Do you sometimes have trouble making decisions because you can't make up your mind what to do or how to do it?   NO YES
86. Do you have higher standards than most people about what is right and what is wrong? NO YES
87. Do you often get angry at other people for breaking rules?   NO YES
88. Have people complained that you are not affectionate enough?   NO YES
89. Do you rarely give presents, volunteer time, or do favors for other people?   NO YES
90. Do you have trouble throwing things out because they might come in handy some day? NO YES

Figure 23–1. Personality Assessment Survey (continued)

REFERENCES

Akhtar S. *Broken Structures: Severe Personality Disorders and Their Treatments.* Northvale, NJ: Jason Aronson; 1992.

American Psychiatric Association. *Diagnostic and Statistical Manual of Mental Disorders*, 4th ed. Washington, DC: American Psychiatric Association; 1994.

American Psychiatric Association. *The American Psychiatric Association's Psychiatric Glossary.* Washington, DC: American Psychiatric Press; 1984.

Bonnivier JF. A peer supervision group: Put countertransference to work. *J Psychosoc Nurs.* 1992; 30:5–8.

Brown GL, Ebert MHM, Goyer PF, et al. Aggression, suicide and serotonin relationships to CSF amine metabolites, *Am J Psychiatry.* 1982;139:741–745.

Brown GL, Linnoila MI. CSF serotonin metabolite (5-HIAA) studies in depression, impulsivity, and violence. *J Clin Psychiatry.* 1990;51(suppl April): 31–43.

Burgess AW, Roberts AR. Levels of stress and crisis precipitants: The stress-crisis continuum. *Crisis Intervention.* 1995;2:31–47.

Coryell WH, Zimmerman MBA. Personality disorder in the families of depressed, schizophrenia, and never-ill probands. *Am J Psychiatry.* 1989;146: 496–502.

Davis J, Janicak PG, Ayd FJ. Psychopharmacotherapy of the personality-disordered patient, *Psychiatr Ann.* 1995;25:614–619.

Dulit RA, Fuer MR, Leon AC, et al. Clinical correlates of self-mutilation in borderline personality disorder. *Am J Psychiatry.* 1994;151:1305–1311.

Erikson EH. *Childhood and Society*, New York: Norton; 1950.

Freud S. The dissolution of the oedipus complex. *Standard Edition.* London: Hogarth Press; 1924;19:72–79.

Freud S. The ego and the id. *Standard Edition.* London: Hogarth Press; 1923;19:3–66.

Freud S. The development of the libido and the sexual organizations. *Standard Edition.* London: Hogarth Press; 1917;16:320–338.

Freud S. Three essays on the theory of sexuality. *Standard Edition*. London: Hogarth Press; 1905;7: 125–243.

Gallop R. Self-destructive and impulsive behavior in the patient with a borderline personality disorder: Rethinking hospital treatment and management. *Arch Psychiatr Nurs*. 1992;6:178–182.

Gunderson JG. The borderline patient's intolerance of aloneness: Insecure attachment and therapist availability. *Am J Psychiatry*. 1996;153:752–757.

Gutheil TG, Gabbard GO. The concept of boundaries in clinical practice: Theoretical and risk-management dimensions. *Am J Psychiatry*. 1993; 150:188–196.

Isometsa ET, Henriksson MM, Heikkinen, ME, et al. Suicide among subjects with personality disorders. *Am J Psychiatry*. 1996;153:667–673.

Kavoussi RJ, Siever LJ. Biologic validators of personality disorders. In: Oldham JM, ed. *Personality Disorders: New Perspectives on Diagnostic Validity*. Washington, DC: American Psychiatric Press; 1991.

Keltner NL, Folks DG. *Psychotropic Drugs*. St. Louis: Mosby-Year Book; 1993.

Kernberg OB. *Borderline Conditions and Pathological Narcissism*. Northvale, NJ: Jason Aronson; 1985.

Kernberg OB. *Severe Personality Disorders: Psychotherapeutic Strategies*. New Haven: Yale University Press; 1984.

Lencz T, Raine A, Scerbo A, et al. Impaired eye tracking in undergraduates with schizotypal personality disorder. *Am J Psychiatry*. 1993;150:152–153.

Linehen M. *Skills Training Manual for Treating Borderline Personality Disorder*. New York: Guilford Press; 1993.

Mahler MS. On the first three subphases of the separation-individuation process. *Int J Psychoanal*. 1972a;53:333–338.

Mahler MS. Rapprochement subphase of the separation-individuation process. *Psychoanal Q*. 1972b;41:487–506.

Mahler MS. A study of the separation-individuation process and its possible application to borderline phenomena in the psychoanalytic situation. *Psychoanal Study Child*. 1971;26:403–424.

Mahler MS. Thoughts about development and individuation, *Psychoanal Study Child*. 1963;18:307–324.

Mann JJ, Stanley M, McBride PA, et al. Increased serotonin-2 and beta-adrenergic receptor binding in the frontal cortices of suicide victims. *Arch Gen Psychiatry*. 1986;43:954–959.

Marin D, De Meo M, Frances A, et al. Biological models and treatments for personality disorders. *Psychiatr Ann*. 1989;19:143–146.

Masterson JF. *Psychotherapy of the Borderline Adult: A Developmental Approach*. New York: Brunner/ Mazel: 1976.

Morrison EF. The evolution of a concept: Aggression and violence in psychiatric settings. *Arch Psychiatr Nurs*. 1994;8:245–253.

Morrison EF. Toward a better understanding of violence in psychiatric settings: Debunking the myths. *Arch Psychiatr Nurs*. 1993;7:328–335.

Siever LJ. Schizophrenia spectrum personality disorders. In: Tasman A, Riba MB, ed. *American Psychiatric Press Review of Psychiatry*. Washington, DC: American Psychiatric Press; 1992;11.

Siever LJ. Biologic markers in schizotypal personality disorder. *Schizophren Bull*. 1985;11:564–575.

Siever LJ, Davis KL. A psychobiological perspective on the personality disorders. *Am J Psychiatry*. 1991; 148:1647–1658.

Sifneos PE. *Short-term Psychotherapy and Emotional Crisis*. Cambridge, MA: Harvard University Press; 1972.

Sifneos PE. Alexithymia: Past and present. *Am J Psychiatry*. 1996;153 (suppl):137–142.

Soloff PH, George A, Cornelius J, et al. Pharmacotherapy and borderline subtypes. In: JM Oldham, ed. *Personality Disorders: New Perspectives on Diagnostic Validity*. Washington, DC: American Psychiatric Press, 1991.

Soloff PH, Lis JA, Kelly T, et al. Risk factors for suicidal behavior in borderline personality disorder. *Am J Psychiatry*. 1994;151:1316–1323.

Stanley M, Stanley B. Postmortem evidence for serotonin's role in suicide. *J Clin Psychiatry*. 1990;51 (suppl April):22–27.

Widiger TA, Corbitt EM, Millon T. Antisocial personality disorder. In: Tasman A, Riba M, eds. *American Psychiatric Press Review of Psychiatry*. Washington, DC: American Psychiatric Press; 1992;11.

CHAPTER 24

WORKING WITH CHILDREN
IN FOSTER CARE

Sandra L. Rosen

*P*lacements estab-
lished in haste may
be mismatched. When
such placements break
down, the child's sense
of rejection is intensi-
fied. Premature place-
ments also unnecessar-
ily burden the social
service agency finan-
cially and otherwise.
On the other hand, hes-
itation in placing a
child may mean ir-
reparable physical
harm.

Chapter Overview

The advanced practice psychiatric nurse may specialize in work with children. Most likely, a percentage of the emotionally troubled youths will reside in foster homes. Whether the clinical nurse specialist chooses to provide therapy to foster children and their families in private practice or takes on the role of case manager at a child welfare agency, the nurse will soon realize the unique needs of foster children, contrasted with those living with their biological parents.

Almost a century ago, in 1909, President Theodore Roosevelt hosted the first White House Conference on the Care of Dependent Children. Three missions were formulated during that meeting:

- Home care is preferred to institutional care.
- Children should not be separated from their parents solely due to financial hardships.
- When parents do not want their children or do not provide an adequate home even in spite of outside financial aid and support, then a carefully selected foster home is to be sought (Simms, 1991a).

These same missions are valued by society today. However, as will be described, current nationwide crises threaten fulfillment. For a more in-depth look at the foster care system in a historical context, the student is directed to Simms (1991a).

The epidemiology statistics concerning foster children are tragic. To address these issues it is particularly helpful to understand the members of the multifaceted system. Maneuvering through the foster care system and collaborating with both the welfare agency and school system require special skill and preparation. This includes gaining insight into the burdens weighing on the natural family, the characteristics of the foster family, and issues facing the child care worker. The school system is another facet deserving exploration. Reasons for placement are examined. In keeping with its far-reaching terror, abuse and neglect receive greater focus in this chapter than do the other causes for out-of-home care.

Both children who have been taken for the first time from their parents and those who have been bounced around from foster home to foster home may display troublesome, albeit normal, signs and symptoms as they struggle to adjust. More disturbing, however, some children may develop an adjustment disorder or depression. Others may demonstrate a conduct disorder. Attention-deficit hyperactivity disorder (ADHD) and learning disabilities are also common in this population. The psychiatric nurse who is able to comprehensively and accurately assess a child's needs and who recognizes the importance of a full team approach is in the best position to work with foster children.

EPIDEMIOLOGY

REASONS FOR PLACEMENT

Over 659,000 children were served by the system during 1993, of which over 461,300 lived in family foster homes (Halfon et al., 1994). Moreover, an estimated 460,00 children were in foster care at end of fiscal 1993 (Halfon et al., 1994). Although a variety of reasons are cited, 75 percent of the children placed in foster care are taken from their homes because of maltreatment or parental inability to provide adequate care (Simms, 1991b). Only about 10 percent are placed because of their own behavioral problems, handicaps, or disabilities. Parental drug use or trade is becoming an increasing reason for placement (Simms, 1991b). Pete C. Strangeways, the Program Director of Services to Intensive Needs Children, Juvenile Justice Center of Philadelphia, reports that almost every family with which they deal has drug or alcohol involvement. He explains that drug problems are especially rampant in families with a child younger than 8 years because of the popularity of cocaine, and adds that prenatal cocaine exposure is very common (personal communication, February 22, 1996). As would be expected considering the frequent stigmatization of infected individuals, HIV-positive children are particularly hard to place (P.C. Strangeways, personal communication, February 22, 1996). Homelessness has also been a growing reason for foster care placement (Simms, 1991b).

THE BIOLOGICAL PARENTS

Most commonly, parents of those children placed in foster care live in poor, inner city neighborhoods. The majority are single-parent homes with below-poverty incomes. More often, the biological parents are black or hispanic. In fact, while 81 percent of the national child population is white, 40 percent of the foster children are nonwhite. As many as one third of the parents also lived in foster homes during their own child-

hoods. High rates of emotional and physical illnesses intertwine with the other hardships. A large number of the families are already known by protective services, the police, or the courts prior to child placement (Simms, 1991a, 1991b).

THE FOSTER CARE HOMES

The Committee on Ways and Means, 1993, recognized that the demand for out-of-home care is increasing rapidly (Usher et al., 1995). At the same time, there is a shortage of foster parents (Benedict and White, 1991; Stehno, 1990). Chicago provides a tragic illustration of this problem: the city uses hospitals to house babies because the child welfare agencies cannot find them homes, and the temporary shelters are already overcrowded (Stehno, 1990). The insufficiency of foster homes is not unique to Chicago but instead is vast and far reaching. "Public and private child welfare agencies *across the nation* [italics added] are facing a crisis that is due in large part to the lack of availability of qualified foster homes" (Chamberlain et al., 1992, p. 387). Strangeways, in speaking about Philadelphia, concurs, and identifies a compounding problem: "all [foster parents] want to work with young kids" (personal communication, February 22, 1996). As the situation stands, while the availability of foster homes is decreasing, more children and adolescents with increasingly complex problems are entering the system (Chamberlain et al., 1992). See Figure 24–1 and Table 24–1 for a description of foster care options.

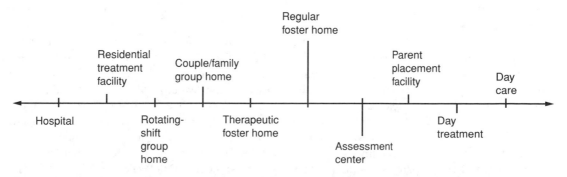

Figure 24–1. Foster care options on a continuum. (From Woolf, 1990.)

TABLE 24–1. FOSTER CARE PLACEMENT OPTIONS

Placement Option	Description
Day care	Least restrictive
Day treatment	Helps parents of children with special medical needs or severe behavior problems. Parental participation is required.
Parent placement facility	Removes the perpetrator, not the victim Assessment and treatment begin quickly
Assessment shelter	Provides smooth transition Length of stay 7 days or less Includes assessment, and intensive crisis management as needed
Regular foster home	For children without behavioral or emotional problems Limited to two placements at a time Variation—risk-adoption program
Therapeutic foster home	At least one adult home on full-time basis employed as supplemental parent Home may have no more than two placements at any time
Couple/family group home (4–6 residents)	Live-in couple—two adults employed full-time Relief staff available For adolescents with minor behavior or emotional problems Helps prepare residents for independent living Three-level system Social worker consultation available
Rotating shift group home (4–10 residents)	For children with moderate behavior or emotional problems Full-time social worker available Children receive daily to biweekly therapy Length of stay 4–8 months
Residential treatment facility (10–15 residents)	Intensive group, individual, and family treatment
Hospitalization	Only for the most severe cases

Information from Woolf (1990).

Recruitment is a long process. Strangeways provides a brief overview. His agency advertises, using newspapers, churches, and fairs. Word of mouth, especially between relatives, is a significant source of referrals. Once an application is made, a home study is initiated. A physical examination, home inspection, and interview are all conducted. This process, ending with a written report, takes a few months. Their foster parent candidates participate in 8 hours of orientation training (P.C. Strangeways, personal communication, February 22, 1996). Simms (1991a) describes a 6- to 8-week training protocol to teach the foster parents about: (1) the agency's philosophy and expectations, (2) problems they may encounter and and how to manage them, and (3) who to contact for needed help. Strangeways adds that 6 hours of training is required annually.

Foster parents range in age from the mid-30s to the late 50s. Their incomes reflect the general population, perhaps skewed toward the lower range (Simms, 1991a; Martin et al., 1992). Surveys show that most foster fathers have blue-collar jobs while foster mothers are less likely to be employed outside the home (Simms, 1991a). Over 50 percent of the foster mothers have incomes under $20,000 (Fein et al., 1990). The "typical" foster family is a couple in a stable marriage with two or more of their own teenage children (Simms, 1991a). The couple usually have underutilized space and want more children (Martin et al., 1992). Many of the foster parents grew up in large families themselves (Simms, 1991a). One study revealed that often couples became foster parents with hopes of finding a child to adopt (Martin et al., 1992). However, locality often alters this "typical" configuration. The contrast is evident in Philadelphia, where, according to Strangeways, two-parent foster families are very rare. Forty-seven per cent of single foster mothers have incomes of less than $10,000 (Fein et al., 1990).

Not only is recruitment of foster homes an issue, but retention is also a significant problem. According to the foster parents who drop out, reasons include deficiency in training, support, and respite care, along with the severity of the children's problems (Chamberlain et al., 1992). Furthermore, when assessed for satisfaction, many foster parents expressed frustration with their foster children's negative behaviors along with difficulties in dealing with those behaviors (Martin et al., 1992). They felt that their knowledge about the children's backgrounds and about agency rules regarding discipline was insufficient. The foster parents want more support in terms of respite care, counseling for behavior problems, medical care, school problems, and simply the costs of providing for children. Therefore, it can be concluded that the basic 6 to 8 hours of orientation is insufficient for prospective foster parents. Benedict and White consider the inadequate training and educating of foster parents a crisis (1991).

Kates and associates (1991) define the "ideal" foster parents not in terms of age or income or any other demographics, but in terms of attitude and behavior. According to these clinicians, the best foster family assumes the role of extended family, viewing themselves as respite care for the temporarily incapacitated parents. Optimally, the couple sees themselves as helpers, as active agents helping the biological family move toward healthy functioning. The all-too-often antagonistic relationship between foster and biological parents is therefore avoided in this ideal situation. Furthermore, the foster parents remain in contact with the child and biological parents after foster care has ended; this minimizes the losses to the child. Advantages of this model are "of reducing parental alienation and noncooperation, of minimizing the disruption of parent–child bonds, and of not subjecting the child to another catastrophic loss when foster care ends" (Kates et al, 1991, p. 589).

KINSHIP CARE

An estimated 10 percent of the 7.7 million children who receive support under the Aid to Families with Dependent Children (AFDC) program are being raised by relatives (Simms, 1991a). Simms states that "in theory," these children will be more comfortable and receive better care than youths placed in nonrelative foster care. However, he then describes a different reality: "In my experience . . . kinship foster families often provide children with considerably fewer opportunities for appropriate care, nurture, and rehabilitation, and cooperate less with the child welfare agency and other professionals than do nonrelative foster parents" (p. 317). Often, the agency's role is less clear in kinship care situations. The result is less monitoring and inadequate family support services (Committee on Early Childhood, Adoption, and Dependent Care, 1993).

PLAN OF CARE

"The process of delivering appropriate health care services to children in foster care is complex" (Halfon et al., 1994, p. 101). Although this population does have an extremely high prevalence of physical, mental, and developmental problems, traditionally it is only when the children become management problems that they receive assessments and treatment by specialists.

This precludes early intervention (Simms, 1991a). Simms lists key points from the Standards for the Health Care of Children in Out-of-Home Care which were developed by the Child Welfare League of America and published in 1988 (Table 24–2). Although the list focuses on physical health and medical care, each point can just as easily be applied to emotional health and mental care services.

ASSESSMENT

Simms (1991b) suggests a health assessment be conducted on every child prior to or within 1 day following placement. Checking height, weight, hemoglobin/hematocrit (anemia), blood lead levels, hearing, and vision are important. In at-risk children, screening for tuberculosis, hepatitis, and/or HIV is also important. Immunization records must be checked, and when unknown, the guidelines developed by the Committee on Infectious Diseases of the American Academy of Pediatrics should be consulted. It is essential to include emotional status and developmental level in the comprehensive evaluation. The Committee on Early Childhood, Adoption, and Dependent Care (1993) notes that in addition to assessing the developmental needs of the children, the family's capacity to meet those needs must be scrutinized.

Assessment of children in foster care demands complex information gathering. The advanced practice psychiatric nurse is encouraged to use the biological parents, past health care providers, foster parents, social workers, and schools (Halfon et al., 1994). However, potential impediments to such a comprehensive evaluation are many. First, usually it is the foster parent who will bring the child. This parent often knows very little about the child; the past history is frequently unknown and at best based on presumptions and third-hand information (Simms, 1991b). Unfortunately, the foster parent rarely brings a history report from the child agency. Adding to the difficulty in accurately assessing medical, emotional, and developmen-

TABLE 24–2. KEY POINTS OF THE STANDARDS FOR THE HEALTH CARE OF CHILDREN IN OUT-OF-HOME CARE DEVELOPED BY THE CHILD WELFARE LEAGUE OF AMERICA, 1988 (Simms, 1991b)

1. Child welfare agencies should identify a core group of individuals who are knowledgeable about foster children and the foster care system.
2. Essential health information should be obtained from the natural parents at the time of placement.
3. All children entering foster care should have an initial health evaluation (including mental status evaluation) before placement if possible, but no later than one working day following placement.
4. A comprehensive medical, developmental, educational, and psychological evaluation should be performed within 30 days of the placement.
5. A specific schedule of prevention-oriented health care activities should be uniformly applied to regular health care of foster children.
6. The activities of other state agencies that provide services to foster children should be integrated with those of the child welfare agency.
7. A standard format should be used at intake to record essential health and background information.
8. A medical passport should be kept with the child and foster parent.
9. Health care providers should be required to submit a record of all encounters with foster children.
10. Foster parents and caseworkers should be provided with written copies of the agency's medical policies and procedures, as well as lists of approved providers.
11. Systems of health care for foster children should offer access during nights and weekends.
12. Agencies should develop consent procedures that enable temporary caretakers to obtain appropriate routine health services for children in their care.
13. Specialized health services should be available for adolescents and chronically ill children.
14. Improvements in the funding of health care for foster children should be undertaken.
15. Transportation should be provided to ensure that foster children have access to all diagnostic and treatment services they require.

tal needs, the foster parent may be conservative in voicing complaints about the child during the first meeting.

> "Over the years, it has become apparent to me that many foster parents fear that their competence is judged by their ability to cope with the children's problems. Wishing to avoid being thought incapable or overly complaining, they may deny the existence of problems to the physician or social worker until the situation becomes intolerable. When the foster parents finally ask for "help," the placement may be in serious jeopardy of failing. Thus, it is very important to pay close attention to any concerns raised by the foster parent" (Simms, 1991b, p. 356).

For these reasons, the nurse therapist is most thorough when she asks the child worker for a case summary, including background information, current goals, and future plans. Table 24–3 provides a few examples of nonleading questions

TABLE 24–3. EXAMPLES OF ASSESSMENT QUESTIONS

To Ask Foster Parents
- When and how did this child come into your care?
- What were the circumstances surrounding this placement?
- Does the child feel abandoned and rejected? How does the child deal with those feelings?
- How well do you think the child is adjusting to your home?
- How comfortable are you in caring for this child?
- Do you think the child feels accepted, nurtured, and secure?
- Does the child exhibit any behaviors that concern you?
- How do you deal with the child's behaviors?
- Do you feel your knowledge of the child's background is sufficient?
- Whose idea was it to bring the child in for an evaluation and counseling?
- Do you agree the child needs help?
- What do you think needs to be done for this child?
- What is the quality of the child's attachment to the biological parents?

- To what extent does the child perceive those parents as people who can be counted on and for whom he or she feels affection?
- Have you had any contact with the biological parents? What were they like?
- What kind of problems do you think the biological parents have?
- Do you know what the agency's long-term plans are for this child?
- In your opinion, do you think the child will be able to return home again?
- Does the child visit with the biological parents? If so, how often and where?
- What is the child's behavior like before and after such visits?
- Do you agree with the visitation setup? If not, how would you change it?
- Have you taken in foster children before?
- What is your impression of the child care agency? Of your child's worker?
- How satisfied are you with the foster parent program/experience?
- Do you understand the agency's rules about discipline?
- Do you get enough support?
- Do you feel you were well prepared for this child's needs?
- Is there information you wish you had but do not?

To Ask Foster Children
- Who do you live with?
- How long have you lived there?
- What happened that you live with (*foster parents*)?
- How do you like living there?
- How is it different from where you lived before?
- What are the rules?
- What kinds of things do you and (*foster parents*) do together?
- Do you see your mom? Dad?
- When do you see them?
- What happens when you see them?
- What is your mom like? Your dad?
- Do you like seeing them?
- If you could choose, where would you like to live the best?
- Do you think you will have to move again? Where will you move to?
- Are there things you do not like about your mom? Dad?
- Do you like living with (*foster parent*)?

that may be posed to the child and the foster parent(s) to aid in assessment.

THE FINDINGS

When children are separated from their parents, they are fearful and anxious. Feelings of loss, rejection, humiliation, and helplessness are expected. Children may feel anger towards the parent for the rejection, and may view the placement as punishment. Children understandably feel helpless; the situation is in fact out of their control. They also fear further rejection and/or punishment (Simms, 1991b; Lush et al., 1991).

The unresolved mourning of separation may translate to the following behaviors: on the lesser end, crying, tantrums, verbal aggression, and school difficulties; and on the more extreme end, destruction of property, physical violence, and threats of suicide (Kates et al., 1991). In a study of 689 foster children in Maryland (Benedict and White, 1991), over 50 percent had some behavior problems—such as aggression, manipulation, withdrawal, or depression—at placement.

The message the child receives is that (1) either the biological parent or the child is bad, and (2) the rescuers are good (Kates et al., 1991). "Because of their attachment to their biological parents or denial of the negative characteristics of those parents and their fear or mistrust of other persons, foster children may choose to be 'bad' " (Kates et al., 1991, p. 587). Furthermore, abused children—having learned to expect harsh, unpredictable punishment as normal—may use negative behavior to gain attention. They may believe punishment is a means of establishing and maintaining contact with adults (Simms, 1991b). When sexual abuse was a component of the child's past, sexual acting-out, such as sexualized behavior often occurs after placement (Simms, 1991b). Colton and colleagues found a high prevalence of behavior problems in placed children (1991, in Mellor and Storer, 1995). When any type of "bad" behavior results in removal from the foster home, children's view of

themselves as bad is further reinforced (Kates et al., 1991). Furthermore, Widom (1991) believes children with multiple placements are prone to delinquency, adult criminality, and violent criminal behavior.

A significant correlation between symptoms of mental illness and the amount of time in reception centers and out-of-home care has been demonstrated by Thorpe and Swart (1992). Halfon and associates (1994) state that approximately 60 percent of foster children have moderate to severe mental health problems. Many are diagnosed with attention-deficit hyperactivity disorder (ADHD). Although disturbed children may be diagnosed with any of a number of illnesses, ADHD has been getting much publicity of late, partly because this is one disorder for which children are often placed on medication; see Table 24–4 for information on Ritalin. Attachment disorders, anger, frustration, aggression, poor school performance,

TABLE 24–4. MEDICATION INFORMATION: RITALIN

Generic Name: Methylphenidate.

Action: Central nervous system stimulant.

Usual Dosage: Initially, 5 mg before breakfast and lunch; increase 5–10 mg each week as needed; Not to exceed 60 mg/day.

Common Side Effects: Decreased appetite, stomach cramps, weight loss, disturbed sleep, abnormal heart rhythms.

Contraindications: Do not give to those with history of epilepsy or other seizures.

Special Instructions: Give last dose by 6 PM, to avoid disturbed sleep.

Signs of Overdosage: Vomiting, agitation, tremors, convulsions, coma, euphoria, confusion, hallucinations, delirium, sweating, flushing, headache, high fever, abnormal heart rate, elevated blood pressure, dry mouth and nose.

Drug Interactions: Interacts with MAO inhibitors and other antidepressants, alcohol, anticoagulants, and anticonvulsants.

Reproduced with permission from Chilnick (1990)

identity problems, concentration problems, poor peer relationships, depression, and psychotic-like behavior have also been observed in deprived foster children and those in group homes (Lush et al., 1991).

PRINCIPLES OF ADVANCED PRACTICE

TREATMENT

Halfon and associates declare, "short-term mental health interventions involving foster parents can help maintain children in foster homes, reduce foster parent turnover, and decrease the probability that a child will need costlier long-term psychotherapy, special education services, or even inpatient treatment" (1994, p. 101). However, obstacles to effective intervention are numerous. For example, Mellor and Storer (1995) cite a lack of resources and training as reducing the effectiveness of therapy. Even when counseling has been scheduled, it is a slow process. Often the foster child demonstrates an inability to form relationships, holds untrue parental images—glorified or denigrated—and is confused about his or her identity (Kates et al., 1991). Since placement undermines the child's senses of trust, mastery, and control, motivation to establish a cooperative relationship with an examiner is compromised (Kates et al., 1991).

Kates and colleagues (1991) identify three primary tasks to include in treatment:

- Tapping into the child's ego resources in order to assist the child with integration of conflicting images and experiences in relation to biological and foster parents and regulate self-esteem.
- Helping the child with early stages of development, because engagement and attachment have been seriously undermined.
- Helping the child with a sense of identity including familial identification.

Moreover, these practitioners believe clinicians working with foster children must focus on the following issues: (1) the child's tendency to split the maternal image into good and bad, (2) the child's inadequate sense of belonging and lack of familial identification, and (3) the child's decreased ability or willingness to form attachments with substitute caregivers.

COLLABORATION WITH OTHER DISCIPLINES

THE CHILD WELFARE AGENCY

Fein (1991) calls for better coordination among the systems affecting foster children. The core system for placed children is the child welfare agency. Three tasks posed to such agencies by the Child Welfare League of America (1975) are the following. These agencies should (1) establish and maintain a system of substitute care for children who have been taken from their parents, (2) aim for finding permanent homes for children to grow up in, and (3) assist children with adjustment to substitute care, along with monitoring their process regarding same. Halfon and associates (1994) note that case management to coordinate services and care by multiple providers is essential.

The advanced practice nurse works closely with child case workers. For this reason, it is important to be aware of major issues facing such workers. For instance, excessive case loads, low salaries, hiring freezes, excessive paperwork, and inadequate work environments are common (Simms, 1991a). Likewise, Mills and Ivery (1991) state that workloads are overwhelming, consisting of extremely difficult cases, with unreasonable time demands, and with little regard for flexibility of the workers' schedules. Stehno also recognizes the problem of overworked, underpaid, undersupported child welfare workers: "The Child Welfare League of America's Standard [case load] is 20. High case loads mean the effective case management is impossible, that workers can do nothing but crisis management, and the workers cope with the impossible by leaving or burning out" (1990, p. 558). To deal with the resulting staff shortages, many agencies hire caseworkers who are not properly trained or without appropriate experience. The Connecticut Department of Children and Youth Services is used as an example, where only 15 percent of the social workers hired hold a bachelor's or master's degree in social work (Simms, 1991a).

Herbert and Mould (1992) analyzed questionnaires of 220 front-line workers of the Department of Social Services in the Canadian Provincial Department of Social Services. Evidence of career dissatisfaction was shown by the gap between assumed and desired roles. The workers rated different roles and identified "agents of social control" and "social brokers" as their two most frequent. However, they felt they *should* be doing "counseling" and "advocacy" most often. Barriers to advocacy included the bureaucracy, large client and organization demands, and their own perceived deficiency of knowledge and skills.

THE SCHOOL SYSTEM

Studies show an extremely high prevalence of educational difficulties when children enter placement (Simms, 1991b). In a longitudinal study of first-time entrances to foster care, 689 children in urban and suburban communities of Maryland were examined (Benedict and White, 1991). Of the 325 school-aged children (defined as age 6 and above), 55 (or 16.9 percent) were already in special education, and another 36 (or 11 percent) needed special education but were still in regular education.

Hopefully appropriate school placement has been achieved or is in the process of being corrected when the foster child is brought to an advanced practice nurse for evaluation and therapy. Reality, however, frequently reveals otherwise. Therefore, as the advanced practice nurse conducts a comprehensive assessment of the new patient, the nurse forms an unofficial estimate of the child's intelligence and educational status, taking into consideration the child's age and developmental level. Sometimes contacting the school psychologist is indicated. The school staff, especially in large cities, may be inadequate for the child's needs, and it is because of such shortages that the path leading to proper educational placement seems a long and winding road, often with detours and dead ends.

The initial step on this path is identification of scholastic difficulties. Yet, despite the high likelihood of educational problems in this population, they are unlikely to be identified or treated. Simms (1991b) identifies numerous possibilities for such underdetection. First, because foster care is seen as "temporary," there is often little motivation to initiate the comprehensive psychoeducational evaluation needed to determine suitable educational placement. Then, diffusion of responsibility about who represents the child at formal educational conferences causes delay. Financial debates also get in the way. Simms asserts, "School systems often balk at underwriting the cost of special educational programming for these children, claiming that the 'educational nexus' [the child's 'home' school district] is responsible for footing the increased costs" (1991b, p. 351). Sometimes, when foster care placement means changes of community and school, the educational records of the child are not transferred to the new school. As a result of these potential delays, decisions about educational placement often take a drastically long period of time. Quite sadly, some children may not be identified as needing intervention even when school performance is obviously inadequate.

To limit detriment to the children, all youths entering foster care should receive not only a comprehensive psychological assessment, but also an educational assessment soon after placement. Moreover, school records must be sent to the new school system promptly. With many child welfare workers on overload, it is frequently the child's therapist who makes the calls and urges action.

ETHICAL AND LEGAL IMPLICATIONS

BUDGETING FOR CARE

Foster parents do receive money from the agencies that recruit them, although not much. For example, in 1990, the average monthly rates paid for foster care in Connecticut fell about 30 percent below the USDA standards for the cost of supporting children (Simms, 1991a). The actual dollar amount varies slightly between agencies. In Massachusetts, the Department of Social Services pays $15 per day per child (Grunwald, 1996). By contrast, foster parents for an agency in Philadelphia typically receive $20 to $25.25 per day per child (P.C. Strangeways, personal communication, February 22, 1996). Another agency in Philadelphia paid $9 to $20 per day in 1992 (Woodall, 1992). Even within one agency, the amount ranges depending on the level of care required for the child. The dollars are intended to be spent solely on the foster child, not used as a source of household income. For this reason, Strangeways explains that his agency has a rule that all their foster homes must have another source of income. Interestingly, according to Chamberlain and colleagues, "caseworkers are often unable to maintain mandated levels of contact with foster parents, and it is not uncommon for foster parents to have trouble getting their reimbursements on time" (1992, p. 388).

The Social Security Act of 1935 expressed a strong federal role in public welfare. However, the amount of money this nation spends on child welfare is devastatingly inadequate. Furthermore, when allocation of federal funds was decreased, the result was greater cost long-term: by spending approximately $102 million less on preventive services in 1989 than 1981, the government spent almost three times more in foster care services (Simms, 1991a). According to Scales and Brunk, prevention is well worth the cost: $3 to $10 is saved for every $1 invested in Head Start and good prenatal care (1990). Despite the consequences of diminished allocation,

in 1990, the social welfare expenditure per child was $1020. This is only 9% of the amount spent per elderly person. In 1990, 20.6% of all children in the United States were poor, compared with only 12.2% of the elderly; "children were the poorest demographic group in 1990" (Ozawa, 1993, p. 518). Moreover, the total social welfare expenditures for all children translated to a measly 5.2% of the federal spending. Again, the amount spent on the elderly was considerably more, at 28.3% (Ozawa, 1993). See Figures 24–2 and 24–3 for a graphic view of the disproportionate amount of money spent on these children.

One fairly new burden to the social welfare system is that some state Medicaid programs limit conditions for which they will reimburse hospitals for inpatient stays. For instance, in Conneticut, Medicaid will no longer pay for children—even those with medical problems—who are hospitalized for social reasons. The Department of Children and Youth Services, already with a tight budget, is now responsible for such costs (Simms, 1991b).

The Massachusetts Department of Social Services has made a stirring plan change, combining managed care and the foster care system. Linda Carlisle, who co-chairs the Child Welfare League of America's managed care committee, recognizes, "I know this is going to be controversial," but reassures, "we're doing the right thing" (in Grunwald, 1996). The new plan is a "capitation" system, which means providers are paid a fixed fee for each child regardless of how much is spent on care. Grunwald describes, "all of them [the youths] have serious emotional problems and most have been unable to function in foster homes," and worries about the impact of the bonuses which are given to providers who keep these abused and neglected youths out of 24-hour residential treatment (1996, p. 1). However, a bonus given whenever a child moves out of *and stays out* of the system for 6 months is supposed to encourage good discharge services to help at-risk youths to adapt to family life. Still, Grunwald continues to argue against the plan, "It is not clear how the financial logic of capitation

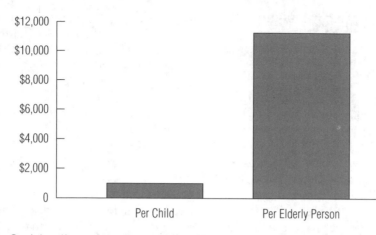
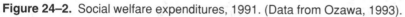

Figure 24–2. Social welfare expenditures, 1991. (Data from Ozawa, 1993).

as it works in health care—in which healthy patients subsidize sick ones by requiring fewer services—would work with youths who all enter the system with major psychological damage" (1996, p. 16). There are in fact differences between this particular managed care system and that of the medical world. Fortunately, treatment is not bound by time limits. The Department of Social Services has veto power over the clinical decision makers, and those decisions are made by nonprofit child welfare agencies, not health

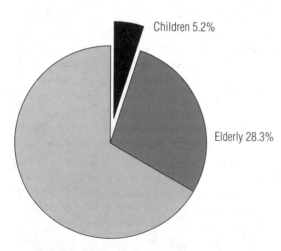

Figure 24–3. Federal social welfare expenditures. (Data from Ozawa, 1993).

maintenance organizations (HMOs). Carlisle says the primary goal is to prepare the children and adolescents for life outside institutions as quickly as possible. This plan went into effect on February 12, 1996, and based on the results, it may influence other states.

ABUSE AND NEGLECT

Interestingly, the first child to receive court protection from abuse was a foster child (Simms, 1991a). It was 1874, and a foster couple was beating and badly mistreating a child. After the court refused to endorse an order to remove her from the home, the child's worker turned to the Society for the Prevention of Cruelty to Animals (SPCA) for help. Finally, the SPCA won the case; the foster parents were jailed for a year; and the child stayed with the worker who had fought for her. A year later, the maiden Society for the Prevention of Cruelty to Children (SPCC) was established to "rescue" children from abusive parents.

The Child Abuse Prevention and Treatment Act of 1974, signed by President Richard Nixon, protects children from physical, mental, and sexual injury as well as abandonment or neglect by their parents or caregivers. The law also mandates professionals having frequent contact with children to report all suspected cases of child abuse or neglect to a public child protective services agency (Simms, 1991a). This category includes registered nurses, social service workers, and mental health therapists. In theory, "mandatory reporting" should minimize prejudices, but tragically bias continues to impact reporting and investigations. For example, Mandel and associates (1994) reviewed studies that compared physician and nurse beliefs about indications of abuse. Although nurses recognized only suspicious injuries (e.g., cigarette burns) as indicators of abuse, physicians considered suspicious injuries, race, and socioeconomic status as signs of abuse. Similarly, in another study, suspiciousness of injury, race, and socioeconomic status predicted whether a physician recognized and reported child abuse, while only suspicious injury predicted nurses' decisions. Amazingly, one physician had even wrongly declared that child abuse does not happen in middle-class families.

"In 1990, the U.S. Advisory Board on Child Abuse and Neglect called the conditions in Children's Protective Services a national emergency" (Rindfleisch and Nunno, 1992, p. 694). According to this same board, in 1989, the estimated incidence of child abuse and neglect was 2.4 million, and 5000 children died from maltreatment by familial and quasifamilial caregivers (U.S. Advisory Board, 1990). Although studies show abused children are much less safe from repeated abuse when remaining with biological parents than when placed in foster care (Simms, 1991b), studies also show that up to 80 percent of the children reportedly abused or neglected are not placed in foster care (Simms, 1991a).

Emotional abuse and neglect receive less attention than physical and sexual abuse. Likewise, although research indicates that chronic emotional neglect means a poor prognosis for normal adult adjustment, there is particular reluctance to remove children living under chronic emotional neglect from their homes (Simms, 1991b). Craft and Staudt (1991) conducted a study of lay citizens and protective service workers from metropolitan and rural communities in a midwestern state. The researchers found that whether one lives in a rural or urban neighborhood does not significantly influence the decision to report a situation as neglect. In other words, they found considerable agreement among the respondents as to what should be reported as neglect. On the other hand, there was less agreement amongst workers as to what would be substantiated in urban versus rural communities. The working definition of neglect appeared to vary from community to community, although not so much because of differences in values between the populations, but because of other factors, such as worker characteristics and case loads, juvenile court expectations, and services available.

The mandatory reporting law has increased the number of abuse cases reported for investigation (Mills and Ivery, 1991). In the United States in 1991, an estimated 2,694,000 children were reported to child protective services agencies (National Center on Child Abuse Prevention Research, 1992). That translated to 42 per 1000 children, and a 40 percent increase over 1985 (NCCAPR, 1992). A report of suspected abuse is given to a social worker to investigate. Simms (1991a, p. 306), however, warns that "an intake worker can decide to dismiss the allegations outright at the time of the report, without gathering any corroborating information or evidence, if the worker believes there is no merit to the report." Mandel and associates (1994) cite two crucial facets of a thorough child abuse and neglect investigation: developing numerous possible hypotheses and searching for uncontaminated information. At the conclusion of the investigation, the worker may (1) dismiss the complaint, labeling it invalid or unsubstantiated; (2) offer recommendations, referrals, or direct services to the family with the goal of protecting the child in the home; (3) use legal means to supervise the child in the parents' home; or (4) remove the child and place him or her in a foster home or institutional setting (Simms, 1991a).

Children returned to their biological parents may be reabused. Between 25 and 33.3 percent of the children are abused or neglected again after being returned to their parents and reenter the foster care system within 1 to 2 years. For this reason, Simms believes "adoption appears to be the best long-term option for abused and neglected children" (1991b, p. 362). Another option, especially for older children, is long-term foster care.

PLACEMENT AND REUNIFICATION

In the 1970s, a movement towards permanency in placement led to passage of the Adoption Assistance and Child Welfare Act of 1980 (Public Law 96-272). According to this law,

> In each case, reasonable efforts will be made (A) prior to the placement of a child in foster care, to prevent or eliminate the need for removal of a child from his home, and (B) to make it possible for the child to return home. (Public Law 96-272, section 471, as cited in Simms, 1991a, p. 306)

Emphasis, therefore, is on preplacement prevention, reunification, and supportive services (Simms, 1991a). Unfortunately, in low-income communities, services for strengthening and supporting the families to prevent foster care placement are inadequate (Stehno, 1990). Likewise, states lack the funds to provide needed intensive home-based services (Fein, 1991). A double bind is established because the law must be followed to receive federal monies. To demonstrate accordance with Public Law 96-272, for each foster child, the child welfare agency writes a care plan documenting that placement (1) is in the least restrictive setting, (2) is in the child's best interests, and (3) is close to the biological parents' home. This detailed plan of care for the child also includes the services required to facilitate reunification or adoption (Simms, 1991a). As a means of reevaluation, case reviews occur every 6 months. The biological parents are invited, and for a number of reasons the psychiatric nurse therapist should also attend. The case review provides an opportunity for the nurse to meet the child's team and for sharing and negotiation of ideas.

Repeated studies show visitation to be the strongest predictor of the child's return to the biological parents' care (Simms, 1991b). Benedict and White (1991) conclude from the various length-of-stay studies that regular and frequent visiting relate to shorter foster care stays. Parental visitation may be a stressful experience. Sometimes, the child demonstrates deteriorating behavior after a visit, which in turn causes concern for the foster parents (Fein, 1991). Foster parents who note their children becoming upset before and after contact with their biological parents may recommend that the visits be discontinued and they may exert subtle or overt pressure on workers to suspend visits (Simms, 1991b). Simms suggests a change in visit location or an increase in supervision to decrease foster parent concerns, but cautions against suspending visits. A visitation schedule should be developed by the child's team. The Committee on Early Childhood, Adoption, and Dependent Care (1993) warns that weekly or sporadic visits "stretch the bounds of children's sense of time and do not allow for a psychologically meaningful relationship with estranged biologic parents" (p. 1008). There are times, however, when either a decrease in frequency or temporary suspension of visits is indicated, such as when the child is very frightened of the parents or if the parents act inappropriately during the visits.

Hess and Folaron (1991) note the impact of ambivalence on permanency planning for foster children. They recount a 3-year study funded by the United States Department of Health and Human Services to demonstrate a Professional Review Action Group (PRAG) model for reviewing cases of disrupted family reunification. Forty cases were studied. The PRAG project staff hypothesized that parental ambivalence, whether verbal or behavioral, about reunification would affect the success of reunification when it did occur. Results of the study included information about contributions to ambivalence (see Table 24–5). The conclusion of the PRAG group was that "in the 40 cases reviewed, this interpretation [that reunification is the successful

TABLE 24–5. REASONS FOR AMBIVALENCE IN THE BIOLOGICAL PARENTS

- Poverty
- Parental readiness
- Personal experiences/histories (own childhood abuse)
- Child characteristics (temperament, handicaps, behaviors)
- Child feelings toward return (only 44% of 16 children of ambivalent parents who expressed a placement preference said home was their placement of choice)
- Parent–child relationship (multiple past separations, parentified children)
- Parental role during placement (allowed to visit but only at special times under special directions, temporary caregivers doing a better job)
- Practitioners' expectation (practitioners expect that all parents want and deserve at least one chance at reunification and sometimes ignore parental messages of ambivalence or renouncement)
- Agency policy and the legal process (staff ambivalence, insufficient policy and directives)
- Agency/community resources (increased cases without increased staff, high staff turnover)

Data from Hess and Folaron (1991).

outcome] of current federal and state mandates appeared to severely jeopardize individual children's safety and well-being" (in Hess and Folaron, 1991).

Simms (1991a) makes clear that although all parents deserve the chance to receive needed assistance, sometimes success is unlikely. In such circumstances, the appropriate actions must focus on alternative permanency. Reunification becomes nearly impossible when a child worker has great difficulty in trying to help the biological parents. A number of biological parents are resistant to meeting with the social worker (50 percent), miss appointments (almost 50 percent), or are tardy for meetings (33 percent). The biological parents who do allow contact may be defensive and not willing to discuss personal problems. Research indicates that biological parents suffer from higher rates of mental illness, but often they do not follow through on referrals.

Supportive, practical help—with housing, employment, day care—is what is most utilized.

TERMINATION OF PARENTAL RIGHTS

Termination of parental rights (TPR) is a last-resort action; indicators that TPR may be appropriate include the following: the child welfare agency demonstrates that reasonable efforts to help the family have failed; without good cause, the parents have not visited the child on a regular basis for at least 6 months; the parents have failed to significantly and continuously or repeatedly maintain contact with the child or plan for the child's future although able to do so (not bound by financial or physical constraints) for over 1 year; or the parents, at present and for the future, are unable to provide appropriate care for the child due to their own mental illness or mental retardation (Simms, 1991a).

OUTCOME MEASURES AND EVALUATION

> A review of foster care history reflects a perpetual march down a road of good intentions with the failure to check the quality of the road, and, indeed, whether the interim goals to be accomplished along the way coincide with those of the final destination (Woolf, 1990, p. 76).

It is a careful balance whether to remove the child from the natural home or not, for removal means all the trauma of separation. The Committee on Early Childhood, Adoption, and Dependent Care (1993) warns that

> Any time spent by a child in temporary care may be harmful. Interruptions in the continuity of a child's caretaker are often detrimental. Repeated moves from home to home compound the adverse consequences that stress and inadequate parenting have on the child's development and ability to cope (p. 1008).

Placements established in haste may be mismatched. When such placements break down, the child's sense of rejection is intensified. Premature placements also unnecessarily burden the social service agency financially and otherwise (NCCAPR, 1992; U.S. Advisory Board on Child Abuse and Neglect, 1990). On the other hand, hesitation in placing a child may mean irreparable physical harm. Simms even reports, "Despite all of the problems inherent in the current system, longitudinal studies suggest that most children who enter foster care show improvements in their emotional, developmental, intellectual, and academic functioning, compared with children who remain at home" (1991b, p. 367).

"Based on available national data, the stated permanent plans for these foster children include reunification with parents or relatives (51 percent), long-term foster care (16 percent), adoption (14 percent), or emancipation (9 percent)" (Simms, 1991b, p. 346) (Fig. 24–4). Although most children are either returned to their biological parents or adopted within 1 year of placement, another 25 percent remain in care for 2 years or more. Although about 50 percent remain in their first home, up to 25 percent change homes at least three times (Simms, 1991b)

Fein and colleagues' large study in 1990 found that most placements were actually quite

stable with 66.6 percent of the children having only been in one or two homes, 25 percent of the foster parents planning adoption, and 75 percent of the children expected to remain indefinitely with their foster parents. According to Fein (1991), adoption is considered for 25 to 30 percent of foster children. Adoption rates do vary between localities, however. For example, Strangeways, talking about his agency in Philadelphia, reports a "pretty small number of kids that actually get adopted" (personal communication, February 22, 1996).

FOLLOW-UP AND REFERRAL

The advanced practice nurse therapist working with foster children will suddenly and unknowingly find himself or herself taking the role of case manager and coordinator at times. The nurse will take charge in collaborating with the child welfare agency and school, for as described earlier, these systems are generally short staffed. The nurse therapist must take responsibility for keeping the child care worker abreast of treatment progress and problems via phone calls and case reports and summaries. When a foster parent and child are missing appointments—either cancellations or no shows—the

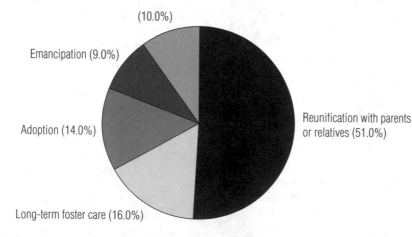

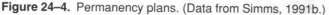

Figure 24–4. Permanency plans. (Data from Simms, 1991b.)

child's worker is often not aware until notified by the therapist.

As already stated, foster children embrace a high prevalence of physical, emotional, developmental, and educational problems; hence, referrals may encompass several different disciplines. Most referrals are made only after consulting with the child welfare worker. Physically, a child may need a "check-up" examination, blood work, vision and/or hearing testing, immunizations; an appointment with a physician or nurse practitioner is then made. Possible developmental delays require further evaluation, which may require the consultation of another discipline such as a speech therapist or school psychologist. Head Start is an excellent program helping numerous youngsters each year. The child may be appropriate for Head Start, but foster parents may be unaware of the program. From using a systems approach, the nurse therapist may make discoveries that lead to suggesting that other family members also seek counseling. Moreover, referrals to support groups and community programs are often utilized.

Due to the circumstances surrounding foster care and its implications, termination of therapy for a foster child demands special care. This child will be losing yet another adult with whom he or she has formed a bond. He or she has learned to count on the therapist who too is "leaving." As always the termination process should begin long before the last meeting. A positive way to initiate the process is for the nurse therapist to tell the child that he or she has enjoyed getting to know the child, and playing and talking together; adding a few concrete examples of noteworthy qualities the child possesses is especially important. By repeating that the child did not do something wrong or bad, the nurse therapist reduces the child's tendency to feel abandoned and rejected again. The nurse therapist explains that the child been doing so very well, and that he or she is proud of the child. The nurse therapist encourages the child to keep up the good work, and lists the positive changes. Even young children who seemingly will not understand the nurse's words should be told the same things. On some level, the child senses the termination. Although the child welfare worker or foster parents may fear the child will quickly and markedly regress to past behaviors just to continue therapy, this rarely occurs. However, because some temporary regression is expected, providing the foster parents with anticipatory guidance is one priority of discharge planning. A mutual sharing during the last session ending with a "gift" exchange is a beautiful way to close; for instance, the child and nurse therapist may color, each making a picture for the other to take home and keep. Tapering frequency of appointments, such as biweekly to weekly to every other week, is often best. A follow-up phone call to both the foster parents and foster child a few weeks after the last session is another idea that the nurse therapist can discuss with the foster parents prior to the final appointment. See Table 24–6 for a list of these helpful hints for termination.

TABLE 24–6. TERMINATION HELPFUL HINTS

- Start the termination process long before the last session.
- Consider a tapering plan, scheduling appointments further and further apart.
- Consider tapering from face-to-face sessions to telephone contacts.
- Provide anticipatory guidance to the foster mother in terms of possible regression and how to handle it.
- Make sure the foster mother knows who to contact in an emergency.
- Make the decision to terminate therapy when both the foster parents and the case worker feel comfortable with it.
- Tell the child that he or she will not be coming anymore. Say you have enjoyed your time together and that he or she did not do something wrong or bad.
- Recount all the progress made with the child. Tell the child how proud you are of his or her behaviors, and encourage the child to continue to do those things.
- Consider a fun activity for the last session. Participate with the child.
- Consider exchanging handmade gifts, such as coloring a picture for each other.

▶ CASE EXAMPLE 1

▶ REASON FOR EVALUATION

Amy is a 8-year-old black girl currently enrolled in regular third-grade classes in an inner city public elementary school. Mrs. Bet seeks evaluation and treatment for her daughter related to behavior problems (arguing with her siblings, not obeying her mother) and very slow development.

▶ BACKGROUND INFORMATION

Mrs. Bet abused free-based crack and alcohol throughout her pregnancy and received no prenatal care. Amy was delivered prematurely at 35 weeks gestation, while her mother was high. From the time of discharge until the age of 6, Amy lived with various relatives. Mrs. Bet was involved in her daughter's care even though they did not live together. Social services has never been involved in this informal kinship care.

Mrs. Bet reports being drug and alcohol free for 2 years and actively involved with both Narcotics Anonymous (NA) and Alcoholics Anonymous (AA). She describes that when she became "clean," she was reunited with her daughter. Presently, Amy lives with her mother, mother's husband, and two siblings (ages 11 and 1). Mrs. Bet shares that although Amy's biological father is unknown, she has led Amy to believe Mr. Bet is her father.

Mrs. Bet describes Amy as in overall good health but "way behind her age." For instance, according to Mrs. Bet, Amy was not walking until age 2, and not talking in sentences of three words or more until age 4. Furthermore, she reports her daughter is completely unable to do her schoolwork. When Amy states she does not like school, her mother adds that last year Amy missed 35 days because she refused to go. Mrs. Bet cannot understand why Amy is passing all her classes despite her great difficulty in reading, writing, and math. Amy cannot add 2 plus 1, tell time, write the alphabet, or read simple words such as "up" and "see." Moreover, she is totally unaware of how to sound out words she does not know.

Reports from school indicate that Amy is well-behaved and attentive, but Mrs. Bet complains that at home her daughter will not obey even the simplest of requests. When asked about disciplining, Mrs. Bet admits that when Amy was younger and she herself was using drugs and alcohol, she used to "beat Amy's bottom." However, Mrs. Bet says she now realizes hitting is "bad," and she will never do it again, adding "it was really the drugs anyway." Mrs. Bet blames herself for her daughter's behaviors, "it's not her fault she's like this; I made her the way she is." She believes, "I have to make up for what I've done," and as a result, does not discipline Amy at all anymore.

Amy is very aware that she is "different." She fears others do not like her, and she denies having any friends. If Amy could make three wishes, she would want "to be smarter, to be beautiful like a model, and to have a big party with lots of friends bringing me presents."

▶ IDENTIFIED PROBLEMS

- Amy is developmentally lagging in reading, writing, and math; perhaps she has a learning disorder.
- Amy is disobedient at home—she has been labeled a "special child" in the family, and is not disciplined.
- Mrs. Bet harbors much guilt about past drug use and its effects on Amy. This interferes with her ability to focus on the here and now and to effectively parent.
- Amy displays poor self-esteem related to "special child" status and also being confused in her classes.

▶ GENERAL GOALS

- Amy will be placed in appropriate school classes—special education.
- Amy will miss no more than 10 days of school this year.
- Amy will demonstrate academic gains this year.
- Amy will establish at least one peer friendship.
- Amy will verbalize good feelings about herself.
- Amy will demonstrate acceptance of parental authority by (1) knowing and following house rules and (2) by complying with requests in a reasonable amount of time.

▶ INITIAL PLANNED INTERVENTIONS

- The nurse therapist will call the school to encourage testing in order to determine proper placement. The Slosson Oral Reading Test, Key Math, Woodcock Reading Mastery Tests, revised, and Wechsler Intelligence Scale for Children III should be included in such testing.
- The nurse therapist will hold family meetings to shift sole focus away from Amy.
- The nurse therapist will explore consequences of not disciplining a child with Mrs. Bet.
- The nurse therapist will discuss methods of disciplining with Mrs. Bet and assist her with limit setting.

- The nurse therapist will provide opportunities for Amy to successfully complete tasks, working towards improved self-esteem.
- The nurse therapist will encourage Amy to talk about the things that bother her and then help her figure out how to deal with her troubles.
- The nurse therapist will monitor scholastic progress by maintaining frequent contact with the school system.

▶ CASE EXAMPLE 2

▶ REASON FOR EVALUATION

Ms. Sten, a new and single foster parent, seeks evaluation and treatment for two sisters, 5-year-old Sarah and 3-year-old Dara. Sarah bruises her own arms and legs by digging at them with her nails and hands. Her concerns about Dara are quite different; this toddler is prone to wild temper tantrums, especially when she gets frustrated. Dara also has a speech problem.

▶ BACKGROUND INFORMATION

Neither their biological mother nor biological father has ever been involved in Sarah and Dara's care. They were bounced around from relative to relative until 18 months ago. At that time, they were turned over to social services by an aunt, because Sarah and Dara were costing the family too much in terms of money and time. The children were placed immediately with Mr. and Mrs. Jacob. These warm, patient foster parents were able to provide a stable home environment. However, tragically, the couple was killed in a car accident almost exactly 1 year after taking in the girls. The children were then placed with Ms. Sten, who applied to be a foster mother with hopes of later adopting. Both children are affectionate towards her. While Dara is extremely needy of attention and fights to have Ms. Sten's full focus on her, Sarah is fearful of getting too close, because she is convinced that Ms. Sten too will one day leave. During the evaluation, Dara hits the nurse therapist's leg repeatedly in an attempt to get her attention. Later in the visit, Dara becomes intolerant over Ms. Sten's attention to the therapist's questions, and she throws a tantrum. In response, Ms. Sten demonstrates good command of the time-out method of discipline she learned in foster parent training.

▶ IDENTIFIED PROBLEMS

Sarah

- Self-inflicted injuries—Sarah denies knowing why she does this and denies remembering what she thinks about while hurting herself.
- Loss of several previous "moms" and "dads"—resulting in fear, grief and identity confusion.

Dara

- Temper tantrums, which include physically aggressive behaviors at times.
- Speech difficulty.
- Loss of several previous "moms" and "dads"—resulting in starvation for love and attention.
- Ms. Sten needs education about the toddlerhood stage of development and expected temper tantrums.

▶ GENERAL GOALS

Sarah

- Sarah will not engage in any self-injurious behaviors.
- Sarah will discuss her feelings about past moms and dads, as well as her current fears during weekly therapy sessions.

Dara

- Dara will be compliant with time-out system.
- Dara will learn to interact and play with others without roughness.

▶ INITIAL PLANNED INTERVENTIONS

The nurse therapist will use play as a way to build rapport and provide a warm, accepting atmosphere in which the children can feel comfortable expressing their emotions.

Sarah

- The nurse therapist will encourage Sarah to talk about her past caretakers.
- The nurse therapist will talk with Sarah about the bruises on her legs and arms. She will provide positive feedback when Sarah does not harm herself.

- The nurse therapist will explore safer outlets for Sarah to express her over-whelming feelings.

Dara

- The nurse therapist will teach Ms. Sten about toddlerhood, including the expected temper tantrums.
- The nurse therapist will reinforce Ms. Sten's use of time-out.
- The nurse therapist will refer Dara for enrollment in the Head Start program.
- The nurse therapist will instruct Ms. Sten to keep Dara separate from other children when needed related to aggressive behaviors.
- The nurse therapist will role model and teach Dara socially appropriate behavior (e.g., how to play "nice," to say "excuse me" to get someone's attention).
- The nurse therapist will make a referral for speech evaluation and therapy.
- The nurse therapist will encourage daily private time for just Ms. Sten and Dara to help meet Dara's inflated attention needs—such as when Sarah is at kindergarten.
- The nurse therapist will be consistent with toy rules during each session, namely, only one toy can be out at a time and must be cleaned up before another toy used. Whoever plays, cleans up.

▶ CASE EXAMPLE 3

▶ REASON FOR EVALUATION

Four-year-old Adam is brought in by his biological mother, Mrs. Tier. This young mother presents as distraught with complaints that she cannot handle her son's behaviors.

▶ BACKGROUND INFORMATION

Adam's biological father was sentenced to prison a year ago. Prior to that, Mr. Tier was abusive towards his son and wife. He was a cocaine user and heavy drinker. When her husband was incarcerated, Mrs. Tier could not manage the debt that her husband had gotten them into, and she lost their home. Unable to provide for herself or her child, Mrs. Tier gave Adam to the social welfare department requesting temporary placement. Approximately a month ago, Adam was reunited with his mother; they currently live in a shelter for women with children. Several behaviors are causing Mrs. Tier great concern: Adam attends an in-house day care at the shelter but fights daily with the other children. Mrs. Tier reports that Adam remembers the abuse the family was subjected to before her husband was put away; he talks about "the hitt'n." He also cries often. Furthermore, since being returned to his mother, Adam has regressed to bedwetting. He bites himself occasionally when he is angry, although never hard enough to break the skin. More often, when Adam is angry, he is physically aggressive towards his mother. In fact, towards the end of the evaluation when Mrs. Tier asks Adam to put the toys away, he refuses by screaming at her. He escalates quickly, kicking his mother and throwing toys at her. Mrs. Tier looks to the nurse therapist with a plea that she cannot handle him. She takes the abuse, while begging Adam to stop. According to the foster mother with whom Adam resided over the past year, his behavior is a drastic change, for she encountered no significant problems with him.

▶ IDENTIFIED PROBLEMS

- Adam is getting into daily fights at day care.
- Adam is resistant to redirection.
- Adam is abusive towards his mother (has been towards self as well).
- Mrs. Tier is not taking control of the situation; she is allowing a 4-year-old to contol her.

▶ GENERAL GOALS

- Adam will clean up the toys he plays with during weekly therapy sessions.
- Adam will listen and obey his mother's redirection.
- Adam will begin to talk about his feelings in therapy sessions.
- Adam will not start fights at day care.

▶ INITIAL PLANNED INTERVENTIONS

- The nurse therapist will help Mrs. Tier learn limit setting techniques, safe passive restraint and appropriate methods of disciplining her son.
- The nurse therapist will use play therapy to help Adam express his fears and anger safely.
- The nurse therapist will make a referral for a therapeutic day care.
- The nurse therapist will not allow Adam to take out a toy until he has put away the one he is abandoning.

▶ CASE EXAMPLE 4

▶ REASON FOR EVALUATION

Seven-year-old Rachel was placed in her first foster home 6 months ago and is struggling to adjust. Her foster mother, Mrs. Smith, is doing likewise. According to Mrs. Smith, Rachel throws a temper tantrum—dropping herself on the floor and screaming—whenever she does not get her own way or is asked to do something she does not want to do. Every morning, Rachel gives her foster mother a hard time about getting out of bed and ready for school. In the evening, the same thing happens regarding taking a bath and going to bed. The tantrums are embarrassing for Mrs. Smith when Rachel throws them in public. Mr. Smith works long hours and rarely encounters Rachel's behavior problems.

▶ BACKGROUND INFORMATION

Rachel's biological father is dead; he shot himself while her mother was pregnant. Her biological mother is a drug addict; she has checked herself into rehabilitation programs numerous times, but has never successfully remained drug free. Each time her mother was an inpatient, Rachel stayed with her Aunt Michele and Uncle Bob and their children. Six months ago, her mother was kicked out of a drug rehabilitation unit after Michele smuggled in drugs during a visit. At that time, Rachel was taken from her mother and aunt and placed in the Smiths' care. Her biological mother is allowed a supervised visit with Rachel for 1 hour every 2 weeks at the child welfare agency. Unfortunately, her mother has only shown up for about 40 percent of these visits. Rachel is a bright child, achieving excellent grades in regular education. However, in the classroom she often gets in trouble for talking to her peers instead of listening to the teacher or doing her work. Except for the tantrums, Rachel is described as energetic, animated, and affectionate.

▶ IDENTIFIED PROBLEMS

- Rachel engages in demanding, attention-seeking behavior—temper tantrums— and is resistant to redirection.
- Rachel has not had a consistent caregiver.
- Visitation by her biological mother has been sporadic and is perceived by Rachel as further abandonment.

▶ GENERAL GOALS

- Modest goals are initially set in the context of a behavior plan, such as:
    Rachel will bathe once per week without a struggle.
    Rachel will go to bed at her 8:30 PM bedtime once per week without a struggle.
    Rachel will get up in the morning once per week without a struggle.
- Rachel will talk about her feelings related to separation from her family in weekly sessions with the nurse therapist.

▶ INITIAL PLANNED INTERVENTIONS

- A behavior plan will be constructed. Colorful sticker stars are used at home to keep track of appropriate behavior.
- The nurse therapist will discuss management techniques for problem behaviors with Mrs. Smith.
- The nurse therapist will teach Mrs. Smith how to use the time-out procedure.
- The nurse therapist will recommend to Mrs. Smith that she limit Rachel's extra public appearances (shopping malls, supermarket) for the time being.
- The nurse therapist will encourage Rachel to talk about her feelings related to separation from her mother and visits with her mother.
- The nurse therapist will work closely with the child welfare agency to determine the benefits versus risks of the current parental visiting schedule and pattern.

REFERENCES

American Psychiatric Association. *Diagnostic and Statistical Manual of Mental Disorders*. 4th ed. Washington, DC: APA; 1994.

Benedict MI, White RB. Factors associated with foster care length of stay. *Child Welfare*. 1991;70: 45–58.

Chamberlain P, Moreland S, Reid K. Enhanced services and stipends for foster parents: Effects on retention rates and outcomes for children. *Child Welfare*. 1992;71:387–401.

Child Welfare League of America. *Standards for Health Care Services for Children in Out-of-Home Care*. Washington, DC: Child Welfare League of America; 1988.

Child Welfare League of America. *Standards for foster family service*. New York: Child Welfare League of America; 1975.

Chilnick LD, ed. *The Pill Book*. 4th ed. New York: Bantam; 1990.

Committee on Early Childhood, Adoption, and Dependent Care. Developmental issues in foster care for children. *Pediatrics*. 1993;91:1007–1009.

Committee on Ways and Means, U.S. House of Representatives. *1993 Green Book: Overview of Entitlement Programs*. Committee print WMCP: 103–18. Washington, DC: U.S. Government Printing Office; 1993:886–887.

Craft JL, Staudt MM. Reporting and founding of child neglect in urban and rural communities. *Child Welfare*. 1991;70:359–370.

Fein E. Issues in foster family care: Where do we stand? *Am J Orthopsychiatry.* 1991;61:578–583.

Fein E, Maluccio AN, Kluger M. *No More Partings: An Examination of Foster Family Care.* Washington, DC: Child Welfare League of America; 1990.

Grunwald M. DSS plan raises fears for children. *Boston Globe.* February 4, 1996; 1, 16.

Halfon N, English A, Allen M, DeWoody M. National health care reform, medicaid, and children in foster care. *Child Welfare.* 1994;73:99–115.

Herbert MD, Mould JW. The advocacy role in public child welfare. *Child Welfare.* 1992;71:114–130.

Hess PM, Folaron G. Ambivalence: A challenge to permanency for children. *Child Welfare.* 1991; 70:403–424.

Kates WG, Johnson RL, Rader MW, Strieder FH. Whose child is this? Assessment and treatment of children in foster care. *Am Orthopsychiatry.* 1991; 61:584–591.

Lush D, Boston M, Grainger E. Evaluation of psychoanalytic psychotherapy with children: Therapists' assessments and predictions. *Psychoanal Psychother,* 1991;5:191–234.

Mandel DR, Lehman DR, Yuille JC. Should this child be removed from home? Hypothesis generation and information seeking as predictors of case decisions. *Child Abuse Neglect,* 1994;18:1051–1062.

Martin ED, Altemeier WA, Hickson GB, et al. Improving resources for foster care. *Clin. Pediatrics,* 1992;31:400–404.

Mellor D, Storer S. Support groups for children in alternate care: A largely untapped therapeutic resource. *Child Welfare,* 1995;74:905–918.

Mills CS, Ivery C. A strategy for workload management in child protective practice. *Child Welfare.* 1991;70:35–43.

National Center on Child Abuse Prevention Research. *Current Trends in Child Abuse Reporting and Fatalities: The Results of the 1991 Annual 50-State Survey.* Chicago: National Committee for the Prevention of Child Abuse; 1992.

Ozawa MN. America's future and her investment in children. *Child Welfare.* 72;1993:517–529.

Rindfleisch N, Nunno M. Progress and issues in the implementation of the 1984 out-of-home care protection amendment. *Child Abuse Neglect.* 1992;16: 693–708.

Scales P, Brunk B. Keeping children on top of the states' policy agendas. *Child Welfare.* 1990;69: 23–32.

Simms MD. Foster children and the foster care system, part I: History and legal structure. *Curr Probl Pediatr.* 1991a;21:297–321.

Simms MD. Foster children and the foster care system, part II: Impact on the child. *Curr Probl Pediatr.* 1991b;21:345–369.

Stehno SM. The elusive continuum of child welfare services: Implications for minority children and youths. *Child Welfare.* 1990;69:551–562.

Thorpe MB, Swart GT. Risk and protective factors affecting children in foster care: A pilot study of the role of siblings. *Can Psychiatry.* 1992;37:616–622.

U.S. Advisory Board on Child Abuse and Neglect. *Child Abuse and Neglect: Critical First Steps in Response to a National Emergency.* Washington, DC: U.S. Department of Health and Human Services; 1990.

Usher CL, Gibbs DA, Wildfire JB. A framework for planning, implementing, and evaluating child welfare reforms. *Child Welfare.* 1995;74:859–876.

Widom CS. The role of placement experiences in mediating the criminal consequences of early childhood victimization. *Am Orthopsychiatry.* 1991;61:195–201.

Woodall M. The foster family: Haven in hard times. *The Philadelphia Inquirer.* August 16, 1992; C1, C8.

Woolf GD. An outlook for foster care in the United States. *Child Welfare.* 1990;69:75–81.

CHAPTER 25

TREATMENT OF COMPLEX SEXUAL ASSAULT

Carol R. Hartman • Ann Wolbert Burgess

*T*he nurse must en-
deavor to under-
stand the patient and
his or her model of the
world. This does not
mean condoning or re-
inforcing, but rather
acknowledging that the
patient's views are not
the nurse's. This is a
validating experience
for the patient and re-
flects that he or she has
been heard.

Chapter Overview

► INTRODUCTION

Multiple studies have reported on different forms of psychological distress associated with experiences of rape and sexual assault (Kilpatrick et al., 1987; Sato and Heiby, 1991; Steketee and Foa, 1987), childhood sexual abuse (Finkelhor, 1988), and childhood physical abuse (Kazdin et al., 1985). Posttraumatic stress disorder (PTSD) is specifically linked to traumatic events and includes symptoms of re-experiencing the traumatic event, avoidance of stimuli associated with the event, and increased autonomic arousal (American Psychiatric Association, 1994). Although PTSD is an acute response to victimization (Burgess and Holmstrom, 1974; Foa et al., 1991), it can also have a long-term outcome or prolonged recovery features.

A perceived life threat, high levels of force, and injury during the rape often increase PTSD symptoms (Finkelhor, 1988; Kilpatrick et al., 1989; Resnick et al., 1993). Sexual assault without a perceived life threat, injury, or high levels of force is often noted when the assault was by a family member or authority figure in cases involving children. Such cases generally unfold over time as an accessory type of relationship in which the perpetrator tries to shape the child to be an active participant in his or her own abuse (Burgess and Holmstrom, 1974; Finkelhor, 1988). Weaver and Clum (1993) reviewed studies examining outcomes in such sexual assault cases and noted two possible patterns. Borderline personality disorder and dissociative disorder significantly discriminated individuals with histories of severe and repeated experiences of childhood physical and sexual abuse from known perpetrators. Similarly, Cole and Putnam (1992), in their literature review of immediate and long-term impact of prolonged sexual abuse, found that victims of incest were significantly more likely than chance to experience somatoform disorders, substance use disorders, and eating disorders, in addition to borderline personality disorder and dissociative disorders.

This chapter focuses on the type of sexual assault in which there are multiple assaults by a perpetrator who stands in a position of power and authority to the child or victim. This type of assault can produce complex responses from the victim. The nature of the responses and the treatment of patients who have had such experiences are discussed.

COMPLEX RESPONSE TO SEXUAL ASSAULT

When there has been repeated sexual assault, symptoms emerge that imply a disruption in the behavior and organization of the individual. Defensive behaviors develop that serve an immediate adaptive purpose, but are dysfunctional over the long term. For example, the individual may use drugs to combat symptoms of PTSD. More to the point are the severe disruptions in the self-system of the individual, such as an inability to self-soothe, an inability to regulate emotions, a lack of a sense of cohesion, a sense of alienation, a deep distrust of others, failure to attach to others, and inability to maintain self-esteem in the face of correction or rejection. These disruptions in the self-system have been identified by Parsons and others as perhaps the most severe aspects of PTSD, and have been referred to as the PTSD of the self-system.

In the production of DSM-IV an effort was made to field test and classify this complex syndrome as a diagnostic category. Although it did not meet the criteria set up by the committee for inclusion in DSM-IV, there is a realization by clinicians that some people respond to traumatic events in complex ways that do not fit neatly within the diagnostic disorder of PTSD nor with the categorization of rape trauma outlined by Burgess and Holmstrom (1974). In fact, many manifestations of childhood sexual assault lead to behavior patterns more often classified as Axis II personality disorders.

A description of the complex post-traumatic stress response that is marked with personality change has been developed by van der Kolk and associates (1996) and Herman (1992):

- Alteration in regulation of affect and impulses
- Alterations in attention or consciousness
- Alterations in self-perception
- Alterations in relations with others
- Alterations in systems of meaning
- Somatization

Associated features include guilt over acts of commission or omission, survivor guilt, and suicide and homicidal intent.

Disillusionment with previously esteemed authority and authority figures often occurs. The disillusionment is accompanied by feelings of hopelessness, sadness, depression, memory impairment, forgetfulness, self-harm, worry about others, and a deep sense of loss. There are also reminders of previous traumatic experiences and a recurrence of post-traumatic experiences. The past is experienced primarily from the standpoint of negative experiences accompanied by some of the symptoms of PTSD.

Other features of complex reactions are increased vulnerability to revictimization by other perpetrators and adoption of distorted beliefs and perceptions of the perpetrator. These features can range from the idealization of the perpetrator and paradoxical gratitude to him or her, to a protec-

tive stance towards the perpetrator and a desire not to shame or humiliate the perpetrator. This can be a consuming preoccupation in the life of the victim.

Accompanying these symptoms is a deep generalized sense of ineffectiveness in dealing with one's environment, which can range from a lack of confidence in one's own judgment to total immobilization or a frozen state. A sense of permanent damage is common and is doubly supported by amnesia for events and extreme states of overinhibition of emotions. Impulsive lack of control, distrust of others, and self-governing of interpersonal relationships are typical, detracting from a sense of pleasure, mastery, and confidence that come from dealing with and relating to other people. The lack of inhibition is also realized in behavior towards others that often parallels the patterns of abuse inflicted on the victim.

The result of this complex response is that experience in the present and the future does not provide the healing and growth that could promote learning for the individual. Rather, it is constantly cast within the filter of distrust and distortions of meaning, both personal and interpersonal, and reacted to with the extreme deviation in inhibition. Given this description of complex responses to sexual assault, we will now turn to principles of practice and therapeutic strategies useful in working with people with this array of symptoms and distortions who seek help through psychotherapeutic efforts.

PRINCIPLES OF TRAUMA TREATMENT

Basic fundamental principles of treatment apply for a trauma patient with complex issues. As previously described, the patient often experiences distortions in the sense of self experienced and may have great distrust with the interpersonal context of the treatment situation. Reflecting on the following treatment principles helps sustain involvement yet maintain objectivity.

- People operate out of their internal maps, and those maps become the interpretive basis for their sensory experiences. With trauma, there is evidence of alteration in the sensory feedback systems that ultimately link with more elaborative cognitive and meaning systems. This alteration is marked by both an over- and under responsiveness that affects the cognitive processing of new information arising externally or internally. A primary issue is managing distrust in the therapy relationship.

- When people act, they are making the best choices for themselves that they can. In short, when a mistake is made, it is made in the context of believing one is doing the right thing. In part, that is why we do not learn from mistakes, because we sincerely believe we are right at the time. It is only dealing with the consequences and the capacity to deal with the consequences in a critical yet nonjudgmental manner that allows for learning and self-correction. The trauma patient vacillates from self-blame to self-denial; the capacity for objective self-reflection has been damaged and needs repair.

- As a listener, the advanced practice nurse needs to respect all communication from the patient for two reasons. First, the APN does not jump to premature judgments regarding the behavior of the patient and its meaning until it is clarified by the patient. Second, from this process, the patient learns to examine his or her behavior for intention, and it keeps the nurse abreast of the many ways meaning is conveyed and disguised both from the patient and the therapist.

- The nurse must endeavor to understand the patient and his or her model of the world. This does not mean condoning or reinforcing, but rather acknowledging that the patient's views are not the nurse's. This is a validating experience for the patient and reflects that he or she has been heard. Further, it is important to remember that the resources for growth and survival reside in the patient and the patient's own personal history. The APN's job is to teach choice, never attempting to usurp the choosing capacities of the individual.

- The person with the most flexibility will be the controlling element in the system. What we see in the examination of symptoms of patients, as well as in their defensive behaviors, is a type of rigidity and redundancy that manifests itself in repetitive behaviors. Rather than accomplishing growth-promoting goals, the repetitive behavior keeps the patient stuck. The nurse needs to remain free from being stuck. This is a challenge with trauma patients because of the horrors of the life events they have endured and because, in the complex responses, their defensive maneuvers with the therapist create a strain on therapeutic empathy.

- In a dyadic exchange a person cannot not respond. Acts of omission are as important as acts of commission.

- Behavior change is hard work and may be overwhelming. If so, the work must be reduced to smaller, attainable steps.

- The outcome of the therapeutic efforts is determined at the behavioral and psychological level of the patient.

PRINCIPLES OF TREATING COMPLEX TRAUMA RESPONSES

The principles of trauma work apply to patients with complex responses to sexual assault, with one major modification. This modification necessitates identifying and managing the patient's defensive structure that has resulted from the early and repetitive trauma experiences. The principles for treating complex trauma responses are outlined in Table 25–1.

MANAGEMENT OF DEFENSIVE PATTERNS

Early childhood abuse triggers the development of defensive behaviors and patterns that can become deeply ingrained personality and characterological traits. The advanced practice nurse needs to assess and identify these patterns in order for therapy to begin. These behaviors develop as a way to protect the patient from inter-

TABLE 25–1. PRINCIPLES FOR TREATING COMPLEX SEXUAL ASSAULT

Management of Defensive Patterns
Stabilization of symptoms
Reducing acting-out behaviors
Strengthening therapeutic alliance

Anchoring for Safety
Personal safety
Environmental safety
Contract for therapy
Patient and therapist commitment
Agreement to change
Identification of interpersonal barriers

Psychoeducation Regarding Complex Trauma Response
Review of diagnostic assessment
Validation of defensive patterns
Ceasing self-destructive and injurious acts
Skill-building strategies

Strengthen Personal Resources
Self-evaluation capacities
Mood regulating capacities
Problem-solving strategies
Social skills
Social network

Surface Trauma Information
Controlled uncovering
Integration of memory fragments
General details

Processing the Trauma
Exposure and reframing
Neutralizing traumatic emotion
Sorting out complex trauma responses
Self-development
Drive integration
Modifying enduring biological sensitivity
Social development
Intimacy
Friendship
Work

Future and Termination
Transferring trauma to past memory
Transference learning
Future goals

personal distress and they can undermine the progress of therapy. The stabilization of symptoms and reduction of acting out behaviors become the first order of business in working with trauma patients with complex responses.

As already indicated in the discussion of complex responses, patients may come to therapy without a clear understanding of the relationship of their behavior to past traumatic events. This is particularly true of patients who experienced chronic childhood sexual abuse. Often they recognize that life has not been happy for them and, as a result, they associate any demands for change on their part as confirmation that they are damaged. Attention to their own behavior is painful and for the most part they expect therapy to validate them and change others.

An assessment needs to be completed and any unsafe behaviors that threaten the therapeutic alliance must be addressed. It can be assumed that the patient is defensively poised not to utilize self-reflection in a constructive way and instead is likely to feel psychologically assaulted or fall into a pattern of severe self-criticism. It is within this context that suicidal and homicidal behaviors have to be evaluated and addressed from the very beginning.

The targeted behaviors to be addressed immediately are suicidal and aggressive behaviors, attachment distortions, behaviors that resist therapy (nonattentive behaviors, noncollaborative behaviors, noncompliance behaviors), and behaviors that discredit the helping environment and the limits of the therapist. A preliminary knowledge of these behaviors reduces burnout for the advanced practice nurse and protects against unnecessary retraumatization and abandonment due to transference and countertransference reactions.

As indicated in the description of the complex responses to trauma, there is often a great deal of disruption in the lives of these patients. This disruption can be manifested primarily in intimate interpersonal relationships or in work accomplishments and relationships. As many of the patients falling into this pattern of complex responses experienced early abuse, there are usually very complicated family relationships. The personal pain and alienation from self and others is often profound and has been responded to with suicide attempts, parasuicide behaviors (nonfatal, intentional self-injurious behavior resulting in tissue damage, self-medication, illness, or risk of death), and/or aggressive, rageful assaults.

Some patients labor under suicidal or homicidal ideation of a vague and unclear nature, and others have a focused plan. Because survivors of trauma are at great risk for suicide or assaultive behavior, it must be the first consideration before any therapy begins. As long as patients are unclear in their commitment to life and are not in agreement to help protect themselves, the progress that can be made in therapy is limited. The burden to both the patient and advanced practice nurse is a key source of stress that can undermine the relationship.

When a person presents with behaviors that convince the nurse and others that suicide or assault is most possible, the focus must be on prevention. If there is a hoarding of drugs, a gun, or suicidal plans, steps must be taken to ensure safety. These steps can involve hospitalization, a restraining order, or the mobilization of persons close to the patient who are willing to be with the patient until the potential for acting on the ideas subsides.

Perhaps the hardest aspect of confronting the depth of pain experienced by the suicidal or homicidal person is recognizing that the life facing the individual is very hard indeed. Taking on the task of assisting the patient in finding a way to a life that is bearable is a heavy responsibility. No one knows what the future holds, but if the patient kills himself or others there is no opportunity to find out.

It is useful to understand that suicide or homicide is thought of as a solution to a variety of problems, as a way of getting away from unbearable pain, seeking revenge, or saving others from suffering. The task of therapy is to move to solutions other than aggression or death. The need to explore the expectations of injurious acts, communications, and ideation is imperative in order to help the patient commit

to behaviors that reduce the risk. Most people do not want to be dead or act out, they want something to be different in their lives and in themselves.

In the face of parasuicidal behavior the results of the acts themselves and the response to them may have a relieving and positive effect. There is a release of negative emotions, accompanied by a sense of relief. This can either help the person recognize that he or she does have choice and control, or it can be a negative reinforcement of parasuicidal behavior. Thus, cutting and cigarette burning of the skin can be injurious and leave scars, but it can also be a desensitization to the acts themselves, leading the way to a more successful suicidal act in the future.

In treatment thus far, two initial points are developed with the patient: (1) suicide or rageful aggression is not a solution; and (2) skills need to be developed to solve problems in a productive manner.

ANCHORING FOR SAFETY

From this position, contracting for safety can begin. The advanced practice nurse discusses personal and environmental safety. The therapist and office setting must be seen as a safe place for the patient to talk and bring problems. Within this phase of treatment, the contract for therapy, the patient/therapist commitment to therapy is made. The patient also makes an agreement to change and identifies interpersonal barriers.

The nurse makes it clear that he or she cannot read minds and cannot rescue the patient from unknown situations. Consequently, the patient must tell the nurse of any self-destructive thoughts or assaultive plans. The fact that the patient and nurse have identified suicide and aggression as maladaptive solutions to life and personal problems provides a prenegotiated position to begin to explore the antecedents to the dysfunctional thinking. The antecedents often reveal the life issue being confronted by the patient.

At times a painful emotional state or other symptoms, such as flashbacks, may be the focus of the aggressive or suicidal action. In these situations, medications may be used for symptom reduction and relief. However, use of medication can evoke a double-edged response from patients. On one hand, it can be seen as a threat that they are incurable, damaged, or marked; on the other, it can be seen and experienced as a relief that there is another method that might help them.

When there is the potential for acting out behaviors such as neglect and abuse of a child, patients need to understand the limits of the practice and the legal requirements faced by the therapist. If this is not discussed in the beginning of therapy and there is need to file a legal report, the patient can suffer additional stress.

Acting out behavior can drive a wedge in the therapy relationship. The therapist defines the limits for physical acts as well as verbal acts (e.g., angry, hostile, threatening, chastising, criticizing remarks regarding the therapist and/or the therapy processes).

The therapist needs to make clear what is needed to conduct therapy efforts; that is, that he or she is not perfect, that mistakes are made, and that the only way both parties can learn is to address these issues and come to some understanding rather than argue and fight. Often an agreement is made not to make a precipitous exit from therapy, allowing at least three sessions to review what is behind the desire to leave, in order to give both therapist and patient time for evaluation.

Medication intervention in the patient with complex responses to sexual assault and trauma tends to be complicated by the patient's defensive behaviors and wishes for a magic remedy mixed with fear of being controlled. Like the issue of suicide, medications and hospitaliza-

tion have to be identified as possible interventions, but ones that require the informed participation and cooperation of the patient. It should be agreed that they are interventions that can only be used if the patient agrees to them. Again, the therapist has to make the therapy issues clear, and the patient has to make clear what his or her expectations (including fears) are of the suggested possible interventions to help with symptoms and problematic behaviors.

A basic fear of patients is to be forced into a hospital and drug regime that is not of their liking or choice. It is important that the therapist make clear at the onset of therapy what steps would be taken to protect the patient. To the extent the patient limits the access of the therapist to important people in the patient's life and information relevant for the patient's protection, such as addresses and phone numbers, the therapist has to be prepared not to start therapy until a workable agreement has been made.

Patterns of attachment can be a barrier to treatment. Because of the high degree of distrust combined with feelings of inadequacy, trauma patients are extremely cautious and dubious. At other times, they react with a clinging attachment. The therapist has to recognize these behaviors and shifts in them.

If the patient cannot keep appointments, therapy cannot proceed. A patient who readily attaches to the therapist often presents with a deferring attitude, never misses appointments, and then begins to make phone calls to the therapist. Often the therapist is the primary support for the patient. Patients' vulnerability and compliance, without understanding that changes in their behavior are for their own benefit, lead to nonproductive therapeutic efforts. There is an idealization of the therapist and the therapy that is usually challenged with the first break in meeting with the patient or disappointing behavior by the therapist.

► CASE EXAMPLE

Jane was referred to the advanced practice nurse because of difficulty at work. She was 38 years old, single, and very angry and reluctant to be coming to therapy. She revealed that she had been in therapy in the past and in fact had been in a day-hospital setting, in which she was accused of plotting suicide with another patient. When her therapist came to her defense, the therapist had been fired from the hospital. Jane eventually entered into another therapy relationship where she focused on behavioral methods for dealing with an unhappy work situation. She felt helped in this setting but still felt depressed. Six months before this referral she broke off another therapy relationship in which the therapist had told her that if she did not either change her job or move out of her present unhappy living arrangement, the therapist could not continue to treat her.

Given this background, Jane was very suspicious of the new therapist and would not provide information regarding her address, phone number, or the names and address of her family. She feared the therapist would suspect that she was suicidal, force medication on her, and trick her into a hospitalization.

Although she agreed to come back for a second visit, she was reluctant to do so. At the second visit, she expressed more of her anger over her right to her thoughts and feelings regarding suicide and her belief no one had the right to decide for her or trick her. She wanted the therapist to trust her, and did not want to trust the therapist to know what was right for her. She denied any specific suicidal plan but did admit to frequent suicidal thoughts and despair over her life. After several visits she agreed to give the therapist her phone number and eventually her address, but she held out against giving information regarding her family.

In this case example we can see the difficulty in establishing trust and a negotiable basis for safety. The past experience of patients with complex trauma responses often involves prior therapies. Hopefully, some were experienced as helpful. When they were not, it presents complications for the new therapist. It is important not to assume that one can rescue the patient from her predicament. In this situation, the commitment to change was difficult for the patient. Because of her past experiences, she felt it was unfair that she was now expected to change, creating a difficult situation from which to embark on a therapy course.

Some patients only come for treatment when there is a crisis. They have a hard time relating to the therapist. The therapist may be a substitute for someone in their lives with whom they are having problems. When that person or another who can substitute for that person comes back into their life, they stop therapy. Often their history reveals that early traumatic events occurred with parental failure to protect. These patients are unable to tolerate the risk of engaging and then being abandoned or not protected; instead, they escape into a multitude of unstable relationships. Unlike the clinging patient, little effort is made by these patients to change their behavior or engage in activities aimed at helping them change. Because of the unstable nature of their relationships, there is often a repetition of primary traumatic experiences and at times an acting out of these experiences with others in their lives, such as their children and spouses.

▶ CASE EXAMPLE

Gisha was in her mid-30s and was referred to the therapist by another patient. Gisha was originally from Germany. She came to this country to get away from her parents and to live a glamorous life with the wealthy and jet-setting people of the world. She came to therapy because of a volatile and unstable relationship with a man from a prominent family who was bipolar and who for years had attempted to treat the mania with alcohol.

Gisha was tall and attractive, with the air of a high fashion model. During childhood, she had developed a fantasy world of glamour, prestige, and money. She had fantasized that she was married to a famous person in her country of origin. This fantasy started in early adolescence and continued in her 20s. She was joined in this fantasy by a girlfriend who also developed a fantasized relationship with a co-famous man to Gisha's. Her friend, when in her early 20s, managed to meet her man and did have a night of sexual intimacy with him. After this experience, Gisha's famous man was killed in an auto accident. In her grief, which she could not share with anyone except her friend, she left her country to come to the United States.

She built a glamorous life for herself for a short period of time. She was in a volatile relationship but believed she loved the man. Her parents came to visit her and she then viewed her life as not good enough, became depressed, and was abandoned by her lover. In the face of this loss, she came to her present state and again started to build her life around her fantasy of glamour. When she feels her relationship with her current lover is smooth, she is no longer depressed or angry. When she feels slighted by him and they fight and there is threat of the relationship ending, she becomes profoundly depressed.

In her country of origin she was raised by parents who had survived World War II and had been subjected to bombing and great deprivation. As they were putting their lives together, Gisha experienced their great emotional volatility and her mother's rage and neglect. Gisha was molested as a child and had witnessed the suicide of two strangers in her community. When she first came to therapy she was offered the chance to talk about herself in her native tongue but she refused, claiming she could not remember her language. This was most revealing, since a main part of her present work situation involved her in being a primary translator.

Her approach to therapy was very hesitant. When she came to appointments she insisted on dealing only with her present relationship. Past history was gathered in a very slow fashion through repeated efforts at coming to therapy and withdrawing when she was re-engaged with her lover.

This went on for over 2 years. As Gisha began to face her life and her sense of herself and became aware that she wanted more out of life, she came to a decision to alter her relationship with her lover. She bought a condominium for herself, prepared to change jobs, and invested more time with her friends. However, as the separation became a reality her depression increased. She finally consented to have a consultation with a psychopharmacologist for antidepressants. The psychopharmacologist was younger than her current therapist, who was approximately the age of her parents. In the face of giving up her lover and recent news that her father had cancer, she used the excuse of a change in her insurance to transfer her therapy to the psychopharmacologist. Several years later she wrote a note to her first therapist saying she missed her and that she was doing fine. She had found a new job and was happy.

In this example we can follow Gisha's effort to avoid contact with and attachment to the therapist. Her need to control the relationship from a distance can be traced to strong emotional issues with her parents and the unprotected experiences of childhood. The degree of pain in her childhood was apparent from her denial that she could speak her language to tell her story, even though her adult work was as a translator. The creation of a fantasized relationship for affection and control does not work for her. Her partners die, they jilt her, and they leave her. If she can replace them she feels better. The patience of the therapist in working with her in and out of therapy paid off in that she could leave the therapist, invest in another therapist, develop further independence, and eventually acknowledge her first therapist, all under her own control.

A focus has been on the establishment of a therapeutic contract in the face of behaviors associated with complex trauma responses that are undermining to a course of therapy and the social network of the patient.

Because of the nature of traumatic events and their impact on the biological, psychological, and social patterns of behavior, it can be seen that in the very beginning of the therapeutic contact, attention to the nature of the therapeutic alliance and a clarification of responsibilities and expectations is particularly important before

work on specific aspects of the traumatic events themselves.

PSYCHOEDUCATION REGARDING THE COMPLEX TRAUMA RESPONSE

The third step is educating the patient with regard to complex trauma response within the context of the review and evaluation of the patient and arriving at a diagnosis. The major objective of the educational aspects of trauma and resultant behaviors helps to validate defensive patterns and move away from a blame framework. Judgmental comments are replaced with assignment of responsibility. Those who raped and abused are responsible for those acts. The patient is responsible for evaluating the impact of those actions on his or her sense of self and behaviors and is responsible for making changes that will help him or her to grow and develop. A delicate balancing act occurs between acknowledgment of negative life events and directing efforts to problem solve in a different manner from the past.

Care must be taken to build the patient's social skills and not to overwhelm the patient with demands to change. Time must be given to the validation of the patient's responses to life events. It takes time to make these distinctions for the patient and it takes careful observation to the reactions of patients for therapists to gauge their pattern of response and determine an appropriate dosage of listening and validating and encouraging change.

When a patient has a great deal of fragmentation, memory disruption, and dissociated states, the individual's sense of being damaged and out of control is intensified and anxiety is increased. An early identification of these behaviors can be most beneficial, but there has to be a counteracting of the negative ideation associated with the behaviors. The fact that the person can observe these behaviors needs to be developed as a strength.

Memory disruption can be addressed in terms of the way it increases with the patient's self-critical and blaming thoughts. Attention to the internal dialogue and noting of these behaviors can be a first step in the development of self-appraisal capacities. Considering these behaviors as maladaptive behaviors associated with negative life events can help to explain experiences that render the person fearful with a sense of inadequacy and a lack of faith in self-determining capacities. It is also important to take the pressure off the patient by countering the notion that every event has to be remembered for the person to feel better. Although avoidance can be a contributor to symptomatic states, excessive focus on negative life events can be an equally destabilizing process.

Memory disruptions and dissociative states have to be understood as processes that are caused by biological disregulation due to alterations in the brain's alarm system and also as psychological defensive operations. Some bodily states of tension and disruption in consciousness will be readily linked to life events, while others will not be. What is important is the development of a capacity to note the onset of these disorganizing states, reduce anxiety surrounding the recognition, and gain some grounding, lessening their influence on present behavior. As noted earlier, the development of self-evaluating capacities is central to development of strategies to interrupt disruptive responses to an awareness of these altered states of consciousness and memory.

► CASE EXAMPLE

Sam, a 29-year-old graduate student, came to therapy because he was beginning to remember sexual abuse that had occurred when he was a teenager. In the past, a movie he had seen in a class on rape and sexual abuse had triggered a profound abreactive state and memory of being raped by a male orderly in a dormitory situation when he was ill with a high fever. He feared he was about to have a similar strong reaction to the fleeting memory he had of being raped by a teacher at a private school where he was a resident.

When he came to see the therapist he was in great distress, fearful of his sense of fragmentation and his inability to remember important events in his life. He believed he was losing his mind and felt helpless and fearful in the face of what was happening to him. He could not tell a story of what was happening to him in a coherent manner. He was aware of having outbursts and periods of time that he could not account for. His anxiety was extremely high, and to some extent he was aware that he did not want to remember his past if it was filled with sexual abuse.

He was pushed and pulled in remembering in the face of other young men from his school coming forward with stories of sexual abuse. Memories came in a fragmented manner. He came to realize he was abused by different teachers. He was in great anguish over his lack of memory for his high school years and he was in pain facing the way he avoided relationships with others. He was fearful and protective of his assailants. He did not want to face them. As memories came back to him, he became more acutely aware of dissociating.

Special techniques for relaxing were developed for him and he was encouraged to note his responses. He began to detail his mounting anxiety and use stress-reducing methods. He began to be less critical of himself and his problems with memory. Eventually there was a court case and he faced his abusers. This process did two very important things for him: (1) his fear was reduced and (2) his awareness of his anger increased. He no longer held himself responsible and he did get validation of his abuse. Although there was possibly more to remember, he had achieved sufficient awareness of numerous events so that he did not have to pursue them in further detail. His productivity in his personal life increased as he prepared to become a father.

The important point in this case is the amount of avoidance manifested by the patient. Even in the face of a flashback several years earlier, the prior memories of his abuse lay buried. In part this was a reflection of the fragmentation of memory induced by being abused as a child and deprived of sleep. There is also a dynamic component in that the abusers were primary father figures for this young man. His deep sense of betrayal by those he wished to love and emulate contributed to his amnesia for the events. The fact that the memories came in bits and pieces caused his greatest terror. He thought he was insane. Early introduction to self-monitoring was begun so he could learn to have control over his recovery from dissociated states and he could pace his own association of personal experiences to past events. This helped him reduce his anxiety over what he observed within himself. When flooded with recollection and fragments, he was exhausted and certainly suffered, fearing there would be no end. But as he gained more control in making decisions about his court case and facing his abusers, his personal sense of fragmentation was reduced and his sense of self was increased.

A review of the diagnosis and of the factors operative at a biological, behavioral, psychological, social, and interpersonal level allows for the staging of treatment efforts and the defining of general goals for treatment. Issues raised during these first two phases of treatment become a source of grounding for the continued therapy. Not only is the plan to open the patient to learning, but there is also an identification of limits of responsibility and a level of insight into behaviors that can be disruptive to the therapeutic process. Both the patient and the therapist can go back to the beginning for review and reorientation, if needed.

During this time, the therapist can introduce general intervention strategies such as medications, hospitalization, family and social supports, and possible group activities that can support some of the strategies that might be needed. Patient expectations and assumptions about these strategies have to be reviewed and obstacles to participating in any of them identified and discussed. Although there may be a reluctance on the part of the patient to participate in these interventions, their possible use in the future is best kept open. In addition to more formal interventions, self-help groups are reviewed at this time with the patient.

If the patients have had experience with these strategies, it is important to detail what helped and what did not. The evaluation of a prior response to treatment can be informative, particularly regarding issues around patterns of attachment and response to treatment, including levels of motivation and commitment. In addition, perceived breaches in prior therapeutic relationships can be evaluated from the patient's perspective, with the therapist keeping in mind how this behavior can be transferred into the present situation.

In summary, the psychoeducation phase introduces the goals of therapy and the possible methods that can foster behaviors to achieve these goals. There is clarification of the reciprocal responsibilities of the patient and therapist. There is a commitment to participate and make efforts towards personal change on the part of the patient with a commitment from the therapist to support and assist the person in this venture. Personal goal setting provides some notion of what would constitute criteria for recovery on the part of the patient; that is, the patient has identified a desired type of outcome and change. To the extent that these phases are negotiated, the therapist knows the limits of the next phases of therapeutic efforts.

STRENGTHENING OF PERSONAL RESOURCES

The fourth step is the strengthening of personal resources. Strengthening personal resources is absolutely essential before trauma information can be dealt with in an intense and potentially resolving manner. If a person does not have the internal resources and/or external supports to counterbalance the negative emotional and psychological aspects of trauma, the chance of simply retraumatizing the patient or driving the patient from therapy is ever present.

What are the essential resources needed to reduce suicidal behavior and decrease behaviors that disrupt therapy or reduce participation in necessary life activities?

Patients with complex trauma responses are challenged in two major areas: the capacity to self-evaluate and to regulate emotional reactions. This reduces the individual's ability to be effective in interpersonal situations. It also means that there is an inability to have a productive self-managing capacity: these individuals cannot soothe themselves; they cannot sustain a good sense of self in the face of distress or disappointment; they cannot maintain a sense of self in the face of attachments and interactions with others; they lack a sense of self cohesion; and they lack a sense of fitting in and belonging (Linehan, 1993). Consequently, key areas of resource building are self-evaluating capacities, mood modifying capacities, and application of these capacities to interpersonal relationships and interpersonal relating.

The objective of self-evaluating capacities is to reduce self-devaluation and increase self-valuation capacities. This aim is accomplished first by having the patient engage in paying attention to thoughts, feelings, and reactions without judging and with more appreciation for being able to note what is going on, even if it is after the fact. This mindfulness gradually takes over during times of intense involvement, but to accomplish this, the patient has to become aware of emotional arousal and numbing and the thoughts and feelings associated with reactions. The patient is often embarrassed and humiliated by strong reactions of rage and panic and demands that others justify their reactions. The arousal to extremes has to be understood as arising out of the dysregulation of the alarm system and as a vacillation between overinhibition and disinhibition. It is not a matter of the emotions being wrong, but rather they overwhelm the patient. The emotional reaction is energy consuming and ineffective in dealing with the associated events.

The first efforts aim at recovering from the extremes of emotions such as rage and panic. This takes time because the chemistry of these emotions takes time to reduce and come back to a stable situation. Because of the trauma history, the restorative process has been altered, making stabilization difficult.

Complementary efforts towards achieving emotional regulation include finding a way to teach relaxation and other self-soothing activities. Attention is paid to pleasurable and restorative activities and to monitoring the amount of stress in the patient's daily life. Finding ways to express emotions before the extremes are triggered involves self-assertion strategies, anger management skills, some basic daily organizational skills, and learning to be self-protective and safe.

The patient needs to be challenged with unexpected situations that demand action. For example, a tire going flat on the car or the basement flooding in the morning when one has to go to work requires dealing with tension and frustration. The patient is taught to relax and deal with thoughts that compound the situation by assaulting a personal sense of self, thoughts such as "everything goes wrong in my life" or "I can-

not handle these situations." Once there is some reduction in the extreme emotional reactions, the patient is better able to define and act upon solutions to the problems.

Management of flashbacks is another part of emotional regulation. Because the recollections are accompanied by a full sense of re-experiencing, flashbacks are addressed first in terms of recovering from the intense emotion. The focus then turns to identifying precursors to the flashbacks as well as recognizing residual negative self-appraisals. Grounding techniques are developed that suit the patient and support from the patient's social network is identified. Note that uncovering of further trauma information is restricted at this time. There must first be a substantial reduction in suicidal behavior, a reduction in therapy-disrupting behaviors, and an increase in a stable and supportive social environment.

Basic attention to nutrition, sleep, and a reasonably ordered environment are all important in increasing positive emotional states and in providing positive experiences to regain balance from distressful situations that lie behind the extreme emotional reactions. These strategies build confidence and tolerance, enabling the patient to endure strong emotion without the cognitive response of dissociation and fragmentation.

Lives devoid of people and material means to bring order, protection, and pleasure often make the change from emotional reactivity to emotional regulation a difficult and prolonged task. Small steps and gains have to be recognized and accumulated to offset these patterns of response.

All of the dimensions of self-management come about as a result of the patient's awareness that learning takes place in increments. There are successes and failures. Failure must be viewed as a positive step, because it does teach if we reflect and learn without punishing self-criticism. Persistence while learning and problem solving is important. Failure helps define areas that need to be modified, such as whether the goal is realistic, whether there was an attempt at too much change, and whether there was a clear analysis of the event and antecedent behaviors, actions, and consequences. A view that willpower is the route to change obscures the learning necessary for change. Willpower merely means the persistence to pursue solutions, even in the face of failure, by converting failure to learning.

Patients have to learn to praise and reward themselves, as well as know how to set up criteria that are workable if they do not follow through. Most often, the consequences of not following though are sufficient. But if there are no immediate negative consequences, there is a tendency to reduce efforts to change. This can be true in the case of changing addictive behavior. Patients must learn to counteract factors that reinforce their lapses in making necessary behavior changes. These lapses, once noted, are usually responded to with negative evaluation, which makes the task impossible, whereas praise for recognizing the lapse and recommitting to the change moves the person through the dilemma of noncommitment.

Situations within the patient's environment need to be examined carefully. Again, in negative environments it is important for the patient to realize the limits of his or her efforts and to gain some understanding of what he or she is facing and what steps need to be taken to reduce the environmental stress. It is not a matter of willpower in many of these stressful situations; rather, it is objectively understanding the limitation inherent in the situation. The difficulty for the patient is changing the patterns of expectations and beliefs from what "should" occur to what is occurring. From this vantage point, the patient can begin to devise measures to deal with the negative situations without self-blame or impulsive rage. Time dimensions can be set, choices can be analyzed, and preparation for changes can be made.

In summary, the development of personal resources to deal with the reactions to overwhelming traumatic events are identified as the key targeted behaviors to be developed. Self-evaluation and mood regulation behaviors are central to development of problem-solving strategies, social skills, and a social network. These targeted areas are vulnerable ones because of the biological changes that occur with trauma as well as the characterological defenses that arise out of traumatic events, particularly those early in life that interfere with the development of these capacities. Change is incremental and is constantly challenged by deeply ingrained beliefs regarding oneself and others and what change, success, and failure mean. While this work is going on, the trauma issues are also being dealt with and addressed at some level. When flashbacks are part of the picture, attention is paid to monitoring them and recovering from the emotional arousal. The same holds true for intrusive thoughts and preoccupation with traumatic events. For those who present with avoidance and numbing, there is still a focused effort with seemingly daily events used to augment emotional awareness and controlled emotional arousal.

SURFACING THE TRAUMA

Once the foregoing principles have been sufficiently developed, attention is directed to surfacing the trauma memories and the trauma story. Eliciting trauma information is a process of controlled uncovering with integration of fragments. This process follows more traditional forms of dynamic psychotherapy. It is important for the patient to be able to tell their story in his or her own words. As the story unfolds, the problems of grief and belief play a big role in the reactions of the patient. It is often very hard for the patient to believe that the event did happen. Many internal reactions can stop the process of uncovering at this time.

Sometimes there is great doubt regarding abusive events, particularly when they occurred early in the life of the patient. Validation of these experiences is most difficult for the patient. If the abuser is a family member, the patient faces the possibility that the individual will deny the accusation and the patient is likely to be fearful that the memory is imaginary. When traumatic events have been out of awareness for a particularly long period of time, their recollection within the therapy process can be disturbing from the standpoint of whether the events really happened and whether there is validation of the events. Most often, the patient and the therapist have to live with the realization that there may be no direct substantiating evidence of the abusive experience.

Deep feelings of self-blame and shame need to be addressed as well as avoidance and moving away from memories that stir strong emotions and usually lead to negative self-appraisals. The avoidance maneuvers are not on a conscious level. Patients can become dazed within a session and not remember what they are talking about; they can go numb and blank, not attributing the prior emotional arousal to stimuli associated with the traumatic events.

Vacillation between intrusive recollections and avoidance responses slows the process of extinguishing the strong emotion embedded in the past traumatic events. Patients can become discouraged in this process if they are not helped to understand that they will remember only what they are ready to remember. Dealing with the memories associated with one abuser may be associated with the uncovering of a variety of events that have been out of awareness. As recollections increase, there is fatigue from the consuming nature of these recollections. The hyperarousal and tension are often accompanied by physiological tension manifested in stomachaches, dizziness, rapid heartbeat, sweating, and interrupted sleep. All create a desire to move away from the past issues, and there is often a premature disengagement from therapy.

It is hypothesized that the biological sensitivity produced by traumatic events bolsters continual repetition of the trauma story without emotional reduction and lessening of the intrusive elements of the traumatic information. In this situation, the person goes over and over the trauma story, and is obsessed with it to such an extent that there is distraction from the demands of daily life and work. In veterans, the phenomenon is believed to be reinforced by disability payments. However, the key to reinforcement may be in the biological release of opioids to block the high emotional arousal associated with the telling of the trauma story.

If the patient can stay with this process long enough, there can be a gradual extinction of the fear reactions associated with recollections. With this reduction there is usually a reframing of perceptions of responsibility. That is, patients can clarify the responsibility of the abuser in their own minds. They can stop blaming themselves and reduce the sense of stigma and shame they associate with the abusive acts.

PROCESSING THE TRAUMA

A series of methods to process and deal with traumatic memories and intrusive thoughts surrounding traumatic events have been developed. Implosion therapy, reported on in the Veterans Administration by Keane and associates (1989), while not without risk of retraumatization, has resulted in the reduction of fear responses to patient-identified traumatic memories. Foa and associates (1991) have had similar results in planned exposures of patients to stories of their rapes. Resnick and associates (1993) have a parallel method of repeated exposure of the patient to the trauma story with specific efforts at reframing negative cognitions associated with the sexual assault event. Their research reports positive results with rape patients.

Other methods devised are eye movement and desensitization and reconstruction (EMDR), devised by Shapiro (1995), and the counting method developed by Ochberg (1996).

In EMDR a basic assumption is made that the processing of trauma information by the brain has become sidetracked. The movement of the therapist's finger in front of the patient, eliciting marked eye movements while focusing on a recurring distressing thought, memory, dream, or problematic relationship and at the same time reframing a negative cognition associated with the experience into a positive one, apparently helps move the stuck information. When this occurs,

► CASE EXAMPLE

Jim is a bright, intelligent man who is a therapist in a highly stressful prison system. He has been in therapy for a number of years. His therapy began with the gradual revelation that he was repeatedly sexually abused by an older brother. The abuse was complicated by the fact that, although his parents were privy to the actions of the older brother, they did nothing to stop the abuse. When Jim made tentative requests for help, he was told to assert himself and take care of the situation himself.

After leaving his family of origin, Jim obtained a college degree and embarked upon a professional career, pushing out of his mind the abuse he endured as a child. He tended to join causes and fight for the underdog. He married an Asian woman after a period of adult years with tentative involvement with the opposite sex. He and his wife had two sons and it was when his sons reached latency age—corresponding to the time his brother began to abuse him—that he began to have memories of the abuse. He held off from therapy because he was afraid to reveal his fear of acting out sexually with his sons. The pressure became so great that he came into therapy and gradually told his story.

Jim moved from a position of avoidance to an obsessive involvement with the details of events between himself and his brother and the dynamics in the family. He became increasingly involved and distracted from his work and family life. This led to a deep depression, during which he needed to be hospitalized. A series of psychotropic drugs were used to relieve his depression and reduce his obsession with the abuse theme.

His depression was linked to his inability to reframe repetition of the abuse issue and its intrusion into his life. However, the telling of the emotionally arousing material was met with a wash of relief after repeating his story. Medications that target the neurotransmission systems associated with repetitive behaviors lessened the obsession and his compulsion to talk about the abuse. Jim regained his life to some extent, but still needs to work on methods of controlling this repetitive behavior pattern.

---

there is increased detailing of the memory and the detailing of subsequent associated traumatic memories. It is hypothesized that the eye movements somehow activate the hemispheres of the brain and allow this beneficial process to begin. Patients report very positive results from this method. There is often a reduction in the intrusive thoughts and there is a perceived reduction in emotional arousal as well as a change in beliefs regarding the event. Much research with this method is continuing. At this point, there is strong support that it does have an positive effect, but the exact mechanisms of how it works are not known. This strategy has to be used within the context of a therapeutic relationship that has addressed the issues raised in the foregoing description of dealing with complex trauma responses.

The counting method devised by Ochberg is also nonintrusive. The patient has usually recounted some aspects of the traumatic events that plague their memories. Within the context of a safe and helpful relationship, the therapist asks the patient to focus on the traumatic event while the therapist counts to 100. No comments are made by the therapist during this procedure. The patient is free to volunteer information, but is not required to explain what he or she is imagining and experiencing. Ochberg suggests that there are possible similarities in his method to the EMDR and that repeated exposure to the trauma helps desensitize the patient to the overwhelming emotions. There is no reported research at this time on this method, although it is being considered in some comparative therapy studies. Other methods also have been used to deal with trauma memories, some within the context of hypnosis and others involving types of visualization strategies.

The important point about treating the trauma information itself is the preparation. If one proceeds too rapidly with the trauma information there can be retraumatization. If one avoids the trauma information, the patient is left struggling with the unresolved information and focusing on the agenda of the therapist. In complex trauma responses this can happen very easily, because the array of upsetting symptoms and experiences and the need of the patient and the therapist to remain in contact overrides the order of therapeutic effort. Long-term treatment can have these confusions. It is imperative that therapists working with patients with complex trauma responses have a team to work with and ongoing consultation. When these very difficult lives are addressed solely by the therapist and the patient, it is often overwhelming for both.

FUTURE AND TERMINATION

At this point in treatment the patient has an integrated appreciation and control of the drive to integration and there is mood stabilization. There has been a sorting out of the issues of sex and aggression and the patient has developed a sense of the future in a positive way. He or she has begun to move out interpersonally, to make plans, and has learned not to withdraw upon disappointment. Work begins on the termination process.

At this phase, patients have the resources to take care of themselves and they know what to do in a wide variety of interpersonal situations. They understand that they can look at their personal reactions; they have more criteria to understand complex interpersonal situations. They have a good sense of self and who they are.

Termination is agreed upon by both patient and therapist and is usually an emotional but positive experience. They terminate with a realistic appraisal, rather than the distortions of the past.

► CASE EXAMPLE

Jasmine came to work with her therapist after a long period of volatile relationships with numerous other therapists, all of whom were angered by her demanding, hostile, and provocative manner. She was assertive, threatened lawsuits, complained at being abused by various treatment situations, and became known as so difficult to work with that no wanted to treat her. As a result, she was assigned to a student.

Jasmine decided to work with the student, who was extremely intuitive and dedicated, as well as enthusiastic. Some calm was brought to Jasmine and her life. Jasmine was living in car, as she was basically homeless and without a job or a means of supporting herself. As they progressed in their work, termination became necessary upon the student's graduation.

As fate would have it, the student joined the staff of the agency and Jasmine returned to the agency for treatment. She was again assigned to the former student, who was now a staff member.

Issues occurred within the agency and Jasmine began to voice multiple complaints against the agency. This created stress in the treatment relationship that was never resolved. The agency sent Jasmine to another division and terminated the therapist's work with her. Both the therapist and Jasmine were infuriated by this arbitrary decision and they agreed to meet outside of the agency under different conditions, although both knew this to be in violation of agency policy.

Work together, though stormy, progressed through the years. Jasmine was given an accurate diagnosis of a seizure disorder and received treatment for it. She finished school and obtained a job, found a roommate, and achieved living arrangements better than the streets, although this was not done without ups and downs in the treatment relationship. Jasmine had an extensive history of sexual and physical abuse. Constant shifts in ego states led the therapist to the eventual consideration and conviction that Jasmine had a dissociative identity disorder.

The focus of the therapy began to be on eliciting the altered states of consciousness to discern the extent of abuse experienced by Jasmine. Rather than addressing the known abuse that was confirmed by Jasmine, the focus was on fragmented memories of bizarre and sadistic experiences not clearly confirmed by Jasmine and terribly frightening in their presentation.

This focus began to increase symptoms and Jasmine's extreme volatility with others persisted, as did her fight with the agency that had rejected her. This extended over several years and aggravated her health condition. As this strategy peaked, the therapist had to absent herself from the therapy because of personal illness, an accident, and deaths in her family. Though she struggled to maintain contact with Jasmine, therapy was disrupted, and with the disruption a deep sense of abandonment and rage increased in Jasmine. Her flashbacks of the abuse increased, particularly with the death of the abuser and further confirmation of the abuse. Her need for the rejecting agency increased as her therapist became distracted by her own personal needs. In addition, Jasmine lost her job and blamed it on the therapist for labeling her as having a multiple personality.

At this point Jasmine fought everyone, yet cried out for help. In her rage she reported her therapist for working with her outside of the agency and threatened a legal suit. The therapist felt very angry with Jasmine and had difficulty working with her. In reality, the therapist was burned out, Jasmine was beside herself with rage, and suffering increasing flashbacks of her earlier abuse.

It took much time in joint consultation for the two to review their work and sort out what was successful and what was not helpful in therapy. Eventually Jasmine worked through her problems with the agency and many of her complaints were addressed. As she gained distance from her therapist and took responsibility for legal assault on the therapist, she did acknowledge the possibility of multiple personality. At the same time, Jasmine emphasized that the actual confirmed abuse needed to be talked about before entering into the confusing area of the extreme states of dissociation.

The therapist gained perspective and has been able to learn from this complex and harrowing experience. Jasmine is in therapy now and is learning to use self-observation and evaluation to modify her extreme emotional responses and to build a new treatment relationship with clearer boundaries.

The seemingly tumultuous therapy provided an experience for healing and development beyond a compromised adaptation. She truly cared about and experienced love and trust with her former therapist. She also experienced and released the rage she felt for all those who did not protect her and care for her as a child. To bring together her great longing to be loved and her fury at not being loved and her ability to retaliate helped heal a division within her sense of self. In the process of honestly and painfully confronting the process of therapy with the therapist, she was able to experience a corrective experience of expressing her deep feelings and learning that neither she nor her therapist need be destroyed by them. She was angered and upset that they could not continue a friendship, and this has taken time to work through. It has been important for the therapist to express her positive interest and regard for Jasmine, but to maintain the termination of the relationship. This experience has brought into play a far less vicious and critical self-evaluative process, which is now operative in Jasmine's efforts to establish a new therapeutic relationship. Her extreme emotions in reacting to the new therapist are much more under her observation and she can now utilize many of the interpersonal skill strategies learned in a variety of self-help groups she participated in and now is much more willing to revisit and not take over. With this increased attention to self-development, she is moving out much more in social relationships with others, including her family, which has been severely dysfunctional.

Sorting out complex trauma responses in the here and now comprises work beyond the level achieved with the working through of trauma information. Self-development is furthered by drive integration and the modifying of enduring biological sensitivity to the residues of the malfunctioning defenses and the trauma response.

This phase of therapy may be ongoing for many years for those who have recovered from severe abuse and trauma. The residue of trauma both in memory and in habit is ever enduring. A reduction in self-blame and shame and the building of a positive philosophy of life helps propel people into the future. Jasmine, for example, was adamant that she would not give up her family. This is extremely important for therapists to understand. Though the parent is abusive and neglectful, the parent may also have been a source of warmth. It is not the therapist's decision to terminate the patient's relationships. The patient has to work them through and make a decision as to what is tolerable and what they believe is necessary.

REFERENCES

American Psychiatric Association. *Diagnostic and Statistical Manual of Mental Disorders. 4th ed.* Washington, DC: APA; 1994.

Burgess AW, Holmstrom LL. Rape trauma syndrome. *Am J Psychiatry.* 1974;131:981–986.

Cole PM, Putnam FW. Effect of incest on self and social functioning. A developmental psychopathology perspective. *J Consult Clin Psychol.* 1992;60: 174–184.

Finkelhor D. The trauma of sexual abuse: Two models. *J Interpersonal Violence.* 1988;2:348–366.

Foa E, Rothbaum B, Riggs D, Murdock T. Treatment of posttraumatic stress disorder in rape victims: A comparison between cognitive-behavioral procedures and counseling. *J Consult Clin Psychol.* 1991; 59:715–723.

Herman JL. *Trauma and Recovery.* New York: Basic Books; 1992.

Kazdin A, Moser J, Colbus D, Bell R: Depressive symptoms among physically abused and psychiatrically disturbed children. *J Abnormal Psychol.* 1985; 94:298–307.

Keane TM, Fairbank JA, Caddell JM, et al. Implosive (flooding) therapy reduces symptoms of PTSD in Vietnam combat veterans. *J Behav Ther.* 1989;20: 245–260.

Kilpatrick D, Saunders B, Amick-McMullan A, et al. Victim and crime factors associated with the development of posttrauamtic stress disorder. *Behav Ther.* 1989;20:199–214.

Kilpatrick D, Saunders B, Amick-McMullan A, et al. Criminal victimization: Lifetime prevalence, reporting to police, and psychological impact. *Crime Delinquency.* 1987;33:479–489.

Linehan MM. *Cognitive-behavioral Treatment of Borderline Personality Disorder.* New York: Guilford Press; 1993.

Ochberg FM. The counting method for ameliorating traumatic memories. *J Traumatic Stress.* 1996;9: 873–880.

Resnick HS, Kilpatrick DG, Dansky BS, et al. Prevalence of civilian trauma and posttraumatic stress disorder in a representative sample of women. *J Consult Clin Psychol.* 1993;61:984–991.

Sato R, Heiby E. Depression and posttraumatic disorder in battered women. *Behav Ther.* 1991;14: 151–157.

Shapiro F. *Eye Movement Desensitization and Reprocessing.* New York: Guilford Press; 1995.

Steketee G, Foa E. Rape victims: Posttraumatic stress responses and their treatment. *J Anxiety Disord.* 1987;1:69–86.

Van der Kolk BA, McFarlane AC, Weisaeth L, eds. *Traumatic Stress: The Effects of Overwhelming Stress on Mind, Body, and Society.* New York: Guilford Press; 1996.

Weaver TI, Clum GA. Early family environments and traumatic experiences associated with borderline personality disorder. *J Consult Clin Psychol.* 1993; 61:1068–1075.

CHAPTER 26

CRISIS INTERVENTION AND PROBLEM-SOLVING WITH BATTERED WOMEN

Albert R. Roberts • Sunny Burman

Crisis intervention is often the critical starting point of a longer journey that will not be culminated until safety is no longer threatened and emancipation and stability are finally achieved. Once the acute problems are addressed, the more chronic difficulties and dilemmas must be assessed.

Chapter Overview

► INTRODUCTION

A study was conducted to learn about the diversity of clinical practice models used by shelter staff in the United States and how the models are incorporated in interventions with battered women. The nature of three intervention formats used in shelters are reported here: intake assessments, counseling, and empowerment strategies. Application of the proposed crisis intervention and cognitively oriented problem-solving practice model will be demonstrated in this chapter through a case example of a battered woman. It will illustrate how this model provides the battered woman with the tools not only to cope with current situations and resulting acute problems, but also to prevent more chronic dysfunction by learning strategies that will reinforce stabilization, healing, and growth.

METHODOLOGY OF A STUDY

A cover letter with a one-page questionnaire was sent in October 1994 to a random sample of shelter directors. Eighty-seven of the 176 shelters (almost 50 percent) responded to this survey. The sample came from the National Organization for Victim Assistance (NOVA) directory and the Office for Victims of the U.S. Department of Justice. The questionnaire began with a case scenario of a battered woman with medical injuries coming to a shelter in acute crisis, with her three children in the middle of the night. The clinical survey collected data in three areas:

1. Types and use of intake forms and assessment protocols.
2. Types and components of crisis counseling and other clinical practice models.
3. Methods of empowering battered women.

FINDINGS

It was found that all of the respondents conduct a basic intake assessment, ranging from a few questions to a seven-page form. The content of the intake forms includes medical injuries, safety needs, demographics, listings of the presenting problem, alcohol and drug use, current abusive incident, prior abusive incidents, prior use of services, and any abuse of children. The respondents indicated that an intake assessment can be delayed as long as 24 hours, until the battered woman in acute crisis is stabilized. Only two of the clinical directors used standardized assessment scales to assess and measure suicide risk, depression, intrusive thoughts and fears, post-traumatic stress disorder, or other psychiatric disorders.

The second part of the survey examined the extent to which shelter staff are likely to use a counseling modality or clinical practice model to intervene with a severely battered woman. The respondents used eight different practice patterns in treating battered women (Table 26–1).

For the most part, respondents showed limited knowledge of basic counseling skills and treatment plans in their responses. They do not seem to understand what constitutes a counseling or practice theory, practice model, or clinical/treatment strategy. It is important for clinicians to assess the safety and stabilize the client, explore and validate feelings, listen actively and reflectively, examine coping skills, empower by exploring options together, and help the client to formulate an action plan. *It is too simplistic and potentially harmful, however, to assume that ventilation, active listening, and referral are sufficient to end the cycle of severe and intense battering.*

TABLE 26–1. PRACTICE MODELS AND TECHNIQUES FOR ABUSED WOMEN

Model	No. Respondents
Provide support by reviewing options and choice and referring to a support group.	28
Explore and validate feelings.	19
Assess immediate needs of clients.	15
Work with client to plan and formulate goals.	14
Short-term crisis intervention.	12
Active listening.	9
Problem-solving method.	8
Referral to community resources and private practitioner.	8

Empowerment is critically important in order for battered women to recover, heal, and lead productive lives in nonviolent relationships. But many severely battered and traumatized women need both empowerment and therapy to survive and thrive. There are no quick fixes or easy solutions. Commitment to escaping permanently from the battering relationship requires a trusting and empathic therapeutic relationship that bolsters ego strengths and re-empowers the survivor through positive reinforcement of small changes as well as large ones (see Table 26–2).

A COGNITIVELY ORIENTED PROBLEM-SOLVING MODEL

After ensuring the safety and survival issues of the battered woman, additional aid is often needed to continue stabilization while helping her resolve major issues and formulate important decisions that will affect her present and future functioning (see Table 26–3). The Roberts's Seven-Step Crisis Intervention Model (1991, 1995) provides guidelines for the crucial stage of early crisis resolution, using an integrated problem-solving approach (see Table 26–4). This critical rehabilitative phase is designed to assist the client in establishing adaptive and constructive coping skills that will reestablish the equilibrium necessary to pursue actions that will overcome the obstacles to personal well-being.

Building on Roberts's crisis intervention model, which provides the foundation for problem-solving, positive change, and empowerment, the client is ready to move toward another stage in the healing and growth-producing process. This sequence can be likened to a progression from the resolution of an acute, debilitating

TABLE 26–2. TYPES OF EMPOWERMENT METHODS USED TO HELP BATTERED WOMEN

Method	No. Respondents
Examine options or choices, and refer to self-help/support group.	38
Explore legal options and encourage client to file criminal charges.	32
Educate about cycle of violence and power/control issues.	24
Provide information about community resources, with numerous referrals, and make first appointment for victim.	24
Reassure client that abuse is not her fault, and correct victim-blaming.	10
Initiate advocacy for welfare or housing.	9
Accompany to court appearances and provide advocacy with judge.	8

TABLE 26–3. CRISIS ASSESSMENT (INCLUDING LETHALITY MEASURES)

First and foremost, the patient needs to be stabilized. It must be determined whether there are, or have been:

- Any guns or rifles in the home; threats to use a weapon on patient.
- Any weapons used in prior battering incidents.
- Any threats with weapons.
- Any criminal history of batterer.
- Need for emergency medical attention by patient.
- Threats or actual killing of a pet.
- Threats of suicide by abuser.
- Batterer's fantasies about suicide or homicide.
- Marital rape or forced sex among cohabitants.
- Increased battering during pregnancy.
- Medical problems as result of pregnancy.
- Medical problems as result of rape (e.g., infections, STDs, HIV infection, unwanted pregnancy, risk to fetus in a pregnant woman).
- Psychological torture (e.g., degradation, forced drug use, isolation of victim, sleep or food deprivation, threats to family of victim).

crisis state to working with clients on sustaining previous advances. At the same time, there is an attending to new modes of learning to reinforce the prolonged acquisition and internalization of survival and actualization skills. Toward this aim, a cognitively oriented, problem-solving model is proposed that will encompass the groundwork of cognitive therapy and problem-solving that has been influential in behavioral and emotional change, as well as the needed alterations in environmental systems that block desired objectives.

To demonstrate the congruence with Roberts's model and the utilization of the concurrent model, a case study is presented. It portrays the difficulties of a battered woman as she struggles with her life of pain and the fears that keep her trapped. Due to her fears she is unable to make constructive decisions that will alter the status quo and provide a sense of hope that change is not only possible, but within her reach.

TABLE 26–4. ROBERTS'S SEVEN-STAGE CRISIS INTERVENTION MODEL

► CASE EXAMPLE

Sandra, a 28-year-old waitress with three children between the ages of 2 and 6 years, had an argument with her intoxicated husband, Luke. Although the argument started out small, it progressed and ended with Luke shoving Sandra and breaking her nose.

After Luke was asleep, Sandra decided she could not take the abuse any longer. She left the house with her three children. At 3:00 AM, Sandra arrived at the center with a bruised face, no money, and fearful that she would be hurt again. She also revealed that this was not the first time Luke had abused her.

► PRELIMINARY ASSESSMENT

The information taken by an intake worker provided important data suggesting the physical harm and emotional turmoil Sandra had experienced in her relationship with Luke. A more detailed history was necessary to ascertain the most appropriate individualized treatment plan for Sandra and her children. Nevertheless, from this brief report, it was hypothesized that Sandra had reached a turning point that was the catalyst for mobilizing her strengths and resources to seek safety measures. It also could provide an opportunity to help her gain the supports, knowledge, and skills that would evoke positive changes and decisions that would prevent future occurrences of domestic violence.

► THE PERSONAL IMPACT OF DOMESTIC VIOLENCE

As Sandra mentioned in the intake, this was not the first time she was abused in her marriage. A more in-depth, structured interview determined the extent and duration of the battering and the deleterious effects on Sandra and the children. Over a 5-year period, she was intermittently brutalized and held captive by fear and the inability to control the inevitable recurrence of her husband's violent episodes.

Sandra was aware of Luke's dysfunctional upbringing as the only child of alcoholic parents. During their short courtship and the early years of marriage, Luke never displayed the kind of rage and bitterness that typified his parents' relationship. Sandra knew that he was never physically harmed at home, but the emotional impact of watching his father physically abuse his mother left wounds that he still felt.

Before the children were born, Sandra and Luke spent "good times" together, often socializing with friends at parties. She drank very little, compared to Luke, yet was always amazed (and somewhat pleased) at "how many he could put away" without showing signs of losing control and becoming "sloppy" drunk. She recalled, with sharp disapproval, how her own father would drink too much at times and become verbally abusive. With pride, she would point out that Luke could "hold his liquor," often becoming more amusing and affectionate. She did not realize that this could change, and described their early years together as "happy and without problems."

With the pressures of raising a family and increasing financial debts, conflicts arose in the marriage. Luke held a steady job as a construction worker, and with Sandra's income and tips as a waitress, they were able to pay their bills and even save a small amount each month. But this was short-lived, as Luke began to gamble heavily. He feared that his job was in jeopardy, as his drinking had begun to interfere with his performance. The escalating stresses particularly affected his relationship with Sandra, often climaxing in loud arguments that catapulted to beatings.

Although he never physically hurt the children, Sandra often feared that he would some day. She also worried that witnessing their father severely injuring her could leave indelible emotional scars. The altercation and resultant bruises that actually triggered her leaving with the children were not as severe as past traumas, in which she sustained a concussion and multiple fractures and bruises. At those times, she fleetingly thought of escaping the pain of living, and occasionally considered taking the children and moving far away. But these fantasies vanished quickly, as she thought, "Where would I go? How can I support the children and myself? Will I be safe anywhere?" So she remained in a fearful, helpless, and untenable position, feeling more and more isolated within herself and incapacitated by escalating depressive symptoms.

At the agency, efforts were made to assess Sandra's safety needs, establish rapport, and identify and prioritize major problems. The worker encouraged Sandra to express her feelings and seek help. An assessment of her coping methods was prompted by the question, "How did you handle those traumatic situations?" It was important to listen empathically and attentively and to acknowledge the intensity of her pain. The barriers and obstacles that undermined the ability to alter her life (lack of funds, perceived supports, and knowledge of available resources) were identified. From this data, possible solutions and their consequences were formulated.

Arriving at an action plan required the development of alternate options and solutions to resolve the crisis (a possible separation and a court-ordered restraining order). Sandra's progress through this intervention phase was supported and monitored closely. With her resolve and determination, she was able to reduce the distressful symptoms of the acute crisis and begin to act on the plan to protect and move on with her life.

THE BATTERING EXPERIENCE

Sandra's anguished experience has many commonalities with other battered women. Avni's (1991) questionnaire of abused women expressed a lengthy range of battering, from 2 to 30 years, with the earliest incident reported during the first month of marriage. Of Sandra's 7 years with Luke, 5 were characterized as abusive. Hamberger and Holtzworth-Munroe (1994) state that victims of battering live in constant terror and stress, resulting in depression, anxiety, and somatic complaints. At the same time, there is a period in which concern, apologies, and assurances of ending the violence are offered, which tend to restabilize the emotional bonds (Walker, 1994). This dubious and precarious reality typified Sandra's and Luke's relationship.

A variety of stresses can increase the potential for violence (Stith and Rosen, 1990). These include the birth of children (Watkins and Bradbard, 1982) and losing a job (or fear of job loss) and concomitant financial instability with a negative impact on an individual's self-esteem (Stith and Rosen, 1990). Add to this the excessive use of alcohol or other drugs, and the frequency and severity of battering (and possible death) are heightened (Walker, 1989). Reviewing Sandra's case report, we can readily identify these factors that might have created the perilous exposure to physical and emotional harm.

This reign of terror can be endured indefinitely. What actually motivates women to escape abusive relationships has been the subject of research by Davis and Srinivasan (1995). Conducting focus groups as a means of learning their subjects' personal experiences, they found several rationales for leaving and seeking help (pp. 57–58):

- Overcoming fear (by finding a way out, perhaps encouraged by a change in attitudes and policies that are more supportive of battered women).

- Children as major catalysts (to protect children from psychological harm).
- Getting older and wiser with time (and the experience and wisdom that follows).

In Sandra's situation, the children definitely influenced her decision, and perhaps the passage of time did, too. There was no evidence of concrete changes in Luke's behavior. These significant operative forces, coupled with the fact that she recognized her vulnerable position, the continued threat of severe violence and possible death, and awareness of her own potential for retaliation substantiated the necessity for taking action.

ROBERTS'S CRISIS INTERVENTION MODEL

Facing her fears and taking control was a self-empowering act that began the journey through and beyond the crisis Sandra was experiencing. An existence of pain and discomfort was being challenged by a shift towards hope and renewal. Assistance in this endeavor was forthcoming once the decision was made to seek help.

Using Roberts' seven-stage model (as previously described), the goal is to assure immediate safety and stabilization, followed by problem-solving and the exploration of alternative options that would culminate in a meaningful action plan. Implicit in this model is a cognitive restructuring of perceptions, attitudes, and beliefs that will confront irrational distortions, misconceptions, and contradictions. The identification of erroneous thought patterns ("I can't make it alone without him") and a redirection to empowering affirmations and beliefs ("If other women have made it, so can I") can enhance self-worth and self-reliance, while reinforcing constructive coping mechanisms. With support, guidance, and acceptance, meaningful solutions that were once unrecognized can become attainable objectives.

A COGNITIVELY ORIENTED PROBLEM

A battered woman's fears and problems are not completely allayed once the immediate crisis has dissipated. If she returns to her partner, the violence will probably recur, particularly if the perpetrator has not received help. If she leaves, the possibility of battering and harrassment, even death, becomes a constant risk. Proceeding successfully through the critical phase of crisis resolution can reestablish a sense of balance, strengthen a much-maligned identity and sense of self, and increase the determination to pattern a life free of turmoil and suffering. But the awareness of vulnerability and helplessness may still remain within the realm of consciousness, provoking an unsettling indecisiveness as to the direction that should be taken. This is often magnified by any disconcerting emotional attachments that still linger.

Given the enormity and depth of the problems encountered, battered women need a continuity of supportive networks and helping services to transcend the horrifying situations they experienced (and may continue to face, if no dramatic changes are made). Crisis intervention is often the critical starting point of a longer journey that will not be culminated until safety is no longer threatened and emancipation and stability are finally achieved. Once the acute problems are addressed, the more chronic difficulties and dilemmas must be assessed. Besides recurrent fears, dysfunctional symptoms of post-traumatic stress disorder and emotional difficulties may intrude into daily routines. These problems must be dealt with in order for the battered woman to regain a sense of adequacy and normalcy.

A cognitively oriented, problem-solving approach is a natural supplement to Roberts's crisis intervention model. It adheres to the basic format, concentrating on behavioral, emotional, and environmental change through the incorporation of cognitive and problem-solving strategies. The integrated principles will be identified,

followed by their application to the assessment and treatment phases of the case presented.

COGNITIVE THERAPY

Cognitive therapeutic methods have been developed from various theories of learning, primarily classical and operant conditioning (Skinner, 1938) and social learning (Bandura, 1977). These theories espouse that behavior is a learned process that occurs through transactions between individuals and their social environments. Through classical conditioning, a response to a paired, repeated stimulus is learned (conditioned); through operant conditioning, a response that is reinforcing (rewarded) will reoccur; and according to social learning theory, learning takes place by modeling (observing and imitating others), as well as through self-reinforcement and evaluations (Longres, 1995).

These theoretical frameworks have set the stage for the adoption of many strategies, such as systematic desensitization to treat anxiety and phobias; aversion therapy to eliminate an undesirable behavior; shaping behaviors by rewarding successive approximations of the desired result; the use of positive and negative reinforcement to increase or reduce targeted behaviors; and role modeling of adaptive behaviors (Longres, 1995). Cognitive restructuring, identifying dysfunctional core beliefs, role plays and rehearsals, realization and stress management training, self-monitored homework assignments, and problem-solving are now widely in use to reinforce the goals of positive learning and change (Beck et al., 1993).

PROBLEM-SOLVING

The problem-solving approach has been a strategic mainstay of many professional disciplines. According to Hepworth and Larsen (1993), problem-solving skills are taught "not only to remedy immediate problems but also to enhance clients' future coping capacities. . . . The principles can be readily transferred from one situation to another" (pp. 434–435). Through effective problem-solving, a range of options can be generated that will enhance decision making; self-reliance, self-esteem, confidence, and self-efficacy can be increased; and tensions, anxiety, and depressive symptoms can be allayed.

The problem-solving model provides a step-by-step framework to intervention planning and implementation. An integral part of any therapeutic process is the initial engaging of the client in a relationship built on trust and rapport. Based on this foundation, the following tasks can be actuated by the mutual effort of both practitioner and client:

1. Assessment developed from the data collected.
2. Problem identification and implications.
3. Goal setting and contracting.
4. Implementation of interventions.
5. Termination and referrals.
6. Evaluation of effectiveness of interventions.

PROBLEM IDENTIFICATION AND CASE IMPLICATIONS

The primary problem, identified by Sandra in the first stage of crisis resolution, was the continuous battering experience she had endured over a 5-year period with no assurance of its stopping. She also realized that the children could be severely damaged by witnessing the battering. Associated with this were fears of continued violence and harassment if she left Luke and not being able to provide for the children and herself without his assistance. Despite the traumas, there existed an underlying attachment to him, which made her ambivalent about ending the relationship. Her lack of self-confidence and low self-esteem and self-worth were also prominent. Through the initial therapeutic process, the immediate crisis was allayed, but lingering trepidations and ambivalence remained that could diminish the gains that had been made. Without additional treatment, anticipatory problems were expected to arise, especially if she were to return to Luke and the violence that would invariably continue.

GOAL SETTING AND CONTRACTING

Preliminary goals were aimed to fortify some of the previous goals made during the crisis resolution phase: (1) continuing to strengthen Sandra's emotional stability, self-esteem and resolve; and (2) empowering her to make desirable, self-assured decisions based on what would promote optimal safety and a better quality of life for her and the children. This would entail helping her to challenge self-defeating thoughts and beliefs that restrain rational decisions; to explore the options and alternatives available; and to recognize and tap into her strengths that would facilitate problem-solving. As therapy continued with Sandra, the assessment and goals were expected to expand, depending on the circumstances experienced. Contracting comprised a verbal agreement to work together on the proposed goals for a period of 20 sessions, after which progress would be evaluated.

IMPLEMENTATION OF INTERVENTIONS

After a brief, but intensive crisis intervention foundation, Sandra was stabilized and acquired the tools to improve her coping and decision-making abilities. Nevertheless, self-doubts and fears still existed that needed qualifying and assuaging. Without sustaining, cognitive explorations of these elements and a dramatic change in emotional and belief manifestations, the depressive and anxiety reactions that were previously noted could result in more debilitating symptoms similar to a post-traumatic stress disorder (PTSD). To allay the possibility of regression and additional problems, the clinician should develop the therapeutic relationship with Sandra based on rapport, trust and empathy.

Sandra began to realize that returning to Luke would be an error in judgment that she would forever regret—the promises to end the battering would continue, but the injuries and subjugation would not cease. Yet her ambivalence about leaving him was influenced by the fears of being autonomous and independent, coupled with an uneasy emotional attachment that lingered. Nevertheless, she did agree on the plan to try a separation; she moved with her children into an apartment that she could afford and obtained a restraining order for added protection. Therapy continued to help her adjust to her new status and setting. An important part of the plan was to bolster her ego strengths and coping skills in order to overcome any difficulties that might occur, while providing supportive structures and resources as needed.

An essential element in the process was the initial turning point that initiated the help-seeking. It was seen as self-empowering and had to be reinforced and supported continuously. Her depression and anxiety were treated with medication until they were markedly reduced. Acknowledging that maladaptive emotional reactions and subsequent behaviors are manifested through distorted thoughts and beliefs, cognitive strategies (Roberts, 1995) were implemented to help Sandra challenge and interrupt these perceptions through reality testing and logic.

The change from her former persona of normalcy, stability and security had been essentially destroyed in the marriage. When this awareness solidified, she became angry and began opening up to new experiences. She had blamed herself for the failing marriage; now she realized that Luke's abusive behaviors and controlling nature were inexcusable and caused most of the friction between them. He had placed her in a defenseless, precarious position—one that provoked fear, isolation, shame and guilt.

She was prompted to participate in a therapy group of abused women who gained strength from one another in their quest to break the destructive bonds they endured. She also joined a self-help support group that included women who left their abusive partners and were managing their lives quite satisfactorily. Many of these women formed relationships that sustained them in moments of apprehension and indecisiveness.

TERMINATION AND REFERRALS

Primary treatment was completed when Sandra stabilized enough to pursue her own goals of independent living with appropriate supports and resources. Referrals were made for legal and financial assistance, and educational guidance was provided at a local academic institution. Follow-up was agreed to, with monthly contacts to determine her current functioning and needs. In addition, it was stressed that any problems and safety concerns would be addressed immediately. It was imperative to clarify this policy so that she would understand that provisions would be available promptly, when necessary.

EVALUATION OF EFFECTIVENESS OF INTERVENTIONS

It should be emphasized that the evaluation of interventions should be an ongoing process. As work with the client continues, issues might arise that were unforeseen, and the action plan must be flexible enough to adjust accordingly. In summarizing Sandra's progress in treatment, problem-solving entailed all the knowledge and skills she had learned from crisis intervention and cognitive therapy. She was able to critically ponder each problem and weigh the consequences of her actions. Without extended therapeutic experience, she might not have been ready to combat detrimental, impulsive responses that would have prevented necessary changes. She was amazed at her own strengths, which were unrecognized before.

She was able to make decisions that could finally end a disastrous relationship and save herself and her children from future turmoil.

SUMMARY

This chapter integrates the findings of a research study and a practice model demonstrating the strategies used by shelters for battered women and a more comprehensive strategic model that is designed to address the many inherent problems of domestic violence. It is suggested that limitations are placed on the helping process by not affording a more intensive, intervention-action plan, utilizing both crisis intervention and cognitively-oriented problem -solving. The dangers involved in battering can be so emotionally and physically devastating that extreme measures must be taken to ensure safety and increase awareness of the dangers involved in remaining in an abusive relationship, while teaching and developing coping skills to resist any repetition of assaults in the future. The critical analysis and consequences of a battered woman's decision should not be treated lightly. If she decides to return to the perpetrator, death or severe and prolonged injuries can occur. Therefore, every effort should be made to help her make an informed decision based on logic, not emotion.

The proposed model can be effectively utilized by generalist practitioners, specialists and professionals in health care agencies and shelters. A multidisciplinary team can assume various responsibilities and tasks in carrying out the rehabilitative stages, from the acute crisis to the more chronic condition with related problems. The goal is to follow the client through the healing and growth phases, empowering her to protect and look after her best interests, while tapping and building ego strengths to prevent recurrent psychological and behavioral incapacitation. It is a present and future-oriented approach to security, healthy functioning and self-sufficiency. With continual support and reality-oriented

feedback, a battered woman who had lost hope can again perceive life with optimism and a renewed sense of determination and be able to strive toward independence and self-fulfillment.

REFERENCES

Avni N. Battered wives: The home as a total institution. *Violence and Victims.* 1991;2:137–149.

Bandura A. *Social Learning Theory.* Englewood Cliffs, NJ: Prentice-Hall; 1977.

Beck AT, Wright FD, Newman CF, Liese BS. *Cognitive Therapy of Substance Abuse.* New York: Guilford Press; 1993.

Davis LV, Srinivasan M. Listening to the voices of battered women: what helps them escape violence. *Affilia 10.* 1995;1:49–59.

Hamberger LK, Holtzworth-Munroe A. Partner violence. In: Dattilio FM, Freeman A, eds. *Cognitive-Behavioral Strategies in Crisis Intervention.* New York: Guilford Press; 1994.

Hepworth D, Larsen J. *Direct Social Work Practice: Theory and Skills.* 4th ed. Belmont, CA: Wadsworth; 1993.

Longres JF. *Human Behavior in the Social Environment.* 2nd ed. Itasca, IL: F.E. Peacock; 1995.

Roberts AR. *Crisis Intervention and Time-limited Cognitive Treatment.* Thousand Oaks, CA: Sage; 1995.

Roberts AR. Conceptualizing crisis theory and the crisis intervention model. In: Roberts AR, ed. *Contemporary Perspectives on Crisis Intervention and Prevention.* Englewood Cliffs, NJ: Prentice-Hall; 1991.

Skinner BF. *The Behavior of Organisms: An Experimental Analysis.* New York: Appleton-Century-Crofts; 1938.

Stith SM, Rosen KH. Overview of domestic violence. In: Stith SM, Williams MB, Rosen K, eds. *Violence Hits Home: Comprehensive Treatment Approaches to Domestic Violence.* New York: Springer; 1990.

Walker LE. *Abused Women and Survivor Therapy: A Practical Guide for the Psychotherapist.* Washington, DC: American Psychological Association; 1994.

Walker LE. *Terrifying Love.* New York: Harper & Row; 1989.

Watkins H, Bradbard M. Child maltreatment: An overview with suggestions for intervention and research. *Family Relations.* 1982;31:323–333.

CHAPTER 27

CARE OF ABUSED PERSONS WHO ARE DEVELOPMENTALLY DISABLED

Virginia Focht-New

*I*mpaired neurologi-
cal pathways slow
information processing,
but usually a person
can understand some, if
not most, information.
The assessment process
must be slowed to allow
for comprehension and
response. Enfield
(1992) recommends
obtaining information
from as many sources
as possible and plan-
ning several time-
limited interviews.
Questions should be
short and concrete and
require brief answers.

Chapter Overview

► INTRODUCTION

Reports of abuse are prevalent in today's society. Pick up a newspaper, or watch the evening news or an afternoon talk show. People agree that abuse must stop. Are we concerned about abuse for everyone? Historically, individuals labeled developmentally disabled, or mentally retarded, have been treated with less concern than others. Is this because they sometimes behave or communicate differently? Unfortunately, many people have been institutionalized because of these differences. Recent surveys suggest an increased risk of abuse among persons with developmental disabilities, especially if they have been institutionalized (Baladerian, 1991; Crossmaker, 1991; Enfield, 1992; Sobsey and Doe, 1991). Abuse ranges from overt physical attacks to more insidious forms of intimidation and neglect.

When people with developmental disabilities seek health care or mental health services as a result of abusive experiences, various challenges are presented. The main concern is communication. The health care provider's preconceived ideas about people with developmental disabilities and what is "normal" behavior may interfere with assessment, intervention, and treatment. Determining the cause of behavioral changes and presenting symptoms in a person with absent or limited communication skills can be confusing and difficult, but these challenges can be met. The varied skills of health care providers make it possible to assess, intervene, and treat abused persons with developmental disabilities. It is often not actual experiences, but the label of "developmental disability," that causes those providing services to quiver at the thought of assessment, intervention, or treatment.

One question often asked is, "What is the functioning level of people with developmental disabilities?" This is a very difficult question to answer regarding some individuals. Most test results are limited by a person's verbal language, or rather lack of expression of language. For instance, many years ago people with cerebral palsy were often institutionalized because they were thought to have a mental incapacity. What many of them really struggled with was a physical disability that made their speech unclear. It is the limitations of the tests that label people and diminish expectations and beliefs about them. Abilities and disabilities vary from individual to individual, for all people of all ages, and across physical and mental disabilities and diseases.

► CASE EXAMPLE

Ryan's story is an example of confused labeling and the result of persistence by caretakers. Ryan's behavior may well have been the result of an abusive experience.

Ryan is a 25-year-old man with a "severe" developmental disability. His communication is limited to high-pitched noises that do not resemble words, and to sign-language words for "drink," "eat," and "please." When Ryan is upset, he responds to people around him by pushing, pulling, and hitting himself and others. On one occasion, his "self-abusive" behavior increased over a 3-day period. Reasons for his behavior were unclear and his caretakers became frustrated. They asked many questions. Was he hungry, sick, hurt, angry, or sad? Finally, after careful observation, they noticed that Ryan's hitting focused in the area of one ear. An appointment was made with the doctor, who discovered that he had an ear infection. Treatment began promptly and Ryan's behavior improved in a day.

If Ryan presented for health care services without the careful observations of his caretakers, he might have been treated with more psychotropic medication for "self-abusive" behavior. It takes thoughtful questioning when information is offered to be aware of what is individually "normal" and then to shake off preconceived ideas in order to assess, intervene, and treat people with developmental disabilities. A deviation from an individual's normal behavior suggests a problem. For Ryan, the problem was an infection.

SETTINGS FOR ABUSE

People with developmental disabilities experience abuse in the same settings as most other people—at home, school, and work. Unlike most others, except the elderly and people with mental health problems, they are likely to reside in institutions or group homes. An institution is typically a large building where hundreds of people live together. A group home is a smaller building, usually a house, with fewer people. Institutionalization is a dynamic of living in a large facility or group home. People in this kind of setting have little choice or self-determination; a person can be institutionalized anywhere.

Institutionalization is an approach where one group of people makes decisions for another. Decisions may include when and where a person goes; what is worn; who is visited; what is eaten; and when, how, and by whom health care is received. Parents, teachers, staff, and health care providers hold powerful decision-making responsibilities for the lives of the people they serve, deciding when people receive assessment, intervention, and treatment and when they do not. It is the "not" that may contribute to abuse.

ABUSE

Abuse is defined by Baladerian (1991, p. 323) as "nonaccidental injury of a person by another or the committing of acts that could result in injury, through acts of commission or omission." Many forms of abuse exist: physical, emotional, psychological, sexual, financial; acts of negligence; and violation of individual rights. Few data have been collected and scant literature written about the abuse of developmentally disabled children and adults. In cases of general child abuse, 29 to 70 percent of children abused have a disability before the abuse occurs (Baladerian, 1991). People with disabilities are perceived to be defenseless and passive, which may lower inhibitions of offenders, simultaneously increasing risk of victimization (Sobsey and Doe, 1991). Victims are chosen because they are unlikely to report or resist the event. To compound the risk, institutionalization limits a person's ability to make decisions for himself or herself and exposes people to a large number of caretakers.

Discovering abuse among people with developmental disabilities, mental health problems or among elderly individuals or children is a similar process. When people with developmental disabilities report abuse they are not always believed. Some caretakers of the disabled devalue the abilities of these individuals, which influences the caretaker's acceptance of the abuse reports. Some people with disabilities cannot verbalize their thoughts or feelings completely, confounding the process of discovery. Recognizing signs and symptoms of abuse is complicated when a person cannot respond verbally to questions. The health care provider must rely on physical evidence and information reported by caretakers. Talk about abuse, injuries of unknown origin, increase in self-abuse, aggressive behaviors toward a specific individual, emotional outbursts when near a particular person, and withdrawal from daily activities or people are some signs and symptoms of abuse that may be seen singularly or in combination. Interpreting these signs and symptoms accurately is a challenge; they may be attributed to a number of other events. The solution is to ask a range of questions to seek a complete picture of contributing factors from as many people as possible.

Institutionalization experiences are compounded by society's devaluing attitudes, stigmatized treatment of the developmentally disabled. "Aggressive" behaviors, self-abuse, and noncompliance are commonly treated with behavior management plans and psychotropic medications. Frighteningly, these behaviors are often the result of current and past abuse. Plan development and decisions about medications typically occur without the input of the individuals concerned, creating passivity rather then empowering individuals to advocate for themselves. Abuse in the lives of people with developmental disabilities has been well hidden by society (Baladerian, 1991). To add to this problem, caretakers establish a relationship that enhances dependency rather than self-determination, leading to increased vulnerability in people receiving services.

► CASE EXAMPLE

Consider the case of eight young men living in a group home. All eight men had challenging behaviors and behavior management programs, and all took large doses of psychotropic medications. Four staff persons worked in the house regularly. A nurse routinely reviewed accident reports for patterns of concern. One month she noticed that there were several individuals with facial injuries of unknown origin and numerous bruises. The staff reported that some of the eight men were increasingly aggressive with each other. The staff also stated that several of these housemates were clumsy and were having accidents around the house. The nurse notified an administrator, and an investigation began. After thorough questioning, it was learned that staff members were wrestling and boxing with the men. These men, who in the past had been placed on programs and medications to reduce their aggressive behavior, allowed the wrestling and boxing to occur without resistance. They were intimidated by the staff, who often made decisions for them and who wrote reports about them. The staff took advantage of the men's silence and hurt them in the process.

ASSESSMENT, INTERVENTION, AND TREATMENT PROCESSES

Assessment, intervention, and treatment of abuse are integrated processes. Each begins at the time of discovery. Health care providers can draw on their existing knowledge and experience for obvious cases of abuse as well as input from people who can reliably communicate. Challenges to health care providers include abused people with slow neurological pathways, existing physical disabilities and limited communication abilities, the lack of communication technology, and their own limiting perceptions about people with developmental disabilities.

► CASE EXAMPLE

Liz's story of abuse by a caretaker is used as an example of assessment, intervention, and treatment in action. Liz is a 28-year-old woman with developmental disabilities, living in a group home. She had been in an institutionalized setting all her life. Caretakers worked varied schedules and often did not stay with the job long. Liz could sometimes come in contact with 10 or more different staff in a year, making continuity and predictability of meeting her needs and getting to know her a difficult task. Liz spent her days at sheltered workshop. In the evening, she helped with household chores, occasionally going to the movies or out to dinner. Left alone, she could not care for herself adequately. Liz had a long history of aggressive behaviors, hitting and kicking people when frustrated. Although Liz could make several sounds, she did not form words. Infrequent gestures, some sounds, and changes in her facial expression or behavior gave her caretakers clues to her feelings and thoughts. A few years ago, Liz's behavior began a subtle change. At first, the staff, who had worked together about a month, did not know why. Then Liz began to have spurts of crying.

At this point, assessment began by the staff. Liz could not say what was happening. She had a history of problem behaviors but there was no staff person available who knew her well enough to help interpret these changes. She did not have involved family members, friends, or housemates who could help get or give information. Staff from work were able to talk about Liz from their experiences. People with developmental disabilities have varying abilities to communicate; but a lack of verbal communication does not equate a lack of comprehension. Asking Liz about her feelings and thoughts gave her an opportunity to try another manner of communicating about what was happening.

Medical histories and records became a focus for information for Liz. What had happened in the past to cause similar behavior? Who had the most accurate information?

At the time of Liz's behavior change, the staff reported they were concerned about interactions between Liz and Ralph, a staff person. At times, Liz was aggressive toward Ralph and would hit him. Later, approaching him with affection, she sat on his lap, laughing. Within a day of the reported staff concerns, Ralph received training about appropriate interactions with Liz and received instructions regarding the agency's abuse policy. Ralph made excuses for Liz's behavior change, saying she had been "aggressive" in the past. Liz's crying increased.

Along with training, Ralph's supervisor observed his job performance carefully. One day later, Ralph was found with Liz in her bedroom. She was upset and crying again. Liz was in a "compromising" position, with her clothes disheveled, and Ralph was adjusting his trousers. Ralph was removed from the job site. Staff whisked Liz off to the emergency room for a rape examination. The police were notified and they began an investigation.

The staff person who accompanied Liz to the emergency room came prepared with information to communicate to the health care providers and police. Liz was not able to speak for herself. Would the health care providers and police be prepared for Liz and her challenges? In fact, they were caring and patient, using the information brought by the staff person, but their ability to elicit further information was affected by a lack of knowledge about people with developmental disabilities and their limited options for effective communication with Liz.

Assessment began at Liz's home when staff researched past problems through medical records and with documented and recalled observations of Liz and Ralph. Intervention began as soon as they felt concern about Ralph's interactions with Liz. Assessment continued in the hospital and treatment for physical effects began as well.

The police completed their investigation and Ralph could not be prosecuted. There was no physical evidence, and Liz could not verbally describe all that had happened. The staff acted as Liz's advocates and helped stop this abusive situation quickly. Liz received minimal (because of her limited communication) counseling for a while afterwards. Ralph was dismissed from his position.

The case example displays a variety of challenges. Forms of communication, perceptions of staff and health care providers, interpretations of behavior, and neurological implications are focal points. Individualizing efforts and broadening the scope of observations can resolve many challenges presented in the assessment, intervention, and treatment process.

Impaired neurological pathways slow information processing, but usually a person can understand some, if not most, information. The assessment process must be slowed to allow for comprehension and response. Enfield (1992) recommends obtaining information from as many sources as possible and planning several time-limited interviews. Questions should be short and concrete and require brief answers. Language used should be familiar to the person and his or her level of development, spoken in a tone of respect. Nonverbal responses are very important and can include facial expressions, posture, body tension, emotional responses (such as crying), tactile defensiveness, activity level, and personal boundaries. Interviews should also assess for low muscle tone, which decreases intensity in a person's facial expression and body language.

When people are institutionalized and change living situations, their records do not always follow them. Histories may be inaccurate, influenced by people's feelings and perceptions at the time of writing. Change in health care providers affects the continuity of information if those providers do not or cannot communicate with each other. Accurate information is a key element in discovering abusive behavior.

An important aspect of assessment, intervention, and treatment is recognition. People who provide care to disabled individuals must be trained to recognize signs and symptoms of abuse. If the cause of changes in a person's behavior is not viewed within the context of the environment, an inaccurate clinical diagnosis may be assigned. People with developmental disabilities may need more time to respond, due to impaired information processing. If someone has no means to talk; is feeling afraid, frustrated, angry, or helpless; and is unable to influence others, then it may be necessary to use actions to attract the attention of someone who can help. People may be ignored for "acting out" because they "just want attention." Instead, caretakers should carefully investigate for causes of behavior change. Behavior as a means of communication is often minimized. This could have happened to Liz and probably had in the past.

ADVOCATES FOR THE DISABLED

Sobsey and Doe (1991) recognize a need for independent advocates for people with developmental disabilities. Advocates are important to an individual who does not communicate clearly and whose comprehension level cannot be determined. Advocates are significant contributors in an abuse investigation, especially if they are not affiliated with service providers. Advocates may be family members, friends, staff persons, housemates, fellow employees, employers, consultants, or others as suggested and agreed upon by the individual. Joyce (1992) states that if a person receiving support requires or wishes to have someone speak on their behalf, because they are unable to fully communicate their wishes, then one or more advocates could be involved in the process. Advocates should know the person well enough to understand and discuss his or her needs and should convey the individual's desires clearly, even if those desires differ from what the advocate thinks may be best for the person. Having more than one advocate increases the understanding of the individual's wishes, needs, and problems. Even when advocates are involved, it is important for others who care about the person to try to understand what the individual is communicating, despite their level of verbal proficiency. Involving several people during assessment, intervention, and treatment increases the reliability of information shared and reduces risks to the person if an "advocate" is also an abuser.

What information is obtained from an advocate? Advocates should be asked the questions that are usually asked of any victimized person. If the abused individual is present during the interview—and the individual should be—respect and tact are required in discussing the person and these very sensitive issues. A written description of what has happened and how present behavior compares with normal behavior is very helpful. Data compiled about behavior change and symptoms of abuse observed over time must be requested when caretakers are involved. Assessments completed by consultants—such as nurses, psychologists, social workers, speech therapists, physical therapists, and occupational therapists—provide valuable interdisciplinary team information. Finally, an assessment is based on observations and questions. Even if the victim does not talk and seems to lack comprehension, staff can trust their observations of a person's behavior to communicate feelings and information.

To determine the best psychological and emotional treatment, providers should consider factors that contribute to symptoms and severity of abuse. The TRIADS checklist developed by Burgess and colleagues (1990) assists in determining severity. The TRIAD checklist evaluates types of abuse, role relationship of the offender to the individual, intensity of abuse, the autonomic response of the individual abused, duration, and style of abuse. Compiled information is used to develop a plan of support.

MEANS OF COMMUNICATION WITH THE DEVELOPMENTALLY DISABLED

Reliance on "talking therapies" limits treatment of developmentally disabled victims. Liz, for example, could not speak. Health care providers need to be educated by family members, advocates, staff, and/or speech therapists in other ways to communicate. Conversation is not the only means to provide and receive information. There are several methods of, and technologies for, communication that may help people with developmental disabilities consider and respond to questions. These methods can be crucial in an alleged abuse investigation. Talking may be supplemented by other types of "language." Sign language is a commonly used form of communication. However, too few health care providers are fluent in signing. Drawing pictures can be a valuable tool, but many institutionalized people were never taught to draw. The use of photographs or sketches can help with an individual who uses gestures to communicate. This idea works well when there are predictable questions and answers. Picture boards or books using pictures from magazines, drawings, or photographs also work well. It may take a little extra time to look through the pictures while asking questions, but the results make the method worthwhile.

FACILITATED COMMUNICATION

Facilitated communication (FC) is a newly recognized means of asking and answering questions. FC did not exist when Liz had her experience, but she does use it now. Facilitated communication involves pointing at letters, words, or pictures with touch resistance of a facilitator. Touch resistance occurs when the person points to a letter, word, or picture with the facilitator pulling the person's hand away from the communication device, giving time for the person to make the next choice. Some people simply use a piece of cardboard with letters, words, or pictures to communicate a message. Others have hand-held pocket-sized keyboards. More sophisticated devices are computerized with a keyboard, tapes to print messages, and voice output.

Bilken (1993) describes FC as physical support that ranges from providing resistance to a person's hand and index finger to periodic taps to the shoulder. Lapos (1993) relates that people are becoming independent in typing. FC was first tried with people labeled autistic. It is thought that autism causes difficulty with focusing thoughts and actions and FC provides needed touch in order to focus thoughts into language (Bilken, 1993). Bilken defines the problem as "developmental dyspraxia" or "an absence or a difficulty with achieving voluntary action."

► CASE EXAMPLE

Jeff had an experience that is a good example of "developmental dyspraxia." A year after he began using FC, Jeff requested a meeting with an administrator from the organization providing him with residential services. Jeff came to the meeting with a friend who helped him through facilitation. He was anxious from the beginning, and had difficulty spelling out words. After several minutes

Jeff began to push his hand against his leg from hip to knee, over and over. The motion became rhythmic, almost hypnotic. At the same time, Jeff typed more clearly. However, he would not answer any questions. Having trouble still, Jeff began singing. Simultaneously, he rubbed his leg, sang a song, and typed out his thoughts and feelings. He was only able to sustain this for 5 minutes. Then he stopped and asked to leave. Two months later, Jeff requested a second meeting with the same administrator. This time his anxiety was less and he typed more clearly.

Wheeler and co-workers (1993) note that FC is useful for individuals who have "profound" or "severe" developmental disabilities. They go on to say that research is recent and limited. Further testing and validation is required. *Facilitated Communication News* (Lapos, 1993), a newsletter from the Central Pennsylvania Susquehanna Intermediate Unit, reports that Pennsylvania now has a database large enough to support research. Bilken (1993) reports that four studies were recently concluded. In addition, the Facilitated Communication Institute is studying progression of individuals toward independence with a second study of individual typing. They are moving toward a double blind study of anxiety during facilitation, which Bilken believes may interfere with validating the use of FC.

Local FC networks are expanding quickly. Groups of trainers, technical assistance and support groups have formed. *Facilitated Communication News* shares stories and letters written by people with FC. Lillian Fisher's letter (1993) is a nice example. An excerpt from Lillian's letter is quite inspiring: "I would like everyone to understand that I am a person and I have an opinion too and I want to share it with you."

Facilitated communication can and should be used in the process of investigating abuse. People who have abused others, who at that time did not have the ability to report abuse, will find the use of FC disconcerting. Others have faith that FC is a vehicle to enhance self-determination in individuals progressing toward independent typing.

► CASE EXAMPLE

The following case illustrates the use of FC, which initiated an investigation of alleged physical abuse. Sarah, age 19, began using FC at age 18½. Sarah was a very active young woman. She had no verbal language. People close to her had long felt that she had greater ability and understanding than she seemed able to demonstrate. Sarah made gradual progress with FC. One day Sarah typed some partial sentences. She typed that she had seen a staff person hit one of her housemates and that this person hit Sarah as well. Sarah was interviewed several times by different people. However, she was reluctant to facilitate with people she did not know well. A number of staff members, including the person who allegedly abused Sarah and her housemates, were also interviewed with no clear indications of abuse. To the best of anyone's knowledge, Sarah had not, in 6 months of using FC, fabricated information. The timing of the alleged abuse could not be determined. Had it happened yesterday or 2 years ago? Sarah did not seem uncomfortable in the presence of the staff person and even showed affection toward this person. Was it something that had happened once and never again? Was she protecting herself? The most pressing question could not be answered clearly: Did Sarah want to continue to have a relationship with the staff person? The decision made was a conservative one. The staff person was transferred to another home to work, with increased supervision. Sarah has not asked to see or speak to the person since then. The staff person has not been involved in any further reports.

Her clarity of communication through the use of FC continues to improve, increasing Sarah's ability to report and perhaps even prevent abuse of herself and others.

PREVENTION AS AN ASSESSMENT, INTERVENTION, AND TREATMENT

Prevention is the key element in assessment, intervention, and treatment. Prevention is especially important because 90 percent of abuse does not result in treatment (Baladerian, 1991). Baladerian says that vulnerability to victimization must be addressed in prevention and balanced with the opportunities to take some risks. Always protecting people from experiences will not protect them from abuse. Keeping people out of institutions, however, does reduce the risk of abuse. Teaching people to comply with therapeutic interventions and requests of caretakers increases the possibility of abuse. Essentially, people are taught to accept things that are helpful— or potentially hurtful. The key is to teach people to balance compliance with assertiveness in following directions and making decisions for themselves. People should be involved in the development of their own therapeutic interventions. Sobsey and Doe (1991) recommend developing a culture that supports victims, eliminates abuse, and supports those people who report

alleged abuse. Everyone should be educated about abuse and what they may do to stop it.

Creating societal, familial, and organizational cultures that support people with developmental disabilities in advocating for themselves minimizes the effects of institutionalization. As long as such people are perceived in a devalued manner, abuse will persevere. Society, families, and service providers have diversified ideas about how people with disabilities learn to live in the world; some are more optimistic than others. Developing a culture that focuses on learning and competence and is influenced by respect for diversity will help these persons to resist and, when necessary, report abuse.

Creating a culture that encourages diversity begins with a set of humanizing principles and goals that are the building blocks of support. Barol (1990) describes goals for professionals in working with the developmentally disabled person. These goals may be applied in all situations including school, work, family, and health care settings. Professionals are responsible to provide adequate, proper, humane, and individualized care; planned habilitation and treatment; and respectful consideration of personal dignity and integrity of a participant (Barol,

1990). It is necessary to include care that is sensitive to cultural differences in the least restrictive or intrusive manner, which is in line with prevailing community standards, and is designed to encourage individual competencies (Barol, 1990). The first step in accomplishing these goals is to believe that individuals with developmental disabilities have the right to understand and to be treated with as much dignity as all other well-respected persons. Change in expectations and attitude contributes to the success in prevention of abuse.

SUMMARY

Living with a label has dramatic effects on people, especially people who have been or are institutionalized. They are economically deprived, have little credibility, lack opportunity for self-determination, depend on others to meet their needs, have limited access to resources, and are taught to be compliant (Crossmaker, 1991). Keeping people from being institutionalized reduces the risk of abuse. Institutionalization is directly related to being labeled disabled. Consider the word "disability." The prefix "dis" is defined as an "absence of" (Webster's, 1988). The word "disability" is defined as an "incapacity." A seemingly more appropriate prefix to the word "ability" is "dys." Webster's (1988) defines "dys" as a difficulty. In persons labeled with developmental disabilities, it is more accurate to define disability as a difficulty with an ability rather then the absence of an ability. When presenting for health care service, such persons have often had labels that become the focus of intervention, rather than underlying factors or past victimization (Crossmaker, 1991).

What do we call people with developmental disabilities? Health care providers often use the term "patients." Residential providers use "resident," "client" or "consumer." Sadly, other people still use "retard," "MR," and "idiot." Many people with developmental disabilities simply want to be described as people—"Sue," "Dave," "Sandy." Labels are often the focus of intervention when people receive health care services. Labels can be changed.

Consider Jeff's situation.

► CASE EXAMPLE

Jeff was a 33-year-old man with developmental disabilities. He often abused himself by pulling his hair. For years, his self-abusive behavior was attributed to chronic anxiety. Jeff did not speak except to repeat other people's words or sing. He had autistic characteristics. A couple of years ago, Jeff tried facilitated communication using a computer. The staff were surprised by the depth of his feelings and observations. At first, he needed a lot of touch resistance, but he gradually became nearly independent in typing, requiring touch to his shoulder only. Over a period of time Jeff's self-injurious behavior dramatically increased. One day the staff sat with him and asked what was wrong. Jeff said that his back hurt. At first the doctor diagnosed him with arthritis in his back, possibly because of an injury or blow to the back. Medication was ordered. Using FC, Jeff persisted in reporting pain. Staff arranged another appointment with his doctor, who ordered further diagnostic tests. Jeff had a kidney dysfunction requiring immediate surgery.

Without Jeff's use of FC, the staff and health care providers could not have made an accurate or timely diagnosis. Anxiety and self-abuse would have continued to be his primary diagnosis until Jeff's medical condition became more serious or even terminal. With his newfound ability to "talk," Jeff became empowered to report accidents and illnesses. He participated in decisions about his care and the staff and health care providers began to respond to him differently. The difference was that they now recognized his abilities because he could "talk" to them. Jeff had been thinking and feeling all along.

Health care providers have the skills required to assess, intervene, and treat abuse in persons labeled developmentally disabled. Abuse is insidious in its presence in our society. Recognizing signs and symptoms of abuse will influence the discovery of abuse in people with developmental disabilities and allow for quick and germane action. Such people can be taught to "speak" for themselves so they are not dependant on others to interpret their actions. Sometimes referrals are not made for treatment because of a belief that individuals with disabilities do not comprehend their experiences and therefore do not have emotions or thoughts to respond to abuse or other experiences. This is a matter of confusing people with preconceived ideas of health care providers and labels.

Underlying cultural beliefs that devalue people are the most difficult to transform, but health care providers do have the capacity to change these beliefs. The ability to treat an abused person with disabilities is limited by perceptions, not skills. As prevention and treatment programs develop, people who receive support services can be empowered to fight abuse through their participation in the development of the programs. Individuals with disabilities must be encouraged to be involved in the development and delivery of the services they receive. These services require attitudes and actions of flexibility, accessibility, and integration.

It is the health care provider who, through his or her own sense of worth, empowers others to take action for themselves. Humanistic principles are the driving force that impart strength and courage to accomplish these actions. The battle to increase self-determination and decrease victimization is ignited through creative communication, assertiveness skills, increased research, expanded literature, and involvement of advocates. People with a wide range of developmental disabilities who have been abused can, with knowledge, support, and respect of their health care providers, be successful in the assessment, intervention, and treatment process.

REFERENCES

Baladerian NJ. Sexual abuse of people with developmental disabilities. *Sexual Disabil.* 1991;9:323–335.

Barol BI. *Values and Ethics for Professionals Serving Persons With Mental Retardation.* Unpublished manuscript; 1990.

Bilken D. Questions and answers about facilitative communication. *Facilitated Communication Dig.* 1993;2:3.

Burgess AW, Hartman CR, Kelley SJ. Assessing child abuse: The TRIADS checklist. *Psychosoc Nurs Ment Health Serv.* 1990;28:6–14.

Crossmaker M. Behind locked doors: Institutional sexual abuse. *Sexual Disabil.* 1991;9:201–218.

Enfield SL. Clinical assessment of psychiatric symptoms in mentally retarded individuals. *Aust NZ J Psychiatry.* 1992;26:48–63.

Fisher L. A whole new life for me. *Facilitated Communication News*. Spring 1993, p. 4.

Joyce S. *Gathering Together: A Collective Approach to Personal Planning with People Who Have Been Labeled*. London, Ontario: Realizations; 1992.

Lapos M. The issue is support. *Facilitated Communication News*. Fall/Winter 1993, p. 2.

Sobsey D, Doe T. Patterns of sexual abuse and assault. *Sexual Disabil*. 1991;9:243–259.

Webster's II New Riverside University Dictionary. Boston: Houghton Mifflin; 1988.

Wheeler, DL, Jacobson JW, Paglieri RA, Schwartz AA. An experimental assessment of facilitated communication. *Ment Retard*. 1993;31:49–60.

CHAPTER 28

PATHS TO SUCCESSFUL STEPFAMILY LIVING

Lou Everett

---

*A*dvanced practice
nurses must recog-
nize that healthy family
functioning involves
much more than the
mere absence of dys-
functional patterns of
interacting; it is con-
ceptualized by a struc-
ture and dynamic that
is unique in kind, direc-
tion, and aim.

Chapter Overview

Adapted with permission from: Everett L. Stepfamilies: An 'ostrich' concept in nursing education. Nurse Educator. *1995;20.*

► INTRODUCTION

With our growing attention to mental health promotion, advanced practice psychiatric nurses should use primary prevention concepts to strengthen and enhance effective family communication. The need for effective communication among members of a new or planned stepfamily is the subject of this chapter. Why the vulnerable population of stepfamilies is often omitted from advanced practice nursing texts may be explained by Clingempeel and associates (1987) who contend that the "nuclear family ideology" has resulted in minimum attention being placed on the structural complexity and heterogeneity of stepfamily forms. Emphasis is placed on the problems and weaknesses rather than the advantages and potential strengths of the stepfamily, and there is a general omission or ignoring of the possibility that satisfactory or close relationships within a remarried family may vary in fundamental ways from those in a nuclear family (Ganong and Coleman, 1994). In addition, others such as Gottman (1995) and Pasley and Ihinger-Tallman (1994) have contributed much to a research base for developing pathways that will lead to successful marriages and stepfamily living.

It is estimated that by the year 2000, the stepfamily will outnumber all other kinds of families in the United States (Glick, 1989). In the 1980s, many social scientists speculated that divorce rates had leveled off, but new data suggest a different conclusion. Gottman and Silver (1995) cite a "1989 study of U.S. Census records by researchers at the University of Wisconsin who found that, based on 1985 data, divorce among recent first marriages stood at a shocking 67 percent . . . two out of every three new couples. Moreover, sixty percent of second marriages end in divorce. According to Glick (1989), one third of Americans were members of a stepfamily.

Issues such as successful stepfamily living may be ignored because clinicians are struggling with reimbursement from health insurance payers (Koldjeski, 1993). In managed care settings, APNs and other health care providers are being asked to demonstrate clinical outcomes. Indeed, clinical outcomes may be documented with relative ease. Divorce, remarriage, and stepfamily living are concepts that nurses must deal with. Many of the stressors that pull at stepfamilies can be handled with greater ease by nurses who know the characteristics of the stepfamily, assessing how these are affecting specific families, and identifying appropriate pathways for interventions.

Stepparents and stepchildren are not legally related to each other; therefore, in managed care settings, it is essential that the nurse remember that the signature of a stepparent is often not acceptable (Visher and Visher, 1991). Knowing that might prevent the embarrassment of stepfamilies in times of stressful situations precipitated by illness. Ramsey (1994) points out that the law tells us "very clearly, for the most part, stepparents do not have a legally recognized status in relation to their stepchildren" (p. 217). Ambiguity of existing law makes the status of the stepparent in our society less clear. With the diversity and complexity of stepfamilies, coupled at times with competing claims of noncustodial parents, the development of any coherent policy is difficult (Ramsey, 1994).

A stepfamily needs assistance in establishing an identity as a new family without losing the important previous values and traditions held by the family of origin (Carson and Arnold, 1996). It is important for nurses to assist stepfamilies to normalize their experiences, but they cannot be viewed as a biological family unit and forced to fit in the typical mold of a nuclear family. Advanced practice nurses must recognize that healthy family functioning involves much more than the mere absence of dysfunctional patterns of interacting; it is conceptualized by a structure and dynamic that is unique in kind, direction, and aim (Koldjeski, 1993). Visher and Visher (1991), pioneers and authorities in shaping the literature on stepfamilies, remind us that even in stepfamilies, stress does not necessarily indicate dysfunction, and pain does not necessarily lead to psychological damage. To the contrary, both can facilitate growth as well as an appreciation for the significance of caring relationships.

Although the stepfamily has unique strengths, it has its issues as well. Research indicates that the relationships are complex, typified by caring but also by struggle (Everett, 1989, 1993, 1995, in press). It is important for nurses to recognize that this emerging family system is characterized uniquely by psychological concepts, structural components of the stepfamily, and cultural concepts that affect the steprelationships of the family (Everett, 1989, 1995).

A multicase phenomenological study was conducted about factors that contribute to stepfather–stepchild relationships (Everett, 1989, 1993, 1995, in press). The initial study included 6 stepfathers, and expanded to include interviews with 50 stepfathers. Two primary factors contributed to a positive stepfather–stepchild relationship: (1) active involvement in teaching the stepchild something mutually valued and (2) a loving relationship between the stepfather and the biological mother of the stepchild. Four main themes affected the stepfather–stepchild relationship: experiences in a parenting role, other relationships within the family, issues that require negotiating, and discipline of the children. Permeating these themes was the problem of lack of negotiation because of ineffective communication.

Many stepfamily members are eager to participate in groups, workshops, and organizations to improve their communication during this time of transition, but lack knowledge of such resources. Although national organizations for stepfamilies are available, as well as local support groups and national organization chapters in many states, the programs seem to be underused simply because many health professionals do not know about them.

When the couple relationship is strong, stepparents are more apt to extend unlimited energy in fostering a positive relationship between themselves and their stepchildren. More primary prevention through education for those who plan to remarry and those who have will facilitate effective communication among all members of the stepfamily. Although the term "stepfamily" is used, it is important to note that concepts in this chapter also apply to couples in long-term relationships who do not marry as well as to same-sex couples.

KEY PATHS OF STEPFAMILY INFORMATION

Visher and Visher (1988, 1991) classify a stepfamily as a normative family—no longer an alternative—with its own challenges and rewards. The majority of people in stepfamilies who seek therapeutic intervention do so during the transition of becoming a member of a new stepfamily. Advanced practice nurses in managed care settings often encounter patients who are members of stepfamilies exhibiting psychophysiological illnesses that often have correlating stress factors originating as stressors in relationships. Often when patients present with various medical problems, the nurse will have opportunities to provide members of stepfamilies with accurate information that will assist them in normalizing their experiences and to support stepfamilies in recognizing that each family progresses at its own rate through the critical pathways.

This chapter presents six key issues that represent pathways to successful stepfamily living: a definition of the stepfamily, characteristics and tasks, the stepfamily cycle, a model of effective communication, information about national organizations, and material resources.

WHAT IS A STEPFAMILY?

Visher and Visher (1979) define a stepfamily as a family in which at least one of the couple is a stepparent. Many problems similar to those found by remarried couples with live-in stepchildren may also be found in remarriages in which the children visit rather than live in the home. Furthermore, many similar situations may also be experienced by couples who have long-term relationships but are not legally married. Because of such experiential similarities, the term "stepfamily" includes the following family patterns, as identified by Visher and Visher (1979, p. xvii) which are similar in that there is an adult couple in the household with

at least one of the adults having a child by a previous marriage:

- Families in which children live with a remarried parent and a stepparent
- Families in which children from a previous marriage visit with their remarried parent and stepparent
- Families in which the couple is not married and children from a previous marriage either live with or visit with the couple

TASKS OF A STEPFAMILY

Visher and Visher (1988, 1991) identify several stepfamily tasks that occur during the transition of becoming a stepfamily: resolving losses and changes, negotiating different developmental needs, establishing new traditions while maintaining some of the old, developing a solid couple relationship while forming new relationships with others, creating a "parenting coalition," accepting ongoing shifts in household composition, and risking involvement despite little societal support. Bounded by environmental characteristics that govern the formation of the stepfamily, children and adults can be expected to progress toward solidity and integration at different rates of speed. Stepfamilies share such characteristics as having begun after many losses and change; incongruent family, marital, and individual cycles; presenting with different expectations from previous families; having a biological parent elsewhere, whether real or in memory; children occupying membership in two households; and a non-existent or ambiguous legal relationship between the stepparent and children.

DEVELOPMENTAL STAGES OF A STEPFAMILY

The stepfamily cycle includes seven stages for individual and family system development. The APN's having knowledge of these stages and sharing them with stepfamilies does much to assist members to normalize their own experiences and decrease feelings of anger, disappointment, and aloneness. These stages include three early stages: fantasy, immersion, and awareness; two middle stages: mobilization and action; and two later stages: contact and resolution (Papernow, 1993).

During the early stages, biological subsystems provide most of the nuturing, rules and rituals, and easy connections, as the family remains primarily divided along biological lines. In the *fantasy stage*, adults in the family long for the healing of wounds left by a previous divorce or death, while children continue to wish to see their parents together again, or even merely to reclaim the relationship with the single parent that had been the child's exclusively before the remarriage.

The *immersion stage* makes it acutely apparent that the stepfamily structure exists, as the stepparent occupies an "outsider" position when compared with the connected biological parent and child (and may sometimes include an ex-spouse). The stepparent often becomes the subject of unanticipated negative and strong feelings. In the *awareness stage*, members begin to clarify myths versus realities, recognizing that it is impossible to move quickly into an instant family without first getting to know the strangers each has joined. Biological parents become more aware of their roles as members of both subsystems.

The middle stages find the stepfamily restructuring itself to strengthen the step subsystems as the stepfamily begins the tasks of loosening old boundaries. In the *mobilization stage*, much discussion occurs between the couple about differences between step and biological family members' needs (Papernow, 1993). These are issues that often provide a focus for negotiation about such topics as meals, chores, and bedtime (Everett, 1989, 1995, in press). With negotiation achieved at last about how the family will function differently, the developmental stage, known as the *action stage*, is achieved (Papernow, 1993).

In the later stages, the *contact stage* clearly defines regular and reliable stepsystem roles

that have emerged as new areas of agreement have been negotiated so that the family might function more easily. Intimacy in step-relationships is now possible. In the *resolution stage*, step-relationships no longer require continued attention, norms have been established, and a stepfamily history has begun to build. Papernow describes an acceptance that some members may feel more inside the family than others, but the stepparent is established now as an "intimate outsider"—intimate enough to be one the stepchild can confide in, and outside enough to provide mentoring and support in issues that are too threatening to discuss with biological parents, such as sex. Step issues, while continuing to arise, no longer threaten the couple or stepparent–stepchild relationship.

Regardless of what developmental stage the stepfamily is experiencing, APNs can do much in teaching remarried couples to refrain from making negative comments about the other natural parent in the presence of children. Stepchildren are much more accepting of their stepparents when they see respect shown to their noncustodial parents. It is difficult for children to accept the divorce of their parents, but it is much less traumatic when parents resolve their differences and treat each other with respect and appreciation as they let go of each other emotionally and learn to co-parent. Each child, except in circumstances that put the child at risk for abuse, needs to be encouraged to maintain relationships with both parents—he or she is a member of two households. It is imperative that children not be placed between the two natural parents and used as persons upon whom to displace anger. A child never needs to be told by a stepparent or natural parent to convey a hostile message to another parent. Children sometimes need support from nurses in learning how to handle such situations by stating: "I would appeciate it if you would tell that to Mom or Dad instead of asking me to."

Many well-intentioned stepparents try too hard to speak for their spouses by communicating messages to their stepchildren that need to be conveyed by the natural parent. A criticism from a stepparent hurts far worse than from a natural parent, because the stepchild feels less secure with the stepparent. Stepparents are sometimes more objective about inappropriate behaviors of their stepchildren than natural parents. Constructive feedback needs to be conveyed directly to the natural parent by the stepparent in privacy, leaving the natural parent the opportunity to handle whatever disciplinary action the couple agree upon that needs to be taken. Although the natural and stepparents may be together when the natural parent discusses the discipline with the child, it is best if the natural parent delivers the discipline.

COUNSELING THE STEPFAMILY

Advanced practice nurses must remember interventions which include education for the stepfamily represents the greatest promise—with premarital counseling being the most effective (Einstein, 1985). Gottman and Silver (1995) have studied 2000 married couples to determine what makes a marriage last. They found that the key is a balance between negative and positive interactions, the magic ratio being 5 to 1! For each negative interaction between a husband and wife, as long as there are five times as many positive interactions, the marriage is likely to remain stable. Couples may resolve differences by adopting various styles, but what is important is how they resolve their differences and that each feels good about the interaction itself. Gottman and Silver identify the disastrous ways a husband or wife might sabotage a mate's attempts to communicate effectively. Ranked in order from least to most hazardous to the relationship, they include criticism, contempt, defensiveness, and stonewalling.

Premarital counseling may be even more important for second or subsequent marriages. Advanced practice nurses must recognize that it is a sign of strength and courage when an individual chooses to seek counseling in order to examine what his or her contributions might have been to the breakup of the former relationship. In examining patterns of resolving conflicts according to Gottman and Silver's findings, individuals may gain insight into how to break old ineffective ways of interacting with one's mate. An objective counselor can help one who experiences the breakup of a marriage to mourn the loss of a biological family unit. The degree to which one can break free of a former mate and continue to co-parent successfully will often determine the success of a future marital relationship as well as markedly affect the adjustment of the children (Einstein and Albert, 1983). Well-meaning friends and relatives often complicate issues because they lack the necessary credentials and skills to guide such an individual. Moreover, they often hold a biased view of the relationship. By actively listening to those who share information about their unresolved issues, advanced practice nurses may intervene through counseling and referrals to organizations or other resources.

"Premarital" counseling for stepfamilies begins when a couple experiences the potential breakup of a first marriage. Although it may initially seem more painful for couples, they owe it to each other and themselves before deciding to separate, divorce, or "call it quits," to spend some sessions together, addressing any hidden agendas they have with each other, any old wounds or grievances that haven't been addressed directly. During the process of counseling, each member of the couple may learn more about what each has contributed to faulty communication patterns or misunderstandings (Satir, 1976). It will assist them in future relationships, and it will help them to become better co-parents even though they may choose to reside separately.

Many individuals who become divorced learn through later counseling that guidance in effectively communicating their feelings could have prevented many of their misunderstandings. Some couples develop an avoidance style of dealing with conflict (Gottman and Silver, 1995), which can sometimes lead to hurt feelings that have been harbored for years. Had both individuals been willing to examine their communication patterns before the breakup, the marriage might have been saved. For example, many men have been socialized not to show feelings openly. Sometimes men need permission to share feelings, or wives need to be taught how to directly ask for what they need to feel loved by their husbands instead of expecting their husbands to read their minds. During the stressful experiences of resolving conflicts and developing healthier pathways in their communication styles, prospective divorcing couples can be provided with much support and encouragement by their advanced practice psychiatric nurse to continue with therapy sessions. Gottman and Silver identify the styles of validating, volatile, and avoidant as potentially viable means of resolving conflicts as long as both partners feel that the interaction is good and they have more positive interactions than negatives. How they resolve the conflict is a key factor in the stability of the marriage.

Should the couple decide to separate and divorce, it can be helpful for individuals to examine what characteristics they desire in a mate, before beginning to date or settle down with one individual. Continuing in therapy with a counselor provides a source of objectivity to assist individuals to recognize when one is about to repeat old patterns of communicating that lead to unresolved conflict and resentment.

In dealing with those who have separated or divorced, APNs can educate individuals who have begun dating again. They need to assess if an individual has been counseled if unresolved grief remains from the lost relationship. Einstein and Albert's *Stepfamily Living Series* (1983) provides excellent interventions to assist individuals to grieve through previous losses. They learn to break free of the previous mate, while continuing to co-parent; establish hope and a link to the future; and plan for remarriage. In addition, the series addresses pitfalls and possibilities and myths and realities of stepfamily living. The series concludes with discipline of children, and using enrichment and encouragement to establish a relationship with members of a stepfamily.

For additional interventions, this author developed five basic steps that can be used as inter-

vention guides to assist adults who wish to bridge the gap between separation or divorce and dating again. By using these guides, many potential stepfamily problems may be prevented.

- Have the adult identify expectations that are realistic and simple for both the adults and the children.
- Have the parent consider a brief initial meeting for the child(ren) to be introduced to the date. Encourage the parent to follow through as promised by keeping it brief; when discipline is required, encourage the natural parent to do this in private; and wait for the child(ren) to ask questions about the date/friend.
- Foster the parent's relationship with the child(ren) between dates. Parents can be supported in showing love and affection, sharing their interests, and keeping clear boundaries (remaining a nuturing parent rather than behaving as a peer).
- Support the adults' directives to have the child(ren) and date/friend convey their own messages to each other whenever possible, which may increase the potential for a friendship between strangers.
- Remind the adults to relax and enjoy discovering what makes them happy. Nurses can explore the probability with the parent who has begun dating again that if the date is someone special, with time the children will likely recognize these qualities; while talking constantly about the date may discourage rather than encourage a friendship between one's child(ren) and the date. The Vishers (1991) encourage both stepparents and natural parents to not only make family time but individual time with each child in the family. It takes time for friendships and love to grow.

Primary prevention of adjustment problems may be done by assisting couples to work through some of the decisions about parenting roles prior to the remarriage.

Issues that require negotiating, such as discipline of the children, need to be addressed before the remarriage. Unfortunately, most couples are so caught up in the romance of the moment that they assume such negotiations will be worked out much more easily than they can be. Most couples do not discuss discipline of the children before remarriage (Everett, 1989, 1995, in press). It seems to be one of the most difficult areas to negotiate in a remarriage, and is best handled initially when the natural parent handles the discipline of the child (Einstein and Albert, 1983).

Advanced practice nurses can inform stepfamily members about the impact that birth order alone might have on any couple (Toman, 1976). An older child, for example, may be responsible for taking care of a younger sibling, often performing tasks for the younger sibling after the child is old enough to perform tasks for himself or herself. When a stepfamily forms and each of the partners has one child, each child will change his or her birth order in the family. Previously both children were the only child with special attention by each parent. Now one of them becomes the older child, while one becomes the younger, requiring each to learn to negotiate their needs in a different manner. Both will compete for power in "bossing" the other child. To teach parents that these role changes are normal in the transitional stages of becoming a stepfamily can decrease their stress when conflict arises.

Workshops on effective communication are useful as a premarital counseling endeavor. Providing stepfamily members rationale for counseling may best be handled by demonstrating through role play the difference between an effective, constructive way to resolve a conflict with one's mate and an ineffective, destructive way. By teaching an effective communication model such as Berne's transactional analysis model (Berne, 1961; Wollams et al., 1976), stepparents will be able to model effective communication patterns to their stepchildren, recognize destructive communication patterns, and make constructive changes in the family's way of dealing with conflict. They will also be more likely to recognize when children need assistance handling conflict. By using effective communication strategies, such as "I statements" to share how one feels, couples are able to communicate angry and hurt feelings in a constructive manner (Gottman and Silver, 1995). Statements that begin with "you" often result in a defensive response, and communication is blocked, with neither partner hearing the other's feelings. Some individuals even need assistance in sharing positive feelings with their mates. Many couples present with sexual problems or different values, but the ultimate problem lies most often in their inability to communicate effectively what each individual needs and thereby how they resolve differences (Gottman and Silver, 1995). Advanced practice nurses need to know that a combination of the nuturing parent, adult, and free child components of the transactional analysis model assists in communicating effectively with respect and love (Berne, 1961; Wollams et al., 1976).

Without counseling, these individuals remarry and often repeat the same ineffective ways of relating. In hospital, community, and social settings, nurses will meet many couples who are divorced who have chosen not to seek professional counseling to assist them in problem solving. Many of these individuals are still hurting and grieving. Nurses must recognize such symptoms, intervene immediately, and make referrals appropriately.

NATIONAL ORGANIZATIONS FOR STEPFAMILIES

Three of the most widely recognized organizations that focus on stepfamily issues are listed in Table 28–1. The Stepfamily Foundation offers both educational and counseling services to members of stepfamilies. Two weekend professional seminars a year are conducted to train professionals to become a part of a stepfamilies counselors' network.

Stepfamily Associates provides workshops and support group meetings for men, women, and couples where stepfamilies can discuss different

TABLE 28–1. NATIONAL STEPFAMILY ORGANIZATIONS

Stepfamily Associates
1368 Beacon Street, Suite 108
Brookline, MA 02146
617–734–8831

Stepfamily Association of America, Inc.
215 Centennial Mall, Suite 212
Lincoln, NE 68508
800–735–0329

Stepfamily Foundation
333 West End Avenue
New York, NY 10023
800–759–7837 or 212–877–3244

concerns. Monthly support meetings are held. The organization assists couples in developing a strong relationship and making space for their children. Sharing their experiences with one another has been beneficial to stepfamily members.

Founded by Emily and John Visher, the Stepfamily Association of America provides support and education through workshops, videos, cassette tapes, books, and pamphlets. There are more than 60 chapters nationwide.

LOCAL SUPPORT GROUPS

Advanced practice nurses might establish local support groups for stepfamilies. Support groups emphasize positive coping skills; they are not designed as "gripe sessions." The local groups can provide an excellent opportunity for single parents to be supported by other group members who have grieved through the early stages of parting from a mate. Having stepparents hear the perspective of a natural parent who is not his or her marital partner may assist couples to work more closely on their own issues. In addition, stepparents who do not have natural children and have never been a parent are given support in the group. Confidentiality forms are signed when a person first begins participating in the group. In a small community or a city of approximately 50,000 people, participants often know each other. Confidentiality assures each person that his or her participation in the group is not shared outside the group with anyone else. If they choose, members may share their telephone numbers and addresses with each other.

SUMMARY

If advanced practice nurses are to be adequately prepared as resourceful clinicians in the work setting and as community resource persons who will meet the needs of contemporary families, they must become more educated about the critical pathways to successful stepfamily living in order to creatively assist stepfamilies in primary prevention of problems instead of leaving such interventions solely up to colleagues in other disciplines. When an APN is the health professional a stepfamily member encounters, it is the responsibility of that clinician to know appropriate avenues for intervention or referral.

Nurses have the ability to assist couples to realize their potential as mates, often through the sharing of mere self-directed material resources. There are many opportunities to use research-based practice strategies as nurses seek to meet the needs of stepfamilies. Community endeavors will reveal opportunities for health promotion and health maintenance of stepfamily living. APNs can have a tremendous impact on that vulnerable population by addressing some of the conditions that precipitate crises, for example substance abuse, marital discord, domestic violence, psychophysiological illnesses, and anxiety disorders. Nurses must become more sensitized to hearing the struggles of stepfamilies as they strive to begin anew, holding on to traditions that are valued, but struggling to let go of those that bring memories of sadness. APNs can take initiatives to intervene promptly and provide referrals. Recognizing that this vulnerable population does not know where to go for resources and sometimes may be embarrassed to admit their concerns, nurses may anticipate their needs.

Advanced practice nurses can assist parents and stepparents to create a more supportive and loving environment for themselves, their biological children, and stepchildren. It is imperative that nurses demonstrate accountability by utilizing their expertise in holistic nursing care and sharing with colleagues in other disciplines this major responsibility to respond to stepfamilies, which by the end of this decade will be the most common family unit in our society.

REFERENCES

Berne E. *Transactional Analysis in Psychotherapy*. New York: Grove Press; 1961.

Carson VB, Arnold EN. *Mental Health Nursing: The Nurse–Patient Journey*. Philadelphia: Saunders; 1996.

Clingempeel WG, Flescher M, Brand E. Research on stepfamilies: Paradigmatic constraints and alternative proposals. In: Vincent JP, ed. *Advances in Family Intervention: Assessment and Theory*. Greenwich, CT: JAI Press; 1987.

Einstein E. *The Stepfamily: Living, Loving, and Learning*. Boston: Shambhala; 1985.

Einstein E, Albert L. *Stepfamily Living Series*. Ithaca, NY: American Guidance Association; 1983.

Everett L. Factors that contribute to satisfaction or non-satisfaction in stepfather–stepchild relationships. *Perspect Psychiatr Care*. In press.

Everett L. Book review of Hanson SM, Heins ML, Julian DJ, Sussman MB, eds. *Single Parent Families: Diversity, Myths and Realities. J Fam Nurs*. 1995; 427–431.

Everett L. Stepfamilies: An "ostrich" concept in nursing education. *Nurse Educator*. 1995;20:29–35.

Everett L. Stepfamilies: The emerging family system. *1993 Nursing Research Congress Abstracts—Advances in International Nursing Scholarship*. Madrid: Sigma Theta Tau International; 1993.

Everett L. Factors that Contribute to Stepfather–Stepchild Relationships. Dissertation, North Carolina State University, Raleigh, 1989.

Ganong LH, Coleman M. *Remarried Family Relationships*. Thousand Oaks, CA: Sage; 1994.

Glick P. Remarried families, stepfamilies, and stepchildren: A brief demographic profile. *Family Relations*. 1989;22:459–463.

Gottman J, Silver N. *Why Marriages Succeed or Fail . . . And How You Can Make Yours Last*. New York: Fireside; 1995.

Koldjeski D. Family mental health. In: Fawcett CS, ed. *Family Psychiatric Nursing*. St. Louis: Mosby; 1993.

Papernow P. *Becoming a Stepfamily*. San Francisco: Jossey-Bass; 1993.

Pasley K, Ihinger-Tallman M, eds. *Stepparenting: Issues in Theory, Research, and Practice*. Westport, CT: Greenwood Press; 1994.

Ramsey SH. Stepparents and the law: A nebulous status and a need for reform. In: Pasley K, Ihinger-Tallman M, eds. *Stepparenting: Issues in Theory, Research, and Practice*. Westport, CT: Greenwood Press; 1994.

Satir V. *Making Contact*. Millbrae, CA: Celestial Art; 1976.

Toman W. *Family Constellation*. 3rd ed. New York: Springer; 1976.

Visher EB. Lessons from remarried families. *Am J Fam Ther*. 1994;22:327–337.

Visher E, Visher J. *How to Win As a Stepfamily*. New York: Brunner/Mazel; 1991.

Visher E, Visher J. *Old Loyalties, Old Ties*. New York: Brunner/Mazel; 1988.

Visher E, Visher J. *Stepfamilies: A Guide to Working With Stepparents and Stepchildren*. New York: Brunner/Mazel; 1979.

Wollams S, Brown M, Huige K. *Transactional Analysis in Brief*. Ann Arbor: Huron Valley Institute; 1976.

CHAPTER 29

CRISIS AND COMMUNITY DISASTER

Marlene Young

If a community de-cides that it wants to have a crisis response team come, NOVA will send a team only if all community leaders are in agreement that the service will be useful. This protocol for out-reach is designed to provide the community with a sense of control over its destiny and to affirm that whatever happens will be guided by leadership from the community, not from the outside.

Chapter Overview

Adapted and reprinted with permission from Young MA. Crisis intervention and the aftermath of disaster. In: Roberts AR, ed. Contemporary Perspectives on Crisis Interventions and Prevention. Englewood Cliffs, NJ: Prentice-Hall; 1991:83–103.

At 9:02 AM, April 19, 1995, in Oklahoma City, the Alfred P. Murrah federal building exploded as a result of a terrorist bomb. At 9:17 AM, NOVA received a telephone call from the attorney general's office in Oklahoma requesting assistance. In the aftermath of the explosion, which killed 168 people and left more than 2000 individuals victimized by the bomb and a city in shock, NOVA sent three teams of crisis intervenors to help with the emotional trauma caused by the crime.

Disasters cause both individual and community-wide crisis reactions. The National Organization for Victim Assistance (NOVA), centered in Washington, D.C., has formed a National Crisis Response Project, designed to address the emotional aftermath of community-wide disasters. The project is based on the premise that immediate intervention can provide communities with tools that are useful in mitigating long-term distress. The intervention techniques used by NOVA have been implemented following disasters that were precipitated by criminal events, as well as natural disasters. Although there are some important differences between natural and manmade disasters, and between those caused deliberately and those caused by accident or recklessness, the commonalities of widespread emotional trauma appear to be more significant than their differences.

This chapter will review the features of crisis and stress reactions in individuals and special issues that are helpful in analyzing crisis situations; explain NOVA's guidelines in providing crisis intervention to such individuals; and describe how those guidelines are applied and adapted in a community-wide disaster.

Although readers may be familiar with the crisis reaction, a detailed understanding of the pattern of the reaction is essential to NOVA's crisis intervention methodology. Teaching survivors and their caregivers elements of the crisis reaction helps them to understand the abnormalities of what they had experienced as normal.

CRISIS, STRESS, AND DISASTER SITUATIONS

CRISIS REACTION

In their everyday lives, individuals exist in a state of emotional equilibrium. They establish their own boundaries for experiencing and expressing happiness, sadness, anger, excitement, and other emotions. Occasional stressors will stretch an individual's sense of equilibrium, but those stressors are usually predictable within the individual's frame of reference, and adequate coping mechanisms can usually be mobilized to deal with the stress.

Trauma, by contrast, throws people so far out of their ranges of equilibrium that it is difficult for them to restore a sense of balance in life. When they do establish a new equilibrium, it will almost always be different than that before the trauma, with new boundaries and new definitions.

Trauma may be precipitated by an "acute" stressor or a "chronic" stressor. Acute trauma-inducing stressors are usually sudden, arbitrary, and often random events. They include many types of crime, terrorism, and manmade and natural disasters.

Among the most common chronic trauma-inducing stressors are interpersonal abuse, developmental stress caused by life transitions, long-term illness, and continuing exposure to disease, famine, or war. Chronic stressors may cause crisis reactions similar to those caused by acute stressors, with some significant differences. Chronic stressors should be noted because they often affect the pre-existing equilibrium, and individuals suffering from chronic stressors are often at higher risk for emotional trauma after an acute stressor occurs. The normal human response to trauma follows a general pattern, characterized by both a physical response and an emotional or psychological response.

The physical response is based on biological instinct and is often not within the individual's control. Physical reactions usually begin with a sense of shock, disorientation, and numbness. The initial response is followed by a state of physical arousal that is triggered by a fight-or-flight instinct. Epinephrine begins to pump through the body. The body may relieve itself of excess materials through regurgitation, defecation, or urination. The heart rate increases. Individuals may begin to breathe rapidly and perspire. Often one sense—sight, hearing, taste, touch, or smell—becomes pronounced, frequently to the detriment of the other senses. This extraordinary sensory experience may well become an intensely vivid memory that, when rearoused, can trigger a re-experiencing of the initial crisis reaction. The immediate physical reaction is typically ended by exhaustion. The body simply cannot sustain the state of extreme arousal for a long period of time. If individuals fail to sleep or rest, they may simply collapse from exhaustion.

The cognitive and emotional reactions to crises are very similar to the physical reaction. The first response is usually one of shock, disbelief, and denial of the trauma, as the mind tries to frame an unthreatening interpretation of the evidence it perceives. There is a sense of a suspension of reality. Not only does the mind refuse to believe what the body is experiencing, but many individuals also feel as though time stops or the world is in slow motion around them.

Shock may last for minutes or weeks. It is usually followed by a turmoil of emotions as time goes on. Emotions engaged may be anger or rage, fear or terror, confusion and frustration, guilt and self-blame, and grief over losses suffered as a result of the crisis. This emotional chaos often precipitates regression to a childlike state in survivors. They are, after all, in a helpless state of dependency on others or on outside forces, a circumstance that they may not have experienced since childhood. This dependency, coupled with the intensity of feelings, is overwhelming, and survivors may want a parent or parent figure to take care of things, just as the child wants the parent to "kiss it and make it better."

Just as the physical reaction results in exhaustion, so does the emotional reaction. Survivors often feel as though they are on a roller coaster of extremes. At one moment, they are besieged with emotion, the next they may simply feel a void or nothingness. In defense, many survivors constrict the range of their emotional reactions to life events, warding off pleasure and pain equally. Over time, many open themselves up to more emotional risks and gains, evolving from traumatized to triumphant, establishing a new equilibrium, and constructing a new sense of self. But some survivors face a lifetime of debilitating stress reactions as a result of the trauma.

LONG-TERM STRESS REACTIONS

Long-term stress reactions tend to take one of four forms: pathological, character changes, post-traumatic stress disorder, or long-term crisis reaction. Only a small percentage of crises resulting from trauma-specific events are associated with pathological reactions. Such reactions may include the development of severe phobias, clinical depression, or multiple personality disorder. Psychotherapy is usually suggested in such cases.

The second type of long-term stress reaction is the development of post-traumatic character changes. Again, these are not common reactions, but they may occur, particularly in survivors of extremely shocking tragedies. Overcontrolling personalities, rigidity of personality, post-traumatic character decline, and extreme behavior change are examples of post-traumatic character change.

The third type of reaction is post-traumatic stress disorder (PTSD). The symptoms of PTSD are often seen in the loved ones of homicide victims, victims of chronic child sexual abuse, survivors of sexual assault, and survivors of catastrophic physical injury.

A final type of long-term stress reaction is one that is not often discussed by mental health practitioners but it has been the reaction that is most often observed in NOVA's work. Referred to as long-term crisis reaction, it simply describes the fact that many victims do not present symptoms of PTSD or other disorders, but are prone to reexperience feelings of the crisis reaction when trigger events recall the trauma. Trigger events may include the following situations:

- Experiencing a physical sensation that is similar to the intense sensory perception that accompanied the initial physical reaction
- Anniversaries of the trauma
- Holidays or birthdays
- Developmental crises or significant life events such as graduations, marriages, divorces, births, and deaths
- Involvement in the criminal or civil justice system as a result of the traumatic event
- Media events or broadcasts that are similar to the trauma
- Memorials of the trauma

ISSUES SURROUNDING DISASTERS

Four points of analysis are helpful in determining whether an event places an individual or community at high risk for trauma: time dimension, spatial dimension, the roles of survivors and the uniqueuess of the trauma. These points can also be useful in determining the key issues that should be addressed in strategies for intervention.

Time Dimension

The first issue is an analysis of the time dimension of the event itself. Time can be broken down into eight phases that may affect a survivor's response:

- Pre-event equilibrium
- Threat of the event
- Warning of the event
- The event's impact
- Inventory after the event
- Time of rescue
- Time of remedial work
- Reconstruction

The pre-event equilibrium is important, because the more stressed that equilibrium, the greater the potential that an additional stressful event will precipitate another crisis. If a trauma is preceded by a period of threat or warning to which the survivors have an opportunity to respond, there is a greater possibility of guilt or self-blame if they did not respond to protect themselves or their loved ones. Conversely, if the victim can take pride in the way he or she used the warning to mitigate the harm, that can be helpful in the reconstruction process. If there is no warning, anger may be a dominant emotion in the immediate aftermath because of feelings of injustice and unfairness.

The time immediately following a crisis is when survivors take inventory of damage and injuries suffered. There is always a stage of inventory taking, even when rescuers appear immediately on the scene. In a medical model, that stage is called triage. If a survivor or rescuer thinks that he or she made a mistake or an inappropriate assessment during the inventory stage, it may contribute to guilt or blame. Such mistakes are not uncommon; under the influence of stress hormones, people can become oblivious to physical injuries, even life-threatening ones.

Actions during the rescue stage or the remedy stage may also lead to guilt or anger. Rescue attempts that fail contribute to frustration and despair. The remedy stage refers to the time after the physical rescue of survivors, when additional resources and services may be provided to help survivors begin to reconstruct their lives. Although it is very common for such assistance to be available in the first hours or days after a traumatic event, it is also general practice for such help to be withdrawn thereafter, which may contribute to feelings of disillusionment and outrage among survivors.

Spatial Dimension

The second issue for analysis is the spatial dimension of the tragedy. This is particularly critical in a community-wide trauma, for it defines and describes the community itself. One factor in the spatial dimension is the proximity of individuals or survivors to the event itself.

A tragedy may be visualized as the center point in a series of concentric circles. The general guideline is that the closer any individual is to the center of the tragedy, the higher the risk for a crisis reaction and for long-term stress reactions. There is a key exception to this guideline, however. The loved ones of victims killed in a disaster must be considered central to the tragedy even if they were not present at the time of the event. The core of their tragedy is different. The death notification is the event of impact, not the actual disaster.

The second spatial dimension is the phenomenon of convergence. Convergence describes the actions of individuals who come to the scene of the tragedy. The more people who converge on the event, the greater the likelihood that the event will be felt as a community-wide trauma. Conversely, when a smaller number of individuals are involved, it is more likely that the event will be experienced as a trauma that happened to specific individuals.

In addition, it is important to examine whether the convergence was positive or negative. In the most obvious terms, positive convergence occurs when those who arrive come to rescue or to help, while negative convergence occurs when voyeurs, vandals, or looters come and contribute to the chaos and damage. Negative convergence may add to feelings of anger, frustration, and loss of faith or trust in humanity. One sometimes encounters these reactions among those who came to the scene as rescuers but rescued no one, serving only to tend to the dead and dying.

Role of Survivors

A third issue to be addressed in the aftermath of tragedy is the roles played by survivors. The more roles the survivors are forced to assume, the higher the risk of trauma.

A victim of a street mugging may have only one role in the event, that of victim of predatory crime—and sometimes without even an eyewitness, as is the case in many purse snatches. However, in a community-wide trauma, it is likely that many survivors will have played multiple roles. A survivor may be injured or not, which is an important differential in itself, but the individual may also be a loved one of someone who was killed in the tragedy, a witness to the event, a rescuer who helped save others, a resident of the neighborhood where it happened, or a caregiver who is responsible for responding to the emotional aftermath of the tragedy in the community. The roles may be further complicated by the survivor's self-perception of how well he or she performed or is performing in any of these roles; obviously, there are almost always major differences in the reactions of rescuers who failed in the rescue attempt and those who were successful. The most dominant role from the survivor's perspective is important to determine, because it may help to assess the individual's most dominant feelings about the event.

Uniqueness of Trauma

The elements that define the uniqueness of the trauma are a fourth issue in the analysis of tragedy. In examining this issue, several features are considered: the extent of personal impact, the type of tragedy, the duration of the trauma, the potential for recurrence, and the ability of individuals to control the impact of the trauma in its aftermath.

Extent. The extent of personal impact can be roughly measured by answering six questions:

- How many people are dead?
- Was there a great deal of carnage, or were a great many people severely injured?
- How much property was destroyed? What was the significance of the property to the survivors?
- Were many people dislocated or relocated from homes, jobs, or schools?
- What was the amount of financial loss, both from the immediate disaster and due to consequent expenses and losses?
- How many people were eyewitnesses to the disaster?

Type. The type of tragedy is defined in several ways, each of which contributes to the understanding of its impact. The cause of the tragedy is one definitive dimension. A natural disaster may cause anger at God but may also be more easily accepted because of the lack of human control over the outcome. An event seen as a manmade accident may raise concerns about human fallibility, blame, and standards for prevention or regulation. A criminal act may cause anger or outrage at human cruelty or, as when drugged or drunk driving leads to multiple deaths, at the driver's wanton and reckless disregard of human life.

The type of destruction experienced in the tragedy is another definitive dimension. Disasters accompanied by flooding or drowning raise concerns about property destruction and bodily disfigurement of those who have died. Fear of water and suffocation may develop in survivors. Catastrophes that involve fire often leave survivors with intense memories of the smell of burning wood or flesh. Burn victims suffer excruciating pain and, at times, mutilation or maiming. Bodies of victims who die in fires are disfigured and often unrecognizable. Survivors may become preoccupied with thoughts of hell or damnation.

Duration. A third issue is the duration of the tragedy. Duration is experienced in three ways, each running on the "subjective time clock" of each victim. The first kind of duration is defined by the length of time a victim or survivor was at the point of impact at the time of the disaster. A victim who is trapped in the wreckage of a train may be at the point of impact for hours, while a victim who was thrown free of the train during the crash may only be at the point of impact for a few minutes before being taken to a hospital or an emergency shelter.

The second kind of duration defines how long survivors' senses are engaged by the disaster. Survivors of arson may have been at the scene of the fire for several hours, but the smell of the burnt building may remain with them for weeks or months after the tragedy if they continue to occupy the premises.

The third kind of duration is defined by the length of time that survivors are involved in the aftermath of the disaster. Thus, a survivor of a disaster caused by criminal attack may be involved in the disaster for years as it works its way through the criminal justice system.

The general guideline is that the longer the survivor is engaged in the disaster in any of these ways, the greater the likelihood for experiencing a severe crisis reaction or long-term stress reactions.

Recurrence Potential. The fourth issue of impact is the likelihood of the disaster's recurring. The greater the perceived chance of recurrence, the more likely it is that survivors will suffer fear as a dominant emotion. The more impossible recurrence seems, the more likely it is that anger will be a dominant emotion.

Control. Finally, it is important to examine the extent to which the survivors have control over the impact of the disaster on their own lives and futures. Catastrophes throw the world of an individual or community out of control. The survivors must confront the chaos of destruction, the rescue response, and lost and interrupted time. The need to reestablish a sense of control is critical to efforts to reconstruct a new equilibrium. Although the disaster itself cannot be controlled, survivors who feel that they are able to control the aftermath and the events that accompany it seem better able to cope.

CRISIS INTERVENTION GUIDELINES

CRISIS INTERVENTION WITH INDIVIDUALS

Understanding of crisis reactions, long-term stress, and special issues in analyzing the emotional impact of disaster helps to structure NOVA's guidelines for crisis intervention. The guidelines address five goals. The first three goals are directed at intervention in immediate crisis reactions, and goals four and five at interventions in long-term crisis reactions

1. Safety and security
2. Ventilation and validation
3. Prediction and preparation
4. Rehearsal and reassurance
5. Education and expertise

Safety and Security
The first goal of crisis intervention is to help the victim reestablish a sense of safety and security. There is a need to provide survivors with safety from physical harm. There is also a need to protect them from unwanted invasions of personal space; to make sure, for example, that a mob of reporters and camera crews does not trespass literally or figuratively on the property of people in distress.

Other safety concerns include avoidance of certain sensory perceptions that might increase the severity of the crisis reaction and the provision of aid to meet basic needs for food, shelter, and clothes. All of these safety and security activities respond to the victims' need for nurturing.

If safety is not an issue for survivors of loved ones who have died in a disaster, security is still a concern. Security should be provided by

ensuring privacy and confidentiality for survivors during death notification or while they await news of their loved ones.

Caregivers who seek to establish safety and security for victims are advised to:

- Make sure that the victims or survivors feel safe or secure at the present moment of intervention. Do not assume that victims feel safe just because they are safe.
- Respond to the need for nurturing. Although victims or survivors do need to begin to make small decisions or take responsibility for some issues in order to regain a sense of self-determination, they also need to be cared for.
- Encourage victims or survivors to relax. Just as physical rest is recommended to deal with physical injury, emotional injury calls for emotional rest.

Ventilation and Validation
The second goal of crisis intervention is to give victims an opportunity to express other feelings and reactions—to "ventilate" and to have their reactions validated. Victims or survivors often experience such intense emotional turmoil that they fear they are going crazy. It is important to help them identify the often competing emotions that make up their turmoil and to give those emotions concrete names and descriptions. Diagramming the normal pattern of a crisis reaction is very useful, because it normalizes the feelings and lets the victims or survivors know that such reactions are legitimate. Some emotions are overwhelming, in part because they are perceived as socially unacceptable. Anger that is expressed as hatred and a desire for revenge, for example, is often perceived as unacceptable. Such feelings are common, and victims and survivors should be reassured that they are normal.

Caregivers can employ the following tools to help victims ventilate and to provide validation.

- Ask the victims or survivors to describe the disaster.
- Ask them to describe where they were when it happened or when they heard about it.

- Ask them to describe their reactions and their response to the tragedy. Avoid asking them to describe or to share their feelings. Words like "sharing feelings" or discussing "emotions" alienate many individuals. Most people, however, can describe their reactions, and those reactions will reveal their feelings.
- List the elements of the crisis reaction (the initial response of shock, disbelief, and denial; the following emotional turmoil and its common components; the eventual reconstruction of a new equilibrium), and have individuals identify where they think they are in the crisis pattern. Draw an emotional roller coaster in which the high points are times of extreme turmoil and the low points are the times of exhaustion and feelings of numbness and depression; ask individuals to identify where they are within those ranges.
- Validate common crisis reactions and useful coping reactions.

Prediction and Preparation

The third goal of crisis intervention is to help the victims or survivors predict the problems, issues, and concerns they will face in the future and help them prepare for dealing with these matters. Such prediction and preparation help victims and survivors regain control over their lives, particularly to restore order in the midst of chaos.

Prediction should include all practical issues that seem relevant: relocation possibilities, financial concerns, legal issues that might arise in the criminal or civil justice system, medical issues, body identification procedures, funeral concerns, media interventions, religious problems, and so forth. When the nurse has no answers, he or she can offer to help the survivor get the information needed.

Prediction should also include giving the survivor a roadmap of normal crisis and stress reactions, while emphasizing that the survivor may experience none of the symptoms described. Prediction should involve the possible reactions of significant others and casual acquaintances, including the common experience of finding warmth and sympathy initially but seeing it give way to the attitude "you should be over that by now." Prediction should also address the problems that might be caused by normal triggering events.

Activities that help victims and survivors prepare for the future, in both practical and emotional terms, contribute to their sense of control. Encourage them to take one day at a time. Plan routines for dealing with each day, and schedule small goals for achievement.

A helpful problem-solving technique is asking victims to identify the three most critical problems they face at the moment and then assisting them in thinking through what they can or cannot do to address them. Some interveners develop a short contract with victims or survivors that if they will take on one task toward the solution of one problem, the intervener will take on a related task, and together they will reach at least a temporary resolution.

Survivors and victims should be encouraged to talk and write about the disaster. Even if they cannot find someone to talk to, keeping a written or oral diary of problems, reactions, and triumphs in the aftermath of disaster can be very useful. Time for memories and memorials should be planned into daily routines.

It is also helpful to identify a person to whom the victim or survivor can turn when special problems arise. Sometimes the person that a victim instinctively, and wisely, turns to is not a close friend or relative. Victims and survivors should be encouraged to eat, sleep, and exercise regularly. Physical exhaustion precipitates emotional exhaustion and further crises.

The last two intervention goals—rehearsal and reassurance; education and expertise—may be used in some cases immediately after a trauma, but they are more useful as additional strategies in the days or weeks after a disaster.

Rehearsal and Reassurance

Victims and survivors should be encouraged to rehearse the event or expected event in the aftermath both mentally and physically and to practice reactions or behaviors that help in coping. Mental rehearsal is a matter of visualizing the event or the expected event and then visualizing reactions. Following those thoughts, individuals are asked to visualize and practice response behaviors that are comfortable for them. At each stage of visualization, the intervener provides comfort and reassurance.

In physical rehearsal, individuals actually role play their reactions or planned behaviors. In some cases, they may want or need to visit the site of the disaster to role play or to think through their responses more completely. Rehearsal and reassurance are not proposed as mental health therapy but rather as a practical way to plan for difficult events. It is similar to the mental and behavioral rehearsal that has been suggested for job candidates prior to an interview.

Education and Expertise
The final goal of crisis intervention strategies is to provide education and ultimately a sense of expertise to the victims and survivors. Information is a critical need in the aftermath of a disaster. Part of that information should address practical issues or strategies of response and potential involvement with institutions with which victims may become involved. Ongoing education and the development of new skills may be very useful in minimizing stress and crisis over time.

One means of providing education for victims and survivors is through homework assignments such as reading and writing. Articles and books on victimization, crisis, stress, and the like are often read eagerly. If victims or survivors are illiterate, an optional method is to provide them with audiotapes or videotapes that cover similar materials. Some victims and survivors find it useful to write letters to institutions that have caused them inconvenience, pain, or grief in the aftermath of disaster.

A variety of skills can be helpful to survivors. Self-assessment skills employed for stress tests, analysis of thinking patterns, and aptitude tests are often revealing and interesting exercises. Relaxation skills can aid survivors in

sleeping and maintaining energy. Communication skills, such as active listening, organization of thoughts, presentation of ideas, and expressing feelings, usually make ventilation more productive. Problem-solving exercises are also useful. Many survivors find the development of new physical activities, such as swimming, dancing, or jogging, both physically and emotionally relieving. Not all survivors will respond to these suggestions, but it is worthwhile to offer them.

In providing crisis intervention and supportive counseling, nurses should involve family members, friends, or neighbors where appropriate. Support networks usually provide the most effective interventions unless they are also impaired by the disaster, and even then it is helpful to urge the members to be patient with one another, knowing that they may not be able to give or get the support they would normally expect of one another.

Finally, the encouragement of peer support group meetings for survivors is advised. The best source of validation of emotional reactions is the knowledge that others exposed to similar horrors reacted in similar ways.

Table 29–1 presents a sample list of phrases that should and should not be used in crisis intervention. It is important to note that the sooner intervention is provided, the more likely it will be effective. It is suggested that crisis intervention take place within the first 24 to 48 hours after a disaster.

CRISIS INTERVENTION IN COMMUNITY CRISES

The principles of crisis intervention can be applied in community crisis situations in a way similar to that used with individuals. NOVA's Crisis Response Project is based on that premise. Both the process used in sending a crisis response team to a community and the procedures that the team follows are designed to address the goals of crisis intervention. When a disaster occurs, NOVA is placed in contact with the community in one of two ways: either the community calls

TABLE 29–1. CAREGIVER VOCALIZATIONS IN CRISIS INTERVENTION

Do Say:
I am sorry this happened to you.
You're safe now (if the person is, indeed, safe).
I'm glad you're here with me now.
I'm glad you're talking to me now.
It wasn't your fault.
Your reaction is a normal response to an abnormal event.
It's understandable that you feel that way.
It must have been upsetting/distressing to see/hear/feel/smell that.
You're not going crazy.
Things may never be the same, but they can get better, and you can get better.
Your imagination can make a horrible reality worse than it is.
Its OK to cry, to want revenge, to hate.

Don't Say:
I know how you feel.
I understand.
You're lucky that you're alive.
You're lucky that you were able to save something.
You're lucky that you have other children/siblings.
You are young and can go on with your life/find someone else.
Your loved one didn't suffer when he/she died.
She/he led a good and full life before she/he died.
It was God's will.
He or she is better off/in a better place/happier now.
Out of tragedies, good things happen.
You'll get over it.
Everything is going to be alright.
You shouldn't feel that way.
Time heals all wounds.
You should get on with your life.

NOVA, or NOVA, on hearing of the tragedy, calls the community and offers assistance.

When NOVA makes the contact, it does so through a local victim assistance program, or if there is none, through other agencies (e.g., police department, sheriff's office, district attorney's office, mayor's office, county commissioner's office, attorney general's office).

No matter how the contact is made, NOVA offers three types of service: sending written materials on how to deal with the aftermath of disaster, sending the materials and providing telephone consultation to leading caregivers in the community, or sending a trained team of volunteer crisis interveners to assist the community.

Should a community decide that it wants to have a crisis response team come, NOVA will send a team only if all community leaders are in agreement that the service will be useful. These initial protocols for outreach are designed to provide the community with a sense of control over its destiny and to affirm that whatever happens will be guided by leadership from the community, not from the outside.

Arrival of Crisis Response Team

The team that is sent to a community will arrive within 24 hours of the disaster, if the community so wishes. That team has three goals:

- To help the community develop an action plan for dealing with the emotional aftermath of the disaster.
- To train caregivers in crisis theory as it applies to disaster.
- To provide immediate care for populations that are at high risk for severe crisis reaction or long-term stress reactions.

The arrival of a team is usually perceived as an act of support and reassurance. The team is seen as an expression of security amid the chaos. The team's role is to serve as adviser to the community and to teach ways to conduct group interventions when necessary. The team (including the local hosts) helps mobilize the community, just as an individual intervener attempts to help an individual in crisis to regain control.

Generally, the team stays in the community for no more than 72 hours. Exceptions have been made to this restriction when tragedies have involved large communities over an extended time. For example, NOVA team members served in Dade County for 7 days after Hurricane Andrew. Team members stayed in Oklahoma City for 12 days and in Kobe, Japan, after the earthquake for 10 days. The 3-day period allows time to accomplish the team's goals but does not promote bonding between community members and team members. In individual crisis intervention, there is a danger that the victim may become dependent on the intervener unless certain boundaries are established; this danger also exists in a community crisis situation. Three days together under those intense circumstances does produce lasting bonds, which reaffirms the sad usefulness of the 72-hour limitation.

Within that time period, ideally, the team will work to complete a clear-cut agenda in conjunction with its community hosts. First, the team will visit the site of the disaster, if possible. It has been NOVA's experience that the site visit is important to the team's understanding of the logistics involved in the disaster, as well as its understanding of the kind of devastation that occurred. For example, when NOVA's team went to Dryden, New York, in the aftermath of the abduction, assault, and murders of two teenage cheerleaders, it was important for the team members to understand that the murders involved the distribution of body parts over a 40-mile radius in the surrounding counties. In addition, when NOVA's teams went to Dade County after Hurricane Andrew, their tours of Homestead, Turkey Point, and other devastated areas gave them a better knowledge of the impact and the scope of the hurricane and the numbers of community members that were involved and at risk for severe crisis reactions.

Second, at some point early on, it is recommended that the team hold a news conference. The news conference serves three purposes: it lets the community at large know of the arrival of assistance, it provides an opportunity to communicate basic information about the emotional aftermath of tragedy, and it may provide an opportunity to notify the community when group discussions will take place to address some of the immediate issues, as well as to advertise which agencies are inviting calls for assistance. The news conference is important because many community members may not understand why they are feeling distressed if they were not at the scene of the disaster or were not its direct vic-

tims. Information from the media can help them understand that their reactions are normal.

Third, the team will meet with community leaders and policy-makers to plan the remainder of the two days. This planning session is critical because it symbolizes the control the community has over its immediate future. The community identifies who will be the lead and auxiliary caregivers to be trained by the team. It plans when and where any community debriefing sessions will take place. It identifies high-risk population groups. It designs an outreach strategy for communicating with all such groups. And it addresses any other urgent issues or concerns such as immediate memorial services or funeral services.

Team Planning Session

The only assertive role that NOVA's team takes during the planning session is to insist that there be a training session for all caregivers who will be involved with the NOVA team over the 2-day period and for any caregivers who will be involved in follow-up care after the team leaves the community. That training session, usually 3 hours long, covers basic crisis and stress theory and crisis intervention guidelines as outlined earlier in this chapter.

The training session has four purposes. First, it provides a forum for nurses and other caregivers who have been exposed to the disaster to express their feelings in a safe context. Second, by reviewing crisis and stress theory, it provides validation for those feelings. Third, it usually provides validation for the services they have already provided. They learn that their natural reactions have been "correct." Fourth, even if the caregivers are familiar with crisis intervention, they may have forgotten their knowledge in the shock of the disaster or may have learned such theories in a different context. It is important that all caregivers use similar words and phrases in communicating with survivors of the disaster. If they do not, they often contribute to the sense of chaos.

The planning session will generate a list of population groups at risk for crisis and stress.

From that list, the planners will identify those with whom the team will be able to meet while they are in the community. Usually, the team tries to meet with groups such as rescuers who have been at the scene of the disaster, victims or survivors, and eyewitnesses. This may include a wide variety of groups: firefighters, law enforcement officers, Red Cross workers, paramedics, emergency medical teams, clergy, teachers, neighbors, and so forth. Much of the remaining agenda after the training session is spent conducting debriefing sessions of those groups. In addition, the planning session usually results in at least one scheduled community-wide debriefing session. The session is an open-to-all session aimed at attracting individuals who have recognized their own distress and their need for help.

NOVA team members generally lead the debriefing sessions, but in most cases, the local caregivers are urged to attend and to serve as immediate and long-term referrals. Team members lead the sessions so that they can model the debriefing process for the caregivers.

Finally, just before the team leaves the community, NOVA recommends that there be another news conference to review what has been done in the community and to convey any lessons learned. In addition, there is usually a final session with local hosts and caregivers to help develop recommendations and strategies for the community to pursue in the weeks, months, and years to come.

The group debriefing sessions are designed to provide the participants with an opportunity to express their reactions to the disaster. Group members help to validate each other's reactions. For some, the debriefings may be sufficient to mitigate severe reactions. Others may need additional sessions or individual help as well. The local caregivers will be the source for that follow-up. The sessions are also designed to begin the process of predicting problems that may arise in the future and to help individuals begin to prepare for them.

The final planning session is devoted to predicting and preparing the community as a whole for the future. For the most part, the team's role is simply one of adviser and resource to community leaders.

Group Debriefing Process

Over the last 20 years a number of group crisis intervention procedures have been developed to deal with different kinds of tragedy. Group defusings are often used to help emergency workers cope with what they have seen at the site of a disaster and continue with their work. Retrospective debriefings may take place months or years after a catastrophe has occurred. In cases where there is an ongoing crisis, such as serial murders or sexual assaults, repetitive debriefing sessions may be helpful to survivors as they confront new issues with media, the criminal justice system, or social repercussions. In most cases, however, a simple model of debriefing follows the steps of individual crisis intervention with a few variations.

It is important to try to arrange debriefings so that they do not conflict with aftermath events such as funerals and memorials. Clearly, the goal is to encourage as many individuals to attend as possible. Night debriefings are usually better for community-wide group meetings, and day debriefings are generally better for people who are employed outside of the home, homemakers, and children. It is advisable to encourage employers to give at-risk employees time off to attend debriefing sessions. Generally, immediate postdisaster group debriefings do not take more than 2 hours each, although in some cases other debriefings may be done as a follow-up.

The location of the debriefing sessions should be designed to promote feelings of safety and security. It is generally not prudent to use a site that triggers reactions to or memories of the disaster (for example, an airport conference room following a plane crash or a school gymnasium following the slaying of a student at the school).

The room for the debriefing should be accessible and comfortable for the group. Seating should be arranged in a horseshoe or a circle, and local caregivers or other team members should be spread around the room. Water should be available, because the intake of water can mitigate physical stress reactions. Boxes of tissues should be available in case there are tears.

NOVA encourages the use of a flip-chart to record the phrases used by participants as the group interaction proceeds. To preserve confidentiality, these records are given to the group at the end of the session or destroyed, depending on the group's decision. No individual's name is attached to any reaction recorded.

Debriefing sessions should be conducted by a debriefing team of two, a leader and an assistant. The leader's role is to conduct the debriefing. The debriefing assistant's role is to provide emotional support to the debriefing leader, to record notes on the flip-charts, to take over if the debriefing leader cannot continue, and to assist individuals who may go into a crisis reaction as a result of the debriefing session itself (although it is better if local caregivers assume this role). The assistant should never be involved in conducting the debriefing unless the leader specifically requests assistance.

Once a group is assembled, the debriefing leader should begin the meeting by introducing the debriefing team and reviewing ground rules for the session. The following rules are essential for preserving the sense of safety and security.

The group is pledged to confidentiality so that people feel they can discuss reactions freely. While expressions of any feelings are legitimate, there must be no physical violence during the session. (At times, individuals may react so strongly that they may try to take out their rage on another group member.)

Individuals may leave the group as they need to, although they are encouraged to stay from beginning to end, and those who leave can expect someone to accompany them for support if they want it. Further, if they do leave, they are encouraged to rejoin the group when they feel they are ready.

The group session is not a critique of how any individuals or institutions behaved during the disaster; rather, it is a discussion of individual reactions.

The team's agenda is to help the group define the crisis reaction, to provide some crisis intervention, and to predict and prepare the group for possible future events. The goal is not to provide individual or group therapy. The announced agenda is to review three things: how the participants reacted or are reacting, how their families or loved ones are reacting, and what they expect in the future.

Opening the Session. To accomplish the aforementioned agenda, the team leader should begin the session with the following type of introduction. The introduction is accompanied by commentary to better explain its use of crisis intervention strategies.

> I am sorry that this plane crash happened here in Midville.

This statement of sympathy is almost a mandatory introductory phrase in the NOVA protocol. It indicates to the listener that the intervener is concerned about the listener and the tragedy. Even though it may seem trivial, many victims have said that the statement of sorrow is very important.

> I know that if I lived here, it would be terribly distressing to me. And even though I live in Center City, it is still upsetting to think that 24 people were killed.

These introductory words are designed to validate in advance feelings of turmoil, and to acknowledge the extent of the disaster and destruction.

> I'm John Jones, a victim advocate with the National Organization for Victim Assistance, or NOVA. With me are Susan Brown, a crisis intervener from Medford, Oregon; and Larry Little, Mary Mays, and Sarah Smith from Midville's Victim Assistance Program. Susan and I are here as members of NOVA's Crisis Response Team Project,

which sends volunteer crisis interveners to help communities in the aftermath of disaster. We have assisted 18 communities since our first response in the aftermath of the Edmond, Oklahoma, post office murders in 1986. Larry, Mary, and Sarah are here to provide follow-up assistance if needed in Midville.

This part is an introduction of the individuals who will be active in the debriefing session and the organization sponsoring them. It includes just enough information to establish the credibility of the project and the intervention.

I want to talk to you today about the impact of this plane crash on Midville. But before we begin our discussion, it is important that everyone here understand some basic ground rules for our talk. First, I think it is important that everyone agrees that this discussion will be confidential between us. That means that no one will report to others what any named individual said about anything. You may want to tell your spouse or a friend that certain things were discussed, or even that someone in the group made a certain remark that you agree or disagree with. But I'm asking you to agree that any such commentary will make no references to names or to specific characteristics that might reveal a person's identity. If you agree with this rule, please nod your head in affirmation.

This rule is very important for ensuring privacy. The experience of NOVA's team debriefing leaders is that when group members are asked to underscore their agreement by nodding their heads, they feel more accountable for maintaining confidentiality, and others feel more trust in their peers.

The second rule is that no matter what your reactions are, you should feel free to tell us about them. But there is an exception to this rule, and that is that you should not express your reactions through physical violence.

That may sound humorous, but I have found that sometimes a tragedy like this can trigger strong anger or a desire for vengeance. Occasionally, that kind of reaction causes individuals to lash out at others without meaning to.

This rule of nonviolence is very difficult to present. NOVA's experience has been that if the rule is presented in the positive manner as a rule of total expression with one exception, it is better received. The rule against physical violence often brings snickers or laughter because no one thinks that such a reaction would happen, but it can, so giving a caution and a reasonable explanation of the caution is a preventive strategy.

The third rule is that you should feel free to go and come as you please. Sometimes people need to get away from the group for a while to collect their thoughts or to think through certain things. If you want to leave for a few minutes, do so. One of our team members will follow you out just to make sure you don't need anything or that if you do, we can help you. We'd like you to return because we think your thoughts and reactions to this disaster are important, but you are not obliged to do so.

Some people have expressed the thought that group debriefings should require that individuals who participate in them stay for the full length of the session. It has been NOVA's experience that it is better to provide participants with the fullest amount of freedom. Any restriction takes away their sense of control. This is a time to help them reestablish their own ability to function as they see fit. At the same time, it is good practice to tell them that someone will be available to talk to them or assist them so that they do not feel stranded if they leave and still need help.

Those are our guidelines; now let me give you some more information that may be helpful. There are water, coffee, and soft drinks on the back table if you would like some refreshments during the session. The bathrooms are located down the hall and to the right. And if you need to smoke, please feel free to do so over in that end of the room. If any of you cannot tolerate smoke, we suggest that you sit over at this end.

Note that in this section, the rules are referred to as guidelines. This softens the impact of the regulation. Also note that permission is given to move about the room, to get refreshments, to go to the bathroom, and to smoke. Once again, this expands the sense of control the group members have over their behavior. At some training sessions, individuals have asked why NOVA allows smoking in debriefing groups. The answer is simple. Although there are good reasons to promote nonsmoking among our general population, we have observed that even reformed smokers may have a need to smoke during intense emotional sessions. We are not encouraging smoking, but it is our view that the time of a disaster is not a time to curb an addiction.

> Now, let me say once again that I'm sorry that the plane crash happened in Midville. It is terrible that so many people were killed and injured. It is terrible that the destruction was so immense. But what I would like you to do at this moment is to think back over the past 48 hours and try to remember the instant when you first saw, heard, or learned of the plane crash. I want you to try to remember where you were, who you were with, and what your reactions were. What do you remember seeing, hearing, smelling, tasting, or even touching at that time?

This is the critical transition to the group crisis work. There are several important factors to this transition. After suggesting that the group think back and remember, the leader should allow a few moments for that to happen. For some, this may be the first time they have allowed themselves to do such thinking. For others, it may be something that has been remembered over and over again. After allowing those few moments,

the leader helps to structure those thoughts by stating what the group should think about. It is important to use the word "reactions" and to talk about physical reactions. These will serve as a lead to other discussions.

> Now, I want to ask for anyone who would be willing to tell me about his or her experience. Where were you? Who were you with? And what were your reactions?

Repeating the questions is useful while someone in the group prepares to respond. In most cases, the leader will not have to wait for a response. However, in the cases where no one responds immediately, the leader should be aware that silence is an ally, not an enemy.

Working With the Group. After the leader has set up the introduction, the group work begins. Usually a number of people will be ready to tell their stories. The normal progression of events will include a description of shock and disbelief, followed by a wide range of conflicting and congruent emotions. It is useful for the group leader gently to interrupt individuals in their discussion of reactions after they have described the shock-and-disbelief stage and their physical reactions. The leader can then proceed to the next person. That type of interruption and progression assists the validation process. However, if an individual seems so consumed by the experience that he or she must continue to describe events up to that very day, the leader should allow the individual to do so. That judgment is subject to the intervener's common sense.

Once the discussion is under way, it is important for the leader to validate all key reactions. Underscore any statements that fit within the crisis reaction framework. For example, if a person says, "I was stunned. I could not believe that it happened," a validating comment would be, "Shock is common in a disaster. How could anyone believe that such a disaster was happening to them?" It is ideal if the group itself does the validation, so that group members say, "I couldn't believe my eyes" or "I felt numb and couldn't move or think." This is the most effective validation because it comes from one peer to another. However, the leader should not be seduced into thinking that she or he should not provide validation if the group does not. Every statement that reflects a normal crisis reaction should be validated.

The leader should keep an eye on the time. After about 30 minutes of introduction and descriptions of shock and disbelief, the leader should move on to reactions of emotional turmoil. If the discussion does not naturally flow in this direction, the leader should ask participants to describe what has happened to them in the aftermath. Again, there should be validation of anger, fear, confusion, grief, self-blame, and other strong emotions.

The second segment of the discussion usually takes longer than the first. One reason is that there is a greater variety of reactions and the emotional content of those reactions is often more intense. After about an hour, the leader should lead the discussion toward questions such as "What do you think will happen tomorrow or next week in your life, and how do you think you will handle it?" This last segment of the session is the predict-and-prepare segment.

In most cases, group participants will accurately predict problems and concerns. In some cases, the leader may have to describe unexpected obstacles. Those obstacles may range from involvement in the criminal justice system (because the disaster involved criminal intent) to media sensationalism.

The leader should remember that an important part of the content at this stage of the discussion is to help survivors to prepare for such issues. As a result, the leader should validate good proposed coping techniques and give the participants a safety net for the future. In most communities, that safety net will develop from the community's mobilization of emotional aftercare. Perhaps there will already be a plan in place for the future. No matter what the stage of preparedness is, the group participants need to know there is a place to turn for help. That is the safety net for their next 24 hours and, sometimes, for the rest of their lives.

In the group debriefing process, the leader needs to be fully prepared for emotional reactions and behavioral symptoms of trauma. Participants may manifest confusion or physical and mental agitation. They may begin to cry or may become withdrawn. They may become angry and irritated. The leader needs to know that such reactions are not directed at him or her personally. The reactions are directed at the disaster but the disaster is not controllable, and the leader is.

The leader should also be prepared for the unexplainable. In most disasters, there are stories of supernatural physical feats, messages from the dead or dying, and visions of death or dying. It is not important whether such events have an explanation; it is important that the individual believes what she or he is describing.

At the conclusion of the group process, the leader should go over the agenda briefly and indicate how it was accomplished. If a flip-chart was used to record reactions, it should be used to review them in the context of normal crisis reactions. Group members will then have confirmed that their statements were reasonable. The leader should ask for any final concerns or questions from the group.

The leader should distribute handouts on crisis reactions, long-term stress reactions, and special issues. Participants need to have something to take home with them. The group should be thanked for their participation and reminded of the confidentiality of the discussion. The ongoing support and interest of the host or leader's organization should be emphasized.

SUMMARY

Understanding the crisis and stress reactions, strategies for crisis intervention, and NOVA's approach to community crisis intervention should demonstrate how closely the theory of crisis and stress can translate into practice.

Disaster occurs far too often in modern life—the disaster of an individual tragedy such as a sexual assault or murder, or the massive destruction of lives and property in a plane crash or multiple slayings. The impact of disasters is exponentially increased by each death, each eyewitness, each injury, each loss.

Thus, it is critical that mental health professionals, clergy, victim assistance workers, and others be prepared to respond to the emotional dimension of disaster. Without appropriate interventions, many individuals may face a lifetime of severe stress reactions. With effective help, most individuals can reconstruct a new life, one that forever carries painful memories of their losses, but one into which they build new hope, pride, and gratification.

SUGGESTED READINGS

Herman J. *Trauma and Recovery*. New York: Basic Books; 1992.

Lystad M, ed. *Mental Health Response to Mass Emergencies*. New York: Bruner/Mazel; 1988.

Raphael B. *When Disaster Strikes*. New York: Basic Books; 1986.

Van der Kolk BA, McFarlane AC, Weisaeth L, eds. *Traumatic Stress: The Effects of Overwhelming Experience on Mind, Body, and Society*. New York: Guilford Press; 1996.

Wilson JP. *Trauma, Transformation and Healing*. New York: Brunner/Mazel; 1989.

Wilson JP, Lindy JD, eds. *Countertransference in the Treatment of PTSD*. New York: Guilford Press; 1994.

Young MA. *Responding to Communities in Crisis*. Des Moines: Kendall Hunt; 1994.

CHAPTER 30

FORENSIC NURSING

Virginia A. Lynch • Ann Wolbert Burgess

*F*orensic nursing
focuses on the
areas where medicine,
nursing, and human
behavior interface with
the law.

Chapter Overview

An 18-year-old woman was found dead in her apartment with her throat slashed. The crime scene indicated that the victim had put up a great struggle, as blood was splattered everywhere. Police arrested three teenagers including a 19-year-old woman and her boyfriend. In exchange for a plea to a lesser charge, the male defendant said that his girlfriend, not he, had been at the crime scene. The prosecution argued that "teenage jealousy" was the motive for the murder. Although the female defendant denied she killed the victim, she provided an alibi for her boyfriend. She was convicted of first-degree murder and sentenced to life without parole.

The forensic nurse trained as a death investigator would be responsible for photographing and gathering evidence at the crime scene. Rules would be followed relating to evidence collection as well as the methods, procedures, and documentation of evidence from the crime scene. At trial, the forensic nurse, as a fact witness, would be expected to know the procedures for labeling, storing, and submitting evidence for forensic examination. The nurse would be expected to know how to provide credible testimony regarding that evidence and a classification of the stab wounds.

In addition, expert witnesses in this case would range from having expertise in the forensic sciences, DNA, crime scene, and profiling to the biopsychosocial areas of rape, battering, and domestic violence.

In this case, 2 years following conviction, a court-appointed attorney filed a federal habeus corpus and was granted a hearing. A new team of defense experts, including one of the authors, was assigned to review the court testimony and file. In this particular case, the advanced practice forensic nurse reviewed the evidence related to the defendant's motivation for covering for the boyfriend, who she now says killed the victim with the female co-defendant. The rationale for her cover-up that put her in the position of being convicted for murder becomes the focus of the expert evaluation of old and new evidence. Attention will be paid to the crime scene photographs as well as factors that played a role in the defendant's passive protective position with the boyfriend.

This chapter discusses forensic nursing in general and specifically outlines how to collect forensic evidence and classify wounds. The advanced practice forensic nurse's role in analyzing and reviewing equivocal death cases is presented, as well as the sexual assault nurse examiner role in forensic nursing, and counseling issues for families of homicide victims.

FORENSIC SCIENCE IN NURSING

Taber's *Cyclopedic Medical Dictionary* defines the "forensic" (Latin *forensis*, a forum) as pertaining to the law, specifically related to public debate in courts of law. Therefore, any subdiscipline of science that practices its specialty within the arena of the law is practicing the principle of forensic science. The interface of law and medicine or nursing produces a medicolegal (meaning legal-medicine) or forensic case. The term "medicolegal" is interchangeable with the word "forensic." Traditionally, the term forensic carried with it a connotation of death, homicide, or murder. That association is because until recently only one kind of forensic science in North America—forensic pathology—had received widespread attention. The forensic pathology subspecialty is mainly concerned with the scientific investigation of death. Clinical forensic practice, on the other hand, is primarily concerned with the survivor of violent crimes or liability-related trauma. Presently, a trend in clinical and community health care involves the awareness and recognition of unidentified or previously unrecognized trauma and the collection of evidence from living patients. Survivors of trauma who require investigation of injuries are the concern of the clinician, not the pathologist. Clinical forensic medicine, originating in the United Kingdom, is now becoming recognized as an essential component of health care in the United States and Canada. Indeed, it has been a respected discipline in public health for 200 years in other parts of the world, including European countries, South America, East Asia, and Russia (Eckert, 1990; Goldsmith, 1986).

DEFINING CLINICAL FORENSIC PRACTICE AND ITS COMPONENTS

In a comprehensive approach to the unmet needs of forensic victims who survive violent crimes and traumatic injuries, new roles are emerging for clinical forensic nursing specialists (Eckert, 1986; Lynch, 1991, 1993a; Smock, 1994; Smock et al., 1993). The forensic nurse has a vital role in cases resulting from intentional or unintentional acts involving criminality or civil action. The medicolegal and psychosocial interaction requires a knowledge of where human behavior interfaces with the law.

Advanced practice forensic nurses are working with crime victims and their families as well as individuals with liability-related injuries resulting from automobile or pedestrian accidents, occupation-related injuries, disputed paternity, medical malpractice and resulting injuries, and food and drug tampering.

In order to establish the foundation upon which forensic nursing is designed, it is necessary to examine the history of clinical forensic medicine, or "living forensics," as it is sometimes called. Forensic nursing's scientific knowledge base emerges from theories of nursing, forensic science, criminal justice, police science, and legal studies. The relative isolation of these disciplines has contributed to the complex tasks and social climate facing emergency care.

Forensic nursing is the application of the nursing process to public or legal proceedings—the application of the forensic aspects of health care to the scientific investigation of trauma. Clinical forensic nursing is defined as the application of clinical nursing practice to trauma survivors or those whose death is pronounced in the clinical environs, involving the identification of unrecognized, unidentified injuries and the proper processing of forensic evidence.

FORENSIC NURSING AND TRAUMA CARE

Traumatic injury is recognized worldwide as a major public health problem. Although each culture may present its own unique drama in types of crime, weapons, and drugs, no age, race, religion, or socioeconomic group is spared from the devastating effect of the trauma such events produce, both physical and emotional. Trauma ranks higher than AIDS, heart disease, and cancer as a cause of hospitalization. According to The American Trauma Society, one reason for concern in trauma care is that for all the reported crimes of human violence, three times as many crimes may be unreported. Statistics indicate that trauma associated with violence is the number-one killer of young Americans between 1 and 44 years of age. These premature deaths cause the loss of approximately 2.2 million potential years of lives (The American Trauma Society, 1993).

SPECIFIC RESPONSIBILITIES IN TRAUMA INVESTIGATION

OBSERVATION AND PRESERVATION OF EVIDENCE

When a patient is admitted for trauma care as a result of suspicious injuries that may be crime-related or self-inflicted, emergency nurses become involved. Nurses must be specifically aware of the manner in which they document the assessment of injury, assist in the collection and preservation of forensic evidence, and coordinate critical data with law enforcement and crime scene officers (Schramm, 1991).

Hospital emergency departments are regularly in contact with essential evidence in criminal cases. The most common types of evidence are clothing, bullets, bloodstains, hairs, fibers, and small pieces of material such as metal, glass, paint, or wood fragments.

The dilemma of gathering evidence in the emergency department is a serious cause of concern in traumatic injury cases. The emergency staff should recognize the importance of recovering possible items of evidence in a legally acceptable manner in the following situations.

- *Medicolegal cases.* A medicolegal case is defined as a treatment situation with legal implications (Mittleman et al. 1983).
- *Suspicious deaths or crime-related injuries.* Suspicious deaths and crime-related injuries are classified as medicolegal cases.
- *Accidents.* It is not always possible to predict if an accident will have medicolegal implications. Yet almost all accidents result in some type of litigation, whether civil or criminal.

Trace and physical evidence are concerns of the criminalist (crime laboratory examiner) and are basically used to establish the facts of a crime. The collection of valuable evidence may have far-ranging consequences for the patient and the accused, as well as for the health care worker. The misinterpretation of physical injuries and evidence, however, may result in an inaccurate opinion (Shaw, 1993). Orris and Lantz (1993) noted that trauma physicians failed to correctly distinguish entrance from exit wounds in more than 50 percent of perforating wound cases.

► CASE EXAMPLE

A young man, admitted to an emergency room with a perforating gunshot wound to the left shoulder, stated that he was shot with a handgun from a distance of approximately 30 feet. Physical examination noted soot around the anterior of the wound and on the patient's shirt. The forensic specialist was aware that the presence of soot surrounding a wound was indicative of a close range of fire. The physical evidence did not support the patient's story. When confronted with these inconsistencies, the patient confessed to self-inflicting his wounds in an attempt to set up a fellow drug dealer so that he would be sent to jail. Without the forensic specialist, the wound would have been cleaned and debrided and all trace evidence, including evidence that would determine the range of fire, would have been lost. The drug dealer could have been falsely arrested and charged with a crime he did not commit (Smock, 1994).

Processing Clothing

It is imperative that nurses in the clinical environment be taught to recognize and preserve vital fragments of trace evidence through the careful handling of the patient's clothing and personal property. Such action has been identified as one of the most important that nurses provide to aid the investigation process. Clothing worn at the time of the incident may, or may not, contain trace evidence useful in linking the victim with the assailant or crime scene.

As noted, missing evidence may be as important as evidence found, as in the William Kennedy Smith case. The woman in that case claimed that Smith had tackled and struggled with her on the lawn of the Kennedy estate and raped her. Forensic scientist Henry Lee testified that grass stains should have been on her panties, but he found none. To emphasize his point, he produced his grass-stained handkerchief, having previously wiped it across the Kennedy compound grass. Smith was acquitted of rape charges.

Careful examination of defects in clothes can be compared with the victim's wounds to provide insight about the type of weapon or wounding instrument. Observe clothing for blood, semen, gunshot residue, or trace materials such as hair or fibers: *document, diagram, photograph, collect, preserve*. The clothing may contain fragments from the assailant and, if the assailant was injured, his or her blood may also be on the victim's clothing. Garments from automobile-pedestrian accidents may display tire impressions or conceal trace evidence such as paint chips or broken glass that could identify the vehicle that struck the victim. Laundry markings may offer a clue to identification or origin of an unknown, unconscious, near-death or deceased individual. Special attention should be applied to the examination and security of clothing from a gunshot victim. As noted in the previous example, gunshot residues surrounding bullet holes in the clothes may de-

termine the distance of the firearm from the victim at the time of firing (range of fire).

As previously noted, missing evidence may make a forensic point. In the O.J. Simpson civil trial, it was reported that criminalist Dennis Fung sounded mystified as he compared the extra-large leather glove tagged as evidence to a photo taken in the police crime lab of the glove that detectives recovered at the murder scene. The photo appeared to depict a rip in the glove over the ring finger, a pebble-sized mark that showed up white against the dark fabric. But the actual glove had no damage on the ring finger and in fact looked relatively unworn. Fung further testified that he was not sure it was the same glove (Simon, 1997). When recalled to testify, Fung did correct this testimony based upon closer examination of the photograph.

Removing clothing should be done carefully to protect any foreign fragments that may be adhering to the clothes. *Do not shake the clothes*. Clothing is frequently cut away during resuscitative attempts. Consequently, the article and/or evidentiary materials may be lost. The cutting of clothing is unavoidable in many life-threatening situations and is necessary to provide immediate access to treatment sites. When this occurs, try to avoid cutting through tears, rips, and holes that may have resulted from the weapon or the assault. *Clothing should never be discarded or thrown on the floor*, as cross-contamination of trace evidence with debris from the treatment environment can result. Due to time constraints during a life-saving intervention, clothing can be placed on a clean, white sheet on an empty trauma table, mayo stand, or the floor in the corner of the room until time permits effective packaging. If a victim can remove his or her own clothes, have the victim stand on a clean sheet or a large sheet of paper. It will collect any trace evidence that may be dislodged. Because the sheet often retains microscopic evidence, it must be placed in a separate paper bag for transfer to the crime laboratory.

In preserving clothes that are moist, they should be hung up to dry in a secure area if possible. If damp clothing is to be retrieved by police, they should be apprised of the damp condition. When stains are present, place clean white paper over stains to avoid cross-contamination. Store each item of clothing in separate paper bags, *not plastic*. Plastic bags are inappropriate because condensation tends to accumulate, and the integrity of the evidence degenerates. Each bag should be sealed and clearly marked with the date, time, and signature or initials of the individual doing the sealing. Fortunately, a hospital is an excellent place to find all manners of containers (bags, bottles, boxes, and tubes) for properly storing evidence.

Documentation

The condition of the patient's clothing including color, type, unusual markings, as well as tears or other damage should be recorded. Occasionally fibers or foreign debris from the crime scene on the victim's clothing may be transferred to the vehicle or assailant. Clothing is often the first circumstantial evidence that may help to identify a missing person, or collaborate an eyewitness statement.

SECURING CUSTODY

Secure custody of personal property must be maintained until it is turned over to the appropriate law enforcement agency. Do not inadvertently release property to family members. Such items should be held for police and generally not returned to the family. In cases, however, where police jurisdiction is doubtful and/or where family members are demanding return of the clothing, a legal opinion may be warranted.

Chain of Custody

The chain of custody begins with the person who collects the evidence, and continues to the individuals having control or custody over evidentiary or potentially evidentiary material or personal property. The chain of custody should be defined in the forensic protocol and generally requires a form of written documentation.

Rules of evidence require a chain of custody for each item recovered from the patient, including trace and physical evidence, laboratory specimens of blood and other body fluids, clothing, and other personal articles. The integrity of every specimen, or piece of evidence, seized must be insured to protect its admissibility in a court of law. Failure to maintain the chain of custody renders potentially important evidence worthless if lost, damaged, or unaccountable from the hands of the nurse to the police officer.

INVESTIGATION OF WOUND CHARACTERISTICS

Investigating undiagnosed trauma often begins with the evaluation of wound pattern characteristics. Detailed documentation of the appearance of the wound may be the identifying factor in determining the type of weapon used to inflict the injury. Wound characteristics constitute evidence that may be obscured by emergency trauma care.

The forensic nurse's documentation should include the location of the injury and approximate measurements of cuts, lacerations, and stab wounds. Diagrams, body maps, or photography help reconstruct injury patterns in subsequent investigations or at autopsy. For patients who survive, or whose wound is excised or extended surgically, later reconstruction of the injury is not possible. The specific importance of reconstruction is magnified when the patient lives for an indefinite period of time and later dies as a result of the injury. Treatment procedures as well as the natural healing process will alter the condition of the wound, thus eliminating the possibility of determining if the wound was inflicted with a single or double-edged blade knife, an entrance or exit gunshot wound, and so forth.

Forensic nurses should have an accurate knowledge of the types of injuries generally resulting in medicolegal cases and be familiar with the appropriate terminology required to describe them. Failure to recognize and describe injuries has confounded the testimony of victim and perpetrator as a defense strategy in the courtroom. The forensic nurse will not only be made to appear unprofessional, but a serious crime may go unpunished. Medicolegal injuries are primarily categorized as follows.

- *Sharp injuries* include stab wounds and incised wounds resulting from penetration or cuts that can reflect patterns or characteristics consistent with the wounding object. It is important not to confuse a cut with a laceration. A laceration is not a sharp injury.
- *Blunt force injuries* usually result from assaults, abuse, accidents, or resuscitative intervention. Abrasions, contusions, lacerations, and fractures are blunt force injuries resulting from the crushing impact of a blunt object against the body. A laceration results only from blunt force impact.
- *Dicing injuries,* generally small and numerous, are most often sustained from motor vehicle accidents. These injuries consist of multiple lacerations caused by contact with shattering tempered glass.
- *Bite mark injuries* remain the patterned injury most frequently unrecognized and unidentified as evidence by nurses when assessing the patient. Human bite marks are indicative of abuse and generally associated with sexual assault. Animal bite marks are usually accidental, but may incur civil or even criminal liability if an animal had been neglected, tortured, or trained to cause an injury or if a dangerous animal escaped captivity by negligence, a deliberate act, or other illegal action.
- *Patterned injuries* have specific characteristics that reflect the identity of the wounding object

or provide information about the nature of the weapon.
- *Defense wounds* indicate the posturing of a victim in protection against attack. Defense wounds are most often found on the hands and arms, although they may be located on any part of the body that is used as a shield. The injuries can be sharp or blunt depending upon the weapon used. One victim received severe injury to her fingers as she protected her heart from piercing scissor blows.
- *Hesitation wounds* are usually superficial, sharp force wounds self-inflicted in the survivor of suicide and accompany a deeper, fatal incision in the decedent. Hesitation marks are generally straight wounds perpendicular to the lower arms found at the wrist, elbow or neck. Scars from hesitation marks may indicate a previous attempt at suicide.
- *Fast force injuries* (usually gunshot) require nurses to be knowledgeable of the mechanics and specifics of gunshot and shotgun wounds in order to recognize the variations of patterns of injury produced by these weapons.

Understanding gunshot wound factors can assist in assessing the extent of injury, provide appropriate nursing care, and anticipate potential problems (Stewart, 1983). The nurse involved in the initial management of a patient must make an assessment based on the wound site, type of weapon involved, and length of time between the injury and emergency care. Cases involving fatal or nonfatal gunshot wounds should be documented regarding the presence or absence of gunshot residue (powder, soot, particles, small punctuate hemorrhages) around the injury. Any bullet or fragments recovered during treatment should be properly packaged and turned over to the crime scene officer in an unaltered condition. Valuable notations should be documented in the charting, for example, the names and addresses of witnesses, the monitoring of procedures or events prior to autopsy, and the safeguards provided clothing and other personal effects (Marsh, 1978). By implementing forensic protocol that emphasizes cooperation with the criminal justice sector, nurses are initiating a critical link in trauma systems that will provide for increased coordination and services.

SUDDEN AND UNEXPECTED DEATHS IN THE CLINICAL AREA

Deaths occur in the hospital environment on a regular basis: dead on arrival, during trauma treatment, in the operating room, delivery room, nursery, and surgical intensive care or recovery room, among others. If these deaths occur as a result of trauma or unknown causes, they require investigation. Generally, any death that occurs during the first 24 hours after admission is reportable to the medical examiner/coroner system regardless of the history.

If death occurs during trauma treatment, the trauma room suddenly becomes a scene of legal inquiry and will be carried as the place of death on the death certificate regardless of where the initial incident occurred. The death scene must then be protected until the body and evidence have been removed at the completion of the medicolegal investigation. The delivery room is a frequent scene of death. If the patient dies as a result of abuse or an accident, this death must be reported and investigated, and evidence must be retained.

Maintaining an index of suspicion is essential when considering criminal activity as a cause of sudden and unexpected death. Evidence preservation, careful documentation of the circumstances surrounding the death, as well as the decedent's social and medical history may form the basis for problem solving when the cause of death is not obvious.

The critical factor in sudden and unexpected death is whether the initiating cause is natural or unnatural. The cause of death is the injury, disease, or combination of the two, that initiated the sequence of disturbances, brief or prolonged, that produced the fatal termination. Note the word "initiated," and that causes may not be immediately fatal, as with carcinoma or a stab wound. Manner of death is the fashion or circumstance in which the cause of death arose. In the United States we have five options: natural, accident, homicide, suicide, or undetermined. Mechanism of death is the physiological derangement or biochemical disturbance incompatible with life that is initiated by the cause of death. Clearly, if the mechanism is initiated by a cause, the two cannot be the same. They are in effect final common pathways out of life. Mechanisms include cardiac arrest, respiratory arrest, and cardiopulmonary arrest. Forensic pathologists characterize cardiac arrest as "the diagnosis of the diagnostically destitute!" (Besant-Matthews, personal communication). It is clear that many physicians and nurses fail to distinguish between cause and mechanism.

A classic instance is when a patient brought into the hospital dies shortly thereafter, and the physician on duty indicates that the cause of death is cardiac arrest. However, this is not a cause, and has no place on a death certificate. Coronary artery disease is a reasonable cause of death, whereas cardiac arrest is not a cause at all but a mechanism. In fact, many death certificates specifically state not to enter cause of death as cardiac or respiratory arrest, shock, or heart failure.

Most deaths that occur in hospital or long-term care facilities are explained or expected because of age or disease, and are classified as natural deaths. These deaths are exempt from investigation by a legal agency and are routinely handled by the attending physician who is willing to certify the death due to natural causes. Often deaths that are expected may be unexplained by pathology and remain inconclusive in the investigation of the medical diagnosis. Sudden death, by definition, implies that death was not expected. Sudden natural death primarily involves three vital systems: cardiovascular, respiratory, and the central nervous system. The term sudden death commonly means less than 5 minutes, frequently with instantaneous immobility (Butt, 1993). Unexpected deaths, in the absence of suspicion, should fall within the jurisdiction of the medical examiner or coroner if no recent medical attention for a natural disease is documented. In contrast, all unexpected deaths that are unnatural usually include trauma, either intentional or unintentional; suicide, self-inflicted injury with the intention of taking one's own life; and homicide, injury inflicted by another with intention to kill and all require re-porting to a legal agency. If the death should occur during medical treatment attended by a physician, these cases remain notifiable due to the circumstances of the death.

EQUIVOCAL DEATHS

Equivocal or questionable death is a challenge for forensic nurses. The questions that arise in the investigation of equivocal cases is whether the death was suicide, accidental, or homicide, as in the death of 43-year-old crime novelist Eugene Izzi on December 7, 1996.

► CASE EXAMPLE

Eugene Izzi was found hanging from a Chicago high-rise building in a bullet-proof vest. An 800-page manuscript on three computer disks found in his pants pocket focused on a Chicago mystery writer marked for death by members of a secret Indiana militia. Although many of Izzi's friends remained convinced he was murdered, police had two theories. The first was that Izzi committed suicide but made it look like the near-murder in his own novel. That theory is supported by bizarre clues found at the crime scene: Izzi was found hanging from a rope tied to the leg of a chair of his metal desk; he was wearing a bulletproof vest and had brass knuckles and a can of mace in his pocket; a loaded .38-caliber revolver was found on the floor in his office. Medical evidence of bruises found on the inside of his thighs were explained as coming from his straddling the window ledge for a period of time before jumping. Also, he was being treated by a psychiatrist and using medication for depression. But those same facts could support a second theory, that Izzi's death was an accident that occurred while he was attempting to experience for himself a scene from his forthcoming novel. He may have attempted to hang himself to infuse in his new novel realistic details about hanging from a noose. A murder theory supports that he was forced out the 14th-story window by militia members and skinheads he had been investigating for an upcoming novel and who he said had been stalking and threatening him. In his unpublished manuscript the writer recovers from the fall from the window and hoists himself back up the rope to his office. There, he grabs a loaded gun and shoots the militia men dead (O'Brien and Martin, 1997).

SEXUAL FATALITY: ACCIDENT OR HOMICIDE?

► CASE EXAMPLE

A 30-year-old single woman was found dead in her locked apartment. She was nude and lying supine on a blanket on the bedroom floor. A pillow beneath her buttocks elevated them. Her legs were slightly spread, and her arms were by her sides. A blouse was lodged in her mouth and covered her face. Next to the body was a dental plate belonging to the victim. Near her left foot were an empty beer can, an ashtray, and a drinking glass. Neither the body nor the scene exhibited signs of a struggle. The victim's clothes and purse (containing her keys) were on her bed. A vibrator and leather-bondage materials were found in her closet. The door was locked with a spring bolt. The autopsy report indicated that she had choked to death.

► ANALYSIS

Although the body condition was consistent with either masturbation or sexual activity with a partner, the victim's sexual paraphernalia were found in her closet, not near her body. The leather-bondage items in the closet suggest previous sexual bondage activity. Although we are familiar with several confirmed autoerotic fatalities involving mechanical airway obstruction, none involves the insertion of a gag to such a depth in the oropharynx. Consultation with forensic pathologists confirmed our suspicions that it would be next to impossible for one to asphyxiate oneself in such a manner. Although the door was locked and the victim's keys were in her purse, the lock was spring-activated and would have locked on closing. The victim's willing participation is suggested but not proved by the absence of defense injuries, signs of struggle, or alcohol or drugs in her body. In sexual acts involving bondage or manual restraint between consenting partners, one partner depends on the other for release, thereby allowing that person wide latitude in the act. We concluded that the death occurred during sexual activity that included use of the gag and at least one other person. It is not possible to determine whether the other person(s) intended to kill the victim. Thus in our opinion the manner of death was homicide, but we are unable to determine whether it was murder or manslaughter (Hazelwood et al., 1983, p. 148).

FAMILY REACTION TO HOMICIDE

Sudden and unexpected death inevitably brings with it victims by extension: the family, partners, friends, and colleagues. In this area as well, forensic nurses have made a significant contribution (Burgess, 1975; Lynch, 1988, 1991, 1993a). A pilot study that described the general reaction areas of family members of homicide victims is included to assist the advanced practice nurse in providing counseling (Burgess, 1975).

ACUTE GRIEF PHASE

Within the acute grief phase, the immediate thoughts of family members include preoccupation with the loss of their family member and their horror at the manner in which the family member died. Following these thoughts, there is an urgency in wanting to know the facts: who did it, who is the murderer. These questions correlate with the style of attack and the way in which the assailant gained access to the victim.

Two main styles of attack may befall murder victims: the blitz attack and the confidence attack. The blitz attack occurs without prior interaction of any kind between assailant and victim. It is difficult for the family of the victim to come to terms with the attack because they can find no reason for the crime. In one case an engineer was shot as he walked across the parking lot to his car at the end of a working day. No clues, evidence, or suspects were found.

The confidence attack is a more subtle set-up than the blitz; the assailant gains access to the victim under false pretenses by using deceit and betrayal. Thus the assailant and victim interact prior to the attack. The assailant may already know the victim and thus have developed some kind of relationship, or may establish a relationship as a prelude to the attack. Like the confidence man, the assailant encourages the victim's trust and then betrays this trust. Betrayal may be within a short period of time or over a longer time. The victim may be captured in three ways: verbally, through an established relationship, or by a controlling relationship over time, as in spousal abuse.

The interaction or relationship that a homicide victim has with the assailant adds a complicated dimension to the dynamics of the case. For example, one daughter said that she could accept her father's death but not the way in which he died. The style of attack in this homicide was captured-over-time. The father was killed by contract and his family, except for the daughter, had resigned themselves to his violent death by the Mafia.

When an assailant with an established relationship is also known to the family, the family has to deal with feelings about their own relationship with the assailant. One niece remarked that her uncle had befriended the man who killed him; she kept asking how the assailant could do such a thing.

If there is no suspect in a homicide case, the family must give considerable time and energy to working with the police to help determine leads, to describe the victim's life prior to the homicide, and to help reconstruct events during and following the homicide.

In cases where the style of attack is not clear cut and the assailant never apprehended, there is no feeling of closure to the crime. Families have been known to go through the incident themselves as part of the settlement process. In one case, the family went to the deserted area in the country where the victim's body was found and tried to act out the scene. A cousin said, "I tried to imagine how he did it and why she couldn't get away. She must have been in so much pain. I can't stand to think about it. This might sound morbid to you but it was just something I had to do."

Another immediate reaction families describe is a wish to physically do something about the crime. An overwhelming feeling of helplessness may trigger this wish for action, usually against the assailant. Families will describe feelings of outrage, anger, and aggression toward the assailant. The father of a murdered daughter said, "I am overwhelmed with rage. I would kill him if I could." A brother who talked of his tremendous feelings of revenge repeated how he wished to "get his hands on the guy." Later, during the trial, the brother became preoccupied with the defendant's hands, hoping he would come near enough to him to be able to choke him.

The next set of questions that arise regard those reality issues the family must complete. Homicide involves all the activities that are part of the grieving process, including funeral or memorial services.

NOTIFICATION OF OTHERS

In a natural death, the family and friends take responsibility for notifying other people of the death and funeral plans. A homicide, however, usually receives media coverage, which may further complicate the grieving process. Families report receiving unwanted calls and letters because of the publicity given the murder.

VIEWING THE VICTIM

Someone has to identify the body; this can place an added psychological burden on the family member to whom this task falls. In one family, the daughter was the only person who felt psychologically strong enough to identify the body. She said when first told the news, she screamed. When she had to identify her father, she was sick to her stomach. Many medical examiner offices now use a videotape of the body to ease the psychological shock of direct confrontation with the murdered family member.

FUNERAL ACTIVITIES

One of the duties that occupies the family's time in the first week following a homicide is attending to the funeral details and arrangements. Such decisions as whether to have an open cas-

ket may need to be made. This may depend on the physical appearance of the body and it can be a difficult decision for the family. Families must take into account how newspaper reporting has handled the situation, in terms of what people's fantasies may be. Families must also take into account the wishes, if they are known, of the victim. In one case, the victim had previously requested having an open casket when he died. This wish heavily influenced the family decision even though the victim had been badly beaten and bruised.

PHYSICAL SIGNS AND SYMPTOMS

Families are numb and confused and will describe a number of physical concerns. Insomnia, sleep pattern disturbances, headaches, chest pain, palpitations, and gastrointestinal upsets are quite common. Medications may need to be prescribed. People will describe not feeling or remembering much about the first weeks and even months.

REACTIONS OVER TIME

Following the acute grief period, families have to deal with their own psychological reactions and they have to deal with the sociolegal issues involved with the crime of homicide.

PSYCHOLOGICAL ISSUES

The family has to go through the process of grief work. This process moves the person from being preoccupied with thoughts of the lost person, through the painful recollection of the loss experience, to the final step of settling the loss as an integrative experience.

Some family members contrast the victim with the crime. As one widow said, "He hated violence . . . and he died by it."

Settlement of the "if only" reaction is important to some people. As the family learns the details of the homicide, they begin to say, "If only I had done such and such this wouldn't have happened."

Dreams and Nightmares

Dreaming of the lost person in terms of wish-fulfillment is documented in bereavement studies (Parkes, 1972). Wish-fulfillment dreams are seen in survivors in terms of trying to save the victim. One person described a dream where she tried to warn her cousin not to go with the murderer and woke up in the middle of the dream crying.

Phobic Reactions

Phobic reactions are common with family members and develop according to the specific circumstances surrounding the events of the crime. One sister of a victim of an unsolved murder developed the fear of having people walk behind her, and she would not even allow her boyfriend to walk behind her.

Families become very aware of the potential for a crime occurring and cope by adding protective measures. Families will take special precautions to protect themselves by getting permits to carry weapons and have security systems installed in their homes.

Identification With Tragedy

Identification with the lost person is a way some people deal with the painful loss. One sister immediately began sleeping in her dead sister's bed and began wearing her sister's clothes. There is a searching out for people with similar experiences.

Role Change

Death forces people into sudden role changes for which they have little preparation. Loss of a wife changes a husband to a widower; loss of an only child or an only uncle or cousin can totally eliminate the role the survivor held. Being forced into assuming a new identity and giving up an important role adds a difficult dimension to the grief process.

SOCIOLEGAL ISSUES

The Court Process

All homicide cases will involve some degree of police and court procedure. There will be investigations to find the murderer. This entire process has a major effect on the grief reaction and crisis settlement. There are many feelings evoked during the process, but one of the hardest to bear, if the case goes to court, is the impersonal attitude of court and the participants.

Concept of Blame

Murder undermines one's faith in the world as an ordered and secure place. Blaming someone for a tragedy is a less disturbing alternative than facing the fact that life is uncertain. It allows people to continue to be in control by putting the responsibility onto another person. Not to be able to explain a situation makes people feel helpless.

People look for a target onto which to project their feelings, and the main target is usually the assailant. Families want justice and the assailant prosecuted. Some people believe in capital punishment, others in prison. Some state that the assailant is mentally ill and should be psychiatrically treated.

Another target is the criminal justice system. Families can become angry at the police for being unsuccessful in finding the assailant. Other people focus on the court process and become angry at judges for "letting criminals right out the door." And the victim can be blamed. This concept holds that no victim is entirely innocent but rather participates to some degree in the crime.

AVOIDANCE BY OTHERS

People have a conscious need to settle the incident, to make some sense out of what happened, to explain it to themselves, to classify it along with other life events, and to make it somehow "fit" into their reorganized lifestyle. Families who had strong emotional support through a social network or through crisis counseling tend to have a good chance of settling the acute crisis period and dealing with the long-term reactions. However, there are some people who have difficulty processing the crisis because of the manner in which outside people treat them in regard to the situation. One case is where people deliberately avoid the family and, consequently, are not supportive.

The second situation is where people unwittingly avoid the family, and thus offer no support.

Deliberate Avoidance

To be acknowledged as a victim involves people validating the crime as a crime. One type of situation in which people have considerable ambivalence over accepting the homicide as a bona fide crime occurs in the style of attack: controlled over time. In such situations, the victim has a long-standing relationship with the assailant. In one case, the victim belonged to a drug ring, and because he "squealed" to the federal agents, he received little recognition as a human being who had been murdered. In this case, the girlfriend had great difficulty grieving because no one acknowledged that her boyfriend was "worth it." The couple had been seen by an advanced practice psychiatric nurse prior to the murder, and the young woman sought the nurse out after the crisis specifically because she had no one else in whom she could confide. The young woman talked regularly with the nurse and was able to reorganize her life after many months.

Unwitting Avoidance

A murder may well be acknowledged in some situations but for some reason the family receives no support in dealing with the crisis and grief. In a situation in which a 19-year-old woman was murdered in a field between her home and her workplace, the family received no intervention. They withdrew as a family and perceived outside people as being hateful and "observing them as animals in a cage." They felt on display because of media coverage and angry about everyone who was talking about them. Six years after the murder, the younger sister, who was then 19, came to a college mental health center complaining that she was "falling apart" and not in control of herself. The advanced practice nurse diagnosed the situation as unresolved homicide-grief, because the woman was unable to discuss with equanimity a death and homicide that occurred 6 years previous and gave a history of failure to grieve at the time of the sister's death. With the nurse as a supportive listener, the young woman immediately began to discuss the death with intense emotion. Within several sessions, she was able to resolve her grief. This freed her to move onto other therapy issues.

The violence in our society will undoubtedly place added dimensions on advanced practice nurses in psychiatric and mental health nursing and in forensic nursing. Crisis work often involves the nurse initiating counseling, rather than waiting for an individual to seek services. One would hope that victim services would be extended to families of every reported crime as one positive step for primary prevention.

NEW ROLES FOR FORENSIC NURSES

SEXUAL ASSAULT NURSE EXAMINERS

A contemporary role in forensic nursing recognized as a new occupational opportunity is the independent contractor in forensic services. Western Nurse Specialists (WNS) (Battiste-Otto, 1995) is one example of this innovative approach. WNS is a privately owned corporation formed of nurses to serve law enforcement agencies in gathering forensic evidence and to advance nursing science in the forensic arena through the Institute of Forensic Studies in Nursing Education and Research. The WNS center, a research and evidence collection facility, contracts with police agencies to gather genetic evidence (blood, semen, tissue, hair, saliva) and other trace and physical evidence in cases of crime-related interpersonal violence.

To date, WNS operates five Sexual Assault Response Team sites in California and recently opened the first privately owned sexual assault examination center in the United States. Each site has the equipment and supplies necessary to complete a detailed evidentiary examination of patients associated with sexual assault, battering, and abuse. These facilities presently employ 75 forensic technicians and nurses specifically skilled in the evaluation of trauma associated with forced sexual contact and maintain the state-of-the-art equipment necessary to document and preserve necessary evidence. These sites provide a one-stop specialized, dedicated center for rapid, sensitive examination and treatment of the client, prescription of medication, and collection of evidence. Each forensic nurse sexual assault examiner is a registered nurse educated in the forensic sciences, skilled in forensic techniques, and qualified as an expert witness in court. Forensic nurse examiners are responsible for case management of sexual abuse victims in coordination with police and rape crisis centers. This privately owned company, which has been based in Redlands, California, since 1990, is an independent contractor of forensic services provided by nurses to 70 law enforcement agencies. These services include the collection of blood-alcohol samples and urine drug screen materials, removal of taser darts, conducting of pre-booking exams, collection of reference samples from sexual assault suspects, and the provision of on-call service 24 hours a day to document and preserve evidence from victims and perpetrators of sexual assault and domestic violence. When contacted by the police, WNS sends out a team of phlebotomists (blood extraction specialists) to the scene to collect the evidence from suspects in custody. The victims are transported to the examination center.

Western Nurse Specialists maintains a comprehensive quality assurance program, and is continually exploring avenues of advancement in contemporary technology. WNS forensic nursing specialists practice under the guidelines established by the Office of Criminal Justice Planning for the State of California. The center employs a Director of Clinical Forensic Medicine, who validates the nurse's forensic technique for quality assurance, consults when complex medical management problems occur, and provides direct patient care when appropriate. The comprehensive preparation of each WNS nurse requires an intensive curriculum in medicolegal examination, and instruction and competency in the use of the colposcope. This instrument is a binocular microscope with variable magnification and photographic capability used to document microscopic genital abrasions.

The colposcope can transmit images onto a color monitor, a camera, or via telephone lines to a monitor in a courtroom or even a hospital in another state. The new WNS research center also has a light staining microscope, designed to enhance the image of sperm and make it easier to detect. Studies published in the *Annals of Emergency Medicine* (June 1992) noted a significant correlation between successful prosecution and presence of physical findings, making colposcopic photodocumentation an essential component of effective examinations.

A private facility permits victims and law enforcement officers to circumvent the hospital emergency department, thus avoiding the delays often encountered in that setting. Furthermore, most emergency personnel often lack the time, equipment, or training to gather evidence necessary for a consultation. An added benefit is that physicians and emergency department staff, faced with increasing numbers of acute medical problems, are spared the additional burden of a lengthy evaluation and continuing responsibility of litigation associated with forensic cases. Police officers are out of circulation for a shorter period of time and can usually avoid the hospital emergency department altogether. A private facility provides timely and subjective examinations, which decrease the stress and humiliation of the experience for the victim. Accordingly, this comprehensive method contributes not only to the efficiency and effectiveness of forensic science, but encourages victims to report sexual offenses with confidence that they will be accorded justice through a thorough and empathic system.

Counties that subscribe to forensic nurse examiners find that public prosecutors advocate the use of forensic nurses in order to facilitate sexual assault prosecution. Physical evidence that is unequivocally documented and clearly presented is generally not contested in court, resulting in a plea bargain to charges and average annual savings of $40,000 per case in court costs to the prosecution. Currently, WNS also operates in specially designated spaces at four other sites in Southern California. These sexual assault response sites, and the preceptorship program that provides didactic and internship components, provide a model program that will, hopefully, be replicated throughout the United States, as well as in other areas of North and South America where they are notably absent.

FACILITATORS OF ORGAN TRANSPLANTATION

Death is difficult under any circumstances. Yet, there is a need for the survivors of a tragic loss—the victims by extension—to transform the loss into a positive outcome: the anatomical gift of life. Multiple organ and tissue recovery for transplantation is recognized as an important aspect of trauma care. Knowledge of the legal framework of organ donation, familiarity with brain death criteria, and confident skills in requesting consent are areas where the forensic nurse can make a significant difference. In cases where the patient dies, death is impending, or brain death is impending or declared, the donor candidacy status must be considered and evaluated. In determining eligibility for organ/tissue donation (solid organs, eyes, bone, skin), the legal disposition of the body must first be defined, and consent for donation by the family must be obtained. Determining the legal status of the case as well as obtaining consent is generally the responsibility of the nursing staff. This can become a difficult situation for most nurses, who may feel that this task is an intrusion during a period of great personal turmoil and crisis. The aftermath of sudden and unexpected death is often a stressful period for the hospital staff involved in direct communication with the grieving family regarding consent. This calls for expertise in both crisis counseling and medicolegal issues, one that must meet the legal requirements while at the same time providing emotional support to the grieving family.

Nationwide, over 31,000 people await lifesaving or life-enhancing organ transplants. However, according to recent studies only 14,000 organs from 4500 donors are available annually (Shafer et al., 1994). A significant proportion of states now require hospital staffs to ask for organ-tissue donations when a patient dies under certain circumstances.

In systems where a regional organ procurement organization is designated by law to work with specific hospitals, the agency provides a transplant coordinator who assumes full responsibility of request and coordinates the anatomical recovery and organ allocation. The organ transplant coordinator (OTC) is a nurse skilled in specific areas such as determination of candidacy for organ donation, donor and family assessment, restrictions, cultural/religious beliefs, and the legality of administrative procedures. Legal requirements in a case of sudden and unexpected death provide the state or county medical examiner or coroner with the ultimate jurisdiction of the body. Yet, with the increased emphasis on procurement of tissue and organs, a conflict between the officiator of death and the organ/tissue transplant coordinator is emerging in jurisdictions lacking essential cooperation and clear-cut policies. Previously, forensic cases could not be processed for organ retrieval prior to autopsy and documentation of premortem injury. In recent years laws have been passed that give the organ transplant coordinator greater access to cases that are potential candidates for procuring tissue and solid organs. This identified conflict has created a lack of coordination, resulting in a breakdown in the system. Without the proper channels detailing necessary medicolegal protocol, the judicial process could be compromised. However, a comparative analysis of the medical examiner and coroner cases that were denied release for procurement indicated that as many as 2979 people were denied transplants from 1990 to 1992 (Shafer et al, 1994). Considering that lives are lost with each nonrelease of organs, it is in the best interest of public policy that lifesaving or life-enhancing organs and tissue for transplantation be maximized.

To avoid any potential conflicts of interest as well as meeting the needs of the grieving and bereaved, the re-education of the OTC in forensic nursing would allow for the designation of a forensic transplantation specialist. This liaison would be skilled in the scientific investigation of injury and death, and the collection and preservation of evidence, and could act as clinical investigator representing the medical examiner or coroner in much the same way that hospice nurses in certain jurisdictions are deputized and act as investigators at the time of an anticipated death. The Joint Commission on Accreditation for Healthcare Organizations guidelines have specific standards for specially trained members of the bioethics staff to act as counselors for the families of potential donors and to interface with the appropriate agencies. A forensic nurse transplantation specialist would be an ideally qualified clinician to ensure compliance with these requirements. This specialist, in an advanced nursing practice role at the administrative level, would be in a position to coordinate the legality concerning organ donor matters. As an expert in both legal issues and sensitivity to the deceased family, a forensic nurse could be utilized to provide consultation as necessary, staff education, and immediate interventions in the emergency department setting. As a nurse manager, the forensic nurse position could provide an opportunity to create or advance existing protocol with greater emphasis on the coordination and cooperation between organ/tissue procurement and the medical examiner/coroner system.

If the system is properly organized, all stand to gain; the medical examiner or coroner will acquire more diagnostic information and will no longer have reason to fear loss of evidence through removal of tissues and organs. In an ideal system, forensic documentation begins before the official pronouncement of death, where features of injury are being recorded that would otherwise have been overlooked or lost. As a result, more

tissue and organs would be released by the medicolegal authorities. With the growing need for anatomical gifts to meet the demands of medical science, recipients and legal protocol require mutual consideration. The forensic nurse liaison represents a comprehensive action plan building an effective alliance between the regional organ procurement organization and local officiators of death that will protect forensically significant evidence, provide more complete clinical data, and establish collaborative strategies that could increase the availability of transplantable organs.

SUMMARY

The forensic nursing role has been expressly designed to provide solutions to some of the most urgent concerns in our society. Forensic nursing focuses on the areas where medicine, nursing, and human behavior interface with the law. Existing problems are great and multifaceted, and call for new solutions. The application of forensic science to contemporary nursing practice reveals a wider role in the investigation of crime and the legal process that contributes to public health and safety. The responsibility of the forensic nurse is to provide continuity of care from the health care institution or the crime scene to courts of law . . . from trauma to trial.

REFERENCES

Battiste-Otto F. Aiding justice: Forensic RN's combine nursing and criminal sciences. In: Proceedings of the 47th Annual Meeting of the American Academy of Forensic Sciences, Seattle, 1995, p. 100. Abstract.

Burgess AW. Family reaction to homicide. *Am J Orthopsychiatry.* 1975;45:391–398.

Butt J. Sudden death and police investigation. *Alberta Province Medical Examination Manual,* 2nd ed., Calgary; 1993.

Eckert, W. Forensic sciences and medicine, the clinical or living aspects. *Am J Forensic Med Pathol.* 1990;11:336–341.

Eckert W, et al. Clinical forensic medicine. *Am J Forensic Med Pathol.* 1986;7:182–185.

Goldsmith MF. US forensic pathologists on a new case: Examination of living persons. *JAMA*. 1986; 256:1685–1691.

Hazelwood RR, Dietz PE, Burgess AW. *Autoerotic Fatalities*. New York: Simon & Schuster; 1983.

Lynch V. Forensic nursing: An essential element in managing society's violence and its victims. *ASTM American Society of Testing & Materials Standardization News*, April 1995a.

Lynch V. Role of the forensic nurse specialist in the identification of sexual assault trauma. In: Proceedings of the 47th Annual Meeting of the Academy of Forensic Sciences, Seattle, 1995b, p. 100. Abstract.

Lynch V. Forensic aspects of health care: New roles, new responsibilities. *J Psychosoc Nurs Ment Health Serv*. 1993a;31:11.

Lynch V. Forensic nursing: Diversity in education and practice. *J Psychosoc Nurs Ment Health Serv*. 1993b;31:11.

Lynch V. Forensic nursing in the emergency department: A new role for the 1990s. *Crit Care Nurs Q*. 1991;14:3.

Lynch V. Biomedical investigation as a mental health nursing role. In: Lancaster J, ed. *Adult Psychiatric Nursing*. 3rd ed. New Hyde Park, NY: Medical Examination Publishing; 1988.

Marsh T. A nurses' guide to sleuthing (Or, how to collect evidence, hospital style). *RN*. 1978;41:48–50.

Mittleman R, Goldberg H, Waksman D. Preserving evidence in the emergency department. *Am J Nurs*. 1983;83:1652–1656.

O'Brien J, Martin A. Writer's death similar to manuscript scene. *Boston Globe*, January 9, 1997, p. A3.

Orris KC, Lantz PE. Interpretation of fatal multiple and exiting gunshot wounds by trauma specialists. Paper presented at American Academy of Forensic Sciences, Boston, February 1993.

Parkes C. Bereavement: Studies of Grief in Adult Life, New York: International Universities Press, 1972.

Schramm C. Forensic medicine: What the perioperative nurse needs to know. *Am Operating Room Nurs J*. 1991;53:3.

Shaw A. Don't be so sure its child abuse. *Med Economics*. March 8, 1993:79–93.

Shafer T, et al. Impact of medical examiner practices on organ recovery in the United States. *JAMA*. 1994;261:23–30.

Simon S. Glove retakes center stage at Simpson trial. *Boston Globe*, January 9, 1997, p. A3.

Smock W. Development of a clinical forensic medicine curriculum for emergency physicians in the USA. *J Clin Forensic Med*. 1994;1:27–30.

Smock W, Nichols G, Fuller P. Development and implementation of the first clinical forensic medicine training program. *J Forensic Sci*. 1993;38:4.

Smock W, Ross C, Hamilton F. Clinical forensic medicine: How ED physicians can help with the sleuthing. *Am Health Consult*. 1994;5:1.

Stewart C. Nursing management of gunshot wounds to the head. *J Neurosurg Nurs*. 1983;15:5.

Swanson C, Chamelin N, Territo L. *Criminal Investigation* 6th ed. New York: McGraw-Hill; 1995.

The American Trauma Society. Domestic Violence: Battered Women, Children, and Elders. Upper Marlboro, MD, 1993.